MICROBES AND MALIGNANCY

MICROBES AND MALIGNANCY

Infection as a Cause of Human Cancers

Edited by
JULIE PARSONNET, M.D.

Departments of Medicine and of Health Research and Policy
Stanford University School of Medicine

New York　　Oxford
OXFORD UNIVERSITY PRESS
1999

Oxford University Press

Oxford   New York
Athens   Auckland   Bangkok   Bogotà   Buenos Aires   Calcutta
Cape Town   Chennai   Dar es Salaam   Delhi   Florence   Hong Kong   Istanbul
Karachi   Kuala Lumpur   Madrid   Melbourne   Mexico City   Mumbai
Nairobi   Paris   São Paolo   Singapore   Taipei   Tokyo   Toronto   Warsaw

and associated companies in
Berlin   Ibadan

Copyright © 1999 by Oxford University Press, Inc.

Published by Oxford University Press, Inc.
198 Madison Avenue, New York, New York 10016

Oxford is a registered trademark of Oxford University Press

Library of Congress Cataloging-in-Publication Data
Microbes and malignancy : infection as a cause of human cancers /
edited by Julie Parsonnet.
p.   cm.   Includes bibliographical references and index.
ISBN 0–19–510401–3
1. Microbial carcinogenesis.   I. Parsonnet, Julie.
[DNLM: 1. Neoplasms—etiology.   2. Neoplastic Processes.
3. Infection—microbiology.   4. Infection—parasitology.
5. Infection—complications.
QZ 202 M6257 1999]
RC268.57.M53 1999   616.99′4071–dc21
DNLM/DLC   for Library of Congress   98–22168

9 8 7 6 5 4 3 2 1

Printed in the United States of America
on acid-free paper

ACKNOWLEDGMENTS

When my brothers and I were children, my parents built book shelves in the dining room so that, during our dinner conversations, we wouldn't have to run to another room to find the reference we needed to bolster our side of a debate. In retrospect, I now think this need to have information at hand was the driving force behind the books each of my parents later authored. I, too, like to have information at hand and have been sorry to find no book on infection and cancer, my primary field of interest. By editing this work, I have followed my parents' example. I am grateful to them for giving me a sense of inquisitiveness and for teaching me that if I want something done, I had better try doing it myself.

Many people have contributed substantially to this work. In particular I would like to thank Sandra Horning, Patrick Moore, Yuan Chang, Bruce Ames, Harry Greenberg, David Relman, and Paul Basch for their thoughtful conversations on the book's contents. Doug Owens earns many brownie points for directing me to Lyn Dupre, who did a beautiful job copyediting the manuscript. I am, as always, indebted to Rosario Villacorta, for her technical support and unwavering good humor throughout the process of putting the pages together. My husband, Tony Alfrey, provided clear-headed editorial advice when I struggled to crystallize ideas into words. His constant support and encouragement make all my work possible.

Finally, I would like to dedicate this book to the post-doctoral fellows, students, and research assistants who have worked with my group and kept me inspired.

Stanford, Cal.   J.P.

.

CONTENTS

III INFECTIONS AND CANCER: PARASITES AND BACTERIA

CONTRIBUTORS

BRUCE N. AMES, PH.D.
Division of Biochemistry and
   Molecular Biology
University of California, Berkeley
Berkeley, CA

WILLIAM A. BLATTNER, M.D.
Professor and Associate Director
Division of Epidemiology
Institute of Human Virology
University of Maryland School of
   Medicine
Baltimore, MD

YUAN CHANG, M.D.
Associate Professor of Pathology
Department of Pathology
College of Physicians and Surgeons of
   Columbia University
New York, NY

STEPHAN CHRISTEN, PH.D.
Department of Biochemistry and
   Molecular Biology
University of California Berkeley
Berkeley, CA

RAYMOND T. CHUNG, M.D.
President
Harvard Medical School
GI Unit
Massachusetts General Hospital
Boston, MA

SAMUEL M. COHEN, M.D., PH.D.
Professor and Chairman
Department of Pathology and
   Microbiology
University of Nebraska Medical School
Omaha, NE

TORY M. HAGEN, PH.D.
Assistant Professor of Biochemisty and
   Biophysics
Oregon State University
Linus Pauling Institute
Corvallis, OR

LORNE J. HOFSETH, PH.D.
Cancer Control Research Unit
British Columbia Cancer Agency
Vancouver, B.C. Canada

PETER M. HOWLEY, M.D.
Department of Pathology
Harvard Medical School
Boston, MA

DR. PETER G. ISAACSON, D.M.,
   F.R.C. PATH
Department of Histopathology
University College London Medical
   School
London, UK

NOBUYUKI ITO, M.D.
Nagoya City University
Nagoya, Japan

JUDITH E. KARP, M.D.
Marlene and Stewart Greenbaum
   Cancer Center
University of Maryland Medical
   Systems
Baltimore, MD

T. JAKE LIANG, M.D.
National Institute of Diabetes,
   Digestive, and Kidney Disease
National Institutes of Health
Bethesda, MD

KARL MÜNGER, PH.D.
Associate Professor
Department of Pathology
Harvard Center for Cancer Biology
Harvard Medical School
Boston, MA

JULIE PARSONNET, M.D.
Associate Professor
Departments of Medicine and of
    Health Research and Policy
Stanford University School of
    Medicine
Stanford, CA

NANCY RAAB-TRAUB, PH.D.
Lineberger Cancer Research Center
University of North Carolina
Chapel Hill, NC

DAVID A. RELMAN, M.D.
Stanford University School of
    Medicine
VA Palo Alto Health Care System
Palo Alto, CA

WILLIAM S. ROBINSON, M.D.
Professor
Department of Medicine/Infectious
    Disease
Stanford University School of
    Medicine
Stanford, CA

MIRIAM P. ROSIN, PH.D.
Environmental Carcinogenesis
    Laboratory
Department of Kinesiology
Simon Fraser University
Burnaby, BC Canada
    and
Cancer Control Research Unit
British Columbia Cancer Agency
Vancouver, BC Canada

DAVID B. SCHAUER, PH.D.
Division of Toxicology
Massachusetts Institute of Technology
Cambridge, MA

MARK K. SHIGENAGA, PH.D.
Division of Biochemistry and
    Molecular Biology
University of California, Berkeley
Berkeley, CA

TOMOYUKI SHIRAI, M.D.
Professor and Chairman
Department of Pathology
Nagoya City University Medical School
Nagoya, Japan

WITAYA THAMAVIT, D.V.M.
    M.SC.
Department of Pathobiology
Faculty of Science
Mahidol University
Bangkok, Thailand

MITSUAKI YOSHIDA, PH.D.
Professor
Department of Cellular and Molecular
    Biology
Institute of Medical Science, University
    of Tokyo
Tokyo, Japan

HARALD ZUR HAUSEN, PROF.
    DR.
Deutsches Krebs Forschungszentrum
Heidelberg, Germany

ABBREVIATIONS

3NT 3-nitrotyrosine
4HNE 4-hydroxynonenal
5HMdU 5-hydroxymethyl-2′-deoxyuridine
8HdG 8-hydroxy-2′-deoxyguanosine
AdE1A or **AdE1B** adenovirus E1 proteins
AFB1 aflatoxin B1
AIDS acquired immunodeficiency syndrome
AT ataxia-telangiectasia
ATase alkyltransferase
ATL adult T-cell leukemia
ATM gene mutated in ataxia telangectasia
BAPN -aminoproprionitrile
BL Burkitt's lymphoma
BLV bovine leukemia virus
BPV bovine papillomavirus
BrdU bromodeoxyuridine
Cdk cyclin-dependent kinase
CGD chronic granulomatous disease
CIF cellular interference factor
CIN cervical intraepithelial neoplasia
CIS carcinoma *in situ*
CKI cyclin-dependent kinase inhibitor
CL chemiluminescence
cNOS constitutive nitric oxide synthase
CNS central nervous system
CREB cyclic AMP-response element binding protein
CREM cyclic AMP-response element modulator protein
CRPV cottontail rabbit papillomavirus
CTL cytotoxic T lymphocyte
DEN diethylnitrosamine
DHBV duck hepatitis B virus
DHEA dehydroepiandrosterone

DHPN dihydroxy-di-n-propylnitrosamine
DLCL diffuse large cell lymphoma
DMN dimethylnitrosamine
DNA-PK DNA-dependent protein kinase
E6AP E6–associated protein
EA early antigen of Epstein-Barr virus
EBER Epstein-Barr virus encoded RNA
EBNA Epstein-Barr virus nuclear antigens
EBV Epstein-Barr virus
ELISA enzyme-linked immunosorbent assay
EM extensive metabolizer
ESR electron spin resonance
EV epidermodysplasia verruciformis
GADD growth arrest DNA damage-inducible gene
GCR G-protein coupled receptor
GM-CSF granulocyte-macrophage colony-stimulating factor
GSH glutathione
GSHV ground squirrel hepatitis virus
GST glutathione-S-transferase
GVHD graft vs. host disease
H2O2 hydrogen peroxide
HAM human T-cell leukemia virus-1-associated myelopathy
HBcAg hepatitis B core antigen
HBeAg heptatis B e antigen
HBIG hepatitis B immunoglobulin
HBsAg hepatitis B surface antigen
HBV hepatitis B virus
HCC hepatocellular carcinoma
HCV hepatitis C virus

HCV hepatitis C virus
HD Hodgkin's disease
HHV8 human herpesvirus 8
HIV human immunodeficiency virus
HLA human leukocyte antigen
HNO2 nitrous acid
HNO3 nitric acid
HOCl hypochlorous acid
HPV human papilloma virus
HSV herpes simplex virus
HTLV human T-cell leukemia virus
HVR hypervariable region
HVS herpesvirus saimiri
IFA immunofluorescence assay
IFN interferon
Ig immunoglobulin
IL interleukin
IM infectious mononucleosis
iNOS inducible nitric oxide synthase
IPSID immunoproliferative small intestinal disease
IQ 2-amino-3-methylimidazo-(4,5-f)quinoline
IR internal repeat
IRES internal ribosome entry site
IRF interferon regulatory factor
ISG interferon stimulated genes
KS Kaposi's sarcoma
KSHV Kaposi's sarcoma-associated herpesvirus
LANA latency-associated nuclear antigens of Kaposi's sarcoma-associated herpesvirus
LMP latent membrane protein of Epstein-Barr virus
LOH loss of heterozygosity
LPS lipopolysaccharide (endotoxin)
LTR long terminal repeat

MALT mucosa associated lymphoid tissue
MCD multicentric Castleman's disease
MCP-1 macrophage-attracting protein-1
MCV molluscum contagiosum virus
MDA malondialdehyde
MeIQ 2-amino-3,4-dimethylimidazo(4,5-f)quinoline
MeIQx 2-amino-3,8-dimethylimidazo(4,5-f)quinoxaline
MHC major histocompatibility complex
MN micronuclei
MoAb monoclonal antibodies
MPO myeloperoxidase
N2O3 nitrous anhydride
NAC N-acetyl-l-cysteine
NHL Non-Hodgkin's lymphoma
NMA NG-methyl-l-arginine
NO• nitric oxide
NO2• nitrogen dioxide
NO2- nitrite
NO2Cl nitryl chloride
NO3- nitrate
NOS nitric oxide synthase
NPC nasopharyngeal carcinoma
•OH hydroxyl radical
1O2 singlet oxygen
O2-• superoxide anion radical
O6-MedG O6-methyldeoxyguanosine
OHL oral hairy leukoplakia
ONOO- peroxynitrite anion
ONOOH peroxynitrous acid
ORF open reading frame
PBMC peripheral blood mononuclear cells

PCNA proliferating cell nuclear antigen
PCR polymerase chain reaction
PEL primary effusion lymphoma
PhIP 2-amino-1-methyl-6-phenylimidazo(4,5-b)pyridine
PIK phosphatidylinositol kinases
PIN penile intraepithelial neoplasia
PMA phorbol 12-myristate 13-acetate
PMN polymorphonuclear leukocyte (neutrophil)
pRb retinoblastoma tumor suppresser protein
PTHrP parathyroid hormone-related protein
PTL post-transplant lymphoma
PTLD post-transplantation lymphoproliferative disorders
PUFA polyunsaturated fatty acid
R2NH secondary amine
rDNA ribosomal DNA
RdRp RNA-dependent RNA polymerase
RIBA recombinant immunoblot assay
RNH2 primary amine
RNOS reactive nitrogen oxide species
ROS reactive oxygen species
RS Reed-Sternberg cell of Hodgkin's disease
RSV Rous sarcoma virus
RT-PCR reverse transcriptase-polymerase chain reaction
SCID severe combined immunodeficiency

SIL squamous intraepithelial lesion
SOD superoxide dismutase
STAT signal tranducer and activator of transcription proteins
STLV simian T-cell leukemia viruses
STP (herpesvirus) saimiri transforming proteins
SV40TAg large tumor antigen of simian virus 40
TBARS thiobarbituric acid reactive substances
TBP TATA binding protein
TG thymidine glycol
TNF tumor necrosis factor
TPA 12-O-tetradecanoyl-phorbol-13-acetate
TR tandem repeat
TRAF TNF receptor-associated factors
Trp-P-2 3-amino-1-methyl-5H-pyridol[4,3-b]indole
Trp-P-2(NHOH) 3-hydroxy-amino-1-methyl-5H-pyrido[4,3-b]indole
TSP tropical spastic paraparesis
VCA viral capsid antigen of Epstein-Barr virus
VLP viruslike particles
VV variola virus
WHV woodchuck hepatitis virus
XLP X-linked lymphoproliferative disease
ZEBRA BamHI Z fragment encoded Epstein-Barr virus replication activator gene

MICROBES AND MALIGNANCY

Introduction

JULIE PARSONNET

> Cancer is caused by chemicals in the air we breathe, the water we drink and the food we eat. Cancer is caused by bad habits, bad working conditions, bad government and bad luck—including the luck of your genetic draw and the culture into which you were born. . . . Granting even that viruses may play a heretofore undiscovered role in . . . cancer, it is probably fair to say that undue attention has been given to this particular collection of agents. The same could be said for infectious agents more generally.
>
> Robert N. Proctor[1]

> Infectious agents probably represent the most important cause of human cancer after tobacco smoking. . . . Recognition of this fact may have enormous implications for the prevention and treatment of cancers associated with these agents.
>
> Paula Pisani et al[2]

Over the past two centuries, a considerable proportion of medical research has been devoted to understanding cancer and its causes. Only in recent years, however, could we finally define the disease. We now know that cancer is a disease of uncontrolled cell growth resulting from an accumulation of mutations within a cell's genome. Yet, we are far less sophisticated in understanding why it occurs. Many people, like Robert Proctor (see above), blame our modern lifestyle.[3] Indeed, there is some truth to this view. In many countries, this past century of industrialization has brought with it almost a doubling of life expectancy. Because cancer is a disease of older people, we can expect a rapidly growing, aging population to bring with it an epidemic of malignancy. Currently, a full one third of the U.S. population can expect to acquire some form of cancer by the

3

age of 75.[4] But industrialization is blamed for much more than the problems that accrue naturally when we live longer. It is assumed to be the prima facie cause of malignancy. Daily, in the news media, we hear of tumors "caused" by electromagnetic fields, cellular telephones, and pesticides. There are community reports of cancer clusters, usually assumed to be due to groundwater contamination, power lines, or air pollution; these outbreaks rarely prove to be anything but the statistically expected blips within populations. Certainly, industrial chemicals can be carcinogenic to people who work with them, but the benefits of industrialization far exceed the cancer risks. Leading epidemiologists estimate that environmental pollution contributes to, at best, 2% of fatal cancers, and occupational exposures account for a similar portion.[5] As for living near power lines or power plants, or drinking chlorinated water, there is as yet no consistent evidence that doing so causes malignancy. No one would argue that pollution should be ignored; in terms of cancer prevention, however, it makes the most sense to be vigilant about the three major preventable causes of cancer: tobacco use (30% of all U.S. cancers); high fat, high calorie, low vegetable, low fruit diets (30% of all U.S. cancers); and infection, the focus of this book[4]

The role chronic infections play in carcinogenesis is frequently overlooked. This blinkered vision is somewhat surprising given that infections are among the best-understood causes of cancer. Since 1901, the Nobel prize has been awarded four times for research directly related to cancer (1926, 1966, 1975, 1989); in each case, the prize involved a discovery relating infectious agents to malignancy. The dominance of infectious diseases in Nobel cancer awards affirms the fundamental insights into carcinogenesis provided by this research. Moreover, the field of chronic infection as cause of cancer is increasingly fruitful over time. During the past 15 years alone, four new microbial causes of human cancer have been discovered—*Helicobacter pylori*, hepatitis C virus (HCV), papillomavirus, and human herpes virus 8 (HHV-8). These microbial pathogens now add to a panoply of previously identified pathogens that cause malignancy.

The popular and professional lack of interest in infection would be understandable if the associated cancers were rare. But, in fact, infections are linked to some of the most important cancers worldwide.[2] *Helicobacter pylori* causes gastric cancer, the second most important cause of cancer death worldwide. Papillomavirus causes the vast majority of cervical cancer, the second most important cause of cancer among women. Liver cancer, caused by the hepatitis viruses, ranks sixth in worldwide cancer incidence. Taken together, between 15% and 20% of cancers of known etiology (a higher proportion in developing countries) have been attributed to underlying infection (Figure I.1). This statistic does not take into account the many cancers for which an etiology has not yet been discovered. So why are these agents largely ignored by the average person and even by many physicians and scientists? Certainly, it is not for want of concern about health. Rather, the interest in infectious diseases as a cause

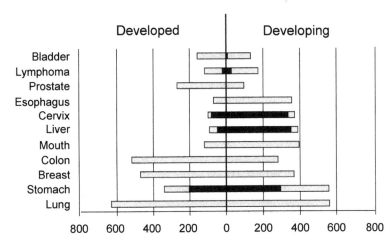

Figure I.1. Estimated number of cancer cases (in thousands) in 1990 in developed and developing countries (adapted from Pisani et al.[2]). Gray bars represent total number of cancer cases; black bars represent the number of cases attributable to infection. Note that a greater proportion of infection-related cancers occur in developing countries. Additional cancers of the colon, bladder, lung and other organs may be directly attributable to infection but no precise number can be quantified.

of cancer seems to parallel the history of infectious diseases—a history fraught with hairpin twists and turns.

THE HISTORY OF INFECTIOUS DISEASES AND CANCER

According to Jacob Wolff,* an early twentieth century medical historian and advocate of the parasite hypothesis of cancer, a contagious etiology of cancer was first proposed in the sixteenth century, when European physicians noted clusters of cancer within families.[6] The distinguished Portuguese physician Lusitanus "proved" person-to-person spread when a mother with ulcerating breast cancer transmitted the disease to all three of her daughters. Similarly, a Dutch physician, Tulpius, documented cancer transmission between a woman and her servant. Examples in which fetuses were afflicted with tumors identical to those of their mortally afflicted mothers confirmed the widely held notion that cancer behaved much like syphilis, a disease known to be infectious but for which a causative pathogen had yet to be identified.

---

*The Science of Cancerous Disease from Earliest Times to the Present , a comprehensive tome written in 1907 by Jacob Wolff and translated eight decades later (Science History Publications, USA 1989), provides a detailed overview of cancer theories from ancient times to 1900. Included in this work is a chapter entitled "Theories of Parasitism" (pp. 433–590), from which much of the early history presented here is derived.

By the mid-eighteenth century, many doctors assumed cancer to be a contagious disease. The German physician Lorenz Heister warned his colleagues to use caution when operating on cancer patients to avoid contact with "the blood which is infected by the cancer virus."[7] In 1773, Bernard Peyrilhe, noting that fever often accompanied cancer, also theorized that tumors were caused by a transmissible infection. In experiments to test this hypothesis, he injected fluid from a human breast cancer into a dog. According to Wolff, "the dog howled a great deal and Peyrilhe's servants tired of listening to this and drowned the dog, so Peyrilhe could not follow the result of his interesting experiment." Despite this abrupt termination to his laboratory career, Peyrilhe advocated using an antiseptic—carbonic acid—to treat cancer. When Langebeck successfully concluded Peyrihle's experiment, the parasite theory received its first major boost. He, too, injected tumor cells into a dog but this time, at necropsy, found multiple cancerous nodules in the dog's lungs. This highly debated result was the first "documented" transplantation of a tumor. Langebeck concluded that tumor cells were themselves autonomous organisms that replicated and grew in their mammalian host until they formed a tumor.

Two important developments in the latter half of the nineteenth century boosted the infectious theory of malignancy. In the 1850s, Virchow recognized the cell as the "ultimate formal element of any living phenomenon" and proposed that all cells grew from other cells (*omnus cellula e cellula*). From this principle, he concluded that cancer derived from human cells, rather than from foreign invaders, and that irritation caused human cells to grow aberrantly (the irritation theory of cancer). Later in the century, Leeuenhoeck, Pasteur, and Koch revolutionized science by identifying a hidden world of organisms that caused human illness, beginning the golden age of microbiology. Enthusiastic microbe hunters subsequently presumed all illnesses to be caused by infectious agents, leading them to vigorously seek the "cancer germ." By the end of the century, numerous instances of cancer contagion between husband and wife or patient and caretaker (termed cancer à deux) had been reported. In response to these cancer clusters, public health officials were often called to investigate and disinfect "cancer houses." When Virchow and other researchers reported that bladder cancer in North Africa arose in the setting of *Schistosoma haematobium* infection, the "parasite theory" and "irritation theory" converged into a unified premise.[8,9] This was further supported when Askanzy reported an association between *Opisthorchis felineus* and liver cancer.[9]

The true age of infection and cancer, however, began as the twentieth century dawned. Microbe hunters from two separate laboratories, in 1908 and 1911, extracted from animal tumors cell-free filtrable agents ("filtrable" indicating they were smaller than bacteria) that caused cancer when injected into healthy animals. The first of these filtrable agents, described by Ellerman and Bang, caused chicken leukemia; this discovery was largely ignored and soon forgotten because leukemia was then thought to be a form of inflammation rather than a malignancy. Soon thereafter, however, Peyton Rous showed that a cell-free filtrate from a chicken sarcoma, when transmitted to another chicken, rapidly caused tumor formation in that second animal. This remarkable work was oppugned for decades by the leaders in cancer research. According to Rous, a typical remark came from a leading British oncologist who exclaimed, "But my dear fellow, don't you see, this can't be cancer because you know its cause!"[7] Even 30 years after Rous's discovery, Ewing proclaimed in his classic oncology textbook that "all the phenomena of the chicken sarcomas may be explained as the result of the action of intrinsic cell products, and at no time is it necessary to introduce the idea of an extrinsic virus."[10] Those who conceded that Rous's discovery might be valid argued that chickens were too distant from mammals to make the discovery more than an interesting curiosity.[11] Discouraged, Rous turned to other productive, and less contentious, research pursuits; it wasn't until the 1950s that his filtrable agent was again studied with any serious intent.

Although leading oncologists incorrectly condemned the Rous sarcoma virus, there remained much room for criticism of the parasite theory. The innumerable false leads provided grist for the mill. Toward the beginning of the twentieth century, yeasts were thought to cause cancer because they were seen frequently in malignant tissue. A British pathologist, H. H. Plimmer, reported that a microaerophilic yeast caused cancer when injected in animals, a finding never substantiated.[12] Numerous investigators proposed that pleomorphic bacteria caused malignancies in plants, animals, and humans. Unfortunately, most of these bizarre bacteria were impossible to cultivate in vitro. Tuberculosis, the scourge of the day, was also presumed to cause 'scar carcinomas" of the lung, an hypothesis that endured through the 1980s but was ultimately discarded.[12,13] Still other scientists concluded that almost all tumors could be explained by parasitic infection, ranging from roundworms to flukes.[14] Along this line, the most famous misstep was that of Johannes Fibiger. In 1913, after noting a high frequency of papillomatous neoplasms in the stomachs of rats obtained from a sugar mill, Fibiger experimentally induced metastatic stomach cancers (Figure I.2) by infecting the animals with a nematode he named *Spiroptera neoplastica* (also variably called *Spiroptera carcinoma* or *Gongylonema neoplasticum*). This series of experiments not only validated the parasite theory of malignancy but also represented the first induction of cancer in an experimental system. In presenting Fibiger with the Nobel prize, Professor W. Wernstedt, Dean of the Royal Karolinska Institute, emphasized the momentousness of this research, stating it was "possible, for the first time, to change by experiment normal cells into cells having all the terrible properties of cancer. It was thus shown authoritatively not that cancer is always caused by a worm, but that it can be provoked by an external stimulus."[15] Following years of unfulfilled promise, Wernstedt claimed that this celebrated discovery "marked the beginning of a new era, of a new epoch in the history of cancer."

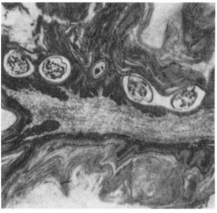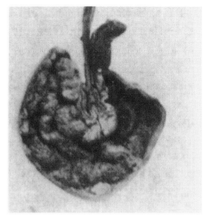

A   B

Figure I.2. Johannes Fibiger won the Nobel prize in 1926 for demonstrating that a nematode, *Spiroptera neoplastica* (shown in microscopic section in a rat's stomach in A), caused gastric cancer in rats. The papillomatous lesions attributed to the worm, however (B), later proved to be neither malignant nor caused by the parasite; rather, they are now thought to have resulted from dietary deficiency.

But this era was not to be. Within a decade of Fibiger's Nobel prize in 1926 and his death from colon cancer in 1928, the work was proved false. Investigators could not replicate his findings. Rats and mice fed *Spiroptera neoplastica* developed no tumors. Several investigators conducted in-depth experiments over several years and ultimately concluded that dietary deficiency induced the papillomatous, nonmalignant lesions that Fibiger had observed[16,17] Fibiger had fed his rats white bread and water, a diet devoid of numerous nutrients. This deficient diet fostered not only an exaggerated papillomatous response to the parasites in the stomach but also caused regenerative lung and lymph node lesions that Fibiger had incorrectly diagnosed as metastases. With these refutations, the parasite theory—always a source of some skepticism—fell from favor. Behan, the author of a leading cancer textbook of the 1930s, reflected the opinion of many oncologists when he discounted the parasite hypothesis as having "too many improbabilities to be scientifically acceptable".[18]

Many of the arguments against infection as a cause of cancer would seem illogical today. For example, it was prevalently believed that all cancer was caused by one specific type of exposure; there was no multifactorial theory of cancer as there is today. Thus, if infection did not cause one tumor type, it caused no tumors. In a critical experiment that purportedly repudiated the bacterial hypothesis, coal tar caused cancer when applied to a rabbit's ear.[18] Because coal tar killed germs but caused cancer, the anti-infection theorists concluded that germs could not cause malignancy. In his 1934 textbook, *The Origin of Cancer*, Dr. Lockhart-Mummary put forth four additional arguments against an infectious etiology of cancer, all of which could easily be refuted today: (1) a virus could not cause sarcoma in chickens because it "does not correspond to what is known about other viruses or known infective agents"; (2) although improved hygiene had led to decreased mortality from acute infectious diseases, cancers had increased, suggesting that infection was not involved; (3) tumors did not act like infectious diseases; (4) twins often developed the same tumors, suggesting a hereditary cause of cancer.[19]

Another basis for denouncing the infection hypothesis was the inability of investigators to achieve the supreme standard for disease causation: meeting Koch's postulates.* To test Koch's postulates, investigators destroyed cancer cells under conditions that would not kill bacteria or viruses, then transplanted the disrupted cells into animals. Cancers were not induced, arguing against the ongoing presence of a transmissible agent (interestingly, although the Rous sarcoma virus fulfilled most of Koch's postulates, it was discounted as an exceptional case that could not refute the many failures). Parasites were also discarded as a cause of cancer despite the numerous epidemiologic links that had been reported in humans and animals. Even supporters of Virchow's irritation theory of cancer denounced the parasite hypothesis, claiming that, at most, infectious agents only indirectly caused cancer by causing irritation. Because it was thought that any cause of cancer must be smaller than the cancer cell itself, parasites simply did not fit into the prevailing belief system.[9] Borrel had earlier tried to circumvent this argument by maintaining that viruses within the infecting parasites were the true cause of malignant transformation.[9] This view had no experimental support, however, and was given short shrift.

Prominent clinicians also contested the contagion hypothesis. They noted that no doctor had ever contracted cancer by cutting himself while operating on a tumor. Moreover, the purported rarity of simultaneous occurrences of penile cancer in men and cervical cancer in their wives was thought to disprove contagion (1 in 130 to 140 wives of men with penile cancer had cervical cancer—a ratio that would be considered to place the women at high risk today).[18] The previously popular concept of cancer houses was also dispelled using the same statistical arguments that are used to dismiss the significance of cancer clusters today.[9] By 1940, despite the discovery of the first two mammalian oncoviruses (the Shope

---

*In Koch's postulates, to prove an infectious agent caused disease, a scientist must:
  1. Find the agent in all cases of disease.
  2. Isolate the agent and grow it in the laboratory.
  3. Show that the laboratory-grown agent causes disease when given to animals.
  4. Reisolate the agent from the sick animals.
Today, it is understood that Koch's postulates cannot be met for most chronic infections, and even for some acute infections.[28]

rabbit papillomavirus and Bittner's milk-transmitted mouse mammary tumor virus), infectious causes of cancer had fallen into almost complete disrepute.

In the 1950s, the miraculous developments of antibiotics, anti-tuberculosis chemotherapy, and effective vaccines for polio and measles galvanized researchers to pursue the promise of infectious diseases research. Scientists were finally able to isolate and cultivate pure viruses and, with the increasing accessibility of electron microscopy, were able to see these viruses. In 1953, Watson and Crick reported the structure of DNA, one of the greatest discoveries of the modern age. This breakthrough surmounted a critical impediment to our understanding of the nature of viruses; these organisms could now be classified based on their genetic content. In 1957, scientists at the 24th Meeting of the Society for General Microbiology finally achieved a consensus about what a virus was.[20]* Charlotte Friend, a cancer virologist, describes the dramatic shift in climate that occurred in the mid-1950s. In 1956, when she first presented her research on a mouse leukemia virus at the national meeting of the American Association of Cancer Research, she says "the virologists in the audience sprang into action to disown what I had cautiously called a 'virus-like agent'; it could not be a virus because it induced a frankly malignant disease. The pathologists were equally vocal in disclaiming the disease as malignant because it was obviously induced by cell-free filtrates."[21] By the next year's meeting, Friend reports that her "colleagues were more receptive" to viral oncology research. And well they should have been! Between 1951 and 1972, 26 mammalian oncoviruses—although only one human oncovirus (Epstein-Barr virus)—had been discovered. This final confirmation of Rous's long-challenged belief resulted in his winning the Nobel prize in 1966, a mere 55 years after his initial discovery.

In the 1960s, viral oncology continued apace. In their Nobel prize research, Temin and Baltimore identified the key reverse transcriptase enzyme in oncogenic retroviruses, including the Rous sarcoma virus. At the same time, epidemiological evidence emerged suggesting that some cancers were transmissible. In 1963, Baruch Blumberg (who won the Nobel prize in 1976) and colleagues identified hepatitis B surface antigen, a serologic marker for active hepatitis B infection. Subsequent epidemiological work from Blumberg's group established hepatitis B as an important cause of liver cancer worldwide. Simultaneously, numerous studies

---

*Scientists at the 24th Meeting of the Society for General Microbiology argued about whether a virus was a microorganism or a chemical molecule. According to A. Grafe, after much debate, viruses were defined as strictly intracellular and potentially pathogenic entities with an infectious phase, and as

1. possessing only one type of nucleic acid
2. multiplying in the form of the genetic material
3. unable to grow and to undero binary fission
4. devoid of a Lipmann system (processes involved in intermediary metabolism).[20]

This definition still holds today.

reported higher rates of cervical cancer in multiparous, married women than in nulliparous, unmarried women. Women with early age of "sexual debut" and second wives of men whose first wives had died of cervical cancer were also found to be at higher risk of this malignancy. Taken together, these data strongly suggested a sexually transmitted cause for cervical cancer.* The organism responsible was sequentially thought to be a syphilitic spirochete (1950s), trichomonas (1960s), herpes simplex 2 (1970s), and ultimately human papillomavirus, the currently accepted culprit (see Chapter 6).[22]

Research on infectious diseases slowed in the 1970s; Surgeon General William H. Stewart, reflecting the tenor of the times, declared that it was "time to close the book on infectious diseases".[23] The war was thought to have been won. Then, in the 1980s, the emergence of the human immunodeficiency virus epidemic once again brought infections to the research forefront. It became apparent that infectious diseases were far from defeated. In the 1990s, several highly publicized outbreaks of new infectious diseases, the publication of several popular books on "emerging pathogens," and international threats of biological warfare aroused collective consciousness to the microbial world. Included in the broad category of emerging pathogens was an impressive array of infectious agents, many of which chronically colonized the human body and led to long term disability. The new herpesviruses (including HHV-6 and HHV-8), human papillomaviruses (HPVs), *Helicobacter pylori*, hepatitis C infection—all common, chronic infections with the potential to cause long-term disability—added to the legacy of chronic HIV. Moreover, infectious agents began to be implicated as causes of nonmalignant chronic conditions including ulcerative colitis, Crohn's disease, rheumatoid arthritis, sarcoidosis, multiple sclerosis, and even atherosclerosis. This renaissance of interest in infection as a cause of chronic disease has led to a burgeoning discipline—the systematic search for occult infections in common diseases.

The rapid advances in molecular biology have now shifted research attention toward understanding the molecular chain of events involved in mutagenesis, DNA repair, and carcinogenesis. This incorporation of molecular microbiology and human oncogenesis resulted in the most recent Nobel prize in cancer research in 1989. Bishop and Varmus, for the first time, recognized the relationship between a retroviral oncogene and a normal human gene (a protooncogene), *src*. Their research was the springboard for the rapid discovery of many of the human and viral oncogenes discussed in this book. Interestingly, with Bishop and Varmus's work, a half century of research on infection and cancer came full circle.

---

*Dr. Rigoni-Stern, an Italian physician who lived in the mid-nineteenth century, is widely credited as being the first person to note the transmissible nature of cervical cancer, but this attribution is now known to be apocryphal. His only published work makes no specific mention of cervical cancer; it notes only that the ratio of breast to uterine cancer is higher in nuns than in other women.

The virus on which Bishop and Varmus based their discoveries was the long-maligned Rous sarcoma virus.

OUTLINE OF THIS BOOK

The chapters in Part I of this book present general mechanisms by which infections might lead to cancer. Infections that cause cancer run the gamut from viruses to large, multicellular parasites. One feature that they have in common is that they all persist for years in their host. The ways in which microorganisms establish their niche and hang on to it are described in Chapter 1.

With few exceptions (e.g., *H. pylori* and gastric lymphoma, and bacteria in colon cancer), infections are thought to cause cancer via one of two pathways: either by causing inflammation or by more directly causing cell transformation. The inflammation pathway hearkens back to the mid-nineteenth century irritation hypothesis of Virchow. Virchow speculated that chronic irritation established the setting in which cells would grow abnormally. Indeed, prior to the advent of antibiotics, physicians commonly witnessed such events. For example, chronic osteomyelitis, left surgically untreated, often resulted in epidermoid cancers of the draining sinus tracks. Similarly, chronic skin ulcers, whether from specific infection (such as *Mycobacterium ulcerans*) or from chronic venous stasis or decubitus ulceration, could lead to aggressive skin cancers. Today, we have experimental evidence of the irritation or inflammation theory. When irritative foreign bodies are deposited beneath the skin of mice and the animals are exposed to additional mutagens, cancers develop in the site of the foreign body at far greater frequency than would be expected without the foreign body in place. Anti-inflammatory agents can mitigate against this occurrence.[24]

How does infection-induced inflammation lead to cancer? There are several leading hypotheses. First, inflammation is invariably accompanied by formation of reactive oxygen and nitrogen species that can damage DNA, proteins, and cell membranes. A detailed description of this process is given in Chapter 2. Second, infections that cause inflammation typically induce an unremitting cycle of cell damage, necrotic cell death, and compensating cell proliferation. This process and its influence on mutagenesis is detailed in Chapter 3. Specific organisms that are thought to cause cancer primarily by inducing chronic inflammation include schistomomal parasites (Chapter 12), the liver flukes (Chapter 13), *H. pylori* (Chapter 14), and probably hepatitis B and C (Chapters 9 and 10). Several other pathogens, not included in this volume, might also act by this pathway, including mycoplasma in the lung, *Mycobacterium ulcerans* in the skin, *Salmonella typhi* in the biliary tree, and chronic bacterial infections of the urinary bladder, bone, and skin. Unfortunately, not enough information is yet available about these latter processes to warrant full chapters on each. General mechanisms for inflammation and cancer presented in Chapters 2 and 3, however, likely pertain to these infections as well.

Directly oncogenic pathogens, all of which are viruses, induce cancer by mechanisms markedly different from those of the inflammatory pathogens. Although some of these pathogens may cause a moderate degree of inflammation, their carcinogenic effects appear to be largely unrelated to this inflammatory process. Instead, the viruses alter the cell cycle and immortalize host cells by inserting active oncogenes, inhibiting tumor suppressor genes, or mimicking growth factors. The oncogenic potential of these viruses is discussed in detail in Chapter 4. Unlike the cancers related to inflammation, cancers from oncogenic viruses do not seem to arise in proportion to the duration of infection; indeed, many of these viruses can cause cancer quickly. For example, in HIV-infected patients, HHV-8 is resident in the host for only a short time before cancer occurs. Similarly, in Africa, Burkitt's lymphoma occurs in young children, suggesting a short incubation period for Epstein-Barr virus. Also, in contrast to inflammation-related malignancy, immunosuppression may be the key to emergence of many of these viral cancers. For example, HPV infection leads to cervical cancer more frequently in HIV-positive patients than it does in women without HIV.[25] Similarly, EBV- and HHV-8-related cancers almost exclusively occur in immunocompromised hosts. The mechanisms by which immunosuppression affect tumor progression are detailed in Chapter 5.

Chapters in Part II describe specific pathogens and these pathogens' associations with cancer. Each provides information on the epidemiological evidence for the association between infection and disease as well as information on probable mechanisms of carcinogenesis. Chapters 15 and 16 conclude the book with conceptual perspectives on bacterial infection as a cause of lymphoma and colorectal cancer.

SUMMARY

At any given time, there are more microbes in the human body than there are human cells. Thus, humans are constantly exposed to infectious agents. It is naive to believe that these organisms inhabit us for our own good. In fact, germ-free animals can live up to twice as long as identical animals living in conventional conditions.[26,27] This extension of life is equal to that seen with calorie restriction, suggesting that chronic colonization of the animal with microbes induces the same metabolic wear and tear on the host as does the average diet. In my mind, it is useful to think of the microbial world in our body as analagous to human life on earth. Clearly, without intending to do so, we damage our environment. We pollute the air and oceans, kill off co-inhabiting species, and even cause planetary overheating. Although not everything we do is bad—indeed some of our undertakings may be beneficial—there is no doubt that many of our activities soil our nest. Why should microbes be any smarter? They cannot see the long-term consequences of their behavior. Moreover, in the case of malignancy, many thousands of microbial generations will transpire before damage to the host is evident. Can humans envision the damage we will have wrought on earth after thousands of generations' time? In many respects, the inflammation theory of infection and cancer paints a beautiful picture of evolution in microscopic form. The microbes chronically, and possibly inadvertently, harm the host, causing cell damage and cell death. The only cells that can survive this foreign onslaught are those that mutate to protect themselves, eventually developing unrestricted cell growth. Thus, some infection-related cancers could be considered an unsuccessful evolutionary response to an alien microbial threat.

We must acknowledge, however, that most people who have oncogenic infections do not get cancer. They escape because, with rare exception, cancer is multifactorial in origin. The fact that only a minority of cigarette smokers—even of heavy cigarette smokers—develop cancer does not mitigate the tremendous importance of cigarette smoking as a cause of malignancy. The same can be said of exposure to microbial mutagens. Most chronic infections may be relatively benign; given these infections' ubiquity, however, their final toll on human life can be extremely high. From a scientific perspective, it is important to understand why cancer occurs in infected hosts. From a public health perspective, it is more important to understand why cancer does *not* occur. What can we do to protect people from dying of infection-related malignancy? Certainly, we are a long way off from establishing a society of germ-free humans. Instead, it makes sense for us to strive to identify those cofactors—be they environmental or genetic—that permit oncogenesis. It is with this thought in mind that I have put together this book on infection and cancer. It is my hope that the information presented here will inspire researchers to learn how to modulate the complex coexistence of microbes and humans.

REFERENCES

1. Proctor R. Cancer Wars. New York: BasicBooks; 1995.
2. Pisani P, Parkin DM, Munoz N, Ferlay J. Cancer and infection: estimates of the attributable fraction in 1900. Cancer Epidemiol Biomarkers Prev 1997;6:389–400.
3. Varmus H. An historical overview of oncogenes. In: Weinberg RA, ed. Oncogenes and the Molecular Origins of Cancer. Cold Spring Harbor: Cold Spring Harbor Laboratory Press; 1989:3–44.
4. Willett WC, Colditz GA, Mueller NE. Strategies for minimizing cancer risk. Sci Am 1996;275:88–95.
5. Trichopoulos D, Li FP, Hunter DJ. What causes cancer? Sci Am 1996;275:80–87.
6. Wolff J. The Science of Cancerous Disease from Earliest Time to the Present. Bethesda: Science History Pub; 1989.

7. Waterson AP, Wilkinson L. An Introduction to the History of Virology. Cambridge: Cambridge Univ. Press; 1978:

8. Rather LJ. Cell theory and the genesis of tumors, 1852–1900. In: The Genesis of Cancer. Baltimore: Johns Hopkins University Press; 1978:118–179.

9. Oberling C. The Riddle of Cancer. New Haven: Yale University Press; 1944.

10. Ewing J. Neoplastic Diseases. Philadelphia: Saunders; 1932:852

11. Vogt PK. Peyton Rous: Homage and appraisal. FASEB J 1996;10:1559–1561.

12. Wainwright M. The return of the 'Cancer Germ'. SGM Quarterly 1995;22:48–50.

13. Flance IJ. Scar cancer of the lung. JAMA 1991;266:2003–2004.

14. Meyer W. Cancer; Its Origin, Its Development and Its Self Perpetuation. New York: P.B. Hoeber; 1931:

15. Wernstedt W. Presentation speech for the Nobel prize in physiology or medicine, 1926. In: Nobel Foundation, ed. Nobel Lectures: Physiology or Medicine, 1922–1941. Amsterdam: Elsevier Publishing Co.; 1965:119–121.

16. Passey RD, Leese A, Knox JC. Spiroptera cancer and dietary deficiency. J Pathol Bacteriol 1935;40:198–205.

17. Cramer W. Papillomatosis in the forestomach of the rat and its bearing on the work of Fibiger. Am J Cancer 1937;31:537.

18. Behan RJ. Etiology. In: Cancer. St. Louis: C.V. Mosby Co.; 1938:54–114.

19. Lockhart-Mummery JP. The Origin of Cancer. London: J&A Churchill; 1934: 28–37.

20. Grafe A. A History of Experimental Virology. Berlin: Springer-Verlag; 1991: 158–159.

21. Friend C. The coming of age of tumor virology: Presidential Address. Cancer Res 1977;37:1255–1263.

22. Aurelian L. Herpesviruses and cervical cancer. In: Phillips LA, ed. Viruses Associated with Human Cancer. New York: Marcel Dekker; 1983:79–124.

23. Garrett L. The Coming Plague. New York: Penguin; 1995:33.

24. Robertson FM, Ross MS, Tober KL, Long BW, Oberyszyn TM. Inhibition of pro-inflammatory cytokine gene expression and papilloma growth during murine multistage carcinogenesis by pentoxifylline. Carcinogenesis 1996;17: 1719–1728.

25. Sun X, Kuhn L, Ellerbrock TV, Chiasson MA, Bush TJ, Wright TC. Human papillomavirus infection in women infected with the human immunodeficiency virus. N Engl J Med 1997;337:1343–1349.

26. Snyder DL, Pollard M, Wostmann BS, Luckert P. Life span, morphology, and pathology of diet-restricted germ-free and conventional Lobund-Wistar rats. J Gerontol 1990;45:B52–58.

27. Tazume S, Umehara K, Matsuzawa H, Aikawa H, Hashimoto K, Sasaki S. Effects of germfree status and food restriction on longevity and growth of mice. Jikken Dobutsu 1991;40:517–522.[Abstract]

28. Fredricks DN, Relman DA. Sequence-based identification of microbial pathogens: a reconsideration of Koch's postulates. Clin Microbiol Rev 1996;9:18–33.

I
MECHANISMS OF INFECTION-INDUCED MALIGNANCY

1

Chronic Host-Parasite Interactions

DAVID A. RELMAN

The traditional understanding of an infectious disease involves a one-sided, intrinsically unstable relationship between an aggressive microbial agent and an unwilling animal host or victim. An uncompromising drive for microbial self-replication leads inevitably to tissue damage and overt disease. The host is lucky to survive; the invading microorganism leaves, having increased in number, in search of new susceptible hosts. This paradigm evolved and spread rapidly in the first half of the twentieth century, heavily influenced by the well-documented societal impact of acute infectious diseases such as bubonic plague on human history, and by the emerging but monochromatic perspective of bacteriology.

In stark contrast, during these years—and still to this day—chronic infections were relatively ignored. Perhaps this oversight should not be so surprising. In part, the situation can be explained by inadequate methods of microbial detection and characterization. But, to paraphrase Sergei Winogradsky, a pioneering environmental microbiologist of the early twentieth century, chronic infections, by their nature, draw little attention to themselves.[1] In a more balanced long-term relationship between microorganism and host, overt damage is less apparent and signs of disease are more subtle. Evidence of a microorganism may be missed. In fact, because of the dependence of the microbial agent on poorly characterized host factors, it may be impossible to reproduce in the laboratory the conditions necessary for the agent's propagation, and hence it may be difficult to detect or identify that agent.

The establishment and maintenance of long-term host-parasite relationships require that each participant "understand" and adapt to its partner. Communication and sensing are important aspects of adaptation, and are discussed in a later section of this chapter. Cell cycle control and cellular proliferation signaling pathways are frequent targets for parasite adaptive responses. In addition, nonspecific immune surveillance mechanisms create selective pressures on these relationships and force accommodation. When Darwin discussed the evolution of communities, he explained that his concept of the "Struggle for Existence" also reflected the "dependence of one being on another" for the preservation of the individual, as well as for the more important purpose of generating successful progeny.[2] This theme is well-illustrated by molecular phylogenetic analyses of endosymbiotic relationships, in which coevolution of host and endoparasite is a common finding.[3,4] Perhaps the most extreme examples of chronic infections giving rise to mutualism over an evolutionary timescale are those putative ancestral infections that may have generated eukaryotic subcellular organelles, such as mitochondria and chloroplasts[5,6] (see later discussion).

Needless to say, long-term dialogues between microorganism and host are subject to misunderstandings, with adverse consequences for either participant. Error-prone nucleic acid replication processes, recombinational events, new secondary infections, misinterpreted environmental signals, aging host immune defenses and cellular maintenance systems, and other host-dependent environmental changes can all lead to an imbalance in a precarious relationship. Because the process of establishing this relationship often involves stimulation and/or subversion of normal host cell growth responses, it directly follows that dysregulated or unregulated host cell growth—that is, cancer—might result. Many of these features of chronic infections—codependence, sensing, and long-term adaptation—do not conform well to traditional paradigms for microbial infection. The definition of a virulence factor becomes clouded. In particular, the details of microbe-host interactions associated with carcinogenesis, described in this volume, force us to broaden our concepts of microbial causation and pathogenesis.

THE SPECTRUM AND NATURE OF CHRONIC HOST-PARASITE RELATIONSHIPS

The language of chronic infections finds many of its origins in the study of long-term viral infections. Viral persistence denotes a spectrum of long-term subcellular relationships that includes chronic infections (productive of infectious particles) on the one hand, and latent infections (nonproductive) on the other hand. Dormancy is sometimes used in place of latency, in the context of long-term bacterial infections. When we look carefully, the distinctions between these types of infections become less meaningful: most persistent viral infections fit neither end of the spectrum, because most chronic infections (e.g., hepatitis B infections) include some degree of viral integration into the host cell genome, and most latent infections (e.g., herpes simplex virus infections) include some degree of viral shedding. The exact level of viral gene expression and assembly is heavily dependent on host species, host cell type, and the state of host immune surveillance. For example, Epstein-Barr virus (EBV) can be found in pharyngeal epithelial cells and in B cells from all seropositive asymptomatic humans. On average, one out of 100,000 peripheral B cells is infected and maintains a nonactivated phenotype, although the numbers vary from one individual to another.[7] In any healthy individual, the number tends to remain stable with time. Viral genes that are expressed preferentially during latency are the subject of intense scrutiny. Whether EBV-infected cells occasionally proliferate or enter a lytic cycle in order to compensate for cell loss due to cytotoxic T lymphocyte–mediated killing is unclear. A different kind of steady state, characterized by rapid virus-mediated cytolysis and compensatory host cell regeneration, is found in some chronic viral infections (e.g., human immunodeficiency virus [HIV] infection[8]), whereas there is little if any host cell turnover in other types of infection. During acute or reactivated disease and neoplastic transformation, this balance is thrown into disequilibrium.

Chronic infection of a host by bacteria, fungi, or parasites may involve adoption of a metabolically inactive (or dormant) state (e.g., *Coxiella burnetii*), differentiation into a spore or cyst (e.g., *Coccidioides immitis*) (see Figure 1.1), formation of a specialized intracellular compartment (e.g., *Toxoplasma gondii*), and/or inducement of the host to form a protected anatomic structure such as a granuloma (e.g., *Mycobacterium tuberculosis*). The molecular details of these host-pathogen interactions are understood less well than are those in the chronically virus infected cell. We do know that specific microbial gene expression patterns are associated with various temporal phases of host infection and with maintenance of a quasi-equilibrium state between pathogen and host. Some of these genetic responses are described in a later section of this chapter.

What might be some of the possible advantages of chronic host-parasite infections for each of the two participants? One can approach this question from an individual- or a population-based perspective. Long-term persistence within a host permits a microorganism to wait for more favorable growth conditions. It may also facilitate microbial dissemination through increased numbers of contacts with other potential hosts over time and space, assuming that the microbe is mobile. Levin describes the "within-host evolution" of acute, host-destructive virulence properties by certain pathogens as "short-sighted" for the species as a whole, although it may confer immediate, locally selective advantages.[9] With the definition of a *pathogen* as any microorganism whose strategy for replication, persistence, and transmission mandates some degree of clinically manifest host damage,[10] we might argue that the difference between those pathogens that establish acute versus chronic host-pathogen relationships is simply a difference in long-term survival strategy.

The advantages of a chronic infection to an individual host are difficult to discern. Protection against superinfection by related organisms and against more frequent neoplastic transformation are theoretical considerations.[11] The postulated beneficial roles of the endogenous, or "normal," microbial (bacterial and fungal) flora of higher order hosts include

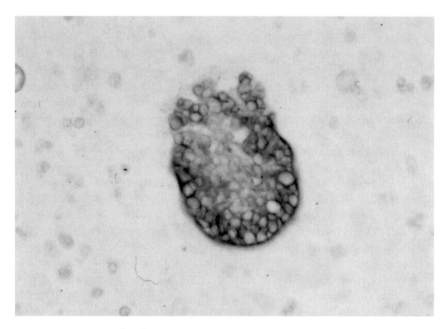

Figure 1.1. *Coccidioides immitis* causes a chronic pulmonary infection with the creation of cavities or nodules in approximately 5% of hosts. Organisms persist as a thick-walled spherule with little host inflammatory response. After years, in some cases, rupture of the spherule (as seen here) releases its pro-inflammatory endospores with subsequent disease reactivation. (Gridley stain, ×400)

synthesis of nutrients and vitamins, resistance against colonization by foreign or opportunistic microbes, and immune system stimulation. Data are most compelling in support of the first two roles.[12,13] Those members of the colonic flora that synthesize vitamins K and B complex, for example, might be viewed as true mutualistic symbionts, whereas those members with no apparent beneficial or harmful effects constitute commensals. Although most members of the commensal flora are rare causes of disease and are not usually defined as primary pathogens, over a broader time scale it may be more difficult to define the differences among pathogenic species that establish chronic relationships with their hosts, opportunistic pathogens, and commensal species. The long-term interplay between pathogen and host may also affect host genetics and population fitness. In fact, an evolutionary perspective might suggest that chronicity is a more highly evolved form of host-parasite relationship.

Intimate associations of pathogen and host sometimes have an important influence on immediate offspring and fecundity. The alpha-proteobacteria, which include the rickettsia-like organisms, are prime examples of pathogens that establish relationships of this type with invertebrate hosts. Transmission of these pathogens from a female arthropod to the eggs in her ovaries, and hence to her offspring (transovarial transmission), or from one arthropod stage of development to the next (transstadial transmission), maintains these microorganisms in nature. *Rickettsia rickettsii*, the cause of Rocky Mountain Spotted Fever; *Rickettsia typhi*, the cause of endemic typhus; and closely related organisms[14] are maintained by these mechanisms in tick and flea populations, respectively. When introduced into an accidental host such a human being, these pathogens induce acute disease. Other rickettsia-like bacteria also form endosymbiotic relationships with their insect hosts by infecting gonadal tissue[15], and, by doing so, give rise to a phenomenon called *cytoplasmic incompatibility* that is responsible for insect reproductive isolation and sex ratio distortion. Insect endosymbionts also enhance nutrient acquisition by their hosts and influence individual fitness positively.[16]

From a broad perspective, it seems likely that all chronic host-pathogen interactions bear evolutionary implications; in fact, numerous studies provide evidence of host-pathogen coevolution. A seminal study examined *in vitro* adaptation of virus and host cell to each other using the murine reovirus infection model.[17] After passage of virally infected murine L cells for approximately 1 year, reovirus isolates were more efficient at establishing persistent infection in uninfected L cells, and the adapted host L cells were more resistant to wild-type virus infection but more competent in the propagation of adapted virus.[17] In individual hosts, Wolinsky and colleagues showed that patients with slower rates of disease progression harbor populations of HIV-1 variants that have more genetic heterogeneity.[18] They proposed that HIV-1 sequences encoding cytotoxic T-lymphocyte epitopes exhibit adaptive evolution in some patients under the selective pressure of host cellular immune responses, leading to slower rates of $CD4^+$ T-cell loss. With a view toward longer time scales, phylogenetic analyses of conserved sequences among the single stranded small DNA viruses—the polyomaviruses, papillomaviruses, and parvoviruses—indicate that these host species–specific viruses may have coevolved with their hosts.[3] These ubiquitous viruses usually cause inapparent and lifelong infection with maintenance of episomal (extrachromosomal, self-replicating) DNA in infected host cells. Evolutionary trees generated from the sequences of conserved viral proteins, and of the host cellular regulatory proteins with which they interact, are congruent. Conversely, the rare members of these viral families that cause acute (versus chronic) disease show evolutionary dislinkage with their hosts. Highly conserved sequences within the host-interaction domains of critical viral proteins, such as the polyomavirus large T antigen, may prove to be central to coevolution. Thus, despite the capacity of these viruses for rapid molecular evolution, persistent infection may require selective genetic stability. At the opposite end of the parasite size spectrum, coevolution is also found with pocket gopher species and their ectoparasites, the chewing lice.[4]

If chronic infections develop into coevolving endosymbiotic relationships, then it would not be too surprising to find that some eukaryotic subcellular organelles may have originated from ancient prokaryotic endosymbioses.[5,6] Analysis of mitochondrial ribosomal DNA (rDNA) sequences from a wide variety of Eukarya reveals a tight line of descent, originating with a single common ancestor also shared by some of the alpha-proteobacteria (e.g., the rickettsiae and ehrlichiae). Chloroplast rDNA sequences suggest that these organelles (chloroplasts) are the descendents of ancestral cyanobacteria, although chloroplasts and cyanobacteria appear to have multiple putative common evolutionary ancestors. Multiple origins of a coevolutionary relationship are also illustrated by the phenomenon of lichen formation: a symbiotic association of fungi with algae.[19] Lichen symbiosis is not a primitive lifestyle; it has arisen at least five times in the evolutionary history of the fungi. Lichen formation may follow from, as well as give rise to, parasitism.

The link between microbial persistence and host cell growth state increasingly shares center stage with immune system interference in discussions about the mechanisms underlying chronic host–microbe relationships. Let us return to EBV as an illustrative example. One of the viral latent gene products, latent membrane protein 1 (LMP-1), induces growth in B cells by mimicking an activated growth factor receptor and transmitting growth signals through the same pathways used by endogenous tumor necrosis factor receptors.[20,21] Immune defense mechanisms may be subverted at the same time. LMP-1 alone has transforming activity in a variety of cell types. Constitutive activation or interference with intrinsic host cell growth-associated processes may also create opportunities for malignant transformation, especially in hosts that have additional underlying risk factors. Babesiosis, or piroplasmosis in the natural animal host, is a chronic parasitic infection associated with lymphoproliferation. Data indicate that the intraerythrocytic pathogen *Babesia microti* may persist in some human hosts as well.[22] In cattle, the intraleukocytic piroplasm *Theileria parva* causes reversible lymphocyte transformation and a rapidly fatal illness[23]; however, early treatment of this infection eliminates the proliferating lymphocyte lineages. Malignant neoplasms are a rare outcome of any persistent infection; one might argue that they are counterproductive and unintended from the perspective of the microbial pathogen.

MECHANISMS FOR ESTABLISHMENT
OF CHRONIC RELATIONSHIPS

What determines whether an infection will result in a short-term or in a long-term relationship? In some instances, the nature of the infectious agent alone dictates the outcome; however, many pathogens are capable of either type of relationship, and for these organisms it is the immunological competence of the host and specific host signals that play a major role. For their part, microbial pathogens send signals and "make requests" of their hosts that often lead to the creation of a specialized niche. *Staphylococcus aureus* is usually considered an agent of acute clinical syndromes; yet, chronic infections are probably far more common, resulting in bony sequestra, thick-walled abscess cavities, or protected bacterial consortia on a foreign body surface. The ability of this organism to behave in this two-faced manner may depend on its use of two-component sensor-response regulator systems to detect and transduce host environmental signals.[24] These signals create a signature for any given host environment and stimulate a coordinated expression pattern of bacterial genes encoding virulence-associated products such as secreted toxins, adherence factors, and immune-modulating factors. Pathogens that usually establish long-term host relationships often limit their interactions to the immediate environment, induce the formation of protective and sequestered anatomic compartments, and act in a discrete manner. Host-pathogen signaling and microbial subversion of host immune defenses are two mechanisms by which chronic infections are established and maintained. These mechanisms will be discussed in more detail later in this chapter.

Host-pathogen signaling, or cross talk, is a two-way, dynamic process that begins within seconds after a pathogen enters the host. Some of the cues and responses that take place within its earliest phases determine the fate and nature of the ongoing infection. However, the process of gaining access to the host, or of creating its preferred niche, may be a complicated one for a microorganism and require passage through a number of diverse environments. Transient or local environmental fluctuations may occur (e.g., dietary changes, alterations in endogenous microflora, local disease). In addition, more global and lasting changes in the host habitat may supervene (e.g., chronic underlying systemic disease, drug-induced immunosuppression, aging). The resulting microbial responses may convert an acute infection into a chronic infection, or a chronic one into an acute one.

Alterations in microbial phenotype *in vivo* may also take place late in the course of infection. Changes in antigen expression are particularly well documented and are thought to be selected in some cases by host immune responses.[25,26] *Borrelia burgdorferi*, the agent of Lyme disease, changes its antigenic profile during chronic stages of human disease,[27] as well as while dwelling within its tick vector.[28] Contact with a host cell surface is also a critical microbe-modulating stimulus. For instance, *Yersinia* attachment to host cells activates a contact-dependent specialized *Yersinia* secretion system that delivers a group of potent cytotoxins (Yops) directly into the host cell cytoplasm; the secretion system also then rids the bacterium of a transcriptional repressor, thereby enhancing Yop expression.[29] *Yersinia* species are responsible for intestinal infections, as well as for plague. In another example, PapG-mediated P-pilus attachment of uropathogenic *E. coli* to its cognate receptors on host cell surfaces in the urinary tract induces expression of an *E. coli* sensor protein, AirS/BarA, that controls bacterial responses to iron limitation.[30,31] Thus, bacterial attachment to a uroepithelial surface receptor activates an iron acquisition system that is critical for bacterial growth in iron-deficient urine. Although *Yersinia pseudotuberculosis* and uropathogenic *E. coli* are not primarily chronic disease agents, they illustrate the phenomenon of specific adaptive microbial gene responses to host cell contact.

Bacterial responses associated with later stages of host infection reflect the stress of nutrient deprivation and increased competition for limited resources. One response mechanism involves modification of RNA polymerase binding specificity through the substitution of alternative sigma factors (binding subunits), and, hence, transcriptional activation of new sets of bacterial genes. Some bacteria (e.g., *Pseudomonas*) are capable of sensing their own local population density, using quorum sensing systems; upon reaching a critical population density, these bacteria activate specialized sets of genes that in some cases provide tissue-invasive properties. Other bacteria respond to nutrient limitation by forming a metabolically-inactive spore. Although some of these responses can be induced *in vitro*, it has been much more difficult to identify the precise, relevant *in vivo* cues. Certain cytokines enhance microbial persistence and latency. For example, interferon gamma may induce persistent chlamydial forms.[32] However, a more precise understanding of microbial responses *in vivo* at the subcellular and transcriptional levels is likely to follow from the recent development of sensitive and selectable gene expression–reporter systems.[33,34] For example, these systems may permit identification of mycobacterial genes that are preferentially expressed (and repressed) during bacterial dormancy within the host.[35]

In any two-way relationship, attribution of causation can be problematic. In the creation of a conducive local environment for a long-term infection, host responses to microbial stimuli are of importance equal to microbial responses. The results of these host responses are readily observed at a macroscopic level: inflammatory cell infiltrates, abscesses, granulomata, and even angiogenesis.[36] But the molecular details and the timing of these subcellular events are more obscure. Local cytokine expression is one component of the host response that is likely to play an important role in this process. Mucosal and epithelial cytokine responses have been characterized for a number of microbial pathogens. The gastric pathogen *Helicobacter pylori* induces expression of interleukin-8 from gastric epithelial cells and mucosal macrophages; expression levels are associated with gastritis severity and with certain bacterial gene products.[37–39] Uropathogenic *E. coli* provoke both IL-8 and IL-6 expression by urothelial cells.[40] However, it is not clear how IL-8, a chemoattractant and activator of neutrophils, might promote bacterial persistence. Cytokine expression patterns in more sequestered anatomic sites are less well studied.

Changes in host cell receptor numbers and function also have been associated with both acute and chronic infections. These sorts of changes affect leukocyte homing, migration of other cells such as fibroblasts, growth factor responses, and binding interactions of pathogens with host target cells.

A third form of host cell response is characterized by cytoskeletal rearrangement and intracellular kinase-mediated signaling. Acute intestinal pathogens elicit a variety of morphologic epithelial cell responses including membrane ruffling[41] and "attaching and effacing" lesion (or pedestal) formation.[42] Pedestal formation, for example, follows bacterium secretion of a bacterial protein into the host cell, subsequent tyrosine phosphorylation, and then its use as a bacterial receptor, and is associated with inositol triphosphate and calcium fluxes.[43] It seems likely that some of these early morphologic responses are also required for microbial persistence. As our tools become more sophisticated, the language of the dialogue between parasite and host will become more easily heard and understood.

An essential requirement for the establishment of a long-term relationship by a microorganism within an animal host is a mechanism for avoiding or subverting protective host immune responses. The wide variety of mechanisms by which microorganisms subvert and avoid innate and acquired immune defenses in the course of long-term infections speaks to the importance of this aspect of chronic microbial disease. Various comprehensive reviews cover this issue.[44-46] The diversity and complexity of these mechanisms suggests that they have evolved over long periods of host-microbe interaction. Of course, mechanisms of immune system subversion are not specific to chronic host-parasite relationships. Many acute, fulminant relationships involve widespread disruption of host immune functions. However, subtlety and precision of targeting are more common to the subversive activities of microorganisms that typically establish long-term relationships with their host.

Avoidance of immune recognition can be achieved by microorganisms in a number of ways[44-46]: 1) drastically reduce expression of all potential antigens by adopting a latent or dormant form of existence (e.g., Epstein-Barr virus; (2) persist within a cell type, such as a neuron, that bears few major histocompatibility complex (MHC) molecules (e.g., herpes simplex virus); or (3) continuously vary dominant antigenic proteins (e.g., borrelia, trypanosomes). Other strategies that involve an active microbial role include down-regulation of host MHC expression or association of microbial antigens with MHC (adenovirus), down-regulation of host accessory molecules used for antigen recognition (*M. tuberculosis*[47,48]), inhibition of stimulatory cytokines or up-regulation of suppressive cytokines, interference with complement activity, and, of course, destruction of essential immune response cells (HIV). Some of these activities have been only inferred from finding microbial genes similar to known proteins, or defined with *in vitro* assays; few have been confirmed with engineered isogenic mutants employed in relevant models of infection.

Selective targeting by some microbial pathogens preserves the integrity of host immune defenses and promotes long-term coexistence. In their quest to orchestrate a conducive environment for long-term persistence, some pathogens have evolved specific mechanisms for altering patterns of host cytokine activity. $CD4^+$ (or T helper, TH) T-cells are capable of two fundamentally different cytokine expression patterns. TH1 cells express interleukin (IL)-2 and interferon gamma (IFN-γ); they are responsible for controlling some types of intracellular infection and for promoting delayed-type hypersensitivity. TH2 cells express IL-4 and IL-5, and promote efficient antibody production. Microbial pathogens—especially those that replicate in an intracellular compartment—tend to suppress TNF, IL-1, and IL-2 activity, and convert TH1 to TH2 host responses.

Microorganisms that depend on their ability to down-regulate host immune responses often express multiple gene products for this purpose, and target multiple arms of the immune system. Many of the best-characterized examples of microbial interference with the host immune system involve the poxviruses, a family of large double-stranded DNA viruses. As a family, the poxviruses cause a wide spectrum of acute and chronic diseases: variola virus (VV), now extinct in the wild, was responsible for smallpox; molluscum contagiosum virus (MCV) causes chronic skin papules with little if any inflammatory response. As acute disease agents, some poxviruses block IFN activity within infected host cells, as well as secrete their own soluble form of a type I IFN receptor with high binding affinity and broad species specificity.[49] IFN is an important component of the host defenses against systemic poxvirus infection. Presumably, the vaccinia virus soluble IFN receptor competitively inhibits host IFN action, because a vaccinia mutant strain with a deletion of the receptor gene is substantially less virulent than the wild-type strain in a murine intranasal infection model.[49]

The published MCV genome sequence suggests multiple additional mechanisms by which this human-adapted poxvirus may subvert the immune response and thereby persist in the host.[50] The MCV genome sequence predicts at least 163 gene products, 104 of which appear to be shared by variola virus and are involved for the most part in the replication and makeup of MCV.[50] The remaining 59 predicted MCV genes are believed to dictate the nature of the virus–host cell interaction and are nonessential for viral replication *in vitro*. Some appear to encode factors expressed early in infection that may modify host defenses. For example, one open reading frame is predicted to encode an MHC class I molecule with deficient peptide binding activity that may competitively inhibit the functions of the host MHC proteins. In addition, MCV encodes a predicted protein that may act as a chemokine antagonist, with sequence similarity to human macrophage inflammatory protein 1b, but devoid of the monocyte activation domain. Of course, an overly aggressive or unrefined microbial strategy for immune subversion may lead to global immunosuppression with secondary opportunistic infections and possible death of the host. The ehrlichiae are obligate intraleukocytic bacteria that disrupt leukocyte function; opportunistic infections complicate the more se-vere cases of ehrlichiosis in both animals and humans.[51-53]

DETECTION OF PREVIOUSLY UNIDENTIFIED CHRONIC HOST-PARASITE RELATIONSHIPS AND CHARACTERIZATION OF GENE RESPONSES

Given their intimate relationship with, and dependence on, the host cell and environment, it should not be surprising that many microorganisms with long-term host relationships are difficult to propagate or purify in the laboratory. The lack of purified microorganism is one reason they have resisted detection and identification. Other reasons stem from the organisms' frequently inactive metabolic state and their low antigenicity. The development of genetic sequence–based approaches for microbial identification and detection directly from host specimens has eliminated reliance on microbial phenotypes. The screening of recombinant expres-sion libraries was one of the first successful—albeit laborious—methods for identifying an occult microbial pathogen (hepatitis C virus).[54] This method makes use of a patient's antibodies to identify pathogen-specific gene products being expressed by one or more recombinant vectors within a large collection. With an approach known as consensus or broad range PCR, phylogenetically useful sequences, such as that of the small subunit ribosomal RNA gene, are amplified directly from host tissues. One uses PCR primers that recognize highly conserved flanking se-quences found within broad groups of microorganisms—for example, all known bacteria.[55-58] The selection of these primers requires few initial as-sumptions about the nature of the putative pathogen. The more variable regions of the amplified product sequence are used to infer evolutionary relationships between the microorganism under investigation and those previously characterized. A different approach, known as *representational difference analysis*,[59] integrates subtractive hybridization methodology with nucleic acid amplification. By mixing together two complex pools of nu-cleic acid, one from an infected host specimen and the other from an uninfected matched specimen, one can then amplify and isolate pieces of DNA or RNA that are unique to the infected pool—that is, that come from the putative pathogen.

In the past decade, sequence-based approaches have revealed a number of previously uncharacterized, persistent microbial pathogens. They in-clude *Bartonella henselae* (the agent of bacillary angiomatosis), *Tropheryma whippelii* (the agent of Whipple's disease), hepatitis C and G, and human herpes virus 8 (the agent of Kaposi's sarcoma; see Chapter 8).[57,58] Endo-symbionts have been revealed in fleas[14] and in other insects.[15] These and other molecular approaches are opening the door to a world of previously unrecognized chronic infections that may play critical roles in the maintenance of host nutrition, control of cell growth, host adaptation to altered environments, and resistance to microbial pathogens. Reflecting an imbalance intrinsic to many long-term host–parasite relationships, a number of human chronic idiopathic inflammatory diseases may also turn out to result from previously unrecognized chronic infections. Such diseases might include inflammatory bowel disease, sarcoidosis, coronary artery disease, rheumatoid arthritis, Wegener's granulomatosis and, as this book suggests, malignancies of as yet unknown etiology. Persistence of an intact microorganism may not be necessary in all of these cases. Novel approaches for detection of gene responses also promise insights into the mechanisms of microbial persistence. Reporter molecules, such as the green fluorescent protein, facilitate rapid and sensitive detection of genes that are expressed within relevant *in situ* host environments.[34,35] High-density microarrays of oligonucleotide probes will allow us to assess, in a comprehensive fashion, local human gene responses in chronically infected tissues.[60,61]

Reliance on molecular approaches for direct detection of microorganisms in idiopathic disorders and for identification of expressed genes *in situ*, however, will require revised criteria for proof of a causal association.[62] The intimate nature of the relationship between host and pathogen in a long-term infection is especially difficult to assess for evidence of causation because of codependence and the subtlety of the effects one exerts on the other.

The next decade will witness the elucidation of some of the subtleties in long-term microbial infections. The signals and cues that allow chronic infections to become established and then maintained will be identified in some cases. Miscommunications that lead to "inappropriate" host cell responses, such as malignant transformation, will be described in more detail. Previously unrecognized microbial pathogens will be detected in association with chronic idiopathic diseases, and the complex process of assessing causality will be undertaken. An exciting consequence of these endeavors will be the elucidation of fundamental biological processes, such as the control of mammalian cell growth, by virtue of an understanding of how microorganisms and host cells have learned to live together.

REFERENCES

1. Ward DM, Bateson MM, Weller R, Ruff-Roberts AL. Ribosomal RNA analysis of microorganisms as they occur in nature. In: Marshall KC, ed. Advances in Microbial Ecology. 12th ed. New York: Plenum Press; 1992: 219–286.
2. Darwin C. On the origin of species (First ed.). London: John Murray, 1859: 490.
3. Shadan FF, Villarreal LP. Coevolution of persistently infecting small DNA viruses and their hosts linked to host-interactive regulatory domains. Proc Natl Acad Sci USA 1993;90:4117–21.

4. Hafner MS, Sudman PD, Villablanca FX, Spradling TA, Demastes JW, Nadler SA. Disparate rates of molecular evolution in cospeciating hosts and parasites. Science 1994;265:1087–90.

5. Fox GE, Stackebrandt E, Hespell RB, et al. The phylogeny of prokaryotes. Science 1980;209:457–63.

6. Gupta RS. Evolution of the chaperonin families (Hsp60, Hsp10 and Tcp-1) of proteins and the origin of eukaryotic cells. Mol Microbiol 1995;15:1–11.

7. Miyashita EM, Yang B, Lam KM, Crawford DH, Thorley-Lawson DA. A novel form of Epstein–Barr virus latency in normal B cells in vivo. Cell 1995;80:593–601.

8. Perelson AS, Neumann AU, Markowitz M, Leonard JM, Ho DD. HIV-1 dynamics in vivo: virion clearance rate, infected cell life-span, and viral generation time. Science 1996;271:1582–1586.

9. Levin BR, Bull JJ. Short-sighted evolution and the virulence of pathogenic microorganisms. Trends Microbiol 1994;2:76–81.

10. Relman DA, Falkow S. A molecular perspective of microbial pathogenicity. In: Mandell GL, Douglas RG, Bennett JE, eds. Principles and Practice of Infectious Diseases. New York: Churchill Livingstone, 1994: 19–29.

11. Berns KI. Parvovirus replication. Microbiol Rev 1990;54:316–329.

12. Mackowiak PA. The normal microbial flora. N Engl J Med 1982;307:83–93.

13. Madigan MT, Martinko JM, Parker J. Brock—Biology of Microorganisms. Upper Saddle River, N.J.: Prentice Hall, 1997: 986.

14. Azad AF, Sacci JJ, Nelson WM, Dasch GA, Schmidtmann ET, Carl M. Genetic characterization and transovarial transmission of a typhus-like rickettsia found in cat fleas. Proc Natl Acad Sci USA 1992;89:43–46.

15. O'Neill SL, Giordano R, Colbert AM, Karr TL, Robertson HM. 16S rRNA phylogenetic analysis of the bacterial endosymbionts associated with cytoplasmic incompatibility in insects. Proc Natl Acad Sci USA 1992;89:2699–2702.

16. Richards FF. An approach to reducing arthropod vector competence. ASM News 1993;59:509–514.

17. Ahmed R, Canning WM, Kauffman RS, Sharpe AH, Hallum JV, Fields BN. Role of the host cell in persistent viral infection: coevolution of L cells and reovoirus during persistent infection. Cell 1981;25:325–32.

18. Wolinsky SM, Korber BT, Neumann AU, et al. Adaptive evolution of human immunodeficiency virus-type 1 during the natural course of infection (see comments). Science 1996;272:537–542.

19. Gargas A, DePriest PT, Grube M, Tehler A. Multiple origins of lichen symbioses in fungi suggested by SSU rDNA phylogeny (see comments) (published erratum appears in Science 1995 Jun 30;268(5219):1833). Science 1995;268:1492–1495.

20. Kieff E. Epstein–Barr virus—increasing evidence of a link to carcinoma (editorial; comment). N Engl J Med 1995;333:724–726.

21. Mosialos G, Birkenbach M, Yalamanchili R, VanArsdale T, Ware C, Kieff E. The Epstein–Barr virus transforming protein LMP1 engages signaling proteins for the tumor necrosis factor receptor family. Cell 1995;80:389–399.

22. Falagas ME, Klempner MS. Babesiosis in patients with AIDS: a chronic infection presenting as fever of unknown origin. Clin Infect Dis 1996;22:809–812.

23. ole-MoiYoi OK. Casein kinase II in theileriosis (comment). Science 1995;267:834–836.

24. Parkinson JS. Signal transduction schemes of bacteria. Cell 1993;73:857–871.

25. Lacey BW. Antigenic modulation of Bordetella pertussis. J Hyg (Camb) 1960; 58:57–93.

26. Brunham RC, Plummer FA, Stephens RS. Bacterial antigenic variation, host immune response, and pathogen-host coevolution. Infect Immun 1993;61: 2273–2276.

27. Craft JE, Fischer DK, Shimamoto GT, Steere AC. Antigens of *Borrelia burgdorferi* recognized during Lyme disease. Appearance of a new immunoglobulin M response and expansion of the immunoglobulin G response late in the illness. J Clin Invest 1986;78:934–939.

28. Schwan TG, Piesman J, Golde WT, Dolan MC, Rosa PA. Induction of an outer surface protein on *Borrelia burgdorferi* during tick feeding. Proc Natl Acad Sci U S A 1995;92:2909–2913.

29. Pettersson J, Nordfelth R, Dubinina E, et al. Modulation of virulence factor expression by pathogen target cell contact (see comments). Science 1996;273: 1231–1233.

30. Nagasawa S, Tokishita S, Aiba H, Mizuno T. A novel sensor-regulator protein that belongs to the homologous family of signal-transduction proteins involved in adaptive responses in *Escherichia coli*. Mol Microbiol 1992;6:799–807.

31. Zhang JP, Normark S. Induction of gene expression in *Escherichia coli* after pilus-mediated adherence (see comments). Science 1996;273:1234–1236.

32. Beatty WL, Byrne GI, Morrison RP. Morphologic and antigenic characterization of interferon gamma-mediated persistent *Chlamydia trachomatis* infection in vitro. Proc Natl Acad Sci USA 1993;90:3998–4002.

33. Cubitt AB, Heim R, Adams SR, Boyd AE, Gross LA, Tsien RY. Understanding, improving and using green fluorescent proteins. Trends Biochem Sci 1995; 20:448–455.

34. Valdivia RH, Falkow S. Fluorescence-based isolation of bacterial genes expressed within host cells. Science 1997; 277:2007–2011.

35. Kremer L, Baulard A, Estaquier J, Poulain-Godefroy O, Locht C. Green fluorescent protein as a new expression marker in mycobacteria. Mol Microbiol 1995;17:913–922.

36. Cockerell CJ, LeBoit PE. Bacillary angiomatosis: a newly characterized, pseudoneoplastic, infectious, cutaneous vascular disorder. J Am Acad Dermatol 1990;22:501–512.

37. Crabtree JE, Wyatt JI, Trejdosiewicz LK, et al. Interleukin-8 expression in Helicobacter pylori infected, normal, and neoplastic gastroduodenal mucosa. J Clin Pathol 1994;47:61–66.

38. Sharma SA, Tummuru MK, Miller GG, Blaser MJ. Interleukin-8 response of gastric epithelial cell lines to Helicobacter pylori stimulation in vitro. Infect Immun 1995;63:1681–1687.

39. Ando T, Kusugami K, Ohsuga M, et al. Interleukin-8 activity correlates with histological severity in Helicobacter pylori-associated antral gastritis. Am J Gastroenterol 1996;91:1150–1156.

40. Svanborg C, Agace W, Hedges S, Lindstedt R, Svensson ML. Bacterial adherence and mucosal cytokine production. Ann N Y Acad Sci 1994;730:162–181.

41. Francis CL, Ryan TA, Jones BD, Smith SJ, Falkow S. Ruffles induced by *Salmonella* and other stimuli direct macropinocytosis of bacteria. Nature 1993;364: 639–642.

42. Knutton S, Baldwin T, Williams PH, McNeish AS. Actin accumulation at sites

of bacterial adhesion to tissue culture cells: basis of a new diagnostic test for enteropathogenic and enterohemorrhagic *Escherichia coli.* Infect Immun 1989; 57:1290–1298.

43. Kenny B, DeVinney R, Stein M, Reinscheid DJ, Frey EA, Finlay BB. Enteropathogenic E. Coli (EPEC) transfers its receptor for intimate adherence into mammalian cells. Cell 1997; 91:511–520.

44. Marrack P, Kappler J. Subversion of the immune system by pathogens. Cell 1994;76:323–332.

45. Smith GL. Virus strategies for evasion of the host response to infection. Trends Microbiol 1994;2:81–88.

46. Zinkernagel RM. Immunology taught by viruses. Science 1996;271:173–178.

47. Pancholi P, Mirza A, Bhardwaj N, Steinman RM. Sequestration from immune CD4+ T cells of mycobacteria growing in human macrophages. Science 1993;260:984–986.

48. Gercken J, Pryjma J, Ernst M, Flad H. Defective antigen presentation by Mycobacterium tuberculosis-infected monocytes. Infect Immun 1994;62:3472–3478.

49. Symons JA, Alcami A, Smith GL. Vaccinia virus encodes a soluble type I interferon receptor of novel structure and broad species specificity. Cell 1995;81: 551–560.

50. Senkevich TG, Bugert JJ, Sisler JR, Koonin EV, Darai G, Moss B. Genome sequence of a human tumorigenic poxvirus: prediction of specific host response-evasion genes. Science 1996;273:813–816.

51. McDade JE. Ehrlichiosis—a disease of animals and humans. J Infect Dis 1990;161:609–617.

52. Dumler JS, Bakken JS. Human granulocytic ehrlichiosis in Wisconsin and Minnesota: a frequent infection with the potential for persistence. J Infect Dis 1996;173:1027–1030.

53. Bakken JS, Krueth J, Wilson-Nordskog C, Tilden RL, Asanovich K, Dumler JS. Clinical and laboratory characteristics of human granulocytic ehrlichiosis. JAMA 1996;275:199–205.

54. Choo QL, Kuo G, Weiner AJ, Overby LR, Bradley DW, Houghton M. Isolation of a cDNA clone derived from a blood-borne non-A, non-B viral hepatitis genome. Science 1989;244:359–362.

55. Lane DJ, Pace B, Olsen GJ, Stahl DA, Sogin ML, Pace NR. Rapid determination of 16S ribosomal RNA sequences for phylogenetic analyses. Proc Natl Acad Sci U S A 1985;82:6955–6959.

56. Relman DA, Loutit JS, Schmidt TM, Falkow S, Tompkins LS. The agent of bacillary angiomatosis. An approach to the identification of uncultured pathogens (see comments). N Engl J Med 1990;323:1573–1580.

57. Relman DA. The identification of uncultured microbial pathogens. J Infect Dis 1993;168:1–8.

58. Gao S-J, Moore PS. Molecular approaches to the identification of unculturable infectious agents. Emerg Infect Dis 1996;2:159–167.

59. Lisitsyn N, Lisitsyn N, Wigler M. Cloning the differences between two complex genomes. Science 1993;259:946–951.

60. Schena M, Shalon D, Davis RW, Brown PO. Quantitative monitoring of gene expression patterns with a complementary DNA microarray (see comments). Science 1995;270:467–470.

61. Chee M, Yang R, Hubbell E, et al. Accessing genetic information with high-density DNA arrays. Science 1996;274:610–614.
62. Fredricks DN, Relman DA. Sequence-based identification of microbial pathogens: a reconsideration of Koch's postulates. Clin Microbiol Rev 1996;9:18–33.

2

Chronic Inflammation, Mutation, and Cancer

STEPHAN CHRISTEN, TORY M. HAGEN,
MARK K. SHIGENAGA, AND BRUCE N. AMES

Phagocyte-derived oxidants protect the host during infection by incinerating invading pathogens; they can also damage the DNA, proteins, and lipids of host cells. This oxidative damage contributes in the short term to cell injury, necrosis, compensatory cell proliferation, and mutation. In the long term, it increases the risk of cancer. Oxidants produced by nonphagocytic cells may also contribute to these processes. In this chapter, we describe important mechanisms of carcinogenesis and present a brief overview of the relationship between chronic inflammation and cancer. We then discuss in depth the role of phagocyte-derived oxidants in carcinogenesis associated with inflammation. In particular, we describe the use of biomarkers of oxidative damage to study the relationship between carcinogenesis and damage caused by inflammatory oxidants. Finally, we review current knowledge of how dietary antioxidants and other strategies can minimize the risk of cancer due to chronic inflammation.

OVERVIEW OF CARCINOGNESIS AND INFLAMMATION

Mechanisms of Carcinogenesis

Mutations

Mutations in several critical genes are required for tumor formation.[1] Exposure of target cells to mutagenic conditions, such as the release of oxidants by phagocytes and compensatory cell proliferation, will increase the probability of these cells developing the mutations necessary for tumor development. The tumor suppressor gene *p53*, for example, is one of several genes that, upon mutation, increase the probability of further mutation, and thus cancer. *p53* mutations are found in about one half of all human tumors. p53 protein guards a cell-cycle checkpoint, and its inactivation by mutation allows cell division to proceed despite the presence of DNA lesions (damaged bases or chromosome breaks). Any oxidative mutagen produced as a consequence of phagocyte activation causes an increase in lesions over the already existing endogenous lesions.[2] Thus, the mutagenicity of a particular lesion depends on its rate of excision by the DNA repair system, and the increased probability that a mutation occurs when the cell divides.

DNA is oxidized because antioxidant defenses are not perfect. The number of oxidative hits to DNA per cell per day is estimated to be about 100,000 in the rat and roughly 10 times fewer in humans, because of their slower metabolic rate.[2a] DNA repair enzymes efficiently remove most but not all of the lesions formed. Thus, oxidative lesions in DNA accumulate with age; so, by the time a rat is old (26 months), it has about 7×10^4 DNA lesions per cell—about three times the numbers seen in a young rat.[2,2a] Similar increases in the accumulation of oxidative lesions are observed in virus-induced hepatitis, a chronic inflammatory disease that also is associated with an increase in specific mutations[3] and a markedly increased risk of developing hepatocellular carcinoma.[4,5] An increase in mutations also occurs during normal human aging.[6]

Cell Division

Chronic inflammation caused by either infectious or noninfectious agents is associated with increased cell division in areas adjacent to inflammatory foci and tissue injury. Cell division is a critical factor in mutagenesis because it converts DNA lesions to point mutations, deletions, or translocations (this is discussed more fully in Chapter 3).[7-10] The cells that appear to be most relevant for cancer are the stem cells, which, unlike their daughter cells, are not discarded. An increase in the rate of division of stem cells increases mutation and hence increases the incidence of cancer. As expected, cancer in nondividing cells is rare. Increased cell division is not only observed in chronic inflammatory diseases but also can be caused by such diverse conditions as increased levels of endogenous hormones,[11] excess calories, or exposure to chemicals at doses causing chronic cell division.[10,12-15] An increase in mutagenesis will be multiplicative when both the rate of DNA lesions *and* cell division are increased simultaneously. This effect is observed in chronic inflammatory diseases, such as the transgenic mouse model of hepatitis described later in this chapter.

Cell cycle checkpoints prevent division of cells that have too many DNA lesions and thus inhibit the formation of mutations. However, like DNA repair, this defense is not perfect. Lesions in transcribed genes are sensed by the transcription apparatus that synthesizes mRNA.[16,17] The presence of lesions appears to induce DNA repair and also to arrest cell division at a cell cycle checkpoint. A possible mechanism may be that p53 protein, which controls the G_1 to S checkpoint, is associated with replication protein A (RPA).[18,19] When DNA damage occurs, the repair protein RPA appears to bind to single-stranded DNA, thereby releasing p53 protein.[18,19] This in turn causes a block of cell division at the checkpoint, preventing conversion of lesions to mutations.[20] Because p53 is involved in triggering apoptotic cell death,[21] a higher level of DNA lesions may also induce apoptosis.[22]

Cell Injury

Chronic inflammation leads to chronic cell killing and compensatory cell division. Surviving cells injured by the barrage of oxidants and other inflammatory mediators suffer genomic damage that increases the probability of mutation[23,24] Thus, during chronic inflammation, cell division and DNA lesions are increased concurrently, leading to multiplicative interactions that can result in higher mutation rates than are caused by either condition alone.

Chronic Inflammation and Cancer

Chronic inflammation can be due to infectious agents or to other chronic stimuli of the immune system. Here, we present only a brief overview of how certain pathogens are involved in carcinogenesis, as this material is presented in detail in other chapters of this book. We also present briefly induction of cancer by noninfectious, particulate irritants such as asbestos and silica to illustrate the carcinogenic effect of chronic inflammation per se. It has been estimated that chronic inflammation caused by chronic infections cause about 21% of new cancer cases in developing countries and 9% in developed countries.[24a]

Chronic Inflammation Caused by Infectious Agents

A direct causal relationship between chronic infection and cancer was at first difficult to establish. The difficulty was in part due to the lengthy latency period—often years—between onset of the infectious disease and the appearance of cancer. Also, factors other than inflammation influence the progression to neoplasia. Moreover, many infectious diseases are species specific, which limited the use of animals to model the effect that chronic infection plays in human carcinogenesis. However, it is now clear that certain chronic infectious diseases are strongly associated with specific types of cancer. The strongest association between chronic infection and cancer has been established between chronic infection with hepatitis B virus (HBV) and liver cancer (see Chapter 9). The risk does not appear to be directly associated with the virus itself in that the HBV genome does not contain any known oncogenic sequences, and integrated HBV genomic sequences only rarely activate cellular protooncogenes.[25–28] Instead, the increased risk of carcinogenesis is associated with the severity of the host immune response to virus-infected cells, and with the duration of infection.[29-31] Epidemiological evidence associating the inflammatory response with increased risk of cancer is bolstered by evidence from transgenic animal models that mimic chronic active human HBV infection.[5] Human hepatitis C virus (HCV)—although structurally different from HBV[32,33]—also increases the risk of hepatocellular carcinoma (see Chapter 10). HCV infection probably accounts for a significant proportion of patients with hepatocellular carcinoma with no serological markers for infection with HBV.[33] Recent studies have shown that 75% to 100% of hepatocellular carcinoma patients without circulating antibodies to HBV have serological markers for HCV. Moreover, the risk of developing hepatocellular carcinoma is significantly and synergistically increased in patients co-infected with HCV and HBV.[33]

Other chronic infectious diseases also have been shown to increase the risk of cancer. For example, persistent parasitic infection by schistosomes[34-36] or liver flukes[37,38] currently afflicts over 300 million people worldwide, particularly in developing countries with poor sanitation (see Chapters 12 and 13). Chronic inflammation associated with infection is apparently not a response to the parasite itself, but instead occurs at the sites where eggs are deposited.[39-41] Egg deposition results in activation and recruitment of monocytes and other leukocytes, followed by chronic ulceration of infected and surrounding tissue.[42-44] Often, epithelial cell hyperplasia ensues, followed by periductal fibrosis.[45] Another example is chronic infection with *Helicobacter pylori*, a bacterium that colonizes and inflames the gastric mucosa (see Chapter 14). Infection is associated with duodenal ulcer disease, gastritis, and stomach cancer,[46-48] again, especially in developing countries.

Chronic Inflammation Caused by Noninfectious Irritants

Chronic inflammation as a result of the host immune response to certain noninfectious agents also increases the risk of developing cancer. Chronic inhalation of inorganic dust (asbestos, silica, quartz dust) leads to pneumoconioses or to chronic interstitial lung diseases,[49-52] resulting in decreased transfer of oxygen to the blood. Of these irritants, only asbestos significantly increases the risk of developing lung cancer.[53,54]

Asbestos, a commercial name given to a group of silicates, does not appear to be directly genotoxic.[12] Rather, the risk of cancer arises from the inability of the lung to effectively remove the mineral fibers from the mesothelium—chronic irritation of the lung results. Needlelike asbestos fibers greater than 8 μm in length appear to be the least effectively removed from the lung and are most associated with asbestos-induced pulmonary fibrosis and development of malignant mesotheliomas.[55-57] The inability of the lung to remove long fibers appears to be a key component in the overall risk of development of lung cancer. Other small spherical mineral irritants that can be cleared readily from the lung do not cause an increased risk of pulmonary cancer,[58,59] although they induce an acute inflammatory response.

Asbestos causes a chronic interstitial lung disease that typically results in the recruitment and activation of phagocytes to the site of fiber deposition (described more fully below). Increased oxidant formation by infiltrating phagocytes contributes to the alveolar epithelial injury and pulmonary fibrosis.[60-62] Like the infectious diseases cited previously, this constant cell injury and regeneration in the presence of high levels of phagocyte-derived oxidants appears to be a likely causal event in the development of asbestos-induced mesotheliomas.

Carcinogenic Mechanisms Shared by Infectious Agents and Noninfectious Irritants

Although the infectious and noninfectious agents mentioned earlier are all different in nature, and each causes distinct pathophysiological processes, disease progression follows several common paths. Both invading pathogens and irritants cause persistent inflammation that often lasts for years. Apparently, chronic inflammation is required to increase the risk of cancer, because drugs or antioxidant therapies that are effective in treating the primary disease can substantially reduce or eliminate the incidence of cancer (described more fully later).

Chronic inflammation may result in a level of tissue damage and scarring that exceeds a certain threshold that is necessary for neoplasia to occur. For example, the risk of hepatocellular carcinoma in chronic active hepatitis is high only after inflammation has caused fibrosis or cirrhosis of the liver. Also, the risk of developing cholangiocarcinoma after *Schistosoma japonicum* infection drops significantly if treatment with praziquantel is begun prior to bile duct obstruction and can be sustained sufficiently to prevent reinfection. Furthermore, tissue scarring correlates with the degree of the host immune response.

The resultant cell death and compensatory cell proliferation promotes oxidative DNA damage and, ultimately, mutations in the presence of phagocyte-derived oxidants. Thus, carcinogenesis due to infection and chronic inflammation likely results *indirectly* from the host immune response to an invading pathogen and not *directly* because of the pathogen itself.

FORMATION OF OXIDANTS DURING THE HOST IMMUNE RESPONSE TO MICROBIAL AND VIRAL INFECTION

Inflammation and Activation of Phagocytes

The Inflammatory Process

Inflammation is normally characterized by three main responses: (1) the affected area is supplied with an increased volume of blood; (2) increased capillary permeability is caused by retraction of the endothelial cells, which allows soluble molecules such as inflammatory mediators and particles to traverse the endothelium; and (3) circulating peripheral blood leukocytes—which include polymorphonuclear leukocytes (PMNs), monocytes, and lymphocytes—migrate out of the capillaries into the surrounding tissue.

After traversing the endothelium, leukocytes migrate toward the site of infection in response to chemotactic factors that diffuse into the tissue. These chemotactic factors are thought to diffuse to the adjoining capillaries where they induce adherence of passing cells to the endothelium and initiate their migration of these cells into the subendothelial space. Complement activation at the site of inflammation causes the deposition of complement fragments onto invading microorganisms (opsonization), a process that greatly facilitates the recognition of foreign cells by recruited phagocytes. Recognized foreign cells are then taken up by the phagocytes in a receptor-dependent process. The phagosomes formed fuse with lysosomes to form phagolysosomes. In the phagolysosomes, the ingested organisms are killed by a battery of microbicidal agents such as activated proteases and potent oxidants formed during the respiratory burst (see references 63–67 for review).

Inflammation is also initiated by the recognition of foreign antigens (e.g., those expressed on the surface of virus-infected host cells) by antigen-presenting cells. This function is mainly carried out by resident tissue macrophages (e.g., Kupffer cells in the liver), which when activated can also release cytotoxic oxidants. The extent of the inflammatory response and the type of immune response elicited depend primarily on how a particular antigen is presented to the infiltrating lymphocytes, and what subsequent pathways are induced by these cells. When an infection cannot be resolved quickly, or the control of the immune response is out of balance, the resulting chronic inflammation can cause extensive tissue damage. This is thought to be, in part, the result of the constant release of phagocyte-derived oxidants. Oxidant-mediated cytotoxicity is enhanced by the potential release of redox-active metals from intracellular stores, and by the activation of proteases.[65,68,69]

The Respiratory Burst

Stimulation of phagocytic cells (PMNs, eosinophils, and mononuclear phagocytes) leads to a respiratory burst: a massive increase in non-mitochondrial oxygen consumption.[70,71] This increased consumption is a result of one-electron reduction of oxygen by the plasma membrane–associated NADPH oxidase to the free radical superoxide anion ($O_2^{\cdot-}$). $O_2^{\cdot-}$ is a weak oxidant[72,73] that can participate in reactions that lead to the formation of more potent oxidants. Reduction of $O_2^{\cdot-}$ by one or more electrons effectively lowers the spin quantum number of ground state oxygen, thus eliminating its spin restriction and significantly enhancing its reactivity toward organic molecules.[74]

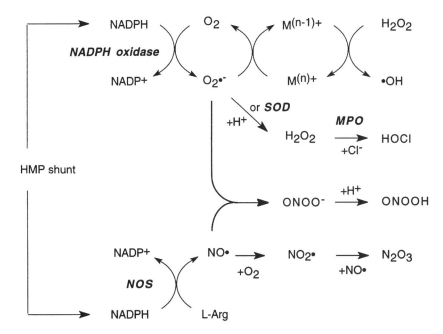

Figure 2.1. Oxidant formation by activated phagocytes. Univalent reduction of molecular (ground-state) oxygen initiates the formation of molecules with lower spin quantum number, thereby eliminating its spin restriction and effectively increasing its reactivity towards organic molecules (see ref. 74). Note: Reactions are not balanced. See text for abbreviations.

The respiratory burst is triggered either by phagocytosis of insoluble particles[70] or by direct stimulation with soluble agents such as immune complexes,[75,76] viruses such as influenza and Sendai,[77,78] an array of pro-inflammatory chemotactic agents such as bacterial formylpeptides,[79,80] complement fragment C5a,[81] platelet-activating factor,[82] and leukotriene B$_4$.[83] The respiratory burst is also stimulated by the tumor promoter phorbol 12-myristate 13-acetate (PMA).[83] This membrane-soluble molecule directly and nonspecifically activates protein kinase C, which is involved in the signal transduction pathway of several of the stimuli mentioned above. Reducing equivalents for the reduction of oxygen in the form of NADPH are obtained from enhanced glucose metabolism through the hexose monophosphate (HMP) shunt (Figure 2.1).

In addition to direct activators, bacterial endotoxin (lipopolysaccharide; LPS), interferon gamma (IFN-γ), and tumor necrosis factor–α (TNF-α) have been shown in vitro to prime phagocytes for enhanced production of O$_2$·⁻. Priming is induction of a cellular state of enhanced NADPH oxidase activity, where O$_2$·⁻ production needs to be triggered by a second factor, such as PMA.[84-86] When phagocytes adhere to physiological matrixes, however, IFN-γ and TNF-α can stimulate both a massive and a prolonged release of $O_2^{\cdot -}$, without the need for a second signal.[87] With interleukin 1 (IL-1), the proinflammatory IFN-γ and TNF-α play a central role in the activation of the various cells involved in the inflammatory response in vivo.

IFN-γ—produced, for example, by T cells—is a potent activator of mononuclear phagocytes. One of the most important effector functions is the induction of an array of antimicrobial and antitumor host defense mechanisms within these cells.[88,89] In mice, injection of monoclonal antibodies against IFN-γ, the lack of functional IFN-γ receptors,[90] or disruption of the IFN-γ gene[91] severely impairs the antimicrobial host defense. Antimicrobial and antitumor activity appear to be mediated, at least in part, by the induction of several rate-limiting enzymes. They include NADPH oxidase;[84] indoleamine 2,3-dioxygenase, which initiates tryptophan degradation along the kynurenine pathway;[92] and nitric oxide synthase (discussed later).[67]

TNF-α, which shares many activities with interleukin 1, is a potent activator of PMNs. It augments phagocytic activity, increases cytotoxicity to microorganisms, stimulates degranulation, acts as a chemoattractant, inhibits PMN migration, and causes PMN adhesion to endothelial cells (see reference 93 for review). Thus, the release of proinflammatory cytokines and other inflammatory mediators by activated phagocytes plays an important role in the tissue injury observed during inflammation.[69,94] Proinflammatory cytokines are under the control of the transcription factor NF-κB, a factor modulated by oxidative stress (see reference 95 for review). Therefore, oxidants may contribute to tissue damage not only directly but also indirectly by disturbing the antiprotease-protease balance and by deregulating normal cellular functions.[94]

The significance of in vivo $O_2^{\cdot -}$ generation by NADPH oxidase is demonstrated by the enhanced susceptibility of patients with chronic granulomatous disease (CGD) to certain types of bacterial infections (reviewed in reference 96). Phagocytes of CGD patients are defective in certain parts of the NADPH oxidase complex. Hence, they do not respond with increased formation of $O_2^{\cdot -}$ on stimulation. However, antimicrobial activity can be restored in macrophages from some CGD patients by treatment with IFN-γ, indicating that multiple, overlapping antimicrobial pathways coexist (reference 97 and references therein). Conversely, overexpression in transgenic mice of cytosolic superoxide dismutase (SOD), which converts $O_2^{\cdot -}$ to hydrogen peroxide (H_2O_2), significantly reduces the microbicidal and fungicidal activity of isolated macrophages, mimicking the reduced antimicrobial and antiviral defense system in patients with Down syndrome, a condition associated with overexpression of cytosolic SOD.[98] Again, this observation suggests that the formation of $O_2^{\cdot -}$ is important for microbicidal activity in vivo. Biochemical evidence for the presence of increased levels of oxidants under in vivo inflammatory conditions will be presented later in this chapter.

Biochemistry of Oxidants

Superoxide-Derived Oxidants

$O_2^{\cdot-}$ formed during the respiratory burst and released into phagolyso-somes or into the extracellular medium can either react with itself (*i.e.*, dismutate) to form H_2O_2—a more potent oxidant than $O_2^{\cdot-}$ itself—or react with other molecules such as nitric oxide (NO•). Associated with the respiratory burst are temporary changes in pH that result in a prolonged drop to more acidic values in the phagolysosomal vacuole[99,100] and the release of protons into the extracellular space.[101] Both of these events may result in an increase in the rate of spontaneous dismutation of $O_2^{\cdot-}$ (Figure 2.1). Conversion of $O_2^{\cdot-}$ to H_2O_2 is even more rapid when catalyzed by SOD. There are several forms of SOD which, depending on their sub-cellular locations, differ in their metal composition in the catalytic center.

Despite its low reactivity, $O_2^{\cdot-}$ is a potentially hazardous compound in biological systems because it can participate in the transition metal–cata-lyzed Haber-Weiss reaction and generate the far more reactive hydroxyl radical (•OH). The rate constant for the formation of •OH from $O_2^{\cdot-}$ and H_2O_2 (Equation 1)—originally proposed by Haber and Weiss[102]—is vir-tually zero in aqueous solution:

$$H_2O_2 + O_2^{\cdot-} \rightarrow O_2 + \cdot OH + OH^- \tag{1}$$

The reaction requires the presence of a redox-active transition metal (M^{n+}) (*e.g.*, Fe^{3+} or Cu^{2+}), which catalyzes the overall reaction between $O_2^{\cdot-}$ and H_2O_2[103,104] according to reactions 2 and 3:

$$M^{n+} + O_2^{\cdot-} \rightarrow M^{(n-1)+} + O_2$$
(reduction of transition metal) \qquad\qquad (2)

$$M^{(n-1)+} + H_2O_2 \rightarrow M^{n+} + \cdot OH + OH^-$$
(Fenton reaction) \qquad\qquad (3)

Net reaction: $O_2^{\cdot-} + H_2O_2 \rightarrow O_2 + \cdot OH + OH^-$
(metal-catalyzed Haber-Weiss reaction) \qquad\qquad (1)

Fenton chemistry, however, does not necessarily involve the formation of free •OH.[105] H_2O_2 also can react with reduced transition metals bound to macromolecules such as DNA to form activated metal complexes (*e.g.*, ferryl or perferryl radical) that can cause extensive and site-specific dam-age.[106,107] DNA damage can be observed, for example, when mammalian cells are exposed to either chemically generated or phagocyte-derived $O_2^{\cdot-}$ and H_2O_2 in vitro, an effect dependent on the availability of intracellular iron.[108]

Transition metals necessary to catalyze the formation of •OH (or of intermediates with similar reactivity) are normally tightly bound to specific binding proteins and are thus not immediately available for redox reactions. Certain conditions may attain, however, under which transition metals can be mobilized. For example, in vitro, iron can be released from ferritin by reductants such as $O_2^{-\cdot}$, a process that may contribute to the toxicity of PMN-derived oxidants to endothelial and other cells. Again, toxicity in the target cells, is dependent on the availability of intracellular iron.[68,109] In vivo, increased free iron is observed in primary hemochromatosis, a condition associated with high mortality from hepatocellular carcinoma (see reference 110 for review). Investigators have recently documented the in vivo formation of $\cdot OH$ using a secondary spin trapping technique and electron spin resonance (ESR) spectroscopy in rats whose diets have been supplemented with nonheme iron.[111] These results indicate that the mammalian storage capacity of transition-metal binding proteins can be exceeded under certain conditions.

Hypochlorous Acid and Chloramines

In addition to NADPH oxidase, PMNs and monocytes (but not macrophages) contain the heme protein myeloperoxidase (MPO), which generates oxidants more powerful than $O_2^{-\cdot}$ or H_2O_2. MPO utilizes H_2O_2 and halides as substrates to form highly reactive hypohalous acids. Because Cl^- is the major halide present in plasma and in other extracellular fluids, hypochlorous acid (HOCl) is probably the most predominant hypohalous acid formed by MPO under physiological conditions (Equation 4).

$$H_2O_2 + Cl^- + H^+ \rightarrow HOCl + H_2O \qquad (4)$$

Another important oxygen-dependent cytotoxic mechanism is the MPO-initiated formation of $\cdot OH$ or the highly electrophilic singlet oxygen ($^1O_2$) via reaction of HOCl with H_2O_2.[74,112] Also, HOCl can deaminate cytosine in DNA to 5-chlorouracil, a promutagenic lesion. MPO-mediated production of HOCl is an extremely effective antimicrobial, antiviral, and cytotoxic mechanism in vitro.[113–115] MPO with acid hydroxylases, elastase, and cationic proteins is present at high concentrations in the primary (azurophilic) granules of PMNs.[63] On stimulation with particulate stimuli, phagocytes release the contents of these granules either into phagolysosomes or into the extracellular space.

The reaction of HOCl with primary amines (RNH_2) can result in the formation of chloramines,[116] relatively long-lived oxidizing species that are also moderately mutagenic (Equation 5):

$$RNH_2 + HOCl \rightarrow RNHCl + H_2O \qquad (5)$$

HOCl and chloramines have been proposed to inactivate α_1-proteinase inhibitor and α_2-macroglobulin in vivo, thereby allowing the proteases released from stimulated PMNs to cause degradation of host tissue.[65] Other powerful oxidants, such as peroxynitrite (see below),[117] also have been shown to inactivate protease inhibitors in vitro. Patients with an inborn MPO deficiency, however, do not display compromised resistance to infection. This observation suggests that HOCl-mediated killing of microorganisms may not be a major pathway used by activated phagocytes,[96] or that other pathways may compensate for the defect in this particular defense mechanism. All oxidants derived from the NADPH oxidase-initiated pathway described so far, including $O_2\cdot^-$ and HOCl, will be referred to here collectively as reactive oxygen species (ROS).

Nitric Oxide, Its Autoxidation Products, and Peroxynitrite

Another mechanism by which phagocytes exert cytotoxicity is through the formation of NO• by nitric oxide synthase (NOS). Briefly, this enzyme exists in inducible (iNOS) and constitutive (cNOS) forms, and is present in many cell types (see reviews in references 118 and 119). Inducible forms are present, for example, in macrophages, smooth muscle cells, and hepatocytes, and are induced by exposure to LPS or cytokines such as IFN-γ.[118] NOS induction during an ongoing host immune response in humans or other mammalian species can be assessed directly by measurement of iNOS gene expression, or indirectly by measurement of the increase in urinary excretion of NO_2^- and nitrate (NO_3^-) (see reference 121 for review). NO_2^-, the principal autoxidation product of NO• in solution, often is not detected in biological samples, such as plasma, because it rapidly reacts with oxyhemoglobin to form NO_3^- and methemoglobin.[121] The use of NO_2^- as a biomarker for the formation of reactive nitrogen oxide species (RNOS) will be discussed more fully below. Although NO• is a well documented effector molecule in stimulated rodent macrophages, its role in human mononuclear phagocytes and PMNs in general has been somewhat controversial. Recent reports have now confirmed, however, that induction of iNOS can be observed in human monocytes or macrophages isolated from patients who have infectious or inflammatory diseases.[122,123] Increased formation of NO• and expression of iNOS also has been observed in both rodent and human PMNs elicited in vivo or stimulated in vitro by a combination of proinflammatory agents.[124]

A large array of biologically important processes, such as vasodilation, platelet aggregation, long-term synaptic potentiation and cytotoxicity, has been attributed to the L-arginine-NO biosynthetic pathway. For example, the cytotoxic effects of activated macrophages against certain microbes and tumor cells in vitro have been shown to depend on the formation of NO•, an effect mediated in part by inhibition of mitochondrial respiratory enzymes.[67,125,126]

Similar to $O_2\cdot^-$, NO• is only moderately reactive and reacts with a small range of molecules only. The chemistry of NO• and how it relates to physiological processes have been reviewed extensively.[127,128] NO• readily reacts with both protein-bound heme and nonheme iron. NO• binding to the heme iron of guanylate cyclase, for example, is responsible for activation of this key regulatory enzyme. It is involved in smooth muscle cell relaxation—possibly the principal physiological function exerted by NO•. NO• also acts as a high affinity inhibitor for many oxidases and oxygenases.

NO• reacts with iron–sulfur clusters to form relatively stable iron–nitrosyl complexes that can lead eventually to the destruction of the cluster. This process might be partly responsibly for the inactivation of crucial metabolic enzymes, such as mitochondrial aconitase and NADH-dependent oxidoreductases, in cells exposed to NO•. Iron-nitrosyl complexes are paramagnetic and can be detected by ESR. Thus, ESR is a useful approach to measure the formation of NO• both in vitro and in vivo.

NO• can also act as a chain-terminating agent. It readily reacts with other radicals, such as lipid peroxyl radicals, thereby inhibiting initiation or propagation of radical chain reactions, such as those involved in lipid peroxidation.[129]

In the gas phase, NO• reacts readily with oxygen to form the potent oxidant nitrogen dioxide radical (NO_2•) (Equation 6). However, this reaction is slow in aqueous solution.[130] Therefore, the short half-life of NO• under physiological conditions cannot be explained completely by oxidation of NO• by molecular oxygen.[131] The short half-life is most likely a result of the near diffusion-controlled reaction with O_2^- to peroxynitrite, for SOD has been shown to increase the life span of NO• under physiological conditions.[131] NO_2• gas decomposes in aerated water to form a mixture of NO_2^- and NO_3^- through the formation of the corresponding conjugate acids: nitrous acid (HNO_2) and nitric acid (HNO_3). However, NO_2^- is the only product found when NO• is allowed to decompose in aqueous solution. It appears that the NO_2• formed during the oxidation of NO• by molecular oxygen rapidly reacts with NO• to form the potent nitrosating species nitrous anhydride (N_2O_3), the anhydride of HNO_2 (Equations 7and 8).[132,133]

$$2NO• + O_2 \rightarrow 2NO_2• \tag{6}$$

$$NO• + NO_2• \leftrightarrows N_2O_3 \tag{7}$$

$$N_2O_3 + H_2O \leftrightarrows 2HNO_2 \leftrightarrows 2NO_2^- + 2H^+ \tag{8}$$

Both HNO_2 and N_2O_3 N-nitrosate secondary amines (R_2NH)[134,135] to form products (Equations 9 and10) that can be highly mutagenic and carcinogenic.[136,137] These nitrosating species can also react with primary amines. In the case of DNA bases, this reaction can result (via deamination) in the direct formation of mutagenic DNA lesions.[137]

Both activated macrophages[138] and PMNs[139] have been shown to nitrosate secondary amines in vitro. These cells may therefore be responsible for some of the endogenously formed N-nitrosamines that can be detected in vivo. Some of the nitrosating species responsible for their formation appear to be derived from the guanidino-moiety of L-arginine, implicating NOS in their formation. Their precise identity remains to be determined, however. It appears plausible that under conditions of increased production of NO•, such as when macrophages or PMNs are activated and NO• can escape reaction with O_2^{-}, N_2O_3 may be formed.

$$R_2NH + HONO \rightarrow R_2N\text{-}NO + H_2O$$
(under acidic conditions)   (9)

$$R_2NH + N_2O_3 \rightarrow R_2N\text{-}NO + NO_2^{-} + H^{+}$$
(primarily at physiological pH)   (10)

A third mechanism by which NO• exerts oxygen-dependent cytotoxicity is the formation of peroxynitrite (Eq. 11) (see reference 140 for review). We will refer to peroxynitrite as both the reaction product of O_2^{-} with NO•, the peroxynitrite anion (ONOO-), and its conjugate acid, peroxynitrous acid (ONOOH). The pK_a of peroxynitrite is about pH 7. Once protonated, peroxynitrite decomposes with a half-life of seconds, as a result of isomerization to NO_3^{-} (Equation 12).[141]

$$NO• + O_2^{-} \rightarrow ONOO^{-}$$ (11)

$$ONOO^{-} + H^{+} \rightarrow ONOOH \rightarrow NO_3^{-} + H^{+} \text{ or } ONOOH^{*}$$ (12)

Peroxynitrite anion readily oxidizes sulfhydryl groups.[142] Peroxynitrous acid (or its proposed activated form $ONOOH^{*}$; see Equation 12) is a potent oxidizing and nitrating species with •OH- and NO_2•-like character.[140,143] Even though homolytic fission of ONOOH to •OH (and to NO_2•) has been questioned,[143] ONOOH initiates oxidation reactions similar to those observed with •OH, such as hydroxylation of phenolic molecules, peroxidation of lipids, and oxidation of sugars and DNA bases.[140] Although peroxynitrite also effectively nitrosates sulfhydryl groups,[140] we do not know whether this reactive species is involved in the formation of N-nitrosamines (see above).

Both the formation and subsequent reactions of peroxynitrite can occur in the absence of free transition metals. This makes peroxynitrite an interesting candidate for a biologically relevant oxidant, because elevated levels of both O_2^{-} and NO• are formed concurrently by activated phagocytes in vivo. We can use the ability of peroxynitrite to ortho-nitrate phenolic substances, such as tyrosine or its analog 4-hydroxyphenylacetic acid, to estimate the amount of peroxinitrite formation. This approach is the basis for various in vitro and in vivo assays that measure free or protein-bound 3-nitrotyrosine (3NT). For example, PMA-activated rat alveolar macrophages readily nitrate exogenous 4-hydroxyphenylacetic acid, indicative of the formation of a nitrating species such as peroxynitrite.[145] Results from recent immunohistochemical and analytical studies that measured 3NT will be discussed further below. All oxidants derived from the

NOS-initiated pathway—including NO•—will be collectively referred to here as RNOS.

Evidence for the In Vivo Formation of Phagocyte-Derived Oxidants

High reactivity and short half-life make studying the roles of ROS and RNOS in physiological and pathological processes difficult. For example, •OH is so reactive that it will diffuse only a few micrometers before reacting with another molecule, so it is virtually impossible to measure this species directly in vivo.[146]

Indirectly, we can assess oxidative stress—a period of significant oxidant formation before the occurrence of substantial damage[147]—by measuring the consumption of endogenous antioxidants. Interpretation of such data can be difficult, however, because of the possibility of tissue redistribution or mobilization of endogenous antioxidants and the presence of inducible antioxidant pathways. We can also assess progressive oxidative stress, which may lead to oxidative damage, by measuring the products formed from the reaction of a putative oxidant with a particular biological target molecule. The application of measuring such biomarkers in assessing the role of oxidant formation in vivo will be discussed below. Measuring oxidatively modified target molecules often provides valuable information on the nature of the biomolecular damage and that damage's possible detrimental physiological consequences. However, this damage may not be oxidant specific, so the exact cause cannot always be identified. To define and control the underlying mechanisms of damage related to the formation of oxidants in vivo, we must use direct measurement of oxidants. Thus, both direct and indirect lines of evidence need to be obtained before the involvement of oxidants in physiological or pathological processes can be established firmly.

Experimental data on the formation of ROS and RNOS under inflammatory conditions is scarce. Recent technological advances, however, have permitted the development of methods that can detect certain reactive species in vivo. One approach is probe-assisted chemiluminescence (CL), which detects the oxidant-induced light emitted from an excitable reporter molecule. Another approach is ESR, which measures paramagnetism exhibited by molecules with unpaired electrons (*i.e.*, radicals), either directly (direct ESR) or indirectly after reaction with chemically defined target molecules that stabilize the radical character (spin-trap ESR). Unfortunately, ESR cannot be used to detect diatomic radicals in solution, excluding the possibility of directly measuring many of the ROS/RNOS in vivo.[148] Although spin-trap ESR yields structural information about the reactant and has greater specificity than CL, CL is more sensitive and easier to use.

Chemiluminescence Detection

Chemiluminescence (CL) is the emission of light that occurs when excited species relax to ground state. Cellular CL in the visible range was first observed by Allen and colleagues in phagocytizing PMNs (see references 74 and 149 for review). This native or low-level CL is generated by the activation of endogenous substrates by oxidants formed by the activity of NADPH oxidase and possibly MPO. The exact nature of the oxidants and of the excited species has not yet been fully elucidated, but $^1O_2$—which itself does not relax by emission of visible light—has been implicated.[74] To increase the sensitivity of cellular CL, scientists use chemilumigenic substrates or probes to enhance or amplify the native signal produced by cells such as phagocytes. A common probe used is luminol (5-amino-2,3-dihydro-1,4-phthalazinedione). The process that measures oxidant production with this probe is called luminol-dependent CL. It is not clear, however, whether the oxidants responsible for luminol-dependent CL are the same as those involved in the generation of low-level CL. MPO-catalyzed formation of $^1O_2$ may be an important contributor to the overall reaction, but other pathways probably contribute to the signal as well.[74]

Researchers have performed most CL experiments by stimulating isolated phagocytes with particles or soluble factors. Luminol-dependent CL can be detected in whole blood exposed to a variety of phagocyte-specific stimuli, or in phagocytes isolated from various hosts with different kinds of ongoing inflammatory reactions (reference 149 and references therein). For example, luminol-dependent CL has been detected in lung tissue and bronchoalveolar lavage cells of rats exposed to toxic silica particles.[150,151] CL in recovered lung tissue or cells was inhibited by preincubation with SOD or with the competitive NOS inhibitor, N^G-nitro-L-arginine methyl ester, suggesting that peroxynitrite may have been the oxidant responsible for causing the signal. This inference is in line with findings that PMA-induced luminol-dependent CL of isolated hepatic Kupffer cells also depends on the L-arginine–NO synthetic pathway and on the concurrent formation of O_2·⁻.[152]

Increased luminol-dependent CL during inflammation has also been observed in a foot-pad edema model in rats. A cell-mediated hypersensitivity reaction was induced in this model by inoculating previously immunized animals with a second dose of Freund's complete adjuvant.[153] The CL response was partially inhibited by free radical inhibitors such as catalase,[153] an enzyme that detoxifies H_2O_2 by converting it to water and oxygen. Similar observations have been made in biopsy specimens of colorectal mucosa from patients suffering from inflammatory bowel disease[154,155] and of duodenal mucosa from patients suffering from various forms of duodenal ulcer disease.[156] Whenever tested, the CL response was inhibited by azide, taurine, and catalase, suggesting that activated PMNs were primarily responsible for the formation of the CL-generating oxidants. Interestingly, increased duodenal CL was associated with *H. pylori* antral infection, but not with smoking, alcohol, or the use of nonsteroidal anti-inflammatory drugs. Indeed, in a separate study, researchers found that spontaneous CL was increased in biopsy specimens of antral mucosa of patients suffering from gastric mucosal injury and infected with *H. pylori*, but was not found in specimens from uninfected patients, despite the presence of inflammatory cells.[157] This indicates that *H. pylori* stimulated the inflammatory cells to release potentially toxic oxidants, which in turn may be involved in the pathogenic mechanism for gastric diseases.

Direct Measurements

Only a few studies have been done to *directly* measure ROS associated with inflammation in vivo. H_2O_2, which is not a radical species, is chemically quite stable and can be measured readily by its reaction with specific H_2O_2-removing enzymes coupled to an oxidizable chromogenic or fluorigenic substrate. Using this approach, researchers detected increased H_2O_2 in the expired breath of asthmatic children suffering from acute upper or lower respiratory tract disease.[158] From this finding, the investigators proposed that H_2O_2 could be used as a biomarker for airway inflammation. Rats whose heterotopically transplanted bladders were pretreated with the carcinogen *N*-methyl-*N*-nitrosourea and then treated with LPS displayed a significantly increased incidence and number of tumors. This co-carcinogenic effect of LPS was associated with a marked increase in both PMNs and concentration of H_2O_2 in the bladder lumen.[159] Although not directly related to cancer, increased formation of H_2O_2 has also been detected in the lungs of mice suffering from influenza.[160] Murine influenza is associated with massive pulmonary infiltration and can be attenuated by the administration of polymer-conjugated SOD.[161] The relative contribution of the potential sources of oxidants—activated infiltrating phagocytes, the $O_2^{\cdot-}$-generating enzyme xanthine oxidase, or other sources—to the pathology remains to be determined, however.

Finally, there are also reports describing the formation of NO· during inflammatory reactions in vivo. These studies are based on the detection by ESR of the rapid reaction of NO· with chelated Fe^{2+} to form stable nitrosyl complexes (see reference 162 for review). Lai and Komarov[163] monitored the in vivo formation of NO· in the blood circulation of mice undergoing LPS-induced septic shock. Subcutaneous injection of the stable and water-soluble *N*-methyl–D-glucamine dithiocarbamate-Fe^{2+} complex after LPS treatment enabled detection of the characteristic Fe-nitrosyl complex at ambient temperature.[163] NO· formation was also detected in the liver and kidney. However, this methodology cannot elucidate which cell type(s) in a tissue is (are) involved in the formation of NO·.

In vivo formation of NO· in several kinds of inflammatory conditions has also been shown through detection of nitrosylated hemoglobin or nonheme nitrosyl complexes. However this method requires ESR detection at low temperature, and thus is unsuitable for real-time measurements in vivo. Despite this limitation, scientists detected nitrosyl complexes in animals with septic shock,[164,165] in isolated syngeneic murine tumors,[166] and in the liver and whole blood of mice infected with *Corynebacterium parvum*,[167] a bacterium that induces chronic hepatic inflammation, using this method. Some of the NO• detected in the latter model is believed to be derived from activated hepatocytes, as suggested by both the detection of hepatocyte-specific iNOS mRNA, and the increase in plasma and urinary NO_2^- and NO_3^- in infected rats.[168] Coadministration of N^G-methyl–L-arginine (NMA), another competitive NOS inhibitor, attenuated the formation of NO•, but, interestingly, also increased hepatic damage. Using specific ROS scavengers, the researchers concluded that NO• exerts this protective effect through its reaction and elimination of ROS.[169] This example demonstrates that the measurement of one ROS or RNOS does not necessarily provide sufficient information on that reactive species' pathogenic role in tissue damage. The pathophysiological role of oxidants can be assessed appropriately only when specific oxidative damage is measured concurrently *and* when this damage can be alleviated by specific inhibitors *and* when the inhibition has a beneficial effect on the pathological outcome.

GENOTOXICITY OF OXIDANTS

A summary of the genotoxic effects of oxidants produced predominantly by activated phagocytes appears in Table 2.1. Most of these data comes from in vitro experiments, but the genotoxic and carcinogenic effects of ionizing radiation in vivo are well documented, and are primarily mediated by ROS (see, for example, references 170 through 172).

Reactive Oxygen Species

Exposure of Isolated DNA
Oxidants formed from H_2O_2 or activated phagocytes in the presence of either free or DNA-bound transition metals, or of radiolytically generated •OH, cause extensive oxidative damage to the base and sugar moiety of isolated DNA.[173–177] More than 30 different adducts have been identified—for example, 8-hydroxy-2'-deoxyguanosine (8HdG), thymidine glycol (TG), and 5-hydroxymethyl-2'-deoxyuridine (5HMdU).[172,178,179] They are the same products generated by exposure of DNA to radiation, or when whole cells are exposed to pure chemical or cell-derived oxidants.[108,180]

Oxidative damage can lead to single- or double-strand breaks, to point and frameshift mutations, and to chromosome abnormalities (see, for example, reference 177 for review). The type of mutation depends on the host cell in which the DNA was replicated, and on the DNA repair system within that host. The most common point mutations of oxidatively altered DNA replicated in bacteria are C → T transitions, followed by G → T and

Table 2.1 Genotoxicity of oxidants and by-products formed by activated phagocytes

Reactive species	Genotoxicity	Comments	Mutational pattern[a]	Reference(s)
I. ROS				
Superoxide ($O_2^{-\bullet}$) (incl. Fe^{2+} and Cu^+)	+	Transition metal-dependent, can also react with NO• to form ONOO⁻ (see below)	Mainly C → T transitions, CC → TT tandem double transitions, some G → T transversions	177,184,185
Hydrogen peroxide (H_2O_2)	+	Transition metal-dependent	same as above	177,184,185
Hydroxyl radical (•OH)	+ + +	(Role *in vivo* difficult to assess)	same as above	177,184,185
Singlet oxygen ($^1O_2$)	+	(Role *in vivo* difficult to assess)	Mostly G → T transversions	186,187
Hypochlorous acid (HOCl)	+/weak	Strongly cytotoxic[b]		191
II. RNOS				
Nitrite (NO_2^-)	+ + +	Mutagenic only at acidic pH	Mainly C → T transitions	205,208,218
Nitrate (NO_3^-)	Non-mutagenic	Certain bacteria can reduce NO_3^- to NO_2^-		
Nitric oxide (NO•)	weak/ + + +	Formation of reactive intermediate is 1st order in O_2 and 2nd order in NO•	Mainly C → T transitions	209,210,212–214

Nitrogen dioxide (NO₂•)	++	Environmental pollutant. Formed from peroxynitrite *in vivo*?		206,212
N₂O₃	+++	Proposed reactive intermediate of NO•	see NO₂⁻ and NO•	222,223
Peroxynitrite (ONOOH)	+/weak	Strongly cytotoxic,[b] •OH/NO₂•-like properties		
III. SECONDARY PRODUCTS				
Aldehydes (MDA etc.)	++	Formed by the reaction of certain ROS and RNOS with lipids, cytotoxic	G → T, C → T, and A → G substitutions	234,235
Lipid peroxidation, transition metal–induced	++	Due to multiple lipid oxidation products	C → G, followed by G → T transversions	240
Chloramines	+	Relatively long-lived, can be metabolically inactivated, however		227
Nitrosamines	+++	Relatively long-lived species, require metabolic activation		135

[a]Mutational patterns often depend on the conditions of exposure and the DNA-repair system of the host, which may be different in prokaryotic versus eukaryotic cells.
[b]Strongly cytotoxic compounds are usually not very mutagenic *in vitro* but may be more mutagenic *in vivo*—due to, for example, via formation of secondary products.

G → C transversions (see, for example, reference 181). These mutations are not randomly distributed but rather are clustered in hot spots, suggesting that the oxidants or the context of the DNA sequence exhibit some specificity. Using various approaches, researchers have demonstrated that the presence of 8HdG in DNA causes the formation of point mutations—mainly G → T transversions.[182-185] However, other base modifications can also lead to this mutation, so this type of mutation cannot be viewed as a specific marker of oxidatively modified genuine bases.

$^1O_2$, a powerful electrophile that reacts readily with guanine residues, mainly induces G → T and G → C transversions in shuttle vectors replicated in mammalian cells.[186,187] Although $^1O_2$ is a potent cytotoxic agent and exhibits some genotoxicity, mutagenicity to intact cells such as bacteria is weak (see reference 188 for review). Thus, $^1O_2$ is probably only a weak direct mutagen in vivo. Similar to potent oxidants like ·OH, however, $^1O_2$ can induce the formation of secondary products that are more mutagenic (described more fully below).

HOCl reacts not only with essential thiols but also with uracil and cytosine.[189,190] The genotoxicity to cytosine possibly involves the formation of a chlorohydrin intermediate that spontaneously deaminates to form 5-chlorouracil, a thymine analogue. If 5-chlorouracil remains unrepaired, a C → T transition will result during DNA replication. Indeed, both HOCl and its conjugate base OCl⁻ have been shown to be mutagenic in bacteria.[191] Both are also clastogenic, inducing strand breaks in vitro (but not in vivo).[192]

Exposure of Intact Cells

H_2O_2 induces DNA strand breaks also in intact mammalian cells,[108] a process dependent on the presence of free transition metals. Furthermore, reporter plasmids replicated in either *E. coli* or simian CV-1 cells exposed to H_2O_2 contained small and large deletions that appeared to be clustered around C-rich regions.[181,193] Analysis of the point mutations in the *E. coli* plasmid revealed mainly A → T, followed by G → C transversions.[181] This frequent mutation at A·T base pairs in bacterial reversion assays contrasts with the H_2O_2-induced mutations in isolated DNA. This discrepancy could be explained by differences in the cells' repair and/or antioxidant defense systems.

The hypothesis that phagocyte-derived oxidants may play an important role in inflammation-associated carcinogenesis[194] was supported by a series of simple, but elegant experiments by Weitzman and his colleagues. These authors showed that human phagocytes stimulated by either bacteria or PMA in vitro induced a variety of cytogenetic changes in co-cultured cells. This treatment resulted in an increased mutation rate in histidine-requiring *Salmonella*[195] and in elevated sister chromatid exchanges in ovary fibroblasts of the Chinese hamster.[196] In both cases, genotoxicity was not observed when phagocytes from CGD patients were used. Furthermore, addition of SOD, catalase, or low-molecular weight antioxidants inhibited these genotoxic effects.[197,198] Other investigators have also reported increased mutagenicity to bacteria,[199] induction of DNA strand breaks,[108,200,201] and the formation of clastogenic factors (a class of ill-defined molecules)[202,203] in many cell types, including activated leukocytes.

Finally, Weitzman and his colleagues showed that human PMNs can induce malignant transformation in C3H 10T 1/2 mouse fibroblasts. Injection of fibroblasts exposed to PMA-stimulated PMNs into athymic nude mice resulted in the formation of both benign and malignant tumors.[204] Malignant transformation was also observed in an in vitro assay. It is possible, however, that the genotoxicity mediated by these cells could also have been a consequence of RNOS formation, or of the interaction of RNOS with ROS.

Reactive Nitrogen Oxide Species

The genotoxicity of NO_2^-/HNO_2,[205] and of NO• and its autoxidation product NO_2•[120,206,207] has been reviewed extensively. NO_3^- (except when enzymatically reduced by bacteria) is nonmutagenic.[206]

Nitric Oxide and Its Autoxidation Products

In experiments with isolated DNA, acidified NO_2^- deaminates DNA bases containing exocyclic amino groups through formation of the nitrosating species N_2O_3 or HNO_2 itself. Cytosine is deaminated to uracil, adenine to hypoxanthine, guanine to xanthine, and 5-methylcytosine to thymine. Mutations arise if these lesions are not repaired correctly.[205] Autoxidizing NO• in solution has been shown to deaminate DNA bases too, most likely also through the formation of N_2O_3.[137] In contrast to NO_2^-, however, NO• deaminates even at neutral pH. Base substitutions in plasmids treated with either NO_2^-,[205,208] pure dissolved NO•,[209], or NO-donors,[210] are mainly C → T transitions. This pattern is consistent with the deamination of cytosine being the genotoxic mechanism. The minor substitutions induced by these treatments vary, probably as a result of the complex autoxidation kinetics of RNOS. Glycosylase repair of either oxidized bases, or uracil formed from deamination of cytosine, leads to the formation of transient nicks. This process can lead to highly lethal double strand breaks if two nicks are within 14 bases on opposite strands.[211]

Genotoxic effects of acidic NO_2^- and autoxidizing NO• have also been reported in experiments on intact cells, such as bacteria[137,205,212–214] and mammalian cells.[215] The mutagenicity of NO•, however, depends heavily on the conditions of delivery. Conditions that favor the formation of N_2O_3, such as slow release of NO• gas or of NO• derived from NO-donors into solution, appear to be more mutagenic (and cytotoxic) than is administration of a large bolus of dissolved NO• gas or of gas-phase NO•.[132] Despite these differences, the majority of point mutations are C → T transitions. Similar to ROS-induced mutations, these point mutations are not randomly distributed, but rather are clustered in hot spots.

DNA isolated from in vitro stimulated macrophages exhibits a higher rate of deamination and oxidation of guanine-containing residues,[216] suggesting that C → T transitions may not result from deamination of cytosine alone. In fact, it has been recently proposed that the mutagenicity of NO_2^- and NO• could be a result of deamination of guanine, rather than of cytosine.[217,218] Mutagenicity of NO• is weak in certain cells, however. For example, exposure of human bronchial epithelial cells to large doses of NO• derived from a synthetic donor, or produced by the overexpression of iNOS in transfected cells, did not result in detectable deamination of 5-methylcytosine in the *p53* gene, or mutation in the hypoxanthine phosphoribosyttransferase (HPRT) locus.[219]

Although, under experimental conditions, inhaled NO• and NO_2• have been reported to induce mutations in lung cells of exposed animals[212] it is much more difficult to assess the role of phagocyte-derived NO• in causing mutatious in vivo. Gal and Wogan studied mutagenicity of endogenous NO• in transgenic mice carrying a reporter gene of bacterial origin.[220] Injection of these mice with pre-B-cell lymphoma cells, which proliferate in the spleen and lymph nodes, induces increased production of NO• by activated macrophages. The tumor-bearing mice exhibited an elevated mutation frequency in the spleen, an effect largely inhibited by administration of NMA. These results suggest that NO• formed by activated macrophages was responsible for the observed increase in mutation frequency in the target tissue. Further studies will tell if host genes, such as *p53*, are also mutated by endogenous NO•.

Peroxynitrite

Like H_2O_2, peroxynitrite induces strand breaks in isolated DNA[221] or in intact cells,[222] but unlike H_2O_2, peroxynitrite does not require the presence of free or DNA-bound transition metals. Analysis of a shuttle vector exposed to peroxynitrite in vitro and replicated in either *E. coli* or human Ad293 cells revealed the presence of large deletions, insertions, and tandem and multiple mutations.[223] The main point mutations were G → T transversions (60%), followed by G → C and G → A substitutions, and were predominantly clustered around hot spots. However, because peroxynitrite is extremely cytotoxic to bacteria and mammalian cells,[224-226] it exhibits only weak mutagenicity toward intact cells (Christen, Lee, and Ames, unpublished).

Secondary Oxidation Products

Although the high cytotoxicity of ROS and RNOS results in generally low mutagenicity toward intact cells (compared to other mutagens), the formation of these reactive species can lead to the formation of secondary products with lower cytotoxic, but higher mutagenic potential.

Substituted Amines

Substituted amines include chloramines and *N*-nitrosamines. As previously mentioned, chloramines, which are mutagenic to bacteria without the need for metabolic activation,[227,228] are formed by reaction of HOCl with primary amines. Although exogenous administration of chloramines—such as the by-products formed during the disinfection of drinking water—does not appear to be carcinogenic,[229] formation of chloramines during inflammation may still contribute to mutations in host cells.

The mutagenicity and carcinogenicity of N-nitrosamines has been known for decades. N-nitrosamines possibly represent the best-researched class of genotoxic and carcinogenic compounds found in the human diet (see reference 136 for review), and will therefore be discussed only briefly here. They are primarily formed by the reaction of secondary amines with nitrosating species such as N_2O_3, and are metabolized—for example, in the liver—to strongly alkylating electrophiles, which in turn readily react with DNA.[230] Again, the DNA lesions formed can lead to mutations if they are not repaired correctly. N-nitrosamines generally require the presence of a metabolic activation system (microsomal preparation) to be mutagenic to bacteria.[135]

Lipid Oxidation Products

Several chain-cleavage products derived from primary lipid oxidation products react directly with DNA (see references 231,232 for review). Formation of DNA adducts or cross-links can lead to mutation and strand breaks (see, for example, reference 233). These secondary products have been used as in vivo markers for assessing the role of lipid peroxidation in the carcinogenic process. In several studies, saturated aldehydes (such as malondialdehyde [MDA]) and α,β-unsaturated aldehydes (such as 4-hydroxynonenal [4HNE]) have been shown to be mutagenic and genotoxic.[234–238] Exposure of M13 phage DNA to MDA and subsequent replication in E. coli revealed primarily base-pair substitutions.[239] Using a similar approach, researchers showed that nonspecific microsomal lipid peroxidation resulted in G → C, followed by G → T transversions. These mutations were probably caused by yet to be defined lesions and probably were not due to formation of 8HdG.[240]

EVIDENCE FOR OXIDATIVE DAMAGE DURING INFLAMMATION AND CANCER

As described in the previous sections, oxidants appear to play a major role in killing invading pathogens. Individuals or animals whose PMNs or macrophages are defective in the formation of oxidants exhibit impaired antimicrobial activity. An inevitable by-product of targeted killing by competent activated macrophages and PMNs, however, is the leakage of oxidants to neighboring host cells. This leakage leads to the induction and accumulation of oxidative damage, including mutagenic lesions, within these cells. Critical to the argument that oxidants play an important role in chronic inflammation and cancer is the identification and measurement of such oxidatively modified lesions in tissue or in biological fluids from individuals affected by or at risk of the cancer in question. Surrogate biomarkers are useful for such purposes.

A surrogate biomarker is a chemically modified endogenous molecule that serves as a fingerprint of a particular reactive process, but that may not necessarily represent a biologically relevant lesion. Numerous analytical methods have been developed that measure biomarkers of oxidative damage to DNA, proteins, and lipids in biological systems. Representative biomarkers include 8HdG, 5HMdU, and TG for DNA oxidation, protein carbonyls and dityrosine for protein oxidation, and MDA and isoprostanes for lipid oxidation. Methods for measuring biomarkers that reflect inflammation-mediated damage have been introduced recently. For example, protein-bound 3NT and 3-chlorotyrosine represent biomarkers of protein damage induced by RNOS and $HOCl/Cl_2$, respectively.

The availability of these methods has allowed us to study the damage to cellular molecules induced by oxidants, such as those formed during inflammation. Chromatographic techniques—such as the measurement of 8HdG in blood lymphocyte DNA,[241] 3NT in plasma proteins,[242] or MDA in plasma[243]—can quantitatively determine the steady-state level of damage. The quantitation of these biomarkers in urine over a defined period provides an estimate of the rate of oxidative damage and repair in the entire body. For example, quantitation of 8HdG in tissue, together with its excised nucleobase 8-hydroxyguanine in urine, provides a good estimate of the repair of oxidative DNA damage.[244] Measuring steady-state levels and rates of oxidative damage is useful for interpreting the effects of given treatment variables, such as pharmacological intervention, lifestyle habits (*e.g.*, smoking), nutritional deficits, and nutritional supplementation.

We can also use in vivo quantitation of mutations as an indictor of oxidative DNA damage. Human lymphocyte DNA can be analyzed for mutation at the HPRT loci. Mutation at this loci has been shown to be higher in lymphocytes isolated from smokers than from nonsmokers or from ex-smokers.[245] Smoke- or phagocyte-derived oxidants may possibly have contributed to this increased mutation frequency. Assays designed to measure mutations that are diagnostic for oxidative DNA damage[246] have now been developed. The quantitative and qualitative assessment of mutations, and the measurement of biomarkers, can assist us in better understanding the role of oxidative damage in cancer. Evidence that mutations and biomarkers of DNA oxidation are modulated by smoking,[241,245] and by dietary antioxidants such as ascorbic acid[247] illustrate the utility of such an approach for investigating the role of chronic inflammation in human cancer.

Examples of Relevant Biomarkers

Biomarkers frequently used to assess the impact of inflammation on mutation and carcinogenesis include biomarkers of DNA oxidation, lipid oxidation, and RNOS damage.

Biomarkers of DNA Oxidation

Oxidative DNA damage and deamination of guanine residues can be readily observed in DNA isolated from activated macrophages *ex vivo* (see above).[216] This effect probably depends largely on the formation of NO• and its reactive by-products, because the formation of these DNA lesions is attenuated by treating these cells with NMA. Tissue levels of 8HdG are elevated in humans and animals suffering from inflammation.[4,5] This marker is formed by the reaction of DNA guanine residues with various oxidants, such as •OH, $^1O_2$, and peroxynitrite.[248] 5HMdU and TG are formed by oxidative modifications to DNA thymine residues. These two products are elevated in epidermal tissue under the proinflammatory conditions of PMA treatment.[174] The presence of plasma autoantibodies to 5HMdU also suggests that oxidative DNA damage is elevated during chronic inflammation. Indeed, studies by Frenkel and colleagues revealed that autoantibodies to 5HMdU are increased in individuals suffering from neoplasms, inflammatory dermatoses,[249] and systemic *lupus erythematosus*.[250]

Biomarkers of Lipid Oxidation

Conjugated dienes, MDA, 4HNE, and isoprostanes are formed as secondary products of lipid oxidation. All these biomarkers have been shown to be elevated under inflammatory conditions (discussed more fully later). Oxidation of polyunsaturated fatty acids (PUFAs) leads to the rearrangement of *bis*-allylic double bonds and to the subsequent formation of conjugated dienes. Subsequent fragmentation or cyclization results in the formation of products such as aldehydes or isoprostanes, respectively. We can estimate formation of conjugated dienes by measuring their absorption at 234 nm, but this technique is useful for only those studies in which pure lipids are used. The use of this method with biological materials is not advised because other compounds can be present that also absorb at this wavelength (*e.g.*, carotenoid oxidation products).

Investigators have employed various methodologies to measure aldehydes. The most popular is the thiobarbituric acid reactive substance (TBARS) assay for the estimation of MDA. MDA is a chain cleavage product of oxidized PUFA with more than two double bonds. Unfortunately, this measurement suffers from a number of limitations, the most important of which are the artifactual formation of TBARS in extracted biological material, and the lack of specificity for MDA.[251] A new gas-chromatographic technique using mass spectrometric detection provides greater sensitivity and accuracy, and can also detect other lipid oxidation products.[243,252] A similar method has been developed recently for F_2-isoprostanes, a group of unique oxidation products derived from arachidonic acid. This new technique has been employed successfully in several in vivo studies for the quantitative estimation of nonenzymatic lipid oxidation (see reference 253 for review).

Reactive by-products of lipid oxidation produced during inflammation may play an important role in the carcinogenic process. As described earlier, both MDA and enals have been shown to be mutagenic. The MDA-2'-deoxyguanosine adduct is a promutagenic lesion,[239] and has been detected in vivo in liver DNA isolated from disease-free humans.[254] Two other DNA-lipid peroxidation adducts have been detected in Long Evans Cinnamon rats,[255] a rat strain that develops spontaneous hepatitis and hepatocellular carcinoma due to aberrant copper metabolism. In these rats, there was a positive correlation between the two etheno adducts, $1,N^6$-ethenodeoxyadenosine and $3,N^4$-ethenodeoxycytidine, and hepatic copper levels. Moreover, the adduct levels peaked with the appearance of fulminant hepatitis.[255]

Some of the lipid peroxidation products could also be procarcinogenic by acting as chemoattractants, stimulating PMNs to migrate to sites of lipid oxidation, and thereby propagating inflammation.[256] For example, 4HNE, which is derived from ω-6 fatty acids, appears to be formed by activated PMNs in vivo. Rats treated with the nondigestible and chronic irritant polydextran Sephadex G-200, which causes an influx of PMNs to the affected site display increased formation of 4HNE.[257]

Biomarkers of RNOS Damage

Biomarkers of RNOS damage include nitrite (NO_2^-), nitrate (NO_3^-), nitrosamines, and 3-nitrotyrosine (3NT). The latter two biomarkers probably represent the most useful of the four.

NO_2^- and NO_3^- are present at high levels in the diet. However, urinary NO_3^- levels in animals and humans exceed the dietary intake, indicating endogenous formation.[258,259] Urinary excretion of NO_3^- increases during various kinds of inflammatory diseases (reviewed in references 120, 207). This elevated excretion has recently been attributed to an increase in the endogenous formation of NO• due to induction of iNOS. However, an elevation of urinary NO_3^- does not necessarily indicate damage caused by RNOS. As previously discussed, NO• has a relatively short half-life in vivo, which is most likely attributable to rapid oxidation reactions that ultimately lead to the formation of NO_2^- and/or NO_3^-. Because NO• can follow several different pathways, however, the measurement of NO_2^- and NO_3^- in vivo reveals little information on the identity of the intermediates formed.

Nitrosating species formed by activated macrophages produce mutagenic nitrosamines. Mechanistic studies show that the formation of nitrosamines is enhanced more than twofold in the presence of SOD, implicating a reactive species other than peroxynitrite in this reaction.[260] As discussed earlier, N_2O_3, the anhydride of HNO_2, could be responsible for this reaction. Humans infected with *Opisthorchis viverrini* excrete three- to fourfold more nitrosoproline after proline ingestion compared to uninfected individuals.[261] This increased excretion indicates increased formation of RNOS in infected people, presumably through enhanced NOS-mediated formation of NO•. Increased nitrosation was inhibited by ingestion of either ascorbic acid—a potent scavenger of nitrosating species[262]—or other components present in fruits and vegetables.[263]

Studies of chronic inflammation in animal models further point to an increased production of nitrosating species as a consequence of NOS induction. For example, macrophages and eosinophils found at the site of inflammation in Syrian golden hamsters infected with the liver fluke *O. viverrini* exhibit increased cytoplasmic immunoreactivity to NOS.[264] This increased NOS immunoreactivity was associated with an increased excretion of nitrosothizolidine 4-carboxylic acid after oral administration of its secondary amine precursor. Similarly, woodchucks infected with woodchuck hepatitis virus exhibit increased levels of NO_3^- and urinary *N*-nitrosodimethylamine, the latter of which is derived from an endogenous secondary amine.[120,265]

Recent studies designed to examine the role of RNOS in pathological conditions have led to the identification of 3NT in affected tissues. Measurement of 3NT, a stable product of the reaction between L-tyrosine and certain nitrating species, has been pivotal in the documentation of the involvement of RNOS in inflammatory diseases. Detection of 3NT at sites of inflammation-induced tissue injury and cellular localization are often achieved by immunohistochemistry using antibodies specific to the modified amino acid.[266] Alternatively, chromatographic techniques employing high sensitivity detection[242,267] are used to quantitate the levels of 3NT in tissues. This approach is useful, for example, to assess the efficacy of intervention strategies.

Scientists have measured 3NT in a number of inflammatory disease states associated with increased NOS activity, including inflammatory bowel disease,[268] acute lung injury,[269] atherosclerosis,[266] endotoxemia,[270] and zymosan-induced peritonitis.[242] Initially, peroxynitrite was presumed to be the proximate nitrating species. However, recent studies suggest that other RNOS may be formed under inflammatory conditions and cause the formation of 3NT. Thus, peroxidases, such as MPO, mediate the oxidation of NO_2^- to $NO_2^\bullet$, a potent nitrating species.[271] MPO also participates in the formation of the nitrating and chlorinating species nitryl chloride (NO_2Cl), a product generated by the reaction of HOCl with NO_2^-.[272] Other RNOS, such as NO_2^- and NO_2Cl, can also react with tyrosine to produce 3NT; therefore, it is difficult to ascribe the in vivo formation of 3NT exclusively to the presence of peroxynitrite.

Multistage Skin Cancer Model

Many classical two-stage carcinogenic regimens have employed promoters that incite inflammatory reactions. Researchers have used the skin tumor promoter PMA—sometimes also referred to as 12-tetradecanoyl phorbol-13-acetate (TPA)—for decades to investigate the mechanisms of carcinogenesis. In susceptible animal species and strains that have been treated with low levels of mutagens, application of PMA to the skin leads to an inflammatory reaction and oxidative DNA damage.[273,274] The sensitivity of various mouse strains to the proinflammatory effect of PMA correlates with the tumor-promoting activity of PMA in these strains. For example, SENCAR mice, which are more sensitive than C57BL/6 mice to the proinflammatory effect of PMA, are also more susceptible to PMA's tumor-promoting activity. Moreover, PMA-stimulated macrophages isolated from SENCAR mice produce higher levels of oxidants and display greater oxidative DNA damage than do those isolated from C57BL/6 mice. Further studies in SENCAR mice revealed infiltration of PMNs to the areas of the epidermis treated with PMA.[275] This infiltration resulted in marked elevation of the biomarkers of oxidative DNA damage 8HdG, 5HMdU, and TG in the epidermis. Both infiltration and oxidative DNA damage were inhibited by epigallocatechin gallate (a food polyphenol) or tamoxifen when applied before PMA.

Biomarkers in Inflammatory Diseases

Hepatitis

Inflammation, particularly macrophage activation, appears to play a critical role in the pathologies associated with both viral and alcoholic hepatitis. In individuals suffering from chronic hepatitis, liver cirrhosis, and hepatocellular carcinoma due to HBV infection, an increase in 8HdG in DNA has been observed.[4] Levels of serum aminotransferase activity, a marker of liver damage, correlated positively with 8HdG levels in precancerous liver tissue, suggesting an association between cell injury and oxidative DNA damage. A similar association between hepatitis and oxidative DNA damage has been demonstrated in a transgenic mouse model of this disease.[5]

Individuals with chronic HCV infection have been shown to exhibit increased levels of liver MDA and turnover rates of glutathione—a highly abundant intracellular low molecular-weight thiol antioxidant. These changes are accompanied by evidence of hepatic inflammation and steatosis. Higher levels of serum ferritin and of liver iron stores also have been noted; they were found to be higher than those in HBV-infected or uninfected individuals. Scientists have suggested that the increased iron stores in these individuals contribute to the observed oxidative damage.[276]

In experimental alcoholic liver disease, alcohol fed to rats in combination with dietary fats resulted in an increase in conjugated dienes (see comments above, however).[277] This increase was associated with apoptotic and necrotic cell death. Concentrations of BCl-2 protein, a cytoprotective protein with putative antioxidant function, appeared to be highest in bile duct epithelial and inflammatory cells. BCl-2 levels correlated with the number of inflammatory cells and the level of conjugated dienes. Parallel studies in this model of alcoholic liver disease indicated that expression of heat shock protein 70—a protein induced under oxidative stress—was associated with H_2O_2 formation, with an increase in microsomal conjugated dienes, and with the severity of tissue injury in the centrilobular region of the liver.[278]

In a model of alcohol-induced liver disease in micropigs, acetaldehyde and MDA, which colocalized in the perivenous region of the liver, were increased.[279] This increase, which was observed after only 1 month of alcohol feeding, correlated with an elevation in serum aminotransferase activity. After 5 months of treatment, increased intensity of immunoreactivity to these aldehydes was associated with evidence of steatonecrosis and focal inflammation. In terminal biopsy samples isolated after 12 months of treatment, evidence of perivenous fibrosis was observed in most of the animals. This study revealed a distinct sequence of events: proinflammatory lipid oxidation at an early stage, followed by cell injury, then chronic inflammation, and finally fibrosis. Similar events may contribute to the pathology of hepatic viral infections.

The oxidative damage and tissue injury observed in alcohol-induced chronic liver disease may be due largely to phagocyte-derived oxidants. For example, it has been shown in rats that inactivation of Kupffer cells with gadolinium chloride greatly attenuates liver injury, inflammation, and necrosis induced by intragastric alcohol feeding.[280] In a follow-up study, administration of antibiotics lowered the increased levels of LPS caused by the bacterial translocation. This treatment also resulted in the reduction of serum aminotransferase activity and hepatic pathology, suggesting that inflammation contributed to the alcohol-induced damage.[281]

Lung Injury

Chronic lung injury is a frequent outcome of a lifetime of smoking. It is also observed in other chronic lung diseases, such as asbestosis, which likewise predispose the individual to lung cancer. Lung injury by these means appears to be accompanied by an increase in oxidative injury to cell components. This oxidative injury is indicated by marked elevations in lipid peroxidation (measured by TBARS), which may be a direct result of either tobacco smoke–derived oxidants, or of the host immune response to the irritating effects of smoke constituents.[282] Researchers have suggested that an influx of PMNs and macrophages to sites injured or irritated by smoke constituents contributes to oxidative injury in the lungs of chronic smokers, or of experimental animals exposed to smoke. Indeed, even with acute smoke inhalation injury, mobilization of PMNs to the lung and activation of macrophages results in increased lipid oxidation (measured by TBARS and conjugated dienes), protein oxidation (detected as dinitrophenylhydrazine-reactive protein carbonyls), and nitration of tyrosine.[269] Thus, acute lung injury caused by smoke inhalation may model important aspects of the more chronic diseases.

When sheep are exposed to smoke, respiratory distress occurs. Subsequently, MDA levels increase in the airway fluid, but not in the airway mucosal or lung parenchymal tissue. However, under the severe conditions imposed in this animal model, evidence of systemic oxidative stress is also noted, because MDA levels increase in the liver. The systemic effect of smoke exposure suggests the involvement of oxidants from sources other than smoke, such as from inflammatory cells.

As mentioned previously, measurement of F_2-isoprostanes is a powerful tool for detecting nonenzymatic lipid peroxidation in various pathological conditions associated with oxidant formation. For example, plasma levels of F_2-isoprostanes have been shown to be higher in chronic smokers than in nonsmokers.[283] However, short-term smoking does not result in a detectable increase in plasma F_2-isoprostanes. Therefore, it is not clear whether the increase in lipid peroxidation in chronic smoking is caused by smoke constituents directly or by secondary reactions mediated by activated inflammatory cells in the lung or circulation.

Other chronic lung injuries also appear to precipitate the inflammation, oxidation, injury cascade. Silicosis is a chronic lung disease that mainly affects individuals in the industrial workplace. Chronic exposure to silica or other irritants leads to an inflammatory response that involves infiltration of PMNs and macrophages. In an acute model of silicosis designed to provide insight into the chronic disease, rats were exposed to freshly fractured quartz particles.[284] Inhalation of these particles led to an increased number of cells in the bronchoalveolar lavage fluid, pulmonary infiltration of PMNs, increased lipid peroxidation, and evidence of phagocyte activation. In another study in rats, intratracheal instillation of silica led to activation of phagocytes, release of proinflammatory cytokines, and fibrosis.[285] Treatment of these rats with the radical-trapping agent N-tert-butyl-alpha-phenylnitrone reversed the lung histopathological changes, decreased production of oxidants from isolated alveolar macrophages, and inhibited expression of TNF-α.

Parasitic Infections

Infiltration of monocytes and other leukocytes to sites of schistosomal growth results in an elevation of proinflammatory cytokines and oxidants (see Chapter 12). Stimulation of NO• production plays an important role in the host immune response to schistosomal infection. For example, treatment of infected C57BL/6 mice with aminoguanidine, an NOS inhibitor, leads to an increase in worm burden of 30%.[286] The same oxidants responsible for preventing proliferation of these parasites, however, may contribute to genetic damage in host cells. Activated inflammatory cells are shown in vitro to induce micronuclei formation in isolated bladder cells; this type of genetic damage is observed in vivo in exfoliated urothelial cells isolated from individuals infected with S. hematobium. These results suggest that although inflammatory cells—which invade areas of schistosomal growth—produce oxidants directed against the parasite, they inevitably cause chromosomal damage in the host's bladder cells, thereby increasing the incidence of bladder cancer in affected individuals.[287]

Similarly, it has been suggested that chronic inflammation that occurs at the site of *O. viverrini* biliary infection plays an important role in the development of cholangiocarcinoma (see Chapter 13). This is supported by the increased levels of salivary NO_2^-, and urinary and plasma NO_3^- observed in individuals with moderate to heavy liver fluke infection.[288]

Intervention Strategies

It follows from the discussion so far that anti-inflammatory drugs and antioxidants might have a significant influence on the development of cancer associated with chronic inflammation. It is therefore worth speculating whether regimens involving antioxidants that limit cellular oxidative damage, compounds that lower formation of phagocyte-derived oxidants by other means, or therapeutic agents that limit infection can reduce the risk of this class of cancer. To date, there is only limited information available on the effectiveness of such regimens.

Dietary Antioxidants

Large-scale intervention studies are currently under way to address whether dietary supplements of endogenous antioxidants such as ascorbic acid (vitamin C; an important water-soluble tissue antioxidant), β-carotene (a carotenoid with pro-vitamin A and antioxidant activity), and α-tocopherol (the principal form of vitamin E and chain-breaking antioxidant in lipid membranes) can boost the body's antioxidant defenses and effectively reduce the risk of certain types of cancers.[289] Because of the sustained immune response in chronic inflammatory diseases, cellular antioxidant defenses may not be maintained adequately and may therefore compromise the cell's ability to control oxidants or xenobiotics. For example, a recent study revealed that chronic inflammatory bowel disease results in a marked loss of most of the small molecular weight antioxidants in the colon compared to those in noninflamed biopsy material.[290] In biopsy tissue from patients with ulcerative colitis, total glutathione declined by 65%; ubiquinol (coenzyme Q; a cofactor of mitochondrial respiration and important lipid membrane antioxidant) by 75% in individuals with Crohn's disease, and by 90% in patients with ulcerative colitis. Interestingly, levels of α-tocopherol remained unchanged. Significantly lower levels of cellular antioxidants have also been reported in other chronic disease states. For example, cigarette smoking is associated with reduced levels of plasma vitamin C and β-carotene;[192] chronic active hepatitis due to HBV infection with lower plasma ubiquinol levels.[291]

There is considerable evidence that people whose diets are rich in fruits and vegetables have a lower overall risk of cancer compared to individuals with an inadequate dietary intake.[292,293] Fruits and vegetables are a rich source of low molecular-weight antioxidants including ascorbic acid, vitamin E, carotenoids, thiols, and others.[292] High levels of these compounds in the diet may be effective in maintaining adequate cellular antioxidant defenses during a pathophysiological insult. In this regard, it has been reported that workers chronically exposed to asbestos consuming a diet rich in vegetables—especially cruciferous vegetables—had a significantly lower overall risk of developing malignant mesothelioma than coworkers with a low vegetable intake.[293] These results could not be explained by differences in asbestos exposure, indicating that a diet rich in antioxidants may indeed reduce overall cancer risk in chronic inflammatory diseases. Epidemiological studies are under way to assess whether specific antioxidants can prevent asbestos- and smoke-induced lung cancer.[294]

High intake of vegetables has also been shown to decrease the risk of cancers of the colon. In a 1992 study that assessed multiple risk factors, vegetable consumption inversely correlated with the incidence of colon cancer.[295] Eliminating all confounding factors, the study still found a significantly reduced risk of developing colorectal cancer with high fruit and vegetable intake. Similar results have also been reported in other studies.[291]

Calcium and Fatty Acids

Other dietary components besides antioxidant vitamins may influence the risk of cancer. Individuals with a high fat intake have a greater probability of developing colorectal cancer.[296] It appears that certain fatty acids cause colonic epithelial cell toxicity and inflammation in the intestinal mucosa.[297] Whether this contributes to the procarcinogenic effect of fatty acids, however, is not known. In mice, oral administration of calcium significantly reduces colonic epithelial cell damage induced by intrarectal instillation of fatty acids. The beneficial effect of calcium is most likely due to its reaction with the fatty acids to form biologically inert soaps.[298] In humans, dietary supplementation with calcium carbonate substantially reduces colonic epithelial hyperplasia in individuals at risk for developing colonic cancer.[299] These results indicate that calcium carbonate supplementation may lower the risk of colon cancer by reducing fatty acid–induced inflammation.

Conversely, other types of fatty acids may lower gastrointestinal irritation and reduce the risk of cancer. Marine fish oils are rich in PUFA with more than two double bonds, in particular eicosapentanoic acid (20:5) and docosahexaenoic acid (22:6). Individuals who consume high levels of these fatty acids appear to have a lower incidence of colonic cancers.[300] These so-called ω-3 fatty acids are thought to reduce the synthesis of prostaglandins and leukotrienes, and may therefore act as anti-inflammatory agents in the gastrointestinal tract.[301,302] Indeed, they seem to reduce the size and number of chemically induced tumors of the colon in rats.[303]

Anti-Inflammatory Drugs and Synthetic Antioxidants

Like antioxidants, anti-inflammatory drugs may provide a cheap and effective means of lowering the overall risk of certain inflammation-induced cancers. For example, nonsteroidal anti-inflammatory drugs, such as aspirin, significantly reduce the incidence of or rate of death from colorectal cancer.[304-306] Intracellular glutathione levels normally depleted by xenobiotics can be effectively maintained by the thiol-based drug N-acetyl-L-cysteine (NAC).[307] NAC may therefore be an effective means to maintain glutathione-dependent antioxidant defenses in chronic inflammatory diseases and to slow the progression of cancer. NAC has been shown to inhibit spontaneous and chemically induced mutations in bacteria. It also inhibits the development of preneoplastic lesions and lowers tumor incidence in rodents.[307]

More exotic treatments also point to the possible beneficial effects of antioxidants or anti-inflammatory drugs. The efficacy of coadministered polyethylene glycol-conjugated catalase to ameliorate lung damage induced by asbestos was tested in rats.[308] Rats that received the catalase conjugate showed lower overall levels of lung injury, as evinced by decreased infiltration of PMNs into alveoli, lactate dehydrogenase release, and fibrotic scarring of the lungs.

Dehydroepiandrosterone (DHEA), a hormone with antioxidant properties, significantly reduced the levels of $O_2 \cdot$ released by alveolar macrophages obtained from lung lavages of nonsmoking asbestos workers.[309] Because DHEA acts as a noncompetitive inhibitor of NADPH oxidase,[310] long-term supplementation may be effective in reducing inflammation-induced oxidative damage, thereby lowering the risk of cancer.

Although the results of long-term clinical trials are needed, the examples mentioned above indicate that antioxidants and anti-inflammatory drugs may be good therapeutic agents to lower the risk of development of inflammation-induced cancer. The studies examining fruit and vegetable intake are particularly encouraging, because increased intake of foods rich in antioxidants would offer a relatively simple approach to the problem.

A TRANSGENIC MOUSE MODEL OF CHRONIC ACTIVE HEPATITIS B INFECTION

Despite the strong correlation between chronic active hepatitis and cancer, the mechanisms involved in the progression to hepatocellular carcinoma are still not entirely understood. Research has been hampered by the long latency period between onset of HBV infection and cancer, and the lack of suitable animal models that mimic chronic human disease. Recently a transgenic mouse model has been developed in which hepatocytes chronically express the large envelope protein of HBV. These mice develop a necroinflammatory liver disease that inevitably leads to hepatocellular carcinoma.[311-315] Typically, mice up to 2 months old do not exhibit histopathological liver lesions. In mice aged between 2 and 4 months, however, high expression of the large envelope protein results in hyperplastic endoplasmic reticulum that resembles "ground glass" under microscopic examination. With advancing age these mice display biochemical and histopathological evidence of liver cell injury, including high levels of serum glutamate/pyruvate transaminase and the occurrence of necroinflammatory foci. Mice between 6 and 18 months of age generally show evidence of microscopic nodular hyperplasia, reflecting the presence of dysplastic hepatocytes and preneoplastic foci. Animals with signs of microscopic nodular hyperplasia also often show evidence of adenomatous neoplastic tumors. Eventually, the mice develop primary hepatocellular carcinoma. This sequence of disease processes closely resembles the pathophysiological progression seen in human chronic active hepatitis. Thus, this mouse model was used to examine the role of ROS and oxidative DNA damage in the progression to hepatocellular carcinoma.

Analysis of Oxidants and Oxidative Damage

The extent of ROS present in the livers of HBV envelope protein transgenic mice was determined by *in situ* perfusion with nitroblue tetrazolium.[5] This dye is reduced to an insoluble formazan derivative on reaction with $O_2^{-}\cdot$.[316] The blue-colored formazan is readily detectable in tissue sections by light microscopy, and therefore is a useful histochemical marker for the presence of ROS. Tissue slices from the livers of 3-month-old transgenic mice showed extensive staining, whereas those from nontransgenic mice showed no formazan deposition.[5] Formazan deposits in HBV transgenic mice were markedly reduced when the livers were coperfused with SOD. Overall, in the transgenics, the most intense staining occurred around nonparenchymal cells. These cells were histologically compatible with Kupffer cells. Thus, the formazan staining evident in the transgenic mouse livers appears to be due to the presence of increased levels of $O_2^{-}\cdot$, presumably released from activated Kupffer cells.

The formation of oxidants also appeared to result in increased cell death and compensatory cell division. Transgenic mice at least 6 months old had a markedly higher rate of cell division (measured by the bromodeoxyuridine labeling assay) than nontransgenic mice;[5] in transgenic mice older than 9 months, proliferation was 80-fold higher than in nontransgenic littermates. Therefore, livers of transgenic mice exhibited a significantly increased rate of cell division in the presence of high levels of oxidants released by activated immune cells.

To determine whether the associated inflammation resulted in increased oxidative DNA damage, mice at different stages of liver injury were sacrificed, and hepatic 8HdG was measured.[244] Results showed a significant and sustained accumulation of 8HdG exclusively in the transgenic mice, that started early and increased progressively with advancing disease. The most pronounced increase occurred in livers exhibiting microscopic nodular hyperplasia, adenomas, and hepatocellular carcinoma. DNA–protein cross-links, another marker of oxidative DNA damage, were also increased substantially in the livers of transgenic mice compared to their nontransgenic littermates (Hagen and Ames, unpublished). The occurrence of high levels of oxidative DNA damage in the presence of increased hepatocellular proliferation greatly increases the probability of mutation within these cells, ultimately leading to the development of hepatocellular carcinoma.

Effects of Antioxidants

Ideally, oxidative DNA damage should be completely balanced by cellular repair systems. In the transgenic model, however, 8HdG accumulated to high levels in hepatocytes despite the active removal of 8-hydroxyguanine from DNA by glycosylases.[317] This finding suggests that cellular antioxidant or DNA-repair defenses were either overwhelmed by the oxidative environment in the inflamed liver, or functionally compromised by the hepatocytic expression of the viral antigen. It has been demonstrated that transgenic mice have significantly lower hepatic catalase levels than do nontransgenic controls.[318] Furthermore, levels of reduced glutathione were substantially lower in the liver of animals exhibiting microscopic nodular hyperplasia, or during later stages of the disease. These levels could be significantly repleted by the administration of NAC. This repletion apparently protected DNA from oxidative damage (Hagen, Chisari, and Ames, unpublished). Levels of DNA–protein cross-links were also significantly lower in animals supplemented with NAC. In contrast to glutathione, hepatic ascorbate levels were only slightly lower in transgenic mice (Hagen, Chisari, and Ames, unpublished).

A 1994 study reported significantly increased levels of 8HdG in liver samples from humans suffering from chronic hepatitis.[4] Moreover, 8HdG content correlated with disease activity as measured by serum transaminases. In conjunction with our work using transgenic mice, these results make a compelling argument that increased oxidative DNA damage occurs in the liver during chronic hepatitis infection, and that this damage likely is involved in the pathogenesis of hepatocellular carcinoma.

SUMMARY

In this chapter we summarized the evidence that suggests that chronic inflammation is a major risk factor for many human cancers. We described briefly the underlying mechanisms by which chronic inflammation can lead to cancer, and presented existing in vivo evidence for oxidant formation by activated cells and the resultant biomolecular damage. We also presented examples implicating phagocyte-derived oxidants in events leading to mutation, compensatory cell division, and cell injury— all important factors in the progression to cancer. We argued that a significant part of the cell injury involved in the inflammatory response is due to the formation of ROS and RNOS by phagocytes at the site of inflammation.

ROS and RNOS, and the secondary products derived from them, are all mutagenic and cytotoxic. Lipid oxidation products not only damage DNA, thus producing promutagenic lesions, but also could act as chemo-attractants for inflammatory cells. Although less well understood, oxidative damage to proteins could be equally important in the development of cancer associated with inflammation. Functional changes caused by the oxidation of critical thiols or by nitration of tyrosine residues in key regulatory proteins could lead to cell injury and cell death, the latter being a stimulus for compensatory cell proliferation. Oxidative damage to DNA, lipids, and proteins thus generates promutagenic DNA lesions and affects the proliferation of cells prone to mutation, thereby increasing the risk of developing cancer.

Antioxidants were shown to be protective in skin cancer models of multistage carcinogenesis induced by tumor promoters. The mechanism by which these compounds protect is not known; it is plausible that they act by scavenging oxidants that would otherwise damage DNA or cause lipid peroxidation (with subsequent release of mutagenic aldehydes and enals).

The evidence that oxidants contribute to cancer associated with inflammation suggests that antioxidant interventions could be protective. This protection may not only be due to the inhibition of oxidant-induced cytotoxicity and mutagenicity but may also be indirectly due to the reduced activation of NF-$\varkappa$B, preventing up-regulation of proinflammatory cytokines.[319] To date, results from epidemiological and animal studies indicate that interventions with nonsteroidal anti-inflammatory drugs, such as aspirin, are effective in reducing the incidence of colon cancer.

Although epidemiological data—largely based on studies of fruit and vegetable consumption—indicate a protective effect of antioxidants, single antioxidant interventions do not appear to be sufficient to prevent cancer. Fruits and vegetables contain a rich diversity of complementary antioxidants and micronutrients. It is not surprising, therefore, that efforts to mimic the protective effect of vegetables and fruits using a single antioxidant, such as ascorbate or α-tocopherol, have largely failed. Perhaps, intervention trials using multiple combinations of antioxidants and anti-inflammatory drugs may prove to be more effective.

Acknowledgments

This work was supported in part by a fellowship from the Swiss Foundation for Medical-Biological Stipends to S. C., a Sandoz Gerontological Foundation Grant to T. M. H., and by National Institute of Environmental Health Sciences Center Grant ESO1896 and National Cancer Institute Outstanding Investigator Grant CA39910 to B. N. A. The editorial help of Leah Christen-Witton is greatly appreciated.

REFERENCES

1. Vogelstein B, Fearon ER, Kern SE, et al. Allelotype of colorectal carcinomas. Science 1989;244:207–211.

2. Ames BN, Shigenaga MK, Hagen TM. Oxidants, antioxidants, and the degenerative diseases of aging. Proc Natl Acad Sci USA 1993;90:7915–7922.

2a. Helbock HJ, Beckman KB, Shigenaga MK, Walter PB, Woodall AA, Yeo HC, Ames BN. DNA oxidation matters: The HPLC-electrochemical detection assay of 8-oxo-deoxyguanosine and 8-oxo-guanine. Proc Natl Acad Sci USA 1998;95:288–293.

3. Hsu IC, Tokiwa T, Bennett W, et al. p53 gene mutation and integrated hepatitis B viral DNA sequences in human liver cancer cell lines. Carcinogenesis 1993;14:987–992.

4. Shimoda R, Nagashima M, Sakamoto M, et al. Increased formation of oxidative DNA damage, 8-hydroxydeoxyguanosine, in human livers with chronic hepatitis. Cancer Res 1994;54:3171–3172.

5. Hagen TM, Huang S, Curnutte J, et al. Extensive oxidative DNA damage in hepatocytes of transgenic mice with chronic active hepatitis destined to develop hepatocellular carcinoma. Proc Natl Acad Sci USA 1994;91:12808–12812.

6. Branda RF, Sullivan LM, O'Neill JP, et al. Measurement of HPRT mutant frequencies in T-lymphocytes from healthy human populations. Mutat Res 1993;285:267–279.

7. Cohen SM, Purtilo DT, Ellwein LB. Pivotal role of increased cell proliferation in human carcinogenesis. Mod Pathol 1991;4:371–382.

8. Ames BN, Shigenaga MK, Gold LS. DNA lesions, inducible DNA repair, and cell division: Three key factors in mutagenesis and carcinogenesis. Environ Health Perspect 1993;101(Suppl 5):35–44.

9. Ames BN, Gold LS. Chemical carcinogenesis: Too many rodent carcinogens. Proc Natl Acad Sci USA 1990;87:7772–7776.

10. Ames BN, Gold LS. Letter Re: E. Farber, Cell proliferation as a major risk factor for cancer: a concept of doubtful validity. Cancer Res 1995;55:3759–3762. Cancer Res 1996;56:4267–4269.

11. Henderson BE, Ross RK, Pike MC, Casagrande JT. Endogenous hormones as a major factor in human cancer. Cancer Res 1982;42:3232–3239.

12. Moalli PA, MacDonald JL, Goodglick LA, Kane AB. Acute injury and regeneration of the mesothelium in response to asbestos fibers. Am J Pathol 1987; 128:426–445.

13. Columbano A, Ledda-Columbano GM, Ennas MG, Curto M, Chelo A, Pani P. Cell proliferation and promotion of liver carcinogenesis: Different effect of hepatic regeneration and mitogen-induced hyperplasia on the development of enzyme-altered foci. Cell 1990;11:771–776.

14. Cunningham ML, Elwell MR, Matthews HB. Relationship of carcinogenicity and cellular proliferation induced by mutagenic noncarcinogens vs carcinogens. Fundam Appl Toxicol 1994;23:363–369.

15. Cunningham ML, Maronpot RR, Thompson M, Bucher JR. Early responses of the liver of B6C3F1 mice to the hepatocarcinogen oxazepam. Toxicol Appl Pharmacol 1994;124:31–38.

16. Hanawalt P, Mellon I. Stranded in an active gene. Curr Biol 1993;3:67–69.

17. Selby CP, Sancar A. Molecular mechanism of transcription-repair coupling. Science 1993;260:53–58.

18. Li R, Botchan MR. The acidic transcriptional activation domains of VP and p53 bind the cellular Replication Protein A and stimulate in vitro BPV-1 DNA replication. Cell 1993;73:1207–1222.

19. Dutta A, Ruppert JM, Aster JC, Winchester E. Inhibition of DNA replication factor RPA by p53. Nature (London) 1993;365:79–82.

20. Abramova NA, Russell J, Botchan M, Li R. Interaction between replication protein A and p53 is disrupted after UV damage in a DNA repair-dependent manner. Proc Natl Acad Sci USA 1997;94:7186–191.

21. Lane DP. A death in the life of p53. Nature 1992;362:786–787.

22. Venkatachalam S, Denissenko MF, Alvi N, Wani AA. Rapid activation of apoptosis in human promyelocytic leukemic cells by ($+/-$)-anti-benzo [a]pyrene diol epoxide induced DNA damage. Biochem Biophys Res Commun 1993;197:722–729.

23. Yamashina K, Miller BE, Heppner GH. Macrophage-mediated induction of drug-resistant variants in a mouse mammary tumor cell line. Cancer Res 1986;46:2396–4401.

24. Shacter E, Beecham EJ, Covey JM, Kohn KW, Potter M. Activated neutrophils induce prolonged DNA damage in neighboring cells. Carcinogenesis 1988;9:2297–2304.

24a. Pisani P, Parking DM, Muñoz N, Ferlay J. Cancer and infection: Estimates of the attributable fraction in 1990. Cancer Epidemiol Rev 1997;6:387–400.

25. Himeno Y, Fukuda Y, Hatanaka M, Imura H. Expression of oncogenes in human liver disease. Liver 1988;8:208–212.

26. Wang J, Chenivesse X, Henglein B, Brechot C. Hepatitis B virus integration in a cyclin A gene in a hepatocellular carcinoma. Nature 1990;343:555–557.

27. Pasquinelli C, Bhavani K, Chisari FV. Multiple oncogenes and tumor suppressor genes are structurally and functionally intact during hepatocarcinogenesis in hepatitis B virus transgenic mice. Cancer Res 1992;52:2823–2829.

28. De Mitri MS, Pisi E, Brechot C, Paterlini P. Low frequency of allelic loss in the cyclin A gene in human hepatocellular carcinomas: a study based on PCR. Liver 1993;13:259–261.

29. Mondelli M, Eddleston AL. Mechanisms of liver cell injury in acute and chronic hepatitis B. Semin Liver Dis 1984;4:47–58.

30. Thomas HC, Pignatelli M, Scully LJ. Viruses and immune reactions in the liver. Scand J Gastroenterol Suppl 1985;114:105–117.

31. Chisari FV. The role of cytotoxic T lymphocytes and inflammatory cytokines in the pathogenesis of acute viral hepatitis. Gastroenterol Jpn 1993;28 Suppl 4:2–6; discussion 17–19.

32. Hopf U, Moller B, Kuther D, et al. Long-term follow-up of posttransfusion and sporadic chronic hepatitis non-A, non-B and frequency of circulating antibodies to hepatitis C virus (HCV). J Hepatol 1990;10:69–76.

33. Tabor E, Kobayashi K. Hepatitis C virus, a causative infectious agent of non-A, non-B hepatitis: prevalence and structure—summary of a conference on hepatitis C virus as a cause of hepatocellular carcinoma. J Natl Cancer Inst 1992;84:86–90.

34. Iarotski LS, Davis A. The schistosomiasis problem in the world: results of a WHO questionnaire survey. Bull World Health Organ 1981;59:115–127.

35. Webbe G. The six diseases of WHO. Schistosomiasis: some advances. Br Med J (Clin Res Ed) 1981;283:1104–1106.

36. Capron A, Dessaint JP. Immunologic aspects of schistosomiasis. Annu Rev Med 1992;43:209–218.

37. Schwartz DA. Helminths in the induction of cancer: Opisthorchis viverrini,

Clonorchis sinensis and cholangiocarcinoma. Trop Geogr Med 1980;32:95–100.

38. Haswell-Elkins MR, Satarug S, Elkins DB. Opisthorchis viverrini infection in northeast Thailand and its relationship to cholangiocarcinoma. J Gastroenterol Hepatol 1992;7:538–548.

39. Thammapalerd N, Tharavanij S, Nacapunchai D, Bunnag D, Radomyos P, Prasertsiriroj V. Detection of antibodies against *Opisthorchis viverrini* in patients before and after treatment with praziquantel. Southeast Asian J Trop Med Public Health 1988;19:101–108.

40. Chen MG, Mott KE. Progress in assessment of morbidity due to *Schistosoma japonicum* infection. A review of recent literature. Trop Dis Bull 1988;85:R1–R45.

41. Sher A. Schistosomiasis. Parasitizing the cytokine system. Nature 1992;356:565–566.

42. Shindo K. Significance of Schistosomiasis japonica in the development of cancer of the large intestine: report of a case and review of the literature. Dis Colon Rectum 1976;19:460–469.

43. Bhamarapravati N, Thammavit W, Vajrasthira S. Liver changes in hamsters infected with a liver fluke of man, Opisthorchis viverrini. Am J Trop Med Hyg 1978;27:787–794.

44. Wongratanacheewin S, Good MF, Sithithaworn P, Haswell-Elkins MR. Molecular analysis of T and B cell repertoires in mice immunized with Opisthorchis viverrini antigens. Int J Parasitol 1991;21:719–721.

45. Viranuvatti V, Stitnimankarn T. Liver fluke infection and infestation in South-East Asia. In: Popper H, Schaffner F, eds. Progress in Liver Disease. New York: Grune and Stratton, 1972:527–547.

46. Villako K, Siurala M. The behaviour of gastritis and related conditions in different population samples. Ann Clin Res 1981;13:114–118.

47. Parsonnet J. Helicobacter pylori and gastric cancer. Gastroenterol Clin North Am 1993;22:89–104.

48. Sipponen P, Hyvarinen H. Role of Helicobacter pylori in the pathogenesis of gastritis, peptic ulcer and gastric cancer. Scand J Gastroenterol Suppl 1993;196:3–6.

49. Becklake MR. Asbestos-related diseases of the lung and other organs: their epidemiology and implications for clinical practice. Am Rev Respir Dis 1976;114:187–227.

50. Ziskind M, Jones RN, Weill H. Silicosis. Am Rev Respir Dis 1976;113:643–665.

51. Green FH, Laqueur WA. Coal workers' pneumoconiosis. Pathol Annu 1980;333–410.

52. Doll R. Mortality from lung cancer in asbestos workers. Br J Ind Med 1955;12:81–86.

53. Mossman BT, Gee JB. Asbestos-related diseases. N Engl J Med 1989;320:1721–1730.

54. Mossman BT, Bignon J, Corn M, Seaton A, Gee JB. Asbestos: scientific developments and implications for public policy. Science 1990;247:294–301.

55. Wagner JC, Berry G. Mesotheliomas in rats following inoculation with asbestos. Br J Cancer 1969;23:567–581.

56. Stanton MF, Layard M, Tegeris A, et al. Relation of particle dimension to carcinogenicity in amphibole asbestoses and other fibrous minerals. J Natl Cancer Inst 1981;67:965–975.

57. Monchaux G, Bignon J, Jaurand MC, et al. Mesotheliomas in rats following inoculation with acid-leached chrysotile asbestos and other mineral fibres. Carcinogenesis 1981;2:229–236.

58. Davis JM. The pathology of asbestos related disease. Thorax 1984;39:801–808.

59. Lee KP, Trochimowicz HJ, Reinhardt CF. Pulmonary response of rats exposed to titanium dioxide (TiO_2) by inhalation for two years. Toxicol Appl Pharmacol 1985;79:179–192.

60. Lemaire I. Characterization of the bronchoalveolar cellular response in experimental asbestosis. Different reactions depending on the fibrogenic potential. Am Rev Respir Dis 1985;131:144–149.

61. Xaubet A, Rodriguez RR, Bombi JA, Marin A, Roca J, Agusti VA. Correlation of bronchoalveolar lavage and clinical and functional findings in asbestosis. Am Rev Respir Dis 1986;133:848–854.

62. Mossman BT, Marsh JP, Sesko A, et al. Inhibition of lung injury, inflammation, and interstitial pulmonary fibrosis by polyethylene glycol-conjugated catalase in a rapid inhalation model of asbestosis. Am Rev Respir Dis 1990; 141:1266–1271.

63. Klebanoff SJ. Oxygen metabolism and the toxic properties of phagocytes. Ann Intern Med 1980;93:480–489.

64. Murray HW. Survival of intracellular pathogens within human mononuclear phagocytes. Semin Hematol 1988;25:101–111.

65. Weiss SJ. Tissue destruction by neutrophils. N Engl J Med 1989;320:365–376.

66. Spitznagel JK. Antibiotic proteins of human neutrophils. J Clin Invest 1990; 86:1381–1386.

67. Nathan CF, Hibbs JB, Jr. Role of nitric oxide synthesis in macrophage antimicrobial activity. Curr Opin Immunol 1991;3:65–70.

68. Ward PA, Warren JS, Johnson KJ. Oxygen radicals, inflammation, and tissue injury. Free Rad Biol Med 1988;5:403–408.

69. Laskin DL, Pendino KJ. Macrophages and inflammatory mediators in tissue injury. Annu Rev Pharmacol Toxicol 1995;35:655–677.

70. Sbarra AJ, Karnofsky ML. The biochemical basis of phagocytosis. I. Metabolic changes during the ingestion of particles by polymorphonuclear leukocytes. J Biol Chem 1959;234:1355–1362.

71. Babior BM. The respiratory burst oxidase. TIBS 1987;12:241–243.

72. Bielski BHJ, Arudi RL, Sutherland MW. A study of the reactivity of HO_2/O_2^- with unsaturated fatty acids. J Biol Chem 1983;258:4759–4761.

73. Bielski BHJ, Cabelli DE, Arudi RL. Reactivity of HO_2/O_2^- radicals in aqueous solution. J Phys Chem Ref Data 1985;14:1041–1100.

74. Allen RC. Role of oxygen in phagocyte microbicidal action. Environ Health Perspect 1994;102 Suppl 10:201–208.

75. Goldstein IM, Roos D, Kaplan HB, Weissmann G. Complement and immunoglobulins stimulate superoxide production by human leukocytes independently of phagocytosis. J Clin Invest 1975;56:1155–1163.

76. Johnston RB Jr, Lehmeyer JE. Elaboration of toxic oxygen by-products by neutrophils in a model of immune complex disease. J Clin Invest 1976;57:836–841.

77. Mills EL, Debets-Ossenkopp Y, Verbrugh HA, Verhoef J. Initiation of the respiratory burst of human neutrophils by influenza virus. Infect Immun 1981;32:1200–1205.

78. Peterhans E, Grob M, Bürge T, Zanoni R. Virus-induced formation of reactive oxygen intermediates in phagocytic cells. Free Rad Res Comms 1987; 3:39–46.

79. Becker EL, Sigman M, Oliver JM. Superoxide production induced by rabbit polymorphonuclear leukocytes by synthetic chemotactic peptides and A23187. The nature of the receptor and the requirement for Ca^{2+}. Am J Pathol 1979;95:81–98.

80. Simchowitz L, Spilberg I. Chemotactic factor-induced generation of superoxide radicals by human neutrophils: Evidence for the role of sodium. J Immunol 1979;123:2428–2435.

81. Webster RO, Hong SR, Johnston RB, Jr., Henson PM. Biological effects of the human complement fragments C5a and $C5a_{desarg}$ on neutrophil function. Immunopharmacology 1980;2:201–219.

82. Shaw JO, Pinckard RN, Ferrigni KS, McManus LM, Hanahan DJ. Activation of human neutrophils with 1-O-hexadecyl/octadecyl-2-acetyl-sn-glyceryl-3-phosphorylcholine (platelet activating factor). J Immunol 1981;127:1250–1255.

83. Passo SA, Weiss SJ. Oxidative mechanisms utilized by human neutrophils to destroy Escherichia coli. Blood 1984;63:1361–1368.

84. Nathan CF, Murray HW, Wiebe ME, Rubin BY. Identification of interferon-γ as the lymphokine that activates human macrophage oxidative metabolism and antimicrobial activity. J Exp Med 1983;158:670–689.

85. McColl SR, Beauseigle D, Gilbert C, Naccache PH. Priming of the human neutrophil respiratory burst by granulocyte-macrophage colony-stimulating factor and tumor necrosis factor-α involves regulation at a post-cell surface receptor level. J Immunol 1990;145:3047–3053.

86. Humbert JR, Winsor EL. Tumor necrosis factor primes neutrophils by shortening the lag period of the respiratory burst. Am J Med Sci 1990;300:209–213.

87. Nathan CF. Neutrophil activation on biological surfaces. J Clin Invest 1987; 80:1550–1560.

88. Murray HW. Interferon-gamma, the activated macrophage, and the host defense against microbial challenge. Ann Intern Med 1988;108:595–608.

89. Nathan C. Interferon-gamma and macrophage activation in cell-mediated immunity. In: Steinman RM, North RJ, eds. Mechanisms of Host Resistance to Infectious Agents, Tumors, and Allografts. New York: Rockefeller University Press, 1986:165–184.

90. Huang S, Hendriks W, Althage A, et al. Immune response in mice that lack the interferon-γ receptor. Science 1993;259:1742–1745.

91. Dalton DK, Pitts-Meek S, Keshav S, Figari IS, Bradley A, Stewart TA. Multiple defects of immune cell function in mice with disrupted interferon-gamma genes. Science 1993;259:1739–1742.

92. Taylor MW, Feng GS. Relationship between interferon-gamma, indoleamine 2,3-dioxygenase, and tryptophan catabolism. FASEB J 1991;5:2516–2522.

93. Beutler B, Cerami A. Tumor necrosis, cachexia, shock, and inflammation: A common mediator. Annu Rev Biochem 1988;57:505–518.

94. Winrow VR, Winyard PG, Morris CJ, Blake DR. Free radicals in inflammation: Second messengers and mediators of tissue destruction. Br Med Bull 1993;49:506–522.

95. Baeuerle PA, Rupec RA, Pahl HL. Reactive oxygen intermediates as second

messengers of a general pathogen response. Pathol Biol (Paris) 1996;44:29–35.

96. Lehrer RI, Ganz T, Selsted ME, Babior BM, Curnutte JT. Neutrophils and host defense. Ann Intern Med 1988;109:127–142.

97. Murray HW. Interferon-gamma and host antimicrobial defense: current and future clinical applications. Am J Med 1994;97:459–467.

98. Mirochnitchenko O, Inouye M. Effect of overexpression of human Cu,Zn superoxide dismutase in transgenic mice on macrophage functions. J Immunol 1996;156:1578–1586.

99. Jensen MS, Bainton DF. Temporal changes in pH within the phagocytic vacuole of the polymorphonuclear neutrophilic leukocyte. J Cell Biol 1973; 56:379–388.

100. Jacques YV, Bainton DF. Changes in pH within the phagocytic vacuoles of human neutrophils and monocytes. Lab Invest 1978;39:179–185.

101. Takanaka K, O'Brien PJ. Proton release associated with respiratory burst of polymorphonuclear leukocytes. J Biochem 1988;103:656–660.

102. Haber F, Weiss J. The catalytic decomposition of hydrogen peroxide by iron salts. Proc R Soc 1934;Ser. A, 147:332–351.

103. Halliwell B. Superoxide-dependent formation of hydroxyl radicals in the presence of iron chelates. FEBS Lett 1978;92:321–326.

104. Gutteridge JMC, Richmond R, Halliwell B. Inhibition of the iron-catalysed formation of hydroxyl radicals from superoxide and of lipid peroxidation by desferrioxamine. Biochem J 1979;184:469–472.

105. Wink DA, Nims RW, Saavedra JE, Utermahlen WE Jr, Ford PC. The Fenton oxidation mechanism: Reactivities of biologically relevant substrates with two oxidizing intermediates differ from those predicted for the hydroxyl radical. Proc Natl Acad Sci USA 1994;91:6604–6608.

106. Imlay JA, Chin SM, Linn S. Toxic DNA damage by hydrogen peroxide through the Fenton reaction in vivo and in vitro. Science 1988;240:640–642.

107. Luo Y, Han Z, Chin SM, Linn S. Three chemically distinct types of oxidants formed by iron-mediated Fenton reactions in the presence of DNA. Proc Natl Acad Sci USA 1994;91:12438–12442.

108. Schraufstatter I, Hyslop PA, Jackson JH, Cochrane CG. Oxidant-induced DNA damage of target cells. J Clin Invest 1988;82:1040–1050.

109. Ward PA, Till GO, Gannon DE, Varani JA, Johnson KJ. The role of iron in injury of endothelial cells *in vitro* and *in vivo*. Basic Life Sci 1988;49:969–974.

110. Toyokuni S. Iron-induced carcinogenesis: The role of redox regulation. Free Radic Biol Med 1996;20:553–566.

111. Kadiiska MB, Burkitt MJ, Xiang QH, Mason RP. Iron supplementation generates hydroxyl radical in vivo. An ESR spin-trapping investigation. J Clin Invest 1995;96:1653–1657.

112. Ramos CL, Pou S, Britigan BE, Cohen MS, Rosen GM. Spin trapping evidence for myeloperoxidase-dependent hydroxyl radical formation by human neutrophils and monocytes. J Biol Chem 1992;267:8307–8312.

113. Belding ME, Klebanoff SJ. Peroxidase-mediated virucidal systems. Science 1970;167:195–196.

114. Rosen H, Klebanoff SJ. Oxidation of microbial iron-sulfur centers by the myeloperoxidase-H_2O_2-halide antimicrobial system. Infect Immun 1985;47: 613–618.

115. Bortolussi R, Vandenbroucke-Grauls CMJE, van Asbeck BS, Verhoef J. Rela-

tionship of bacterial growth phase to killing of *Listeria monocytogenes* by oxidative agents generated by neutrophils and enzyme systems. Infect Immun 1987;55:3197–203.

116. Grisham MB, Jefferson MM, Melton DF, Thomas EL. Chlorination of endogenous amines by isolated neutrophils. Ammonia-dependent bactericidal, cytotoxic, and cytolytic activities of the chloramines. J Biol Chem 1984;259: 10404–10413.

117. Moreno JJ, Pryor WA. Inactivation of alpha 1–proteinase inhibitor by peroxynitrite. Chem Res Toxicol 1992;5:425–431.

118. Marletta MA. Nitric oxide: Biosynthesis and biological synthesis. TIBS 1989; 14:488–492.

119. Moncada S, Higgs A. The L-arginine-nitric oxide pathway. N Engl J Med 1993;329:2002–2012.

120. Liu RH, Hotchkiss JH. Potential genotoxicity of chronically elevated nitric oxide: a review. Mutat Res 1995;339:73–89.

121. Doyle MP, Hoekstra JW. Oxidation of nitrogen oxides by bound dioxygen in hemoproteins. J Inorg Biochem 1981;14:351–358.

122. Moilanen E, Moilanen T, Knowles R, et al. Nitric oxide synthase is expressed in human macrophages during foreign body inflammation. Am J Pathol 1997;150:881–887.

123. MacMicking J, Xie QW, Nathan C. Nitric oxide and macrophage function. Annu Rev Immunol 1997;15:323–350.

124. Evans TJ, Buttery LDK, Carpenter A, Springall DR, Polak JM, Cohen J. Cytokine-treated human neutrophils contain inducible nitric oxide synthase that produces nitration of injected bacteria. Proc Natl Acad Sci USA 1996;93: 9553–9558.

125. Hibbs JB Jr, Taintor RR, Vavrin Z, Rachlin EM. Nitric oxide: A cytotoxic activated macrophage effector molecule. Biochem Biophys Res Commun 1988;157:87–94.

126. Stuehr DJ, Nathan CF. Nitric oxide. A macrophage product responsible for cytostasis and respiratory inhibition in tumor target cells. J Exp Med 1989; 169:1543–1555.

127. Stamler JS, Singel DJ, Loscalzo J. Biochemistry of nitric oxide and its redox-activated forms. Science 1992;258:1898–902.

128. Butler AR, Flitney FW, Williams DL. NO, nitrosonium ions, nitroxide ions, nitrosothiols and iron-nitrosyls in biology: a chemist's perspective. Trends Pharmacol Sci 1995;16:18–22.

129. Rubbo H, Radi R, Trujillo M, et al. Nitric oxide regulation of superoxide and peroxynitrite-dependent lipid peroxidation. Formation of novel nitrogen-containing oxidized lipid derivatives. J Biol Chem 1994;269:26066–26075.

130. Wink DA, Darbyshire JF, Nims RW, Saavedra JE, Ford PC. Reactions of the bioregulatory agent nitric oxide in oxygenated aqueous media: determination of the kinetics for oxidation and nitrosation by intermediates generated in the NO/O_2 reaction. Chem Res Toxicol 1993;6:23–27.

131. Palmer RM, Ferrige AG, Moncada S. Nitric oxide release accounts for the biological activity of endothelium-derived relaxing factor. Nature 1987;327: 524–526.

132. Tamir S, Lewis RS, de Rojas-Walker T, Deen WM, Wishnok JS, Tannenbaum SR. The influence of delivery rate on the chemistry and biological effects of nitric oxide. Chem Res Toxicol 1993;6:895–899.

133. Lewis RS, Tannenbaum SR, Deen WM. Kinetics of N-nitrosation in oxygenated nitric oxide solutions at physiological pH: Role of nitrous anhydride and effects of phosphate and chloride. J Am Chem Soc 1995;117:3933–3939.

134. Challis BC, Edwards A, Hunma RR, Kyrtopoulos SA, Outram JR. Rapid formation of N-nitrosamines from nitrogen oxides under neutral and alkaline conditions. IARC Sci Publ 1978;1978:127–142.

135. Yahagi T, Nagao M, Seino Y, Matsushima T, Sugimura T. Mutagenicities of N-nitrosamines on Salmonella. Mutat Res 1977;48:121–129.

136. Tricker AR, Preussmann R. Carcinogenic N-nitrosamines in the diet: occurrence, formation, mechanisms and carcinogenic potential. Mutat Res 1991;259:277–289.

137. Wink DA, Kasprzak KS, Maragos CM, et al. DNA deaminating ability and genotoxicity of nitric oxide and its progenitors. Science 1991;254:1001–1003.

138. Miwa M, Stuehr DJ, Marletta MA, Wishnok JS, Tannenbaum SR. Nitrosation of amines by stimulated macrophages. Carcinogenesis 1987;8:955–95

139. Grisham MB, Ware K, Gilleland HE Jr, Gilleland LB, Abell CL, Yamada T. Neutrophil-mediated nitrosamine formation: role of nitric oxide in rats. Gastroenterology 1992;103:1260–1266.

140. Beckman JS, Chen J, Ischiropoulos H, Crow JP. Oxidative chemistry of peroxynitrite. Methods Enzymol 1994;233:229–240.

141. Beckman JS, Beckman TW, Chen J, Marshall PA, Freeman BA. Apparent hydroxyl radical production by peroxynitrite: Implications for endothelial injury from nitric oxide and superoxide. Proc Natl Acad Sci USA 1990;87:1620–1624.

142. Radi R, Beckman JS, Bush KM, Freeman BA. Peroxynitrite oxidation of sulfhydryls. The cytotoxic potential of superoxide and nitric oxide. J Biol Chem 1991;266:4244–4250.

143. Koppenol WH, Moreno JJ, Pryor WA, Ischiropoulos H, Beckman JS. Peroxynitrite, a cloaked oxidant formed by nitric oxide and superoxide. Chem Res Toxicol 1992;5:834–842.

144. Mayer B, Schrammel A, Klatt P, Koesling D, Schmidt K. Peroxynitrite-induced accumulation of cyclic GMP in endothelial cells and stimulation of purified soluble guanylyl cyclase. Dependence on glutathione and possible role of S-nitrosation. J Biol Chem 1995;270:17355–17360.

145. Ischiropoulos H, Zhu L, Beckman JS. Peroxynitrite formation from macrophage-derived nitric oxide. Arch Biochem Biophys 1992;298:446–451.

146. Allen RC. Biochemiexitation: Chemiluminescence and the study of biological oxygenation reactions. In: Adam W, Cilento G, eds. Chemical and Biological Generation of Excited States. New York: Academic Press, 1982:309–344.

147. Sies H. Oxidative Stress: In: Sies H, ed. Oxidants and Antioxidants. 2nd ed. London: Academic Press; 1991.

148. Mason RP, Hanna PM, Burkitt MJ, Kadiiska MB. Detection of oxygen-derived radicals in biological systems using electron spin resonance. Environ Health Perspect 1994;102 Suppl 10:33–36.

149. Van Dyke K. Introduction to cellular chemiluminescence, neutrophils, macrophages, and monocytes. In: Van Dyke K, Castranova V, eds. Cellular Chemiluminescence. Boca Raton, FL: CRC Press;1987:3–22.

150. Van Dyke K, Antonini JM, Wu L, Ye Z, Reasor MJ. The inhibition of silica-induced lung inflammation by dexamethasone as measured by broncho-

alveolar lavage fluid parameters and peroxynitrite-dependent chemilumi-nescence. Agents Actions 1994;41:44–49.

151. Antonini JM, Van Dyke K, Ye Z, DiMatteo M, Reasor MJ. Introduction of luminol-dependent chemiluminescence as a method to study silica inflam-mation in the tissue and phagocytic cells of rat lung. Environ Health Per-spect 1994;102 Suppl 10:37–42.

152. Wang JF, Komarov P, Sies H, de Groot H. Contribution of nitric oxide syn-thase to luminol-dependent chemiluminescence generated by phorbol-ester-activated Kupffer cells. Biochem J 1991;279:311–314.

153. Dowling EJ, Symons AM, Parke DV. Free radical production at the site of an acute inflammatory reaction as measured by chemiluminescence. Agents Actions 1986;19:203–207.

154. Simmonds NJ, Allen RE, Stevens TR, Van Someren RN, Blake DR, Rampton DS. Chemiluminescence assay of mucosal reactive oxygen metabolites in inflammatory bowel disease. Gastroenterology 1992;103:186–196.

155. Sedghi S, Fields JZ, Klamut M, et al. Increased production of luminol en-hanced chemiluminescence by the inflamed colonic mucosa in patients with ulcerative colitis. Gut 1993;34:1191–1197.

156. Davies GR, Simmonds NJ, Stevens TRJ, Grandison A, Blake DR, Rampton DS. Mucosal reactive oxygen metabolite production in duodenal ulcer dis-ease. Gut 1992;33:1467–1472.

157. Davies GR, Simmonds NJ, Stevens TR, et al. Helicobacter pylori stimulates antral mucosal reactive oxygen metabolite production in vivo. Gut 1994;35:179–85.

158. Dohlman AW, Black HR, Royall JA. Expired breath hydrogen peroxide is a marker of acute airway inflammation in pediatric patients with asthma. Am Rev Respir Dis 1993;148:955–960.

159. Kawai K, Yamamoto M, Kameyama S, Kawamata H, Rademaker A, Oyasu R. Enhancement of rat urinary bladder tumorigenesis by lipopolysaccharide-induced inflammation. Cancer Res 1993;53:5172–5175.

160. Buffinton GD, Christen S, Peterhans E, Stocker R. Oxidative stress in lungs of mice infected with influenza A virus. Free Radic Res Commun 1992;16:99–110.

161. Oda T, Akaike T, Hamamoto T, Suzuki F, Hirano T, Maeda H. Oxygen radi-cals in influenza-induced pathogenesis and treatment with pyran polymer-conjugated SOD. Science 1989;244:974–976.

162. Archer S. Measurement of nitric oxide in biological models. FASEB J 1993;7:349–360.

163. Lai CS, Komarov AM. Spin trapping of nitric oxide produced in vivo in septic-shock mice. FEBS Lett 1994;345:120–124.

164. Westenberger U, Thanner S, Ruf HH, Gersonde K, Sutter G, Trentz O. Formation of free radicals and nitric oxide derivative of hemoglobin in rats during shock syndrome. Free Radic Res Commun 1990;11:167–178.

165. Wang QZ, Jacobs J, DeLeo J, et al. Nitric oxide hemoglobin in mice and rats in endotoxic shock. Life Sci 1991;49:L55–L60.

166. Bastian NR, Yim CY, Hibbs JB, Jr., Samlowski WE. Induction of iron-derived EPR signals in murine cancers by nitric oxide. Evidence for multiple intra-cellular targets. J Biol Chem 1994;269:5127–5131.

167. Chamulitrat W, Jordan SJ, Mason RP, et al. Targets of nitric oxide in a mouse model of liver inflammation by *Corynebacterium parvum*. Arch Bio-chem Biophys 1995;316:30–37.

168. Geller DA, Di Silvio M, Nussler AK, et al. Nitric oxide synthase expression is induced in hepatocytes in vivo during hepatic inflammation. J Surg Res 1993;55:427–432.

169. Harbrecht BG, Billiar TR, Stadler J, et al. Inhibition of nitric oxide synthesis during endotoxemia promotes intrahepatic thrombosis and an oxygen radical-mediated hepatic injury. J Leukoc Biol 1992;52:390–394.

170. Hsie AW, Recio L, Katz DS, Lee CQ, Wagner M, Schenley RL. Evidence for reactive oxygen species inducing mutations in mammalian cells. Proc Natl Acad Sci USA 1986;83:9616–9620.

171. Yuan J, Yeasky TM, Rhee MC, Glazer PM. Frequent T:A—G:C transversions in X-irradiated mouse cells. Carcinogenesis 1995;16:83–88.

172. Simic MG. DNA markers of oxidative processes in vivo: Relevance to carcinogenesis and anticarcinogenesis. Cancer Res 1994;54:1918s-1923s.

173. Loeb LA, James EA, Waltersdorph AM, Klebanoff SJ. Mutagenesis by the autoxidation of iron with isolated DNA. Proc Natl Acad Sci USA 1988;85: 3918–3922.

174. Frenkel K, Chrzan K, Troll W, Teebor GW, Steinberg JJ. Radiation-like modification of bases in DNA exposed to tumor promoter-activated polymorphonuclear leukocytes. Cancer Res 1986;46:5533–5540.

175. Imlay JA, Linn S. DNA damage and oxygen radical toxicity. Science 1988; 240:1302–1309.

176. von Sonntag C. The chemistry of free-radical-mediated DNA damage. Basic Life Sci 1991;58:287–317; discussion, 317–321.

177. Feig DI, Reid TM, Loeb LA. Reactive oxygen species in tumorigenesis. Cancer Res 1994;54:1890s–1894s.

178. Dizdaroglu M. Chemical determination of oxidative DNA damage by gas chromatography–mass spectrometry. Methods Enzymol 1994;234:3–16.

179. Breen AP, Murphy JA. Reactions of oxyl radicals with DNA. Free Radic Biol Med 1995;18:1033–1077.

180. Jackson JH, Gajewski E, Schraufstatter IU, et al. Damage to the bases in DNA induced by stimulated human neutrophils. J Clin Invest 1989;84:1644–1649.

181. Akasaka S, Yamamoto K. Hydrogen peroxide induces G:C to T:A and G:C to C:G transversions in the supF gene of Escherichia coli. Mol Gen Genet 1994;243:500–505.

182. Kuchino Y, Mori F, Kasai H, et al. Misreading of DNA templates containing 8-hydroxydeoxyguanosine at the modified base and at adjacent residues. Nature 1987;327:77–97.

183. Shibutani S, Takeshita M, Grollman AP. Insertion of specific bases during DNA synthesis past the oxidation-damaged base 8-oxodG. Nature 1991;349: 431–434.

184. Wood ML, Dizdaroglu M, Gajewski E, Essigmann JM. Mechanistic studies of ionizing radiation and oxidative mutagenesis: genetic effects of a single 8-hydroxyguanine (7-hydro-8-oxoguanine) residue inserted at a unique site in a viral genome. Biochemistry 1990;29:7024–7032.

185. Cheng KC, Cahill DS, Kasai H, Nishimura S, Loeb LA. 8–Hydroxyguanine, an abundant form of oxidative DNA damage, causes G—T and A—C substitutions. J Biol Chem 1992;267:166–72.

186. Costa de Oliveira R, Ribeiro DT, Nigro RG, Di Mascio P, Menck CF. Singlet oxygen induced mutation spectrum in mammalian cells. Nucleic Acids Res 1992;20:4319–4323.

187. Ribeiro DT, De OR, Di MP, Menck CF. Singlet oxygen induces predominantly G to T transversions on a single-stranded shuttle vector replicated in monkey cells. Free Radic Res 1994;21:75–83.

188. Piette J. Mutagenic and genotoxic properties of singlet oxygen. J Photochem Photobiol, B: Biology 1990;4:335–342.

189. Dennis WJ, Olivieri VP, Kruse CW. Reaction of uracil with hypochlorous acid. Biochem Biophys Res Commun 1978;83:168–171.

190. Hoyano Y, Bacon V, Summons RE, Pereira WE, Halpern B, Duffield AM. Chlorination studies. IV. The reaction of aqueous hypochlorous acid with pyrimidine and purine bases. Biochem Biophys Res Commun 1973;53:1195–1199.

191. Wlodkowski TJ, Rosenkranz HS. Mutagenicity of sodium hypochlorite for Salmonella typhimurium. Mutat Res 1975;31:39–42.

192. Anderson R. Assessment of the roles of vitamin C, vitamin E, and beta-carotene in the modulation of oxidant stress mediated by cigarette smoke-activated phagocytes. Am J Clin Nutr 1991;358S-361S.

193. Moraes EC, Keyse SM, Tyrrell RM. Mutagenesis by hydrogen peroxide treatment of mammalian cells: a molecular analysis. Carcinogenesis 1990;11:283–293.

194. Weitzman SA, Gordon LI. Inflammation and cancer: role of phagocyte-generated oxidants in carcinogenesis. Blood 1990;76:655–663.

195. Weitzman SA, Stossel TP. Mutation caused by human phagocytes. Science 1981;212:546–547.

196. Weitberg AB, Weitzman SA, Destrempes M, Latt SA, Stossel TP. Stimulated human phagocytes produce cytogenetic changes in cultured mammalian cells. N Engl J Med 1983;308:26–30.

197. Weitzman SA, Stossel TP. Effects of oxygen radical scavengers and antioxidants on phagocyte-induced mutagenesis. J Immunol 1982;128:2770–2772.

198. Weitberg AB, Weitzman SA, Clark EP, Stossel TP. Effects of antioxidants on oxidant-induced sister chromatid exchange formation. J Clin Invest 1985;75:1835–1841.

199. Fulton AM, Loveless SE, Heppner GH. Mutagenic activity of tumor-associated macrophages in Salmonella typhimurium strains TA98 and TA 100. Cancer Res 1984;44:4308–4311.

200. Birnboim HC. DNA strand breakage in human leukocytes exposed to a tumor promoter, phorbol myristate acetate. Science 1982;215:1247–1249.

201. Chong YC, Heppner GH, Paul LA, Fulton AM. Macrophage-mediated induction of DNA strand breaks in target tumor cells. Cancer Res 1989;49:6652–6657.

202. Emerit I, Cerutti PA. Tumour promoter phorbol-12-myristate-13-acetate induces chromosomal damage via indirect action. Nature 1981;293:144–146.

203. Emerit I. Reactive oxygen species, chromosome mutation, and cancer: possible role of clastogenic factors in carcinogenesis. Free Radic Biol Med 1994;16:99–109.

204. Weitzman SA, Weitberg AB, Clark EP, Stossel TP. Phagocytes as carcinogens: malignant transformation produced by human neutrophils. Science 1985;227:1231–1233.

205. Zimmermann FK. Genetic effects of nitrous acid. Mutation Res 1977;39:127–148.

206. Victorin K. Review of the genotoxicity of nitrogen oxides. Mutat Res 1994;317:43–55.

207. Ohshima H, Bartsch H. Chronic infections and inflammatory processes as cancer risk factors: Possible role of nitric oxide in carcinogenesis. Mutat Res 1994;305:253–264.

208. Routledge MN, Mirsky FJ, Wink DA, Keefer LK, Dipple A. Nitrite-induced mutations in a forward mutation assay: Influence of nitrite concentration and pH. Mutat Res 1994;322:341–346.

209. Routledge MN, Wink DA, Keefer LK, Dipple A. Mutations induced by saturated aqueous nitric oxide in the pSP189 *supF* gene in human Ad293 and *E. coli* MBM7070 cells. Carcinogenesis 1993;14:1251–1254.

210. Routledge MN, Wink DA, Keefer LK, Dipple A. DNA sequence changes induced by two nitric oxide donor drugs in the supF assay. Chem Res Toxicol 1994;7:628–632.

211. Dianov GL, Timchenko TV, Sinitsina OI, Kuzminov AV, Medvedev OA, Salganik RI. Repair of uracil residues closely spaced on the opposite strands of plasmid DNA results in double-strand break and deletion formation. Mol Gen Genet 1991;225:448–452.

212. Isomura K, Chikahira M, Teranishi K, Hamada K. Induction of mutations and chromosome aberrations in lung cells following *in vivo* exposure of rats to nitrogen oxides. Mutat Res 1984;136:119–125.

213. Arroyo PL, Hatch-Pigott V, Mower HF, Cooney RV. Mutagenicity of nitric oxide and its inhibition by antioxidants. Mutat Res 1992;281:193–202.

214. Christen S, Gee P, Ames BN. Mutagenicity of nitric oxide in a new set of basepair-specific *Salmonella* tester strains (TA7000 series). Methods Enzymol 1996;69:267–278.

215. Nguyen T, Brunson D, Crespi CL, Penman BW, Wishnok JS, Tannenbaum SR. DNA damage and mutation in human cells exposed to nitric oxide *in vitro*. Proc Natl Acad Sci USA 1992;89:3030–3034.

216. deRojas WT, Tamir S, Ji H, Wishnok JS, Tannenbaum SR. Nitric oxide induces oxidative damage in addition to deamination in macrophage DNA. Chem Res Toxicol 1995;8:473–477.

217. Schmutte C, Rideout I, W. M., Shen J-C, Jones PA. Mutagenicity of nitric oxide is not caused by deamination of cytosine or 5-methylcytosine in double-stranded DNA. Carcinogenesis 1994;15:2899–2903.

218. Hartman Z, Henrikson EN, Hartman PE, Cebula TA. Molecular models that may account for nitrous acid mutagenesis in organisms containing double-stranded DNA. Environ Mol Mutagen 1994;24:168–175.

219. Felley-Bosco E, Mirkovitch J, Ambs S, et al. Nitric oxide and ethylnitrosourea: relative mutagenicity in the p53 tumor suppressor and hypoxanthine-phosphoribosyltransferase genes. Carcinogenesis 1995;16:2069–2074.

220. Gal A, Wogan GN. Mutagenesis associated with nitric oxide production in transgenic SJL mice. Proc Natl Acad Sci USA; 93:15102–15107.

221. Salgo MG, Stone K, Squadrito GL, Battista JR, Pryor WA. Peroxynitrite causes DNA nicks in plasmid pBR322. Biochem Biophys Res Commun 1995;210:1025–1030.

222. Salgo MG, Bermudez E, Squadrito GL, Pryor WA. DNA damage and oxidation of thiols peroxynitrite causes in rat thymocytes. Arch Biochem Biophys 1995;322:500–505.

223. Juedes MJ, Wogan GN. Peroxynitrite-induced mutation spectra of pSP189 following replication in bacteria and in human cells. Mutat Res 1996; 349:51–61.

224. Zhu L, Gunn C, Beckman JS. Bactericidal activity of peroxynitrite. Arch Biochem Biophys 1992;298:452–457.

225. De Groote MA, Granger D, Xu Y, Campbell G, Prince R, Fang FC. Genetic and redox determinants of nitric oxide cytotoxicity in a Salmonella typhimurium model. Proc Natl Acad Sci USA 1995;92:6399–403.

226. Bonfoco E, Krainc D, Ankarcrona M, Nicotera P, Lipton SA. Apoptosis and necrosis: two distinct events induced, respectively, by mild and intense insults with N-methyl-D-aspartate or nitric oxide/superoxide in cortical cell cultures. Proc Natl Acad Sci USA 1995;92:7162–7166.

227. Shih KL, Lederberg J. Chloramine mutagenesis in *Bacillus subtilis.* Science 1976;192:1141–1143.

228. Silhankova L, Smid F, Cerna M, Davidek J, Velisek J. Mutagenicity of glycerol chlorohydrins and of their esters with higher fatty acids present in protein hydrolysates. Mutat Res 1982;103:77–81.

229. Herren-Freund SL, Pereira MA. Carcinogenicity of by-products of disinfection in mouse and rat liver. Environ Health Perspect 1986;69:59–65.

230. Bartsch HE, Hietanen E, Malaveille C. Carcinogenic nitrosamines: free radical aspects of their action. Free Radic Biol Med 1989;7:637–644.

231. Eder E, Scheckenbach S, Deininger C, Hoffman C. The possible role of alpha, beta-unsaturated carbonyl compounds in mutagenesis and carcinogenesis. Toxicol Lett 1993;67:87–103.

232. Eder E, Sebeikat D, Zugelder JP, et al. DNA adducts of allyl compounds, enals and unsaturated ketones. Significance for mutagenicity and carcinogenicity. IARC Sci Publ 1994;443–447.

233. Vaca CE, Wilhelm J, Harms RM. Interaction of lipid peroxidation products with DNA: a review. Mutat Res 1988;195:137–149.

234. Basu AK, Marnett LJ. Molecular requirements for the mutagenicity of malondialdehyde and related acroleins. Cancer Res 1984;44:2848–2854.

235. Marnett LJ, Hurd HK, Hollstein MC, Levin DE, Esterbauer H, Ames BN. Naturally occurring carbonyl compounds are mutagens in Salmonella tester strain TA104. Mutat Res 1985;148:25–34.

236. Brambilla G, Cajelli E, Canonero R, Martelli A, Marinari UM. Mutagenicity in V79 Chinese hamster cells of n-alkanals produced by lipid peroxidation. Mutagenesis 1989;4:277–279.

237. Canonero R, Martelli A, Marinari UM, Brambilla G. Mutation induction in Chinese hamster lung V79 cells by five alk-2-enals produced by lipid peroxidation. Mutat Res 1990;244:153–156.

238. Esterbauer H. Cytotoxicity and genotoxicity of lipid-oxidation products. Am J Clin Nutr 1993;57:779S–85S; discussion 85S–86S.

239. Benamira M, Johnson K, Chaudhary A, Bruner K, Tibbetts C, Marnett LJ. Induction of mutations by replication of malondialdehyde-modified M13 DNA in Escherichia coli: determination of the extent of DNA modification, genetic requirements for mutagenesis, and types of mutations induced. Carcinogenesis 1995;16:93–99.

240. Akasaka S, Yamamoto K. Mutagenesis resulting from DNA damage by lipid peroxidation in the supF gene of Escherichia coli. Mutat Res 1994;315:105–112.

241. Asami S, Hirano T, Yamaguchi R, Tomioka Y, Itoh H, Kasai H. Increase of a type of oxidative DNA damage, 8-hydroxyguanine, and its repair activity in human leukocytes by cigarette smoking. Cancer Res 1996;56:2546–2549.

242. Shigenaga MK, Lee HH, Blount BC, et al. Inflammation and NO_X-induced nitration: assay for 3-nitrotyrosine by HPLC with electrochemical detection. Proc Natl Acad Sci USA 1997;94:3211–3216.

243. Yeo HC, Helbock HJ, Chyu DW, Ames BN. Assay of malondialdehyde in biological fluids by gas chromatography-mass spectrometry. Anal Biochem 1994;220:391–396.

244. Shigenaga MK, Aboujaoude EN, Chen Q, Ames BN. Assays of oxidative DNA damage biomarkers 8-oxo-2'-deoxyguanosine and 8-oxoguanine in nuclear DNA and biological fluids by high-performance liquid chromatography with electrochemical detection. Methods Enzymol 1994;234:16–33.

245. Ammenheuser MM, Hastings DA, Whorton EB Jr, Ward JB Jr. Frequencies of hprt mutant lymphocytes in smokers, non-smokers, and former smokers. Environ Mol Mutagen 1997;30:131–138.

246. Reid TM, Loeb LA. Tandem double CC—TT mutations are produced by reactive oxygen species. Proc Natl Acad Sci USA 1993;90:3904–3907.

247. Fraga CG, Motchnik PA, Shigenaga MK, Helbock HJ, Jacob RA, Ames BN. Ascorbic acid protects against endogenous oxidative DNA damage in human sperm. Proc Natl Acad Sci USA 1991;88:11003–11006.

248. Inoue S, Kawanishi S. Oxidative DNA damage induced by simultaneous generation of nitric oxide and superoxide. FEBS Lett 1995;371:86–88.

249. Frenkel K, Khasak D, Karkoszka J, Shupack J, Stiller M. Enhanced antibody titers to an oxidized DNA base in inflammatory and neoplastic diseases. Exp Dermatol 1992;1:242–247.

250. Frenkel K, Karkoszka J, Kim E, Taioli E. Recognition of oxidized DNA bases by sera of patients with inflammatory diseases. Free Radic Biol Med 1993; 14:483–494.

251. Gotz ME, Dirr A, Freyberger A, Burger R, Riederer P. The thiobarbituric acid assay reflects susceptibility to oxygen induced lipid peroxidation in vitro rather than levels of lipid hydroperoxides in vivo: a methodological approach. Neurochem Int 1993;22:255–262.

252. Liu J, Yeo HC, Doniger SJ, Ames BN. Assay of aldehydes from lipid peroxidation: gas chromatography-mass spectrometry compared to thiobarbituric acid. Anal Biochem 1997;245:161–166.

253. Roberts LJ 2nd, Morrow JD. The generation and actions of isoprostanes. Biochim Biophys Acta 1997;1345:121–135.

254. Chaudhary AK, Nokubo M, Reddy GR, et al. Detection of endogenous malondialdehyde-deoxyguanosine adducts in human liver. Science 1994;265: 1580–1582.

255. Nair J, Sone H, Nagao M, Barbin A, Bartsch H. Copper-dependent formation of miscoding etheno-DNA adducts in the liver of Long Evans Cinnamon (LEC) rats developing hereditary hepatitis and hepatocellular carcinoma. Cancer Res 1996;56:1267–1271.

256. Curzio M, Esterbauer H, Di Mauro C, Cecchini G, Dianzani MU. Chemotactic activity of the lipid peroxidation product 4-hydroxynonenal and homologous hydroxyalkenals. Biol Chem Hoppe Seyler 1986;367:321–329.

257. Schaur RJ, Dussing G, Kink E, et al. The lipid peroxidation product 4-hydroxynonenal is formed by—and is able to attract—rat neutrophils in vivo. Free Radic Res 1994;20:365–373.

258. Green LC, Tannenbaum SR, Goldman P. Nitrate synthesis in the germfree and conventional rat. Science 1981;212:56–58.

259. Green LC, Ruiz de Luzuriaga K, et al. Nitrate biosynthesis in man. Proc Natl Acad Sci USA 1981;78:7764–7768.

260. Ohshima H, Tsuda M, Adachi H, Ogura T, Sugimura T, Esumi H. L-arginine-dependent formation of N-nitrosamines by the cytosol of macrophages activated with lipopolysaccharide and interferon-gamma. Carcinogenesis 1991;12:1217–1220.

261. Srivatanakul P, Ohshima H, Khlat M, et al. Opisthorchis viverrini infestation and endogenous nitrosamines as risk factors for cholangiocarcinoma in Thailand. Int J Cancer 1991;48:821–825.

262. Mirvish SS. Experimental evidence for inhibition of N-nitroso compound formation as a factor in the negative correlation between vitamin C consumption and the incidence of certain cancers. Cancer Res 1994;54:1948s–1951s.

263. Helser MA, Hotchkiss JH, Roe DA. Influence of fruit and vegetable juices on the endogenous formation of N-nitrosoproline and N-nitrosothiazolidine-4-carboxylic acid in humans on controlled diets. Carcinogenesis 1992; 13:2277–2280.

264. Ohshima H, Bandaletova TY, Brouet I, et al. Increased nitrosamine and nitrate biosynthesis mediated by nitric oxide synthase induced in hamsters infected with liver fluke (*Opisthorchis viverrini*). Carcinogenesis 1994;15:271–275.

265. Liu RH, Baldwin B, Tennant BC, Hotchkiss JH. Elevated formation of nitrate and N-nitrosodimethylamine in woodchucks (Marmota monax) associated with chronic woodchuck hepatitis virus infection. Cancer Res 1991; 51:3925–3929.

266. Beckman JS, Ye YZ, Anderson PG, et al. Extensive nitration of protein tyrosines in human atherosclerosis detected by immunohistochemistry. Biol Chem Hoppe Seyler 1994;375:81–88.

267. Leeuwenburgh C, Hardy MM, Hazen SL, et al. Reactive nitrogen intermediates promote low density lipoprotein oxidation in human atherosclerotic intima. J Biol Chem 1997;272:1433–1436.

268. Miller MJ, Thompson JH, Zhang XJ, et al. Role of inducible nitric oxide synthase expression and peroxynitrite formation in guinea pig ileitis. Gastroenterology 1995;109:1475–1483.

269. Ischiropoulos H, al Mehdi AB, Fisher AB. Reactive species in ischemic rat lung injury: contribution of peroxynitrite. Am J Physiol 1995;75:L158–L164.

270. Wizemann TM, Gardner CR, Laskin JD, et al. Production of nitric oxide and peroxynitrite in the lung during acute endotoxemia. J Leukoc Biol 1994;56:759–768.

271. van der Vliet A, Eiserich JP, Halliwell B, Cross CE. Formation of reactive nitrogen species during peroxidase-catalyzed oxidation of nitrite. A potential additional mechanism of nitric oxide-dependent toxicity. J Biol Chem 1997;272:7617–7625.

272. Eiserich JP, Cross CE, Jones AD, Halliwell B, van der Vliet A. Formation of nitrating and chlorinating species by reaction of nitrite with hypochlorous acid: a novel mechanism for nitric oxide-mediated protein modification. J Biol Chem 1996;271:19199–19208.

273. Lewis JG, Adams DO. Inflammation, oxidative DNA damage, and carcinogenesis. Environ Health Perspect 1987;76:19–27.

274. Wei L, Wei H, Frenkel K. Sensitivity to tumor promotion of SENCAR and C57BL/6J mice correlates with oxidative events and DNA damage. Carcinogenesis 1993;14:841–847.

275. Wei H, Frenkel K. Relationship of oxidative events and DNA oxidation in SENCAR mice to in vivo promoting activity of phorbol ester-type tumor promoters. Carcinogenesis 1993;14:1195–1201.

276. Farinati F, Cardin R, De MN, et al. Iron storage, lipid peroxidation and glutathione turnover in chronic anti-HCV positive hepatitis. J Hepatol 1995; 22:449–456.

277. Yacoub LK, Fogt F, Griniuviene B, Nanji AA. Apoptosis and bcl-2 protein expression in experimental alcoholic liver disease in the rat. Alcohol Clin Exp Res 1995;19:854–859.

278. Nanji AA, Griniuviene B, Yacoub LK, Sadrzadeh SM, Levitsky S, McCully JD. Heat-shock gene expression in alcoholic liver disease in the rat is related to the severity of liver injury and lipid peroxidation. Proc Soc Exp Biol Med 1995;210:12–19.

279. Niemela O, Parkkila S, Yla HS, Villanueva J, Ruebner B, Halsted CH. Sequential acetaldehyde production, lipid peroxidation, and fibrogenesis in micropig model of alcohol-induced liver disease. Hepatology 1995;1208–1214.

280. Adachi Y, Bradford BU, Gao W, Bojes HK, Thurman RG. Inactivation of Kupffer cells prevents early alcohol-induced liver injury. Hepatology 1994; 20:453–460.

281. Adachi Y, Moore LE, Bradford BU, Gao W, Thurman RG. Antibiotics prevent liver injury in rats following long-term exposure to ethanol. Gastroenterology 1995;108:218–224.

282. Chow CK. Cigarette smoking and oxidative damage in the lung. Ann NY Acad Sci 1993;686:289–298.

283. Morrow JD, Frei B, Longmire AW, et al. Increase in circulating products of lipid peroxidation (F2-isoprostanes) in smokers. Smoking as a cause of oxidative damage. N Engl J Med 1995;332:1198–1203.

284. Vallyathan V, Castranova V, Pack D, et al. Freshly fractured quartz inhalation leads to enhanced lung injury and inflammation: potential role of free radicals. Am J Respir Crit Care Med 1995;152:1003–1009.

285. Gossart S, Cambon C, Orfila C, et al. Reactive oxygen intermediates as regulators of TNF-alpha production in rat lung inflammation induced by silica. J Immunol 1996;156:1540–1548.

286. Wynn TA, Oswald IP, Eltoum IA, et al. Elevated expression of Th1 cytokines and nitric oxide synthase in the lungs of vaccinated mice after challenge infection with Schistosoma mansoni. J Immunol 1994;153:5200–5209.

287. Rosin MP, Anwar WA, Ward AJ. Inflammation, chromosomal instability, and cancer: the schistosomiasis model. Cancer Res 1994;1929s–1933s.

288. Haswell-Elkins MR, Satarug S, Tsuda M, et al. Liver fluke infection and cholangiocarcinoma: model of endogenous nitric oxide and extragastric nitrosation in human carcinogenesis. Mutat Res 1994;305:241–252.

289. Boone CW, Kelloff GJ, Malone WE. Identification of candidate cancer chemopreventive agents and their evaluation in animal models and human clinical trials: a review. Cancer Res 1990;50:2–9.

290. Buffinton GD, Doe WF. Depleted mucosal antioxidant defences in inflammatory bowel disease. Free Radic Biol Med 1995;19:911–918.

291. Block G, Patterson B, Subar A. Fruit, vegetables, and cancer prevention: a review of the epidemiological evidence. Nutr Cancer 1992;18:1–29.

292. Block G. The data support a role for antioxidants in reducing cancer risk. Nutr Rev 1992;50:207–213.

293. Schiffman MH, Pickle LW, Fontham E, et al. Case-control study of diet and mesothelioma in Louisiana. Cancer Res 1988;48:2911–2915.

294. Omenn GS, Goodman GE, Thornquist MD, et al. The Carotene and Retinol Efficacy Trial (CARET) to prevent lung cancer in high-risk populations: pilot study with asbestos-exposed workers. Cancer Epidemiol Biomarkers Prev 1993;2:381–387.

295. Thun MJ, Calle EE, Namboodiri MM, et al. Risk factors for fatal colon cancer in a large prospective study. J Natl Cancer Inst 1992;84:1491–1500.

296. Committee on Diet, Nutrition and Cancer. Lipid (fats and cholesterol). Diet, Nutrition and Cancer. Washington, DC: National Academy Press, 1982:73–105.

297. Constantinides P, Kiser M. Arterial effects of palmitic, linoleic and acetoacetic acid. Atherosclerosis 1981;38:309–319.

298. Wargovich MJ, Eng VW, Newmark HL. Calcium inhibits the damaging and compensatory proliferative effects of fatty acids on mouse colon epithelium. Cancer Lett 1984;23:253–258.

299. Wargovich MJ, Isbell G, Shabot M, et al. Calcium supplementation decreases rectal epithelial cell proliferation in subjects with sporadic adenoma. Gastroenterology 1992;103:92–97.

300. Blot WJ, Lanier A, Fraumeni JJ, Bender TR. Cancer mortality among Alaskan natives, 1960–69. J Natl Cancer Inst 1975;55:547–554.

301. Hillier K, Jewell R, Dorrell L, Smith CL. Incorporation of fatty acids from fish oil and olive oil into colonic mucosal lipids and effects upon eicosanoid synthesis in inflammatory bowel disease. Gut 1991;32:1151–1155.

302. Awad AB, Ferger SL, Fink CS. Effect of dietary fat on the lipid composition and utilization of short-chain fatty acids by rat colonocytes. Lipids 1990;25:316–320.

303. Deschner EE, Lytle JS, Wong G, Ruperto JF, Newmark HL. The effect of dietary omega-3 fatty acids (fish oil) on azoxymethanol-induced focal areas of dysplasia and colon tumor incidence. Cancer 1990;66:2350–2356.

304. Rosenberg L, Palmer JR, Zauber AG, Warshauer ME, Stolley PD, Shapiro S. A hypothesis: Nonsteroidal anti-inflammatory drugs reduce the incidence of large-bowel cancer. J Natl Cancer Inst 1991;83:355–358.

305. Kune GA, Kune S, Watson LF. Colorectal cancer risk, chronic illnesses, operations, and medications: case control results from the Melbourne Colorectal Cancer Study. Cancer Res 1988;48:4399–4404.

306. Thun MJ, Namboodiri MM, Heath CW Jr. Aspirin use and reduced risk of fatal colon cancer. N Engl J Med 1991;325:1593–1596.

307. De Flora S, Izzotti A, D'Agostini F, Cesarone CF. Antioxidant activity and other mechanisms of thiols involved in chemoprevention of mutation and cancer. Am J Med 1991;91:122S–130S.

308. Mossman BT, Marsh JP, Sesko A, et al. Inhibition of lung injury, inflammation, and interstitial pulmonary fibrosis by polyethylene glycol-conjugated catalase in a rapid inhalation model of asbestosis. Am Rev Respir Dis 1990;1266–1271.

309. Rom WN, Harkin T. Dehydroepiandrosterone inhibits the spontaneous release of superoxide radical by alveolar macrophages in vitro in asbestosis. Environ Res 1991;55:145–156.

310. Whitcomb JM, Schwartz AG. Dehydroepiandrosterone and 16 alpha-Br-epi-androsterone inhibit 12-O-tetradecanoylphorbol-13-acetate stimulation of

superoxide radical production by human polymorphonuclear leukocytes. Carcinogenesis 1985;6:333–335.

311. Chisari FV, Pinkert CA, Milich DR, et al. A transgenic mouse model of the chronic hepatitis B surface antigen carrier state. Science 1985;230:1157–1160.

312. Chisari FV, Klopchin K, Moriyama T, et al. Molecular pathogenesis of hepatocellular carcinoma in hepatitis B virus transgenic mice. Cell 1989;59: 1145–1156.

313. Chisari FV, Filippi P, McLachlan A, et al. Expression of hepatitis B virus large envelope polypeptide inhibits hepatitis B surface antigen secretion in transgenic mice. J Virol 1986;60:880–887.

314. Chisari FV, Filippi P, Buras J, et al. Structural and pathological effects of synthesis of hepatitis B virus large envelope polypeptide in transgenic mice. Proc Natl Acad Sci USA 1987;84:6909–6913.

315. Dunsford HA, Sell S, Chisari FV. Hepatocarcinogenesis due to chronic liver cell injury in hepatitis B virus transgenic mice. Cancer Res 1990;50:3400–3407.

316. Halliwell B, Gutteridge JMC. Free radicals in biology and medicine. Oxford: Clarendon, 1989:74–75.

317. Kasai H, Chung MH, Yamamoto F, et al. Formation, inhibition of formation, and repair of oxidative 8-hydroxyguanine DNA damage. Basic Life Sci 1993; 61:257–262.

318. Huang SN, Chisari FV. Strong, sustained hepatocellular proliferation precedes hepatocarcinogenesis in hepatitis B surface antigen transgenic mice. Hepatology 1995;21:620–626.

319. Grimble RF. Nutritional antioxidants and the modulation of inflammation: theory and practice. New Horiz 1994;2:175–185.

3

Infection, Cell Proliferation, and Malignancy

SAMUEL M. COHEN

Cancer, a devastating disease, is currently the second leading cause of death in the United States. Although researchers have made considerable progress during the past decades in the early detection and treatment of cancers, prevention continues to offer the best opportunities for reducing the incidence and mortality of cancer. In the United States, cigarette smoking is the single most common cause of cancer, not only of the lung, but also of several other tissues, including the larynx, oral cavity, and urinary bladder. In addition, several other etiologic factors have been identified for specific cancers, including nutrition, hormones, ethanol, and environmental chemicals. During the past decade it has become increasingly apparent that several infectious diseases also contribute significantly to the development of certain types of cancer.

The first evidence that infectious organisms might be related to the causation of cancer was provided by Ellerman and Bang in 1908[1] and by Peyton Rous in 1910,[2] with their demonstration that cell-free extracts were capable of transmitting tumors between chickens. The tumors studied by Rous were ultimately shown to be caused by the RNA virus named after him, the Rous sarcoma virus (RSV). In the ensuing four decades, interest waned in infectious organisms as the causative agent of cancer for several reasons. There were numerous technical difficulties in demonstrating the etiologic relationship for these organisms in animal models and in humans. In addition, the discovery that the parasite *Spiroptera neoplastica* (*Gongylonema neoplasticum*), identified by Johannes Fibiger as the causative agent of stomach cancer, was an artifact of the laboratory dissuaded scientists from pursuing this area of investigation.[2] Fibiger provided evidence that this organism caused stomach cancer in rats, and he argued that infectious organisms could truly be the cause of cancer. He received the

Nobel prize in 1926 for this "discovery," but he died shortly thereafter and only months before his observations were disproved.[2,3] This experience with cancer research soured the Nobel Prize Committee for Physiology and Medicine from awarding further prizes for cancer research until 1966, when it belatedly recognized the seminal work of Peyton Rous and also of Charles Huggins.[3]

In the intervening years of this century, radiation and various chemicals were demonstrated to produce cancer in animals and in humans. Many of these act by directly damaging DNA. It is now well accepted that numerous infections—including a wide variety of organisms such as RNA and DNA viruses, bacteria, and specific parasites (fungi have not been demonstrated to be direct causes of cancer, although they can produce highly carcinogenic toxins, such as aflatoxin and ochratoxin)—also are related to an increased risk of certain types of cancer.[4,5] Unlike chemicals and radiation, however, many of the infectious organisms associated with cancer do not directly interact with DNA of the target tissue, raising questions about the mechanism by which they produce such a deleterious effect on cells.

CELL PROLIFERATION AND CARCINOGENESIS

In 1914, Boveri[6] postulated that cancer was caused by mutations in cells, arising from alterations either of germ lines or, more commonly, of the genetic material of somatic cells. The discovery in 1953 of the structure of DNA and its transmission of genetic information to daughter cells implied that the alterations related to carcinogenesis ultimately involved changes in DNA. During the past four decades, considerable evidence has accumulated strongly supporting the hypothesis that cancer is caused by alterations in specific genes. These genes have been identified as belonging predominantly to two classes: those that act in a dominant manner, called *oncogenes*,[7] and those that require damage of both alleles of a given gene, consistent with a recessive mode of action, called *tumor suppressor genes*.[7,8] It has also become apparent not only that damage to DNA is the ultimate basis for carcinogenesis but also that more than one genetic mistake is required.

A two-hit genetic model for carcinogenesis was originally postulated by Knudson based on his examination of sporadic and hereditary retinoblastomas in children.[9] In sporadic cases, the two alleles of the retinoblastoma gene must both be damaged. The chance of either allele being affected is low; the chance of both being damaged in the same somatic cell is extraordinarily low. In contrast, individuals who have inherited damage to one of the alleles in the germ line need have damage occur in only the second allele of any retinoblast for a tumor to arise. As a consequence, individuals with germ line mutations not only have tumors in both eyes more commonly than individuals with sporadic retinoblastomas, but also frequently have multiple tumors in each eye. In his seminal 1971 publication, Knudson demonstrated that, based on only spontaneous mutations occurring during normal retinoblast DNA replication, DNA alterations could occur in sufficient numbers to explain the rate of retinoblastoma occurrence under these different circumstances.[9]

DNA replication occurs with an extraordinary degree of fidelity, but that fidelity is not 100%. The error rate per DNA replication in human cells containing 3×10^9 nucleotide pairs is in the range of approximately one mistake per cell per DNA replication.[10] Alterations occur predominantly during DNA replication, S phase, although they also occur less commonly between DNA replications. Because DNA replication carries with it a low—but not zero—rate of error, mistakes may occur in the genes related to the development of cancer, leading to an increased risk of that cell developing into a cancer.

Based on the strongly supported assumptions that cancer is caused by multiple alterations in DNA and that DNA replication does not have 100% fidelity, there are ultimately only two ways in which any agent—whether chemical, radiation, or infectious organism—can increase the chance of a cell becoming malignant.[11-13] The agent can either damage the DNA directly, as occurs with genotoxic (DNA-reactive) chemicals or radiation, or increase the number of DNA replications, as occurs with non–DNA-reactive chemicals, hormones, and infectious organisms. Many of the agents that damage DNA directly also increase cell proliferation when exposure is sufficiently high.

Additional research has strongly suggested that there are other factors involved in the association of cell proliferation with carcinogenesis.[11-13] To be related to the development of cancer, the errors that occur during DNA replication must happen in the pluripotential cells of a given tissue. In many tissues, these cells are referred to as the *stem cell population*; for purposes of this chapter, however, we will define pluripotential cells as those cells that can replenish the cellular population of a tissue following damage. Such cells have been well defined in hematopoietic tissues and in some epithelia; in other tissues, the specific cell populations that have these attributes have not been delineated clearly.

This model of carcinogenesis implies that if individuals lived sufficiently long, all would develop cancer of one type or another, because DNA replication errors occur constantly and accumulate over time. However, these errors are extraordinarily rare events, and multiple events must occur in the same cell; thus, the chance of spontaneously developing all of the necessary mistakes in one cell in the usual lifetime of any animal, including humans, remains low. Thus, the hypothesis that most cancers in human populations arise secondary to environmental influences remains likely to be valid.

Until recently, the errors that occurred during normal cell DNA replication were referred to as spontaneous, a term commonly used by scientists that reflected our ignorance. More recently, it has become apparent that these replication errors occur by a variety of mechanisms secondary to routine endogenous processes that occur in cells. These processes include oxidative damage, depurination (and less commonly, depyrimidination), deamination, inappropriate alkylation, nitric oxide interaction with DNA, exocyclic adduct formation, mismatch repair defects, and other processes yet to be identified.[14] Cell processes that increase the rate of any one of these DNA-damaging mechanisms can ultimately lead to an increase in the number of defects occurring during DNA replication. Most of these defects are repaired by a variety of enzymatic processes. The DNA defects that are of importance with respect to carcinogenesis are those that are not repaired and thus are passed on to daughter cells.

A common mistake in interpreting the relationship of cell replication to carcinogenesis has been to focus on rates of cell division, rather than on the actual number of DNA replications.[14,15] It is the latter that is of significance, for it is during each replication that errors can occur. The replication rate is the quotient of the number of cells replicating divided by the total number of cells in the tissue. The total number of DNA replications thus is the product of the replication rate times the total number of pluripotential cells in the tissue. The replication rate can be assessed either by determination of the mitotic rate, or, more commonly, in animal models utilizing various labels of DNA synthesis, such as tritiated thymidine or bromodeoxyuridine (BrdU). Alternatively, replication rate can be determined by measuring one of the many proteins involved in the replication of DNA, such as proliferating cell nuclear antigen (PCNA). An agent can increase the number of DNA replications by increasing either the rate of replication or the number of pluripotential cells present. Increasing the number of cells is a common means of increasing the number of DNA replications occurring per unit time in a variety of preneoplastic lesions, such as adenomatous polyps in the gastrointestinal tract or hyperplastic nodules in the liver. Increasing the number of pluripotential cells and their rate of replication, as frequently occurs in various types of hyperplasia, provides a highly synergistic situation for increasing the number of replications.

Several cellular processes have been identified that can increase the number of replications. They can be divided into two broad categories: those that increase cell births and those that decrease cell deaths.[14] The latter produce an increase in DNA replications because decreasing cell deaths leads to an accumulation of cells in the relevant cellular population. Cell births can be increased either by directly stimulating mitogenesis, which usually involves alterations in hormones and/or growth factors, or by inducing cell toxicity, thereby causing consequent regeneration. Cell deaths can be decreased either by inhibiting apoptosis or by decreasing cellular differentiation. *Differentiation* is a cellular process that removes cells from the pluripotential cell population, dooming the cell in most tissues to eventual death. Considerable research has been done on mechanisms of increasing cell births. Mechanisms for decreasing cell

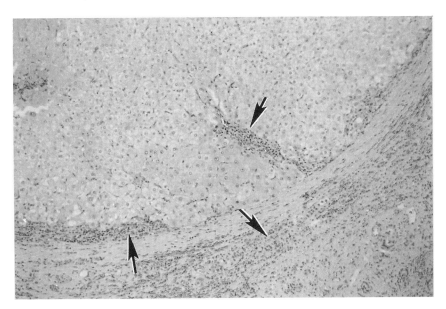

Figure 3.1. Chronic active hepatitis showing nodular hepatocellular degeneration and regeneration with chronic inflammation (arrows) and fibrosis.

death, however, has become an extremely active area of investigation during the past decade, with respect to both differentiation and apoptosis.

NECROSIS AND REGENERATION

Some infectious agents associated with cancer lead to cell proliferation by causing necrotic cell death and consequent compensatory tissue regeneration. Examples are described below.

Hepatitis Viruses

Clinical reactions to hepatitis B[16] and hepatitis C[17] viruses differ considerably across individuals, ranging from no evident clinical signs or symptoms; to an acute, transient illness; to a prolonged, chronic inflammatory state. It is the latter situation that is related to an increased risk of development of hepatomas. Cardinal features of chronic active hepatitis are hepatocellular necrosis and regeneration (Figure 3.1). The liver is normally a relatively mitotically quiescent tissue, with cell turnover rates ranging between 50 and 100 days. However, the liver, like most epithelia, has a tremendous capacity for regeneration.[18] The detailed mechanisms by which these hepatitis B and hepatitis C viruses produce a chronic active toxic phenomenon is described in detail in other portions of this book (Chapters 9 and 10); it suffices to say here that the proliferative rate is increased compared to controls. This increased proliferation obviously carries with it an increase in the number of DNA replications over time, giving rise to an increased risk of the development of liver cancer.

The nonspecific nature of the carcinogenic effect of this chronic active state can be seen in animal models of hepatitis, as well as in other forms of chronic active proliferation in the liver, including cirrhosis, that are known to be associated with an increased risk of liver cancer in humans. If a transgene for the coat protein of the hepatitis B virus is engineered molecularly into mice, a chronic active regenerative process develops in the liver similar to that seen in humans, and it is associated with an increased incidence of hepatocellular carcinomas.[19,20] This process happens without the hepatitis viral X-antigen (a putative oncogene in hepatitis B). Thus, the malignant transformation appears to merely reflect the chronic proliferative state associated with the immune reaction to a foreign antigen leading to cytotoxicity and regeneration. Similarly, the woodchuck hepatitis virus, which does not have an analogous X-protein, readily causes a chronic active inflammatory state in woodchuck livers with cell regeneration and frequent development of hepatomas.[21]

Other causes of chronic active inflammation of the liver, including other causes of cirrhosis, likewise carry with them increased risks of liver cancer.[4,5] In Western countries, chronic inflammation is associated most commonly with alcoholic hepatitis and cirrhosis but can also be related to a variety of other factors, including inherited disorders such as hemochromatosis, alpha$_1$-antitrypsin disease, galactosemia, and Wilson's disease. The common feature of all these disorders is increased hepatocellular necrosis with consequent regeneration and ultimately the development of cirrhosis and increased risk of hepatomas. With some of these disorders, there is a marked sex hormone influence; immunological control mechanisms appear to be involved in others.

Helicobacter Pylori

A situation similar to that seen in hepatitis B and hepatitis C viruses in the liver occurs in relation to *Helicobacter pylori* infection in the stomach (described more fully in Chapter 14).[22] In most individuals, this infection does not produce symptomatic disease, although it occasionally produces dyspepsia and duodenal ulcer disease. In all cases, however, infection with *H. pylori* induces a chronic active inflammatory process, much the same as in the liver with hepatitis. This inflammation can be related to chronic recurrent gastric ulcers or loss of gastric glands (atrophic gastritis). The characteristic features of these conditions again are chronic cellular necrosis and regeneration.

Unlike the liver, the stomach is normally a relatively rapidly proliferating tissue. However, there is also a rapid differentiation of the cells, so they are removed from this pluripotential cell (stem cell) population of the stomach.[23] In chronic inflammatory disorders, including ulceration, the regenerative process tends to carry with it not only an increased rate of proliferation, but also an increase in the proportion (and absolute numbers) of the cells that are in the pluripotential cell population, in contrast to those that undergo differentiation. Conversion of the gastric mucosa to an intestinal type of epithelium—intestinal metaplasia—leads to a type of epithelium that has even more rapid proliferation and can undergo adenomatous change. Such a change consists of an accumulation of cells in the pluripotential cell population of the crypt, rather than continual evolution and differentiation of the cells. Metaplastic and regenerative changes result in increases in proliferative rate and in the number of pluripotential cells. If these increases continue for a sufficiently long period of time, the result may be a marked increase in the risk of gastric carcinoma. It is ironic that in contrast to the rapid acceptance of the carcinogenic nature of the parasite discovered by Fibiger, which proved to be erroneous,[2] acceptance has been extremely slow for the relationship of *H. pylori* not only to the carcinogenic process in the stomach, but also to inflammatory disorders of the gastric mucosa in general.[22,24]

Schistosomes and Other Parasites

Schistosomiasis is one of the most common infections in the world (see Chapter 12). Infection by *Schistosoma hematobium*, a species endemic to the Nile River valley, results in the deposition of the eggs in the wall of the lower urinary tract.[25] The eggs produce a chronic inflammatory disorder with hematuria that usually progresses to squamous metaplasia. Ulceration of the bladder epithelium is common; even without it, however, there is a marked increase in the proliferation of the bladder epithelium. The normal urothelium of the lower urinary tract is of transitional cell type, and, like the liver, is a mitotically quiescent tissue. Also, like the liver, the transitional epithelium responds to chronic toxins with prominent regeneration, markedly increased rates of proliferation along with hyperplasia (an increase in the number of cells). Squamous metaplasia, when present, is associated with the usual high proliferative rate of any squamous epithelium.

The chronic inflammatory state associated with schistosomiasis, like chronic active hepatitis, carries with it a marked increase in the development of cancer—in this case, of the urinary bladder and of the lower urinary tract.[25] In the Nile River valley, bladder cancer is the most common type of cancer. In contrast to other parts of the world, where the preponderance of bladder tumors are of urothelial cell type, there the majority of bladder tumors arising in association with schistosomiasis are squamous cell carcinomas, presumably related to the precursor lesion squamous metaplasia.

Schistosomiasis is the most common of numerous chronic inflammatory states that can be present in the lower urinary tract, all of which are

associated with an increased risk of bladder cancer.[26,27] Such chronic inflammatory states include the presence of neurogenic bladder, as seen in
paraplegics, or the long-standing presence of calculi, diverticuli, or
chronic bacterial infections. All these chronic inflammatory states are
associated with an increase mostly in squamous cell carcinoma. Recent
research by Oyasu and his colleagues[28] suggests that the chronic inflammation in the lower urinary tract is associated with large amounts of inter-
leukin-6 (IL-6) produced by the mononuclear inflammatory cells; the IL-6
acts as a significant growth factor for bladder epithelial cells. Increased
IL-6 augments the large amounts of epidermal growth factor—the major
growth factor stimulus for the bladder—already present in urine.[29]

There is evidence that the chronic inflammatory state seen in schistosomiasis might be related to the synthesis of a variety of nitrosamines in
the acidic milieu of the urine, and that these nitrosamines may contribute
to the carcinogenic process.[30] However, this hypothesis has not been corroborated for nitrosamines that are known to have an effect on the bladder, such as dibutylnitrosamine. Several nitrosamines that can be formed
in the acid milieu of the urine associated with chronic inflammation are
reabsorbed through the damaged bladder epithelium and wall, but are
not necessarily carcinogenic for the bladder epithelium. This has been
described in detail in a variety of studies by Lijinsky and his colleagues.[31,32]

Infection of the lower gastrointestinal tract by *Schistosoma mansoni* and
Schistosoma japonicum—organisms common in the Far East and elsewhere—is associated with the development of carcinoma, in this case, of
the colon.[4,5] This association occurs considerably less frequently than that
between schistosomiasis and bladder cancer. Again, it is the sustained increased proliferation of the colonic epithelium in association with adenomatous changes of the epithelium that provides the mechanism responsible for these cancers.

Chronic biliary tract infections with the liver flukes *Clonorchis sinensis*[4,5,33]
or *Opisthorchis viverrini*[4,5,34] evoke destruction and epithelial regeneration of
the biliary tract, from bile ductules in the liver to the larger ducts leading
to the duodenum (see Chapter 13). Infection with these flukes poses a
significant increased risk for development of cholangiocarcinoma.[35] A specific DNA-reactive chemical carcinogen does not appear to be implicated
in this process, whereas there is obviously increased cell proliferation sustained in the bile ducts and bile ductules.

For all of the examples described here, the common features are
chronic inflammation, cell death, and cell regeneration. A possible chemical mechanism common to these situations could be marked increased
oxidative damage related to the chronic inflammatory state.[36] We must
keep in mind, however, that the major cellular infiltrate in this situation is
composed predominantly of lymphocytes and plasma cells, rather than of
polymorphonuclear leukocytes, although numerous macrophages also
can be involved. The role of oxidative damage in chronic inflammatory
states requires further investigation.

MITOGENESIS

In addition to causing necrosis and cell death, infections can more directly cause host cells to divide. In many instances, this direct influence on proliferation by the infectious agent depends on deficiencies in the host immune system.

Epstein-Barr Virus

Epstein-Barr virus (EBV) infects several cell types, but primarily interacts with B cells.[37] When exposed to a B cell, the virus adheres to the surface through a specific receptor, CD21, triggering a sequence of events leading to mitogenesis.[38] If confronted with specific immunological controls, predominantly affected by T cells, the virus becomes latent in the B cell, and mitogenesis ceases. Without the proper immune controls, however, proliferation continues. Depending on the interaction of the virus with these cells and the immune controls over them, a variety of clinical responses can arise (described more fully in Chapter 7).

Clinically, EBV infection usually produces pharyngitis and, if the infection is more severe, lymphadenopathy, infiltration of the liver and spleen, and a variety of other symptoms and signs, commonly known as infectious mononucleosis.[39] The severity and length of the clinical course is determined by the status of the infected individual's immune system. Ultimately, in most individuals, clinical symptoms resolve and the virus latently persists in the B cells, typically infecting approximately 1% of the total B cell population of the host.

In contrast, if the infection occurs during a time in which the immune response is suppressed, more severe disorders can arise.[4,5] These occur whether immunosuppression is produced by an inherited disorder (e.g., X-linked lymphoproliferative disease (XLP), Wiskott-Aldrich syndrome, or one of a variety of other inherited disorders) or by an acquired immune suppression (whether secondary to immunosuppressive drugs following transplantation or for treatment of autoimmune diseases or secondary to infection with the human immunodeficiency virus [HIV] or malaria). In young children, the severe form of EBV evolves into Burkitt's lymphoma, whereas in older children or in adults, it takes the form of polyclonal lymphoid proliferations that can evolve into oligoclonal or monoclonal lymphomas.[4,5] It is irrelevant what the cause of the immune suppression is: whether a new infection or reactivation of latent infection, the result is poorly controlled EBV infection and B cell mitogenesis.

This type of proliferation does not involve necrosis followed by regeneration, as seen with the diseases described above, such as hepatitis; rather, it involves a direct mitogenic effect that can no longer be controlled by the normal host defense mechanisms—in this case, the immune system.[37,38] It is not surprising that, under these circumstances, there is a markedly increased risk of development of malignant lymphomas.

Immunosurveillance

In the late 1950s and early 1960s, the theory of immune surveillance of neoplasia was put forward to explain a number of perplexing observations[40] (see Chapter 5). Investigators noted that immunocompromised hosts—including humans and other animals—suffered an increased incidence of cancer. Moreover, they observed that mice in which tumors had been transplanted expressed antigens on the tumor surface not seen in normal cells. The investigators thus concluded that the immune system's loss of ability to recognize these alien antigens was a permissive factor in carcinogenesis. Because various viral and chemical agents known to cause cancer also caused immunosuppression, the destruction of immune surveillance was the mechanism by which these agents were thought to induce malignancy.

As additional investigations were performed, however, it became clear that this paradigm was not scientifically sustainable.[5,40] Most of the specific tumor antigens turned out to be virally related and were associated with the various infectious agents under study. Few, if any, tumor-*specific* antigens have been identified in humans; rather, the antigens identified on many tumors were tumor-*associated* antigens. Tumor-associated antigens are human antigens that normally are not highly expressed in adults but are expressed at high levels during embryonic and fetal development. Moreover, the immunosuppressive activity of many of the carcinogenic agents that were tested occurred only at relatively high doses, far in excess of those required to produce neoplasia. Most important, immunosuppressed patients were observed to not have an increased risk of the most common tumors, such as those of the breast, colon, lung, or prostate; rather they had increased risks of developing only very specific tumors. These tumors were malignant lymphomas, particularly those of B cell origin, and certain squamous cell tumors, especially of the cervix and occasionally of the skin and lip.

As described above, the increase in B cell proliferation in immunosuppressed individuals is explained by EBV mitogenesis of the B cells. However, also occasionally immunosuppression can lead to proliferation of B or T cells independent of EBV infection.[41] Exact mechanisms by which this occurs are unclear, but likely reflect various growth control mechanisms that T cells exert over the proliferation and expression of immune cells (see Chapter 5).

The other malignancy that occurs frequently in immunosuppressed patients is squamous cell carcinoma.[42] These tumors are nearly always associated with human papillomavirus (HPV) infection[43] (see Chapter 6). Proliferation of nonmalignant cells infected with HPV is normally held in check by the immune system, at least to a degree. In immunosuppressed individuals, however, proliferation of infected cells proceeds at a much higher rate. Thus, the immune system is not directly designed for surveillance of neoplasia, but rather for infectious organisms (Figure 3.2). It just so happens that some of the infectious organisms that the immune system

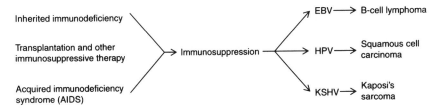

Figure 3.2. Schematic diagram illustrating the relationship between types of immunosuppression and development of specific cancers.

is designed to control occasionally are associated with the development of neoplasia.

Another viral agent associated with a neoplastic process has been discovered in immunosuppressed patients, particularly those with acquired immunodeficiency disease (AIDS): the Kaposi's sarcoma–associated herpesvirus (KSHV or HHV-8). Although the details of its mechanism of action are unknown, it also appears to act as a mitogen to the target cell population, possibly acting by altering the regulation of growth factors and of their receptors.[44] Again, the result is sustained proliferation that is not controlled by the immune system or by other growth control mechanisms. People with an intact immune system appear to be able to suppress the proliferative and therefore the neoplastic activity of this virus, much as they can when infected with EBV and B cells.

EFFECTS ON DIFFERENTIATION

The influence of an infection on proliferation depends on the stage of differentiation of the infected host cell. Moreover, the long-term consequences of this proliferation also depend on the stage of differentiation of the infected host cell. An excellent example of this process is provided by human papillomavirus and squamous cell carcinomas (HPV; see Chapter 6).

It is now well accepted that HPV is the etiologic factor for squamous cell carcinoma of the cervix, and also for carcinomas of certain other squamous epithelia, such as the vulva, penis, lip, and skin[43]; esophagus and the metaplastic squamous epithelium seen occasionally in the lower urinary tract appear to be affected by HPV less readily.[45] It appears that only a selected few of the numerous HPV types (e.g., types 16 and 18) are associated with an increased risk of development of squamous cell carcinoma.[43] The others are more commonly associated with benign proliferations, such as condyloma acuminatum and various types of verrucae (common warts). The reason for the benign versus malignant proliferations associated with different types of HPV is not entirely clear, but may, in part, be related to the layers of the squamous epithelium that are infected.

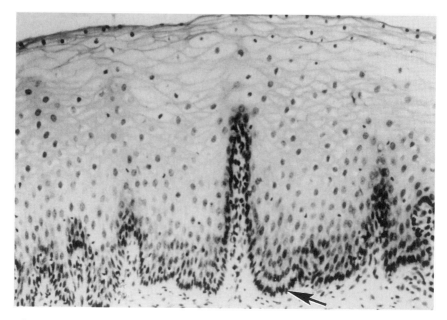

Figure 3.3. Normal cervical squamous epithelium showing a distinct basal layer (arrows) with progressive maturation of keratinocytes to their flattened appearance at the surface.

The squamous epithelium is a stratified, layered epithelium with a pluripotential cell population present in the basal cell layer (Figure 3.3), particularly as part of hair follicles in the epidermis.[46] Basal cells evolve to stratified keratinocytes, which gradually become larger and flatter as they progress to the surface of the epithelium. By the time they reach the surface, their nuclei are completely pyknotic, eventually disappearing before the cell is sloughed from the surface.

If HPV infects cells in the suprabasal layers of the squamous epithelium, benign proliferations occur,[43] as seen in verrucae. As indicated in the introduction to this chapter, for neoplasia to develop, it is essential that proliferation occurs in the pluripotential cells of a given tissue. Because the suprabasal layers are composed of keratinocytes committed to differentiation and on their way to terminal differentiation, they will not give rise to malignant neoplasms. Even if there is increased proliferation in those infected cells, the proliferating cells are simply the wrong cells for malignancy to evolve. The stem cell population of the epithelium is unaffected in these circumstances.

In contrast, certain strains of HPV are able to affect the basal cell layer of the epithelium, particularly in the cervix, and thus have the potential of infecting the appropriate cell population that can give rise to neoplasia.[43] As described previously, the proliferative response in HPV-infected cells partly depends on the immune system and other control mechanisms. However, a major feature of the infection that leads to the

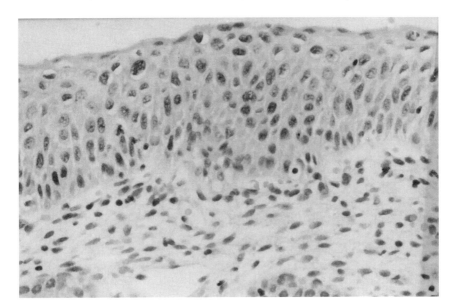

Figure 3.4. High-grade dysplastic cervical squamous epithelium with de-creased maturation of keratinocytes. Chronic inflammation is present in the submucosa.

development of malignancy is that the virus partially inhibits the differen-tiation process of the affected squamous epithelium. Thus, cells resem-bling more the basal cell layer than the superficial cell layers gradually accumulate[4,5] (Figure 3.4). This accumulation gives rise to a morphologic entity, commonly referred to as dysplasia or cervical intraepithelial neoplasia (CIN).[47] Eventually, these abnormal cells occupy the entire thickness of the squamous epithelium, at which time the diagnosis of squamous cell carcinoma *in situ* is made. At this point, the cells are char-acterized by two major features: (1) the cells resemble immature cells in the epithelium, reflecting a block in differentiation, and (2) the cells are proliferating at a rate faster than do the normal squamous epithelial cells. Because differentiation is blocked, more cells remain in the pluripotential cell population; even if they were proliferating at the normal rate, the result would be an increase in the number of cell divisions occurring in this epithelium. Ultimately, in the final step in the neoplastic process, there is invasion of the basal lamina and underlying connective tissue

INTERACTION OF GENOTOXIC CHEMICALS AND INFECTIONS

As indicated in the introduction to this chapter, an agent can increase the risk of cancer either by increasing the number of DNA replications, sev-eral examples of which have just been described for various infectious organisms, or by directly damaging DNA during replication. Agents that damage DNA include various chemicals and radiation of different types, such as ultraviolet and x-radiation.[11-13] A substantial synergy occurs if there is direct DNA damage and increased cell proliferation. Thus, if the rate of DNA damage per replication is increased and the number of replications is also increased, the chance for a mistake to occur that can lead to cancer is increased substantially. Examples of this type of synergy have already been identified in animal models and, in a few instances, in humans.

In parts of China, there are high incidences of hepatoma, largely associated with the hepatitis B and hepatitis C viruses.[48,49] In some of these regions, however, there is also a high exposure to aflatoxin, a genotoxic mycotoxin that is metabolically activated to a reactive intermediate; this intermediate forms highly mutagenic and carcinogenic DNA adducts.[50] In one study, the lifetime risk of hepatoma was 2.5-fold higher in persons with aflatoxin exposure (at an average exposure of one million ng per kg body weight per day) than in those without aflatoxin exposure. In persons with both hepatitis infection and aflatoxin exposure, however, the risk of hepatoma was an astounding 25-fold higher than in those with aflatoxin exposure alone.[51] This massive increase in risk reflects the synergy between the two types of effects on carcinogenesis in individuals exposed to both the virus (a strong, persistent proliferative stimulus) and increased levels of aflatoxin (a DNA-damaging stimulus).[52] A similar synergy between hepatitis virus and aflatoxin has been demonstrated in woodchucks.[21]

Less well documented is the synergy that occurs in women who are infected with HPV and are also cigarette smokers. Cigarette smoke contains large amounts of chemicals that are metabolically activated to reactive intermediates, such as nitrosamines and polycyclic aromatic hydrocarbons; these then form DNA adducts that are mutagenic and carcinogenic.[53] It is unclear which of these chemicals specifically has an effect on the cervix, although cigarette smoke condensate has been shown to act synergistically with HPV in an in vitro model of cervical carcinogenesis.[54] Nearly all women who develop cervical cancer are infected with HPV, and have experienced the proliferative effects of the virus as described earlier. However, women with HPV (a strong persistent proliferative stimulus) who are also cigarette smokers (a potentially strong DNA damaging stimulus) have an increased risk of developing cervical cancer compared with those who have only one of these factors.[55]

In the etiology of stomach cancer, the relationship between specific types of chemicals[56] and *H. pylori*[22] and the ultimate development of neoplasm is not as well delineated. However, two dietary exposures—salt and nitrates—seem to be reasonably well established as contributing to the carcinogenic hazard in certain populations.[56] The carcinogenic mechanism of action for salt is not known but is not related to the formation of DNA adducts and direct mutations. Alterations in the mucus protective layer of the stomach has been suggested. With regard to nitrates, the formation of various nitroso compounds has been implicated in stomach carcinogenesis and has been examined extensively in certain animal models. Some of these compounds are highly reactive, such as N-methyl-N-nitroso-N'-nitroguanidine. The formation of nitroso compounds can occur directly in the acidic milieu of the stomach by the reaction of the nitrite with secondary amines. However, this reaction can be inhibited by a variety of agents present in the diet, such as vitamin C. The exact interaction among these various agents in the etiology of stomach cancer has yet to be determined, but again, the possibility of a synergy between a strongly proliferative stimulus from the *H. pylori* and the direct DNA-damaging effects of the nitroso compounds is a likely possibility.

SUMMARY

It is well accepted that cancer arises as the result of multiple genetic events occurring in the pluripotential cell (stem cell) population. It is also well established that DNA replication has incredible fidelity, but rarely mistakes do occur. Based on these assumptions, cancer risk can be increased by an agent that either directly interacts with DNA, causing mutation, or that increases the number of replications of the DNA, or that does both. Certain infectious organisms have the propensity to cause disease states in which there is increased cell proliferation over prolonged periods, due to necrosis and regeneration, to direct mitogenesis, or to a block in differentiation. Other means of increasing cell proliferation certainly may exist. Interaction with genotoxic carcinogens in specific situations enhances the carcinogenic risk of the infectious process.

The direct or indirect effects of these infectious agents on the carcinogenic process present an opportunity for prevention of carcinogenesis either by treatment of the infection, or, even better, by vaccination against initial infection with the organism. Even in situations where the infectious organism is only one contributor to the carcinogenic process, removing it should greatly reduce the incidences of certain types of tumors worldwide.

Acknowledgments

I gratefully acknowledge the assistance of Denise Miller, Marty Cano, James Wisecarver, and Stan Radio with the preparation of this manuscript.

REFERENCES

1. Ellermann V, Bang O. Experimentelle Leukamie bei Hurnern. Zentralbl Bakteriol 1908; 46: 595–609.
2. Majno G, Joris I. Cells, Tissues, and Disease; Principles of General Pathology. Cambridge, MA: Braun-Brumfield; 1996:815–864.
3. Schlessinger BS, Schlessinger JH, eds. The Who's Who of Nobel Prize Winners 1901–1990. Phoenix, Arizona: The Orynx Press, 1991, Second Edition.

4. Preston-Martin S, Pike MC, Ross RK, Jones PA, Henderson BE. Increased cell division as a cause of human cancer. Cancer Res 1990;50:7415–7421.

5. Cohen SM, Purtilo DT, Ellwein LB. Pivotal role of increased cell proliferation in human carcinogenesis. Mod Pathol 1991;4:371–382.

6. Boveri T. Zur Trage der Entstehung maligner Tumoren. Fisher G, ed. Jena: 1914.

7. Perkins AS, Stern DF. Molecular biology of cancer: Oncogenes. In: DeVita VT Jr, Hellman S, Rosenberg SA, eds. Cancer, Principles and Practice of Oncology. New York: Lippincott-Raven; 1997:79–102.

8. Knudson, AG. Antioncogenes and human cancer. Proc Natl Acad Sci USA 1993; 90:10914–10921.

9. Knudson AG. Mutation and cancer; statistical study of retinoblastoma. Proc Natl Acad Sci USA 1971;68:820–823.

10. Simpson AJG. The natural somatic mutation frequency and human carcinogenesis. Adv Cancer Res 1997;71:209–240.

11. Cohen SM, Ellwein LB. Cell proliferation in carcinogenesis. Science 1990; 249: 1007–1011.

12. Cohen SM, Ellwein LB. Genetic errors, cell proliferation, and carcinogenesis. Cancer Res 1991; 51:6493–6505.

13. Cohen SM, Ellwein LB. Risk assessment based on high-dose animal exposure experiments. Chem Res Toxicol 1992;5:742–748.

14. Cohen SM. The role of cell proliferation in the etiology of neoplasia. In: Bowden GT, Fisher SM, eds. Chemical Carcinogens and Anticarcinogens, Volume 12 of Comprehensive Toxicology, Sipes, I.G., Gandolfi, A.J., and McQueen, C.A. (Series Eds), Pergamon (Elsevier), Amsterdam, 1997:401–424.

15. Greenfield RE, Ellwein LB, Cohen SM. A general probabilistic model of carcinogenesis: analysis of experimental urinary bladder cancer. Carcinogenesis 1984;5:437–445.

16. Beasley RP. Hepatitis B virus—The major etiology of hepatocellular carcinoma. Cancer 1988; 61:1942–1956.

17. Edamoto Y, Tani M, Kurata T, Abe K. Hepatitis C and B virus infections in hepatocellular carcinoma. Cancer 1996;77:1787–1791.

18. Wright N, Alison M. The liver. In: The Biology of Epithelial Cell Populations. Oxford: Clarendon Press;1984:2:880–980.

19. Dunsford HA, Sell S, Chisari FV. Hepatocarcinogenesis due to chronic liver cell injury in hepatitis B virus transgenic mice. Cancer Res 1990;50:3400–3407.

20. Hagen TM, Huang S, Curnutte J, Fowler P, Martinez V, Wehr CM. Extensive oxidative DNA damage in hepatocytes of transgenic mice with chronic active hepatitis destined to develop hepatocellular carcinoma. Proc Natl Acad Sci USA 91:12808–12812.

21. Bannasch P, Imani Khoshkou N, Hacker JH, et al. Synergistic hepato-carcinogenic effect of hepadnaviral infection and dietary aflatoxin B_1 in woodchucks. Cancer Res 1995;55:3318–3330.

22. Correa P. Human gastric carcinogenesis: a multi-step and multifactorial process. First American Cancer Society Award Lecture on Cancer Epidemiology and Prevention. Cancer Res 1992;52:6735–6740.

23. Wright N, Alison M. Kinetic parameters in the gastrointestinal mucosa. In: The Biology of Epithelial Cell Populations. Oxford: Clarendon Press;1984: 634–687.

24. Infection with Helicobacter pylori. In: World Health Organization. IARC

monographs on the evaluation of carcinogenic risks to humans. Vol. 61. Schistosomes, liver flukes and Helicobacter pylori. Lyon, France: International Agency for Research on Cancer, 1994:177–240.

25. El-Bolkainy M. Schistosomiasis and bladder cancer. In: Bryan GT, Cohen SM, eds. The Pathology of Bladder Cancer. Boca Raton, FL: CRC Press;1983:I:57–89.

26. Kawai K, Yamamoto M, Kameyama S, Kawamata H, Rademaker A, Oyasu R. Enhancement of rat urinary bladder tumorigenesis by lipopolysaccharide-induced inflammation. Cancer Res 1993;53:5172–5175.

27. Burin GJ, Gibb HJ, Hill RN. Human bladder cancer: evidence for a potential irritation-induced mechanism. Food Chem Toxicol 1995;33:785–795.

28. Okamoto M, Kawamata H, Kawai K, Oyasu R. Enhancement of transformation in vitro of a nontumorigenic rat urothelial cell line by interleukin 6. Cancer Res. 1995;55:4581–4585.

29. Momose H, Kakinuma H, Shariff SY, Mitchell GB, Rademaker A, Oyasu R. Tumor-promoting effect of urinary epidermal growth factor in rat urinary bladder carcinogenesis. Cancer Res 1991; 51: 5487–5490.

30. Hicks RM, James C, Webbe G. Effect of Schistosoma haematobium and N-butyl-N-(4-hydroxybutyl)nitrosamine on the development of urothelial neoplasia in the baboon. Br J Cancer 1980; 42:730–755.

31. Lijinsky W, Thomas BJ, Kovatch RM. Local and systemic carcinogenic effects of alkylating carcinogens in rats treated by intravesicular administration. Jpn J Cancer Res 1991;82:980–986.

32. Lijinsky W, Thomas BJ, Kovatch RM. Systemic and local carcinogenesis by directly acting N-nitroso compounds given to rats by intravesicular administration. Carcinogenesis 1992;13:1101–1105.

33. Purtilo DT. Clonorchiasis and hepatic neoplasms. Trop Geogr Med 1976;28: 21–27.

34. Kurathong S, Lerdverasirkul P, Wongpaitoon V, et al. Opisthorchis viverrini infection and cholangiocarcinoma. Gastroenterology 1985;89:151–156.

35. Thamavit W, Moore MA, Hiasa Y, Ito N. Enhancement of DHPN induced hepatocellular, cholangiocellular and pancreatic carcinogenesis by Opisthorchis viverrini infestation in Syrian golden hamsters. Carcinogenesis 1988;9: 1095–1098.

36. Ames BN, Shigenaga MK, Hagen TM. Oxidants, antioxidants, and the degenerative diseases of aging. Proc Natl Acad Sci USA 1993;90:7915–7922.

37. Klein, G. Epstein–Barr virus strategy in normal and neoplastic B cells. Cell 1994;77:791–793.

38. Rickinson AB. On the biology of Epstein–Barr virus persistence: a reappraisal. In: Lopez C, et al, eds. Immunobiology and Prophylaxis of Human Herpesvirus Infections. New York: Plenum Press;1990:137–146.

39. Straus SE, Cohen JI, Tosato G, Meier J. Epstein–Barr virus infections: biology, pathogenesis, and management. Ann Intern Med 1993;118:45–58.

40. Schwartz RW. Another look at immunologic surveillance. N Engl J Med 1975;293:181–184.

41. Seemayer TA, Gross, TG, Maarten Egeler R, et al. X-Linked lymphoproliferative disease: twenty-five years after the discovery. Pediatric Res 1995;38:471–478.

42. Penn I. Tumors of the immunocompromised patient. Annu Rev Med 1988; 39:63–73.

43. zur Hausen H. Viruses in human cancers. Science 1993;254:1167–1173.
44. Boshoff C, Endo Y, Collins PD, Takeuchi Y, Reeves JD, Schweickart VL, et al. Angiogenic and HIV-inhibitory functions of KSHV-encoded chemokines. Science 1997;278:290–294.
45. zur Hausen, H. Papillomavirus infections—a major cause of human cancers. Biochim Biophys Acta 1996;1288:F55–F78.
46. Wright N, Alison M. The kinetic organization of squamous epithelium. In: The Biology of Epithelial Cell Populations. Oxford: Clarendon Press;1984: 287–345.
47. Prat J. Female reproductive system. In: Damjanov I, Linder J, eds. Anderson's Pathology, 10th ed. St. Louis, MO: Mosby;1996:2231–2309.
48. Buendia MA. Hepatitis B viruses and hepatocellular carcinoma. Adv Cancer Res 1992;59:167–226.
49. Yen FS, Yu MC, MO CC, Luo S, Tong MJ, Henderson BE. Hepatitis B virus, aflatoxins, and hepatocellular carcinoma in Southern Guangxi, China. Cancer Res 1989;49:2506–2509.
50. Harris CC. Chemical and physical carcinogenesis; advances and perspectives for the 1990s. Cancer Res. 1991;51:5023–5044.
51. Hoseyni MS. Risk assessment for aflatoxin. III Modeling for the relative risk of hepatocellular carcinoma. Risk Anal 1992;12:123–128.
52. Feitelson MA. Biology of hepatitis B virus variants. Lab Invest 1994;71:324–349.
53. Clarke EA, Morgan RW, Newman AM. Smoking as a risk factor in cancer of the cervix: additional evidence from a case-control study. Am J Epidemiol 1982;115:59–66.
54. Nakao Y, Yang X, Yokoyama M, Pater MM, Pater A. Malignant transformation of human ectocervical cells immortalized by HPV 18: in vitro model of carcinogenesis by cigarette smoke. Carcinogenesis 1996;17:577–583.
55. Gram IT, Austin A, Stalsberg H. Cigarette smoking and the incidence of cervical intraepithelial neoplasia, grade III, and cancer of the cervix uteri. Am J Epidemiol 1992;135:341–346.
56. Mirvish SS. Role of N-nitroso compounds (NOC) and N-nitrosation in etiology of gastric, esophageal, nasopharyngeal and bladder cancer and contribution to cancer of known exposure to NOC. Cancer Lett 1995;93:17–48.

4

Viral Oncogenesis

HARALD ZUR HAUSEN

For more than 100 years, researchers have suspected that tumors have an infectious etiology. Successful transmission of warts by cell-free extracts in dogs initially hinted at the infectious causation of a benign tumor in 1898, soon followed in 1907 by similar observations in warts of humans and cattle.[1,2]

In 1911, Peyton Rous[3] successfully transmitted a malignancy from one chicken to another by injecting cell-free extracts from the tumor. His work seemed to signal the start of a new era in cancer research. Although, sporadically, scientists demonstrated the transmissibility of other tumors—such as skin tumors in rabbits, mammary cancer in mice, and renal cancer in leopard frogs—the majority of other attempts were unsuccessful.

A renaissance of the viral hypothesis occurred in the early 1950s, when Ludwik Gross[4] discovered the transmissibility of murine leukemias by infecting newborn animals with tumor extracts. His work ushered in numerous additional studies that eventually led to the identification of RNA-containing viruses (retroviruses) as causative agents for a variety of lymphoproliferative diseases in diverse species, including mice, rats, and cats. Shortly thereafter, DNA-containing tumor viruses were discovered that were potent carcinogens when inoculated into newborn rodents. These viruses included polyomavirus of mice; SV40, a virus originating from cultures of rhesus monkey kidney cells; and human adenovirus types 12 and 18. Unfortunately, attempts in the early 1960s to find these or related viruses in human tumors met with no visible success.

In 1964, Epstein and his colleagues[5] in Bristol, using electron microscopy, observed herpesvirus-like particles in an occasional cell of Burkitt's lymphoma cell cultures. Dennis Burkitt, a British surgeon, first speculated in 1958[6] that this childhood tumor, endemic in certain regions of equatorial Africa, might have a viral origin. His idea was based mainly on his observation that regions with endemic Burkitt's lymphoma coincided with those where malaria was transmitted throughout the year. He suspected arthropod-borne transmission of the putative agent of Burkitt's lymphoma, similar to that of malaria. Despite a gradually increasing interest in the particles found in cultured Burkitt's lymphoma cells, subsequently designated as Epstein-Barr virus (EBV), it took almost 30 years before they were firmly identified as a human tumor virus and before their mode of interaction with human B cells was at least partially understood.

In the meantime, however, new viruses had been linked to human tumors. This correlation was recognized in the 1970s and 1980s with hepatitis B virus and hepatocellular cancer,[7] and with a retrovirus (human T-cell leukemia virus 1 or HTLV-1) in a human leukemia prevalent in coastal regions of southern Japan.[8,9] Although the mechanisms are not entirely clear for hepatitis B virus, specific functions of the viral genome seem to contribute to the malignant conversion of infected cells. Thus, these agents appear to directly provoke human cancer development.

Almost unnoticed by contemporary investigators, another group of viral infections emerged in the late 1970s and during the 1980s: the papillomaviruses. The infectious nature of human and animal warts was demonstrated at the turn of this century (reviewed in ref. 10). Initial experimental attempts to relate these infections to cancer development and to study interactions with other carcinogenic factors were made by Rous and his associates in the 1930s.[11-14] Subsequently, Rous demonstrated in ingenious experiments the carcinogenic potential of a cottontail rabbit papillomavirus in domestic rabbits, and showed the syncarcinogenic activity of tar and of defined chemical carcinogens when jointly applied with the virus infection. The carcinogenic activity of the Shope papillomavirus (later renamed cottontail rabbit papillomavirus, or CRPV) was irrefutably proved in 1961 by Ito and Evans,[15] who induced carcinomas in domestic rabbits with purified CRPV DNA and with DNA extracted from CRPV-induced papillomas and carcinomas.

Two different lines of studies contributed to the development of papillomavirus research. In 1959, Olson and colleagues[16] reported the induction of urinary bladder tumors in cattle by a bovine papillomavirus found in skin fibropapillomas. The same virus was tumorigenic when inoculated into newborn hamsters[17,18] and transformed calf and murine cells in tissue culture.[19,20] Therefore, a second member of the papillomavirus group, besides CRPV, was clearly able to induce malignant tumors.

A second line of investigation into papillomaviruses dates back to 1922, when Lewandowsky and Lutz[21] reported a rare and obviously hereditary verrucosis in humans; people with generalized warts later developed skin carcinoma at sun-exposed sites. This syndrome was named epidermodysplasia verruciformis (EV). Initially, the authors were not aware of the potential infectious origin of the papillomatous plaques and macules covering the affected skin. That etiology was subsequently demonstrated by Lutz[22] and by Jablonska and her colleagues,[23,24] who induced papillomas following intracutaneous autoinoculation of cell-free extracts.

Interest in papillomaviruses blossomed in the latter half of the 1970s. This attention was in part the consequence of a hypothesis that papillomaviruses played a significant role in the etiology of cancer of the cervix.[25,26] Tests to substantiate this hypothesis had established the plurality of papillomavirus types and subtypes.[27-29] In addition, Meisels and Fortin in 1976[30] proposed a papillomavirus origin of koilocytotic atypias, separating the latter from "true" preneoplastic lesions. This scheme represented a valuable diagnostic aid in grading lesions for surgical intervention. The demonstration of papillomavirus particles in typical koilocytes supported Meisels and Fortin's observations.[31-33] Papillomavirus research was also stimulated by the identification of novel human papillomavirus (HPV) types in lesions of patients with EV, particularly in malignant tumors of such patients.[29,34]

A substantial shift in the interest in papillomavirus research occurred in the 1980s. The isolation of new HPV types from genital warts (HPV 6 and 11)[35,36] and subsequently directly from cervical cancer biopsies (HPV types 16 and 18)[37,38] resulted in a rapid expansion of experimental work and also in early epidemiological investigations. It took almost one decade before the causal role of specific HPV types in cancer of the cervix and the respective precursor lesions was more or less generally accepted.[39-42]

At present, the main interest in papillomavirus research has shifted to understanding mechanisms of carcinogenesis: how do genes of these viruses influence cell growth, how do their oncoproteins interact with host cell components, and to what extent is the failure of specific host cell functions related to papillomavirus-induced oncogenesis? The recent recognition of a link between HPV infection and other widespread human tumor types, such as cancers of the skin and of the oropharynx, points to the magnitude of the problem. Papillomaviruses emerge as the most common carcinoma viruses[43] and appear to play a specific role as major cancer pathogens.[44] Simultaneously, successful first attempts to vaccinate animals against their own papillomavirus infections[45] raise the hope for the prevention of specific human cancers based on similar vaccination protocols.

During the past 20 years, it became evident that a direct contribution does not represent the sole mode by which virus infections contribute to the development of human cancers: the emerging AIDS epidemic, resulting from HIV infections and leading to severe immunosuppression, favored the development of B-cell lymphomas, of Hodgkin's disease, of the otherwise extremely rare Kaposi's sarcoma (a pigmented tumor arising from the proliferation of vascular-endothelial cells), and of skin cancers. Because HIV-DNA is not found in these cancer cells, it is likely that this virus contributes indirectly to the emergence of these cancers by reducing immunological defense mechanisms against the oncogenic viruses (as discussed in Chapter 5). Other virus infections (e.g., herpes simplex virus, cytomegalovirus) have been shown to aid persisting tumor viruses (papilloma- and polyomaviruses) by amplifying the genomes of the latter in infected cells.[46,47] This mechanism emerges as a second indirect mode of

interaction by which specific viruses may increase the risk of tumor formation. A third mode may be induction of chronic inflammation (see Chapter 2).

In recent years, additional virus infections associated with certain types
of human tumors have been discovered: they include hepatitis C virus in a
subset of liver cancers, a new herpesvirus (human herpesvirus type 8,
HHV-8) in Kaposi's sarcomas,[48] and approximately 50 novel papillomavirus genotypes in squamous and basal cell carcinomas of the skin.[49-51]
Their mere presence within these tumors does not prove an etiologic
relationship; nevertheless, it represents the starting point for further investigations in this direction. Besides these agents, there exist several additional viral infections in humans that, on transmission to newborn rodents
(mice, hamsters), induce maligant tumors after latency periods of several
months. They include small DNA viruses, widely spread in the human
population and excreted in the urine under conditions of immunosuppression (BK and JC viruses), as well as some types of human pathogenic
adenoviruses, most frequently identified in mild respiratory illnesses.
None of these agents has yet been found consistently in any human cancer. They may, however, be considered as potential human tumor viruses.

If we limit our consideration to only those human cancers with a
proven relationship to specific virus infections, approximately 15% of the
worldwide cancer burden (with substantial geographic variation) emerges
as caused by viruses, among them the second most frequent cancer in
women, cancer of the cervix, and about 80% of liver cancers. This figure
will almost double if other cancers currently associated with specific virus
infections are proved to be caused by such agents. More than 100 years
after initiation of such investigations, virus infections emerge today as one
of the major risk factors for human cancers.

Tables 4.1 through 4.3 summarize our present knowledge of viruses in
human tumors, showing agents directly or indirectly linked to human cancers, those suspected to represent human tumor viruses, as well as potential human tumor viruses (identified by only their tumorigenic properties
for newborn rodents).

GENERAL CONSIDERATIONS OF VIRUSES AS CAUSATIVE
AGENTS FOR MALIGNANT TUMORS

As outlined in the introduction, suspicions that cancer may have an infectious etiology root back for more than one century (reviewed in reference
52), and the first animal data on cancer induction by animal viruses became available approximately 90 years ago.[3,53] Yet, it proved to be extremely difficult to demonstrate a causal involvement of infections in human cancers. There are several major reasons for this difficulty:[54]

- Viruses suspected to be involved in human carcinogenesis are frequently ubiquitous (e.g., EBV, papillomaviruses, hepatitis viruses).

Table 4.1 Viruses directly linked to human tumors

Virus	Acute infection	Tumor
Epstein-Barr virus	infectious mononucleosis	B-cell lymphomas (*after immunosuppression*) Burkitt's lymphoma Nasopharyngeal cancer (Hodgkin's disease) (T-cell lymphomas)
Hepatitis B virus	Hepatitis B	Hepatocellular carcinoma
Papillomavirus types 5, 8, 14, 17, 20, 47	Epidermodysplasia verruciformis (EV)	Skin cancer in EV patients
Papillomavirus types 16, 18, 31, 33, 35, 39, 45, 52, 56, 58 and a few others	Squamous intraepithelial neoplasia, Bowenoid papulosis	Cancer of the cervix Anogenital cancer Cancer of the tonsils Cancer of the nailbeds
Papillomavirus types 6 + 11	Condyloma acuminatum	Verrucous carcinoma (*rare*)
HTLV-1	Smoldering leukemia	Adult T-cell leukemia

Table 4.2 Potential human tumor viruses

Virus	Acute infection	Tumor
Not yet named novel papillomavirus types	Warts, bowenoid lesions	Squamous cell carcinomas + basaliomas of the skin in organ allograft recipients and in immunocompetent patients
HPV16, 18, 33, 57, 73, and others	Papillomas, intraepithelial neoplasias	Cancers of the oral cavity, tongue, larynx, nasal cavity, esophagus ???
Herpesvirus type 8	???	Kaposi's sarcoma ?
Hepatitis C virus	Hepatitis	Hepatocellular carcinoma Low-grade lymphomas ???
JC, BK, and SV40-like polyoma-type viruses	? (PML)	Brain tumors??? Pancreatic islet tumors??? Mesotheliomas???
Human endogenous retroviruses (HERV-K)	?	Seminomas??? Germ cell tumors???
Adenoviruses	Respiratory infections Eye infections	???

Table 4.3 Viruses indirectly involved in human tumors

Virus	Acute infection	Tumor
Human immunodeficiency virus (HIV) I and II	Acquired immunodeficiency syndrome (AIDS)	Kaposi's sarcoma B-cell lymphoma Skin cancer
Herpes simplex virus, cytomegalovirus, varizella zoster virus, HHV	Various symptoms	*Only experimental data available on mutagenic activity and induction of DNA amplification of persisting polyoma- and papillomavirus DNA*

Only a small percentage of infected individuals develops the respective form of cancer.

• The time intervals between primary infection and cancer development are frequently on the order of several decades.
• The arising tumors are commonly monoclonal and, thus, cannot be the result of a systemic infection.
• Chemical and physical carcinogens are frequently suspected to be causally related to the same tumor types.

These observations seem to be incompatible with cancer development as the immediate or sole consequence of an infection. The infection may still be necessary, but clearly it is not sufficient for cancer induction.

Another problem is the frequent reliance on Koch's postulates[55] to affirm a virus as a causative agent in malignant disease. Unfortunately, the propagation of the suspected agent under experimental conditions outside the host and the induction of disease in suitable experimental animals from in vitro cultures cannot be applied to most viruses suspected of playing a role in human tumors, because most of these viruses neither can be propagated under experimental conditions nor are tumorigenic for laboratory animals. The use of seroepidemiological evidence as an additional proof of causation was stressed by Evans[56] as a way to overcome the problems establishing a relationship between viral infections and specific human cancers. This argument was motivated by seroepidemiological data linking EBV to specific human cancers (see review in reference 57). In other tumor virus infections, however—specifically those involving papillomaviruses—these criteria are frequently invalid. For example, a substantial percentage of cervical cancer patients carrying HPV16- or 18-positive tumors appears to be devoid of detectable immune responses to antigens of the respective virus.[58,59] Thus, even seroepidemiology often provides insufficient information to establish proof of a link between viral infection and cancer.

Despite these problems, scientists have attempted to establish criteria that would permit an unequivocal statement of causality for oncogenic viruses. These criteria, which do not apply to infectious agents that act purely by an inflammation pathway, include:[60]

1. Epidemiologic evidence (risk assessment, coincidence of geographic prevalence, seroepidemiology, plausability of relationship) that the infection represents a risk factor for the development of specific tumors.
2. Regular presence and persistence of nucleic acid of the infectious agent in cells of specific malignant tumors.
3. Stimulation of proliferation on transfection of the relevant genome or parts thereof in appropriate tissue culture cells.
4. Demonstration that the induction of proliferation and the malignant phenotype of specific tumor cells depends on effects or functions exerted by persisting DNA furnished by the infectious agent.

The way that these molecular criteria can be met is exemplified with papillomavirus. In cervical carcinoma cells, the genetic activity of the latent papillomavirus genomes has been knocked out in different experimental settings, with a resulting decreased proliferation rate and loss of the malignant phenotype.[61-63] The application of these or similar criteria may turn out to be useful for those viral systems in which position effects of viral DNA integration or specific viral gene functions are suspected to be important for cancerogenesis.

The problem of proving carcinogenicity of oncogenic viruses is further complicated by disparity in the oncogenic potential of specific viral subtypes. For example, within the HPV group, the tumorigenic potential of individual types varies substantially. Therefore, high- and low-risk HPV infections have been proposed.[64] The original definition of high-risk viruses was based on their prevalence in cervical and anogenital cancers. Subsequently, the viruses were classified based on functional properties. High-risk viruses were shown to immortalize human keratinocytes, whereas low-risk viruses failed to do so.[65,66] The observation that the cellular proteins p53 and pRB were bound by high-risk HPV oncoproteins, but not by several low-risk viruses, provided another functional parameter for this differentiation.[67,68] Induction of chromosomal aberrations as the consequence of high-risk viral oncoproteins overriding cell cycle control mechanisms has emerged as the functionally most important distinction between these virus groups.[69-73] Because of their mutational activity, high-risk viruses are apparently able to contribute directly to the progression of latently infected cells and seem to act as solitary carcinogens.[74]

As mentioned, a further complicating issue is that chemical and physical carcinogens are frequently found to cause tumors that under other circumstances have been suspected to be of viral etiology. These premises are not mutually exclusive, however. Interestingly, cancer cells that contain low-risk HPV frequently exhibit modifications in the cellular p53 gene and occur at sites exposed to chemical or physical carcinogens.

Basal cell and squamous cell carcinomas of the skin are one example[50]; squamous cell carcinoma of the larynx following irradiation with x-rays for extensive laryngeal papillomatosis is another example (summarized in reference 75). The role of low-risk HPVs in these malignant conversions has not been clarified. Yet these observations suggest that mutagenic modifications of host cell genes, presumably required to activate the oncogenic potential of these viruses, can be mediated by physical carcinogens. The apparent inability of these viruses to code for mutagenic oncoproteins independently seems to be the main reason for their failure to act as solitary carcinogens and for their dependence on interaction with other mutagenic factors in the generally rare events of malignant development following these infections.[10]

IMMORTALIZATION OF TISSUE CULTURE CELLS BY VIRUSES–THE EXAMPLE OF PAPILLOMAVIRUS

The induction of continuous growth of cells in vitro by virus infection without detectable tumorigenicity of the cells after heterotransplantation into immunosuppressed animals is defined as *immortalization*. Transformation, in contrast, defines continuous growth of cells that on heetrotransplantation under the same conditions form invasively growing tumors.

Immortalization of human cells was initially described for polyoma-type viruses (reviewed in reference 76) and subsequently for a member of the herpesvirus group, EBV.[77] It has also been reported for HTLV-1[78] and more recently for high-risk papillomavirus infections.[65,66] Although polyoma-type viruses were the prime target in studies of immortalization in the 1960s and 1970s, and EBV immortalization of human B cells occurs with unusual efficiency, most recent studies were devoted to immortalization induced by high-risk papillomavirus. They will be discussed in the next section.

Because immortalization is defined under experimental conditions, it is not entirely clear how it correlates with clinical virus-induced lesions. In high-risk HPV infections, however, in vitro immortalization corresponds with at least a proportion of low grade intraepithelial neoplasias as deduced from three observations: (1) immortalized cells in organotypic cultures histologically resemble low-grade intraepithelial lesions (reviewed in reference 79); (2) many clinical low-grade neoplasias, in contrast to high-grade lesions and invasive cancer, reveal a similar restriction of E6/E7 oncogene transcription, as do immortalized cells, when the latter are heterografted into immunocompromised animals[80]; and (3) although difficult, it has been possible to cultivate immortalized lines from some explants of intraepithelial neoplasias.[81–83]

First attempts to immortalize cells by papillomavirus infection date back to 1963 when Black et al.[19] and Thomas et al.[20] demonstrated immortalization of fetal bovine cells by bovine papillomavirus infection. In 1980, Lowy and colleagues[84] showed that only 69% of the genome was required for successful immortalization. Immortalization and transformation of murine cells by human papillomavirus types appeared in 1984 and 1986.[85,86] Similar data quickly followed after transfection of rat cells with HPV16 or HPV18 DNA.[87,88] It became apparent at about the same time that the HPV16 E7 gene cooperates with the *ras* oncogene in the transformation of primary rat kidney cells.[89,90] Only DNA fragments carrying the E6/E7 genes were sufficient for immortalization of these rodent cells.[87]

Immortalization of human cells with HPV16 DNA was first demonstrated in 1987[65,66] and with HPV18 DNA in 1988.[91] Subsequently, a large number of human cell types—including skin, bronchial and kidney epithelium, smooth muscle, and endothelium—have been immortalized by high-risk HPV DNA transfection (reviewed in reference 79). Recent reports describe the immortalization of human prostate[92] and ovarian cells[93] by high-risk HPV DNA. As in the rodent, DNA fragments with the E6/E7 genes are required for immortalization of human cells.[91,94,95]

Althoug viral oncogenes must be expressed for immortalization of cells by high-risk HPV, this expression is clearly not sufficient.[96] There exists good evidence that modifications in specific host cell genes are required. This has been demonstrated by somatic cell hybridization studies, initially performed with cells infected with SV40[97-99] and subsequently with HPV.[100] Only a small fraction of initially infected or transfected cells eventually becomes immortalized; the vast majority of cells, while continuing to express viral oncoproteins or, in the case of HPV transfection, to transcribe E6/E7 message, still undergoes senescence.[98,100] Somatic cell hybridization performed with different clones of immortalized cells has identified four complementing groups of genes required for senescence of either polyomavirus- or papillomavirus-immortalized cells.[97,100] In conjunction with expression of viral T-antigen (SV40) or E6/E7 (HPV), failure of any of these four cellular genes, which are presumably engaged in the regulation of the same signaling pathway, may result in immortalization.[10,101] Other complementing groups are still being sought and may be identified in the future.

The involvement of cellular genes whose failing function in the presence of polyomavirus or HPV oncogenes leads to immortalization points to two predictions: (1) the function of these genes in nonmodified cells interferes with the function of viral oncoproteins, as evidenced by the continued expression of the latter even in cells undergoing senescence, and (2) specific mutational changes—possibly even visible chromosomal aberrations—would be expected for cells to become immortalized. Indeed, specific chromosomal aberrations in HPV-immortalized human keratinocytes, preferentially involving sites on chromosomes 3 and 18, have been reported.[102-105] These data are still difficult to interpret, however, because some of these immortalized cells had converted to malignant growth. It may be relevant, however, that even malignant HPV-positive cells can be converted to senescence by the introduction of chromosome

11,[106-109] chromosome 4,[110] chromosome 2,[111] and chromosome 1.[112] Unfortunately, most of these studies—particularly those involving chromosomes 11 and 2—were performed with malignant lines, rendering impossible interpretation of the relationship between suppressing events and immortalization.

No cellular genes engaged in the prevention of virus-induced immortalization have been definitively identified to date. Researchers have suggested, however, that one of these cellular genes may code for the cyclin-dependent kinase inhibitor $p16^{INK4}$.[113] This protein is up-regulated under conditions of pRB inactivation.[114-116] Because the pE7–pRB interaction results in pRB inactivation, the up-regulation of $p16^{INK4}$ may account for the growth limitation of primary HPV-infected cells resulting in senescence after a prolonged life span. This hypothesis could explain the functional impairment of senescent HPV oncoprotein-expressing cells. In spontaneous immortalization of Li-Fraumeni syndrome, loss of $p16^{INK4}$ expression in fibroblasts has been consistently observed.[117] More studies are needed on $p16^{INK4}$ expression in HPV-immortalized cells to clarify the role of this gene product and of other cyclin-dependent kinase inhibitors in the suppression of immortalization.

It is unlikely that the cellular protein p53 is directly involved in control of immortalization. Mice with a p53 knockout phenotype develop relatively normally with an increased tumor incidence only in later life.[118] Scientists have suggested, however, that p53 plays an important indirect role in the progression of HPV-infected cells to immortalization and even to a malignant phenotype[74]: the inactivation of p53 by the E6 protein emerges as the event responsible for the prevention of the p53-mediated G1 arrest following DNA damage.[69,73] Accumulation of resulting mutations in the course of subsequent cell divisions is probably an important precondition for the eventual selection of cell clones with acquired mutations in cellular genes controlling immortalization. The functionally inactive p53 thus seems to represent the most important progression factor, possibly without a direct role in immortalization and transformation.

The stability of telomere sequences regulated by the telomere polymerase has been proposed to play an important role for cell proliferation and senescence.[119] Indeed, telomere shortening is observed consistently under conditions of cellular senescence whereas activation of telomerase and recovery of telomere length with telomere stabilization occurs in immortalized cells.[120] Telomere shortening is also observed in normal human and precrisis HPV-expressing cells with a recovery of telomere length after immortalization.[121] It will be interesting to analyze the telomerase activity in virally infected and not yet immortalized cells, to better understand the role of telomerase activation for the process of immortalization.

Hormones are supposed to play an important role in in vivo events related to immortalization of HPV-infected cells (see later discussion). High-risk HPVs harbor glucocorticoid responsive elements within the long control region.[122] Glucocorticoids substantially enhance immortalization by HPV 16 but fail to induce the same activity in HPV 11 infections.[123,124]

The hormone-dependent transformation by HPV 16 and ras can be inhibited by a hormone antagonist, RU 486.[125] Although all these studies were performed under tissue culture conditions, they support the clinical finding of marginally increased risk of cervical cancer after long-time oral contraceptive use.[126,127]

MALIGNANT PROGRESSION

The long time interval between acquisition of oncogenic infection and development of malignancy often confounds our ability to detect an association between the two. A substantial time lag exists between primary infection with high-risk HPVs and development of cervical intraepithelial neoplasias, carcinomata in situ, and finally invasive cancer. Cervical HPV infections occur most frequently when women are at a young age, soon after onset of sexual activity. By the age of 16 to 20 years, females in Western countries have high rates of HPV infection.[128,129] The peak incidence of cervical intraepithelial neoplasias occurs between 25 and 35 years, whereas cervical cancer incidence peaks between 55 and 65 years.[130] These data alone suggest that the latency period between primary infection and development of intraepithelial neoplasia averages several years, and that progression to invasive growth requires several decades.[54]

We are beginning to understand the molecular basis for this long time span. In situ hybridization studies[80,131] and analyses of HPV16 E6/E7 transgenic mice[132] frequently indicate an incremental up-regulation of HPV E6/E7 expression at each stage of neoplasia. Conversely, down-regulation of E6/E7 transcription takes place in HPV-immortalized nonmalignant cells after they are heterografted into immunocompromised animals or exposed to human macrophages in vitro.[133-135] At the same time, growth is markedly inhibited. The selective inhibition of HPV18 E6/E7 gene expression in cervical carcinoma cells also results in growth inhibition and loss of tumorigenicity.[61-63] High-risk HPV E6/E7 expression is therefore a prerequisite for continued growth stimulation. This finding suggests a correlation between the quantity of the viral oncogene product and the severity of the lesion because up-regulation of the former occurs in the course of progression. It is currently not known whether the same holds true for polyoma-type viruses. The selective E6/E7 down-regulation that occurs after nonmalignant cells are heterografted into immunocompromised animals shows, moreover, that the regulation of viral oncogene expression differs between immortalized and malignant HPV-harboring cells.

THE CIF CONCEPT

Several observations suggest that infection with the various genotypes of papillomaviruses has accompanied us since the prehominid phase of human development. Some papillomavirus types found in African monkeys and apes are more closely related to certain human genotypes than they are to one another. Obviously, in the course of our evolution we have developed a tight control of these infections that blocks viral activity in cells that are still capable of proliferating.

Assuming that functional papillomavirus oncoproteins are necessary for the malignant growth of HPV DNA containing cancer cells, these considerations led us to propose the existence of a cellular interference factor (CIF).[54,136,137] This posited CIF somehow interferes with the function of potential viral oncoproteins or down-regulates the activity of viral oncogenes in cells that are still capable of dividing, thus preventing the development of cancer. Although this theory has subsequently shifted from single factors to cellular interfering networks with several CIFs, it has nonetheless turned out to be a useful concept. Magnus von Knebel Doeberitz and other scientists[61–63] demonstrated that HPV-positive cervical carcinoma cells depended on the expression of specific viral genes (E6/E7) for the continuation of the cells growth properties. These genes are regularly preserved in these cancer cells and are genetically active.

Interestingly, in the course of malignant conversion, the viral ring molecule frequently (but not uniformly) integrates into host cell DNA, losing its structural integrity and part of the E1, E2, and L2 genes.[138,139] The integrational events result in a prolonged life span of E6/E7 messenger RNA, and thus contribute to a deregulation of the expression of these viral oncogenes. The regular presence and expression of E6/E7 in cancer cells, as initially noted by Elisabeth Schwarz and her colleagues in 1985,[138] were the first hints for an important role of these genes in growth stimulation and carcinogenesis.

Evidence for the existence of a functional control of viral oncoproteins originated from studies of HPV-immortalized human epithelial cells. The E6/E7 genes of high-risk HPVs are able to induce continuous growth of such cells, which, in contrast to most carcinoma cells, remain nonmalignant when injected into immunocompromised (nude) mice.[65,66] After a period of initial growth stimulation, most of the E6/E7-expressing cells go into senescence and eventually die. Only a small, usually clonal population continues to grow and becomes immortalized. As was shown later, the growth of these immortalized clones depends on the expression of the viral oncoproteins.

Why do most of the cells that express the viral oncoproteins go into senescence and die rather than becoming immortalized? A partial answer to this question came from experiments initiated by Pereira-Smith and Smith in 1981.[97] They performed cell fusion studies on SV40-immortalized cells. If cells from an immortalized clone were hybridized to normal human fibroblasts, the resulting hybrid cells regained "mortality"—they underwent senescence and died. Thus, the immortalized phenotype was a recessive trait because, despite continued expression of viral oncoproteins, the cells died when normal cellular genes were expressed. Moreover, hybridization of two different immortalized cell lines also caused cell senescence, suggesting that different clones were immortalized by different recessive mechanisms. Four *complementation groups* were established in these experiments. When cells of one complementation group were hybridized to those of another complementation group, the cells underwent senescence; when cells of the same complementation group were hybridized together, they remained immortal.[98,99] Similar data to these seen with SV40-immortalized cells have later been obtained by another group using HPV-immortalized cell lines.[100] These data demonstrated clearly for the first time that a loss of function of cellular genes is involved in the development of immortalization after these tumor virus infections. This seems to indicate the failure of the function of specific host cell genes that counteract the growth-stimulatory functions of viral oncoproteins. That there are four complementation groups suggests that at least four separate genes are engaged in this type of control.

At this moment, there exist only hints, rather than exact identifications, of the genes involved in this process. Howley and his colleagues showed that the high-risk HPV oncoprotein E6 interacts with the cellular protein p53[68] (see Chapter 5). In this process, p53 is degraded rapidly.[140] The protein p53 controls the execution of repair functions after DNA damage by arresting the cells in a prereplicative (G_1) phase. Its functional failure, mediated in this case by the viral E6 protein, results in a probably random accumulation of mutations within the host cell DNA during each replicative cycle. Presumably, these mutations eventually result in the accidental inactivation of specific genes within individual cells. The loss of the p53 function therefore appears to predispose the infected cell to mutations in specific regulatory pathways. In this interpretation, p53 is not a CIF gene; the absence of its normal function, however, predisposes the HPV infected cell to mutations in CIF pathways.[74]

Cyclin-dependent kinase inhibitors emerge as interesting candidate proteins for the interference with growth-stimulatory functions of viral oncoproteins. The normal cell cycle is driven by cyclins activated by cyclin-dependent kinases. Specific cyclins, for instance, effect the transition of a cell from a quiescent state to DNA replication and subsequent mitosis. The inhibitors play an important regulatory role and physiologically interfere with the function of cyclin/cyclin-dependent kinase complexes. Two cyclins (cyclin E and A) are activated by the high-risk HPV E7 oncoprotein.[141] This seems to explain, in part, HPV E7's growth-stimulatory function. The same viral oncoprotein binds a cellular regulatory protein, pRb, which in its unphosphorylated form binds and blocks an important transcription factor (E2F), required at least for the activation of cyclin A. The stimulation of cyclin A by E7 is therefore at least in part due to the release of E2F from pRb binding and thus is an indirect interaction.

Specific cyclin-dependent kinase inhibitors—p16, p21, and p27—accumulate during cellular senescence. One of them (p16) accumulates also as the consequence of pRb inactivation by E7, because it is negatively regulated by pRb. Another one (p27) has been shown to interact directly with an adenovirus oncoprotein (E1A), and recent observations suggest a similar interaction with high-risk HPV E7. It is therefore likely that genes engaged in the regulation of cyclin-dependent kinases govern the pathway that interferes with the function of viral oncoproteins (we call it the CIF-I pathway). The disruption of these regulatory genes due to mutation appears to be crucial for the unlimited life span—the immortalization—of high-risk HPV genome-harboring cells. That is, immortalization seems to be caused by the loss of a functional control of viral oncoproteins.

If viral oncoprotein functions are unimpaired in immortalized cells, why do these cells not continue to grow and form tumors when they are heterografted into an immunocompromised animal, in contrast to most malignant cells? The answer originated from a set of experiments: when implanted into immunocompromised animals, HPV-immortalized cells, in contrast to malignant HPV-infected cells, drastically reduce the transcriptional activity of the viral oncogenes.[133,134] Frank Rösl and colleagues[135,142,143] showed that this transcriptional repression can be mimicked under tissue culture conditions, when they added human macrophages to such cultures. Specific cytokines, particularly tumor necrosis factor–α (TNF-α),[144] excreted by the macrophages, apparently mediate the suppression of viral oncogene transcription. The intracellular pathway activated in this process is clearly different from CIF-I; it seems to involve at least one dephosphorylating enzyme (protein phosphatase 2A) and apparently, as the final step, a modification of the composition of a transcription factor (AP-1) that is essential for viral genome activity (Frank Rösl and associates, personal communication). This transcription factor usually consists of a pair of homodimeric or heterodimeric proteins (frequently c-jun/c-jun homodimers, or c-jun/c-fos heterodimers) binding to specific sites within promoter regions of a number of genes and activating the transcription. Under conditions of HPV transcriptional suppression, this complex is modified to contain mainly phosphorylated c-jun/fra-I heterodimers, which are apparently directly responsible for the blockade of viral oncogene transcription.

In malignant cells, this regulatory pathway that interferes with viral transcription (here designated as CIF-II) is not functional. Macrophages and TNF-α do not down-regulate viral oncogene transcription in these cells. The signaling cascade from TNF-α receptors, which obviously regulates the composition of AP-1 complexes, is interrupted, permitting the dysregulation of viral transcription and the unimpaired function of viral oncoproteins.

The CIF concept therefore points to the determinant role of viral oncogene products for malignant growth of infected cells. At the same time it points to the existence of two independent regulatory pathways that interfere with the function of viral oncoproteins and with the transcription of viral oncogenes. Progression to cancer is clearly a multistep event, requiring in addition to the uptake of viral DNA the modification of cellular genes engaged in the regulation of two independent pathways (CIF-I and CIF-II). Oncogenic viruses, in addition to their growth-stimulating activity, facilitate this process through mutagenic functions of their oncoproteins.

In addition to the molecular events decribed here, cancer development depends on the nonrecognition of viral antigens and the resulting nonresponsiveness of the host's immune system against the modified cells (see Chapter 5). For example, approximately one half of HPV-positive cervical carcinoma patients have no detectable immunological reactivity to HPV antigens. At present the reason is not fully understood. It is also unclear why the other half, who show some reactivity, cannot control the tumor growth. One interesting clue originates from our experiments, which point to the suppression of the induction of the macrophage-attracting protein-1 (MCP-1) by viral oncoproteins.[135] This suppression may prevent macrophage attraction and the processing of viral antigens by these cells and could represent a special mechanism by which these agents evade immunological control.

On the other hand, the fact that only a limited number of tumor virus–infected individuals eventually develop an infection-related cancer is probably to a large degree because the hosts have functioning immunological control.

The CIF concept seen with HPV and SV-40 may not be applicable to other human tumor virus infections or may be applicable in only a modified form. The complex system, however, should dissuade us from the naive view that solely immunological defense mechanisms protect us against these types of infections and their consequences, and it points to intracellular regulatory networks as a prime defense line in protection against malignant conversion.

CONCLUSIONS

After more than 100 years of intensive research, the role of infectious events in a substantial subset of human tumors has been clearly established. At present, an etiological relationship of virus infections to tumor development can be demonstrated in about 15% of the worldwide cancer burden. Approximately two thirds of these cancers are caused by papillomavirus infections; hepatitis B virus infections dominate in the remaining one third. Although often necessary, neither of these infections is sufficient for the induction of the respective cancer; additional modifications have to occur within the genome of the infected host cell or, as in EBV-induced lymphomas in immunocompromised patients, secondary events have to paralyze the host's immune system.

In addition to the virus infections currently established as etiologic factors in human tumors, there exists an increasing number of agents suspected to play a role in human cancer development. It is therefore likely that the percentage of malignant tumors linked to such infections will increase. The identification of viral infections as major risk factors for cancer development should pave the way for new strategies in cancer prevention, particularly by development of appropriate vaccines.

REFERENCES

1. McFadyan J, Hobday F. Note on the experimental "transmission of warts in the dog." J Comp Pathol Ther 1898;11:341–343.
2. Ciuffo G. Innesto positivo con filtrado di verrucae volgare. G Ital Mal Venereol 1907;48:12–15.
3. Rous P. Transmission of a malignant new growth by means of a cell-free filtrate. Am J Med Assoc 1911;56:198.
4. Gross L. Susceptibility of newborn mice of an otherwise apparently "resistant" strain to inoculation with leukemia. Proc Soc Exp Biol Med 1950;73:246–248.
5. Epstein MA, Achong BG, Barr YM. Virus particles in cultured lymphoblasts from Burkitt's lymphoma. Lancet 1964;1:702–703.
6. Burkitt D. A sarcoma involving the jaws in African children. Br J Surg 1958;45:218–223.
7. Beasley RP, Hwang LY, Lin CC, Chien CS. Hepatocellular carcinoma and hepatitis B virus: a prospective study of 22,707 men in Taiwan. Lancet 1981;2:1129–1133.
8. Poiesz BJ, Ruscetti FW, Gazdar AF, et al. Detection and isolation of type C retrovirus particles from fresh and cultured lymphocytes of a patient with a cutaneous T-cell lymphoma. Proc Natl Acad Sci USA 1980;77:7415–7419.
9. Hinuma Y, Nagata K, Hanaoka M, et al. Adult T cell leukemia antigen in an ATL cell line and detection of antibodies to the antigen in human sera. Proc Natl Acad Sci USA 1991;78:6476–6480.
10. zur Hausen H. Papillomaviruses—a major cause of human cancers. Biochim Biophys Acta Rev on Cancer, 1996;1288:F55–F78.
11. Rous P, Beard JW. Carcinomatous changes in virus-induced papillomas of the skin of the rabbit. Proc Soc Exp Biol Med 1934;32:578–580.
12. Rous P, Beard JW. The progression to carcinoma of virus-induced rabbit papilloma (Shope). J Exp Med 1935;62:523–548.
13. Rous P, Kidd JG. The carcinogenic effect of a papillomavirus on the tarred skin of rabbits. I. Description of the phenomenon. J Exp Med 1938;67:399–422.
14. Rous P, Friedewald WF. The effect of chemical carcinogens on virus-induced rabbit papillomas. J Exp Med 1944;79:511–537.
15. Ito Y, Evans CA. Induction of tumors in domestic rabbits with nucleic acid preparations from partially purified Shope papilloma virus and from extracts of the papillomas of domestic and cotton tail rabbits. J Exp Med 1961;114:485–491.
16. Olson C, Pamukcu AM, Brobst DF, Kowalczyk T, Satter EJ, Price JM. A urinary bladder tumor induced by a bovine cutaneous papilloma agent. Cancer Res 1959;19:779–782.
17. Friedmann J-C, Levy J-P, Lasnaret J, Thomas M, Boiron M, Bernard J. Induction de fibromes sous-cutanés chez le hamster doré par inoculation d'extrait

acellulaires de papillomes bovins et leur transformation maligne par greffes isologues. Compt Rend Acad Sci (Paris) 1963;257:2328–2331.

18. Boiron M, Levy J-P, Thomas M, Friedmann JC, Bernard J. Some properties of bovine papilloma virus. Nature 1964;201:423–424.

19. Black PH, Hartley JW, Rowe WP, Huebner RJ. Transformation of bovine tissue culture cells by bovine papilloma virus. Nature 1963;199:1016–1018.

20. Thomas M, Levy J-P, Tanzer J, Boiron M, Bernard J. Transformation in vitro de cellules de peau de veau embryonnaire sous l'action d'extraits acellulaires de papillomes bovins. Compt Rend Acad Sci (Paris) 1963;257:2155–2158.

21. Lewandowsky F, Lutz W. Ein Fall einer bisher nicht beschriebenen Hauterkrankung (Epidermodysplasia verruciformis). Arch Dermatol Syph (Berlin) 1922;141:193–203.

22. Lutz W. A propos de l'epidermodysplasie verruciforme. Dermatologica 1946; 92:30–43.

23. Jablonska S, Millewski B. Zur Kenntnis der Epidermodysplasia verruciformis Lewandowsky-Lutz. Dermatologica 1957;115:1–22.

24. Jablonska S, Dabrowski J, Jakubowicz K. Epidermodysplasia verruciformis as a model in studies on the role of papovaviruses in oncogenesis. Cancer Res 1972;32:583–589.

25. zur Hausen H, Meinhof W, Scheiber W, Bornkamm GW. Attempts to detect virus-specific DNA sequences in human tumors: I. Nucleic acid hybridizations with complementary RNA of human wart virus. Int J Cancer 1974;13:650–656.

26. zur Hausen H. Condylomata acuminata and human genital cancer. Cancer Res 1976;36:530.

27. Gissmann L, zur Hausen H. Human papilloma viruses: physical mapping and genetic heterogeneity. Proc Nat Acad Sci USA 1976;73:1310–1313.

28. Gissmann L, Pfister H, zur Hausen H. Human papilloma viruses (HPV): characterization of four different isolates. Virology 1977;76:569–580.

29. Orth G, Favre M, Croissant O. Characterization of a new type of human papillomavirus that causes skin warts. J Virol 1977;24:108–120.

30. Meisels A, Fortin R. Condylomatous lesions of the cervix and vagina. I. Cytologic patterns. Acta Cytol 1976;20:505–509.

31. Della Torre G, Pilotti S, de Palo G, Rilke F. Viral particles in cervical condylomatous lesions. Tumori 1978;64:459–463. 32.Laverty CR, Russel P, Hills E, Booth N. The significance of non-condyloma wart virus infection of the cervical transformation zone: a review with discussion of two illustrative cases. Acta Cytol 1978;22:195–201.

33. Meisels A, Roy M, Fortier M, Morin C, Casas-Cordero M, Shah KV, Turgeon H. Human papillomavirus infection of the cervix: the atypical condyloma. Act Cytologica 1981;25:7–16.

34. Orth G, Jablonska S, Jarzabek-Chorzelska M, Rzesa G, Obalek S, Favre M, Croissant O. Characteristics of the lesions and risk of malignant conversion as related to the type of the human papillomavirus involved in epidermodysplasia verruciformis. Cancer Res 1979;39:1074–1082.

35. Gissmann L, zur Hausen H. Partial characterization of viral DNA from human genital warts (condylomata acuminata). Int J Cancer 1980;25:605–609.

36. Gissmann L, Diehl V, Schultz-Coulon H, zur Hausen H. Molecular cloning and characterization of human papillomavirus DNA from a laryngeal papilloma. J Virol 1982;44:393–400.

37. Dürst M, Gissmann L, Ikenberg H, zur Hausen H. A papillomavirus DNA from a cervical carcinoma and its prevalence in cancer biopsy samples from different geographic regions. Proc Natl Acad Sci USA 1983;80:3812–3815.

38. Boshart M, Gissmann L, Ikenberg H, Kleinheinz A, Scheurlen W, zur Hausen H. A new type of papillomavirus DNA, its presence in genital cancer and in cell lines derived from genital cancer. EMBO J 1984;3:1151–1157.

39. Schiffman MH, Bauer HM, Hoover RN, Glass AG, Cadell DM, Rush BB, Scott DR, Sherman ME, Kurman RJ, Wacholder S, et al. Epidemiologic evidence showing that human papillomavirus infection causes most cervical intra-epithelial neoplasia. J Natl Cancer Inst 1993;85:958–964.

40. Muñoz N, Bosch FX, de Sanjose S, Tafur L, Izarzugaza I, Gili M, Viladiu P, Navarro C, Martos C, Asunce N. The causal link between human papillomavirus and invasive cervical cancer: a population-based case-control study in Colombia and Spain. Int J Cancer 1992;52:743–749.

41. Bosch FX, Manos MM, Muñoz N, Sherman M, Jansen AM, Peto J, Schiffman MH, Moreno V, Kurman R, Shah KV. Prevalence of human papillomavirus in cervical cancer: A worldwide perspective. International biological study on cervical cancer (IBSCC) Study Group. J Natl Cancer Inst 1995;87:796–802.

42. Matsukura T, Sugase M. Identification of genital human papillomaviruses in cervical biopsy specimen: segregation of specific virus types in specific clin-icopathologic lesions. Int J Cancer 1995;61:13–22.

43. zur Hausen H. Papillomaviruses as carcinomaviruses. Adv Viral Oncol Klein G, ed. Raven Press, New York: vol. 8, pp. 1–26.

44. zur Hausen H. Papillomviren, die "heimlichen" Krebserreger? Robert Koch Found Bull Commun 1983;6:9–17.

45. Suzich JA, Ghim S-J, Palmer-Hill FJ, White W, Tamura JK, Bell JA, Newsome JA, Jenson AB, Schlegel R. Systemic immunization with papillomavirus L1 protein completely prevents the development of viral mucosal papillomas. Proc Natl Acad Sci USA 1995;92:11553–11557.

46. Schlehofer JR, Gissmann L, Matz B, zur Hausen H. Herpes simplex virus induced amplification of SV40 sequences in transformed Chinese hamster cells. Int J Cancer 1983;32:99–103.

47. Schmitt J, Mergener K, Gissmann L, Schlehofer RJ, zur Hausen H. Amplifica-tion of bovine papillomavirus DNA by N-methyl-N'-nitro-N-nitrosoguanidine, UV-irradiation, or infection by herpes simplex virus. Virology 1989;172:73–81.

48. Chang Y, Cesarman E, Pessin MS, Lee F, Culpepper J, Knowles DM, Moore PS. Identification of herpesvirus-like sequences in AIDS-associated Kaposi's sarcoma. Science 1994;266:1865–1869.

49. Shamanin V, Glover M, Rausch C, Proby C, Leigh IM, zur Hausen H, de Villiers E-M. Specific types of human papillomavirus found in benign prolif-erations and carcinomas of the skin in immunosuppressed patients. Cancer Res 1994;54:4610–4613.

50. Shamanin V, zur Hausen H, Lavergne D, Proby C, Leigh IM, Neumann C, Hamm H, Goos M, Haustein U-F, Jung EG, Plewig G, Wolff H, de Villiers E-M. HPV infections in non-melanoma skin cancers from renal transplant recipients and non-immunosuppressed patients. J Natl Cancer Inst 1996;88: 802–811.

51. Berkhout RJM, Tieben LM, Smits HL, Bouwes Bavinck JN, Vermeer BJ, ter Schegget J. Nested PCR approach for detection and typing of epidermo-

dysplasia verruciformis-associated human papillomavirus types in cutaneous cancers from renal transplant recipients. J Clin Microbiol 1995;33:690–695.

52. Gross L. Oncogenic Viruses, 3rd ed. Oxford: Pergamon;1983.

53. Ellermann V, Bang O. Experimentelle Leukämie bei Hühnern. Centralbl. f. Bakt. Abt.I. (Orig.) 1908;46:595–609.

54. zur Hausen H. Intracellular surveillance of persisting viral infections: Human genital cancer resulting from failing cellular control of papillomavirus gene expression. Lancet 1986;2:489–491.

55. Koch R. 1891. Über bakteriologische Forschung. Verhandlgn. 10. Intern. Med. Congress, Berlin, Vol. 1, p.35.

56. Evans AS. Epidemiological concepts and methods. In: Evans AS, ed. Viral Infections of Humans, Epidemiology and Control. London: Wiley;1976:1–32.

57. zur Hausen H. Oncogenic herpesviruses. Biochim Biophys Acta 1975;417:25–53.

58. Dillner J, Wiklund F, Lenner P, Eklund C, Frederiksson-Shanazarian V, Schiller JT, Hibma M, Hallmans G, Stendahl U. Antibodies against linear and conformational epitopes of human papillomavirus type 16 that independently associate with incident cervical cancer. Int J Cancer 1995;60:377–382.

59. Fujii T, Matsushima Y, Yajima M, Sugimura T, Terada M. Serum antibody against unfused recombinant E7 protein of human papillomavirus type 16 in cervical cancer patients. Jpn J Cancer Res 1995;86:28–34.

60. zur Hausen H, ed. Human pathogenic papillomaviruses. Springer-Verlag, Heidelberg-New York, Curr Top Microbiol Immunol 1994;186:1994.

61. von Knebel Doeberitz M, Oltersdorf T, Schwarz E, Gissmann L. Correlation of modified human papillomavirus early gene expression with altered growth properties in C4-1 cervical carcinoma cells. Cancer Res 1988;48:3780–3786.

62. von Knebel Doeberitz M, Rittmüller C, zur Hausen H, Dürst M. Inhibition of tumorigenicity of cervical cancer cells in nude mice by HPV E6-E7 antisense RNA. Int J Cancer 1992;51:831–834.

63. von Knebel Doeberitz M, Rittmüller C, Aengeneyndt F, Jansen-Dürr P, Spitkovsky D. Reversible repression of papillomavirus oncogene expression in cervical carcinoma cells: consequences for the phenotype and E6-p53 and E7-pRB interactions. J Virol 1994;68:2811–2821.

64. zur Hausen H. Genital papillomavirus infections. In: Viruses and Cancer, PWJ Rigby, NM Wilkie, eds. Cambridge University Press;1986:83–90.

65. Dürst M, Dzarlieva-Petrusevska RT, Boukamp P, Fusenig NE, Gissmann L. Molecular and cytogenetic analysis of immortalized human primary keratinocytes obtained after transfection with human papillomavirus type 16 DNA. Oncogene 1987;1:251–256.

66. Pirisi L, Yasumoto S, Fellery M, Doninger JK, DiPaolo JA. Transformation of human fibroblasts and keratinocytes with human papillomavirus type 16 DNA. J Virol 1987;61:1061–1066.

67. Dyson N, Howley PM, Münger K, Harlow E. The human papillomavirus-16 E7 oncoprotein is able to bind to the retinoblastoma gene product. Science 1989;243:934–937.

68. Werness BA, Levine AJ, Howley PM. Association of human papillomavirus types 16 and 18 E6 proteins with p53. Science 1990;248:76–79.

69. Kessis TD, Slebos RJ, Nelson WG, Kastan MB, Plunkett BS, Hau SM, Lörincz AT, Hedrick L, Cho KR. Human papillomavirus 16 E6 expression disrupts the

p53-mediated cellular response to DNA damage. Proc Natl Acad Sci USA 1993;90:3988–3992.

70. Demers GW, Forster SA, Halbert CL, Galloway DA. Growth arrest by induction of p53 in DNA damaged keratinocytes is bypassed by human papillomavirus 16 E7. Proc Natl Acad Sci USA 1994;91:4382–4386.

71. Hickman ES, Picksley SM, Vousden KH. Cells expressing HPV16 E7 continue cell cycle progression following DNA damage induced p53 activation. Oncogene 1994;9:2177–2181.

72. Slebos RJC, Lee MH, Plunkett BS, Kessis TD, Williams BO, Jacks T, Hedrick L, Kastan MB, Cho KR. p53-dependent G$_1$ arrest involves pRb-related proteins and is disrupted by the human papillomavirus 16 E7 oncoprotein. Proc Natl Acad Sci USA 1994;91:5320–5324.

73. White AE, Livanos EM, Tlsty TD. Differential disruption of genomic integrity and cell cycle regulation in normal human fibroblasts by the HPV oncoproteins. Genes Dev 1994;8:666–677.

74. zur Hausen H. Human papillomaviruses in the pathogenesis of anogenital cancer. Virology 1991;184:9–13.

75. zur Hausen H. Human papillomaviruses and their possible role in squamous cell carcinomas. Curr Top Microbiol Immunol 1977;78:1–30.

76. Shay JW, Wright WE. Quantitation of the frequency of immortalization of normal human diploid fibroblasts by SV40 large T-antigen. Cancer Res 1989;184:109–118.

77. Henle W, Diehl V, Kohn G, zur Hausen H, Henle G. Herpes-type virus and chromosome marker in normal leukocytes after growth with irradiated Burkitt cells. Science 1967;157:1064–1065.

78. Yamamoto N, Okada M, Koyanagi Y, Kannagi Y, Kannagi M, Hinuma Y. Transformation of human leukocytes by cocultivation with an adult T-cell leukemia virus producer cell line. Science 1992;217:737–739.

79. McDougall JK. Immortalization and transformation of human cells by human papillomavirus. Curr Top Microbiol Immunol 1994;186:101–119.

80. Dürst M, Glitz D, Schneider A, zur Hausen H. Human papillomavirus type 16 (HPV16) gene expression and DNA replication in cervical neoplasia: analysis by in situ hybridization. Virology 1992;189:132–140.

81. Schneider-Maunoury S, Croissant O, Orth G. Integration of human papillomavirus type 16 DNA sequences: a possible early event in the progression to genital tumors. J Virol 1987;61:3295–3298.

82. Stanley MA, Browne HM, Appleby M, Minson AC. Properties of a non-tumorigenic human cervical keratinocyte line. Int J Cancer 1989;43:672–676.

83. Bedell MA, Hudson JB, Golub TR, Turyk ME, Hosken M, Wilbanks GD, Laimins LA. Amplification of human papillomavirus genomes in vitro is dependent on epithelial differentiation. J Virol 1991;65:2254–2260.

84. Lowy DR, Dvoretzky I, Shober R, Law M-F, Engel L, Howley PM. In vitro tumorigenic transformation by a defined subgenomic fragment of bovine papilloma virus DNA. Nature 1980;287:72–74.

85. Watts SL, Phelps WC, Ostrow RS, Zachow KR, Faras AJ. Cellular transformation by human papillomavirus DNA in vitro. Science 1984;225:634–636.

86. Yasumoto S, Burkhardt AL, Doniger J, DiPaolo JA. Human papillomavirus type 16 DNA-induced malignant transformation of NIH 3T3 cells. J Virol 1986;57:572–577.

87. Bedell MA, Jones KH, Laimins LA. The E6-E7 region of human papilloma-virus type 18 is sufficient for transformation of NIH 3T3 and rat-1 cells. J Virol 1987;61:3635–3540.

88. Watanabe S, Yoshiike K. Transformation of rat 3Y1 cells by human papillo-mavirus type-18 DNA. Int. J. Cancer 1988;41:896–900.

89. Matlashewski G, Schneider J, Banks L, Jones N, Murray A, Crawford L. Human papillomavirus type 16 DNA cooperates with activated ras in transform-ing primary cells. EMBO J 1987;6:1741–1746.

90. Phelps WC, Yee CL, Münger K, Howley PM. The human papillomavirus type 16 E7 gene encodes transactivation and transformation functions similar to those of adenovirus E1A. Cell 1988;53:539–547.

91. Kaur P, McDougall JK. Characterization of primary human keratinocytes transformed by human papillomavirus type 18. J Virol 1988;62:1917–1924.

92. Rhim JS, Webber MM, Bello D, Lee MS, Arnstein P, Chen LS, Jay G. Stepwise immortalization and transformation of adult human prostate epithelial cells by a combination of HPV-18 and v-Ki-ras. Proc Natl Acad Sci USA 1994;91: 11874–11878.

93. Tsao SW, Mok SC, Fey EG, Fletcher JA, Wan TS, Chew EC, Muto MG, Knapp RC, Berkowitz RS. Characterization of human ovarian surface epithelilal cells immortalized by human papilloma viral oncogenes (HPV-E6E7 ORFs). Exp Cell Res 1995;218:499–507.

94. Schlegel R, Phelps WC, Zhang YL, Barbosa M. Quantitative keratinocyte assay detects two biological activities of human papillomavirus DNA and identifies viral types associated with cervical carcinoma. EMBO J 1988;7:3181–3187.

95. Münger K, Phelps WC, Bubb V, Howley PM, Schlegel R. The E6 and E7 genes of human papillomavirus type 16 are necessary and sufficient for trans-formation of primary human keratinocytes. J Virol 1989;63:4417–4423.

96. zur Hausen H, de Villiers EM. Human papillomaviruses Annu Rev Microbiol 1994;48:427–447.

97. Pereira-Smith OM, Smith JR. Expression of SV40 antigen in finite lifespan hybrids of normal and SV40-transformed fibroblasts. Somat Cell Genet 1981; 7:411–421.

98. Pereira-Smith OM, Smith JR. Genetic analysis of indefinite division in human cells: identification of four complementation groups. Proc Natl Acad Sci USA 1988;85:6042–6046.

99. Whitaker NJ, Kidston EL, Redell RR. Finite lifespan of hybrids formed by fusion of different simian virus 40-immortalized human cell lines. J Virol 1992;66:1202–1206.

100. Chen TM, Peccoraro G, Defendi V. Genetic analysis of in vitro progression of human papillomavirus-transfected human cervical cells. Cancer Res 1993;53: 1167–1171.

101. zur Hausen H. Disrupted dichotomous intracellular control of human pa-pillomavirus infection in cancer of the cervix. Lancet 1994;343:955–957.

102. Smith PP, Bryant EM, Kaur P, McDougall JK. Cytogenetic analysis of eight human papillomavirus immortalized human keratinocyte cell lines. Int J Can-cer 1989;44:1124–1131.

103. Smith PP, Friedman CL, Bryant EM, McDougall JK. Viral integration and fragile sites in human papillomavirus-immortalized human keratinocyte cell lines. Genes Chromosomes Cancer 1992;5:150–157.

104. Klingelhutz AJ, Smith PP, Garrett LR, Mcdougall JK. Alteration of the DCC tumor-suppressor gene in tumorigenic HPV-18 immortalized human kerati-nocytes transformed by nitrosomethyl-urea. Oncogene 1993;8:95–99.
105. Montgomery KD, Tedford KL, McDougall JK. Genetic instability of chromo-some 3 in HPV-immortalized and tumorigenic keratinocytes. Genes Chromo-somes Cancer 1995;14:97–105.
106. Srivatsan ES, Benedict WF, Stanbridge EJ. Implication of chromosome 11 in the suppression of neoplastic expression in human hybrid cells. Cancer Res 1986;46:6174–6179.
107. Saxon PJ, Srivatsan ES, Stanbridge EJ. Introduction of human chromosome 11 via microcell transfer controls tumorigenic expression of HeLa cells. EMBO J 1986;5:3461–3466.
108. Koi M, Morita H, Yamada H, Satoh H, Barrett JC, Oshimura M. Normal human chromosome 11 suppresses tumorigenicity of human cervical tumor cell line SiHa. Mol. Carcinogen. 1989;2:12–21.
109. Koi M, Johnson LA, Kalikin LM, Little PFR, Nakamura Y, Feinberg AP. Tumor cell growth arrest caused by subchromosomal transferable DNA frag-ments from chromosome 11. Science 1993;260:361–364.
110. Ning Y, Weber JL, Ledbetter DH, Smith JR, Pereira-Smith OM. Genetic anal-ysis of indefinite division in human cells: evidence for a cell senescence-re-lated gene(s) on human chromosome 4. Proc Natl Acad Sci USA 1991;8: 5635–5639.
111. Uejima H, Mitsuya K, Kugoh H, Horikawa I, Oshimura M. Normal human chromosome 2 induces cellular senescence in the human cervical carcinoma cell line SiHa. Genes Chromosomes Cancer 1995;14:120–127.
112. Hensler PJ, Annab LA, Barrett JC, Pereira-Smith OM. A gene involved in the control of cellular senescence localized to human chromosome 1q. Mol Cell Biol 1994;14:2291–2297.
113. zur Hausen H, Rösl F. Pathogenesis of cancer of the cervix. Cold Spring Harbor Symp. Quantit Biol 1994;59:623–628.
114. Serrano M, Hannon GJ, Beach D. A new regulatory motif in cell cycle control causing specific inhibition of cyclin D/CDK4. Nature 1993;366:704–707.
115. Otterson GA, Kratzke RA, Coxon A, Kim YW, Kaye F. Absence of p16^{INK4} protein is restricted to the subset of lung cancer lines that retain wildtype RB. Oncogene 1994;9:3375–3378.
116. Yeager T, Stadler W, Belair C, Puthenveettil J, Olopade O, Reznikoff C. In-creased p16 levels correlate with pRb alterations in human urothelial cells. Cancer Res 1995;55:493–497.
117. Rogan EM, Bryan TM, Hukku B, Maclean K, Chang AC, Moy EL, Englezou A, Warneford SG, Dalla-Pozza L, Reddel RR. Alterations in p53 and p16INK expression and telomere length during spontaneous immortalization of Li-Fraumeni syndrome fibroblasts. Mol Cell Biol 1995;15:4745–4753.
118. Donehower LA, Harvey M, Hagle BL, McArthur MJ, Montgomery CA, Jr, Butel JS, Bradley A. Mice deficient for p53 are developmentally normal but susceptible to spontaneous tumours. Nature 1992;356:215–221.
119. Greider CW. Telomeres. Curr Opin Cell Biol 1991;3:444–451.
120. Prowse KR, Greider CW. Developmental and tissue-specific regulation of mouse telomerase and telomere length. Proc Natl Acad Sci USA 1995;92: 4818–4822.
121. Klingenhutz AJ, Barber SA, Smith PP, Dyer K, McDougall JK. Restoration of

telomeres in HPV-immortalized human anogenital epithelial cells. Mol Cell Biol 1994;14:961–969.

122. Gloss B, Bernard H-U, Seedorf K, Klock G. The upstream regulatory region of the human papillomavirus-16 contains an E2 protein-independent enhancer which is specific for cervical carcinoma cells and regulated by glucocorticoid hormones. EMBO J 1987;6:3635–3743.

123. Mittal R, Tsutsumi K, Pater A, Pater MM. Human papillomavirus type 16 expression in cervical keratinocytes: role of progesteron and glucocorticoid hormones. Obstet Gynecol 1993;81:5–12.

124. Pater MM, Hughes GA, Hyslop DE, Nakshatri H, Pater A. Glucocortocoid-dependent oncogenic transformation by type 16 but not type 11 human papilloma virus. Nature 1988;335:832–835.

125. Pater MM, Pater A. RU486 inhibits glucocorticoid hormone-dependent oncogenesis by human papillomavirus type 16 DNA. Virology 1991;183:799–802.

126. Hildesheim A, Reeves WC, Brinton LA, Lavery C, Brenes M, de la Guardia ME, Godoy J, Rawls WE. Association of oral contraceptive use and human papillomaviruses in invasive cervical cancers. Int J Cancer 1990;45:860–864.

127. Muñoz N, Bosch FX, de Sanjosé S, Shah KV. The role of HPV in the etiology of cervical cancer. Mutat Res 1994;305:293– 301.

128. de Villiers E-M, Wagner D, Schneider A, Wesch H, Micklaw H, Wahrendorf J, Papendick U, zur Hausen H. Human papillomavirus infections in women withhout and with abnormal cervical cytology. Lancet 1987;2:703–706.

129. IARC Monograph on Evaluation of Carcinogenic Risks of Humans. Human Papillomaviruses. Lyon: IARC Lyon;1995 vol. 64.

130. de Villiers E-M, Wagner D, Schneider A, Wesch H, Munz F, Micklaw H, zur Hausen H. Human papillomavirus DNA in women without and with cytological abnormalities: results of a five-year follow-up study. Gynecol Oncol 1992; 44:33–39.

131. Stoler MH, Rhodes CR, Whitbeck A, Wolinske SM, Chow LT, Broker TR. Human papillomavirus type 16 and 18 gene expression in cervical neoplasias. Hum Pathol 1992;23:117–128.

132. Arbeit JM. Transgenic models of experimental neoplasia and multi-stage carcinogenesis. Cancer Surveys 1996;26:7–34.

133. Bosch F, Schwarz E, Boukamp P, Fusenig NE, Bartsch D, zur Hausen H. Suppression in vivo of human papillomavirus type 18 E6-E7 gene expression in nontumorigenic HeLa-fibroblast hybrid cells. J Virol 1990;64:4743–4754.

134. Dürst M, Bosch F, Glitz D, Schneider A, zur Hausen H. Inverse relationship between HPV 16 early gene expression and cell differentiation in nude mice epithelial cysts and tumors induced by HPV positive human cell lines. J Virol 1991;65:796–804.

135. Rösl F, Lengert M, Albrecht J, Kleine K, Zawatzky R, Schraven B, zur Hausen H. Differential regulation of the JE gene encoding the monocyte chemoattractant protein (MCP-1) in cervical carcinoma cells and derived hybrids. J Virol 1994;68:2142–2150.

136. zur Hausen H. Cell-virus gene balance hypothesis of carcinogenesis. Behring Inst Mitt 1977;61:23–30.

137. zur Hausen H. Papillomaviruses in anogenital cancer: a model to understand the role of viruses in human cancers. Cancer Res 1989;49:4677–4681.

138. Schwarz E, Freese UK, Gissmann L, Mayer W, Roggenbuck B, zur Hausen H.

Structure and transcription of human papillomavirus type 18 and 16 sequences in cervical carcinoma cells. Nature 1985;314:111–114.

139. Yee C, Krishnan-Hewlett I, Baker CC, Schlegel R, Howley PM. Presence and expression of human papillomavirus sequences in human cervical carcinoma cell lines. Am J Pathol 1985;119:361–366.

140. Scheffner M, Werness BA, Huibregtse JM, Levine AJ, Howley PM. The E6 oncoprotein encoded by human papillomaviruses 16 and 18 promotes the degradation of p53. Cell 1990;63:1129–1136.

141. Zerfass K, Schulze A, Spitkovsky D, Friedman V, Henglein B, Jansen-Dürr P. Sequential activation of cyclin E and cyclin A gene expression by human papillomavirus type 16 E7 through sequences necessary for transformation. J Virol 1995;69:6389–6399.

142. Rösl F, Dürst M, zur Hausen H. Selective suppression of human papillomavirus transcription in non-tumorigenic cells by 5-azacytidine. EMBO J 1988; 7:1321–1328.

143. Rösl F, Achtstetter T, Hutter K-J, Bauknecht T, Futterman G, zur Hausen H. Extinction of the HPV 18 upstream regulatory region in cervical carcinoma cells after fusion with non-tumorigenic human keratinocytes under non-selective conditions. EMBO J 1991;10:1337–1345.

144. Smits PHM, Smits HL, Minnaar R, Hemmings BA, Mayer-Jaekel RE, Schuurman R, van der Noordaa J, ter Schegget J. The trans-activation of the HPV 16 long control region in human cells with a deletion in the short arm of chromosome 11 is mediated by the 55kDa regulatory subunit of protein phosphatase 2A. EMBO J 1992;11:4601–4606.

5
Immunosuppression, Infection, and Cancer

JUDITH E. KARP AND WILLIAM A. BLATTNER

The relationships among immunodeficiency, infection, and cancer have been well documented for several decades. The predisposition to develop neoplasia was perhaps first observed in patients with genetically determined disorders of cellular and humoral immunity; later, not surprisingly, it was seen in patients receiving immunosuppressive therapies for autoimmune disorders and/or transplantation. We see this propensity now in the setting of human immunodeficiency virus (HIV) and acquired immunodeficiency syndrome (AIDS). The malignancies arising in the context of insufficient immune function are frequently of lymphoid origin, most commonly B cells, but also epithelial- (in particular, anogenital cancers, including cervical cancer in women) and endothelial-derived cancers (in particular, Kaposi's sarcoma).

There are three common themes underlying the emergence and perpetuation of the diverse malignancies in these heterogeneous immunocompromised hosts:

1. The absence of protective immune surveillance to recognize and eradicate abnormal clones
2. Disruption of the normal balance between cell proliferation and differentiation that may be augmented by abnormal growth factor expression
3. Chronic antigenic stimulation, sometimes accompanied by infection with "oncogenic" pathogens, which leads to expansion of one or more cell cohorts (Table 5.1).

Moreover, these malignancies may share a common underlying molecular theme—namely, aberrations in the mechanisms associated with the ability of the cell to recognize, respond to, and repair DNA damage. Malfunc-

Table 5.1 Selected potential factors involved in the pathogenesis of malignancies arising in immunologically disturbed states

---

Host factors: disruption of genomic integrity, orderly proliferation, and differentiation
  Oncogene activation or dysregulation (e.g., c-myc, cyclin D1/bc1-1, bc1-2, bc1-6 ras)
  Tumor suppressor inactivation (e.g., p53, Rb, cyclin-dependent kinase inhibitors)
  Cytokine dysregulation (e.g., IL-2, IL-6, IL-10, IL-12, fibroblast growth factors)
  Defective repair of DNA Damage (including insertional mutagenesis)

Infectious pathogens: transformation and chronic antigenic stimulation
  DNA viruses (e.g., EBV, KSHV, HPV)
  Retroviruses (e.g., HTLV-1, HIV)
  Bacteria (e.g., *Helicobacter*)
  Parasitic (e.g, *Strongyloides* in HTLV-1)

---

tions along such pathways, in turn, permit the emergence and establishment of a genetically aberrant clone that can progressively accumulate additional genetic lesions and undergo expansion. AIDS lymphomas exemplify particularly well the multiple interactive mechanisms that may operate, to varying degrees, to effect the emergence and perpetuation of malignant lymphocytes. Uncovering the molecular lesions that cause immune dysfunction, whether inherited or acquired, and elucidating mechanisms that permit malignant transformation in this setting will allow us to develop targeted molecular strategies that may be applicable to the prevention and therapy of cancers in general.

This chapter provides an overview of selected mechanisms that modulate the balance among proliferation, differentiation, survival, and death of lymphohematopoietic cells. The perturbation and dysregulation of these mechanisms by genetic lesions or inflammatory stimuli (including infectious pathogens), in turn, lead to immunodeficiency and cancer.

GENETIC IMMUNODEFICIENCIES: DISORDERS OF DNA REPAIR

Various studies have uncovered diverse mechanisms of DNA repair as being critical to the appropriate generation, maintenance, and expansion of targeted immune responses. In this regard, the rare genetic immunodeficiency syndromes are instructive. For example, the molecular dissection of the defects in ataxia-telangiectasia (AT) and variants of severe combined immunodeficiency (SCID) demonstrate an important relationship between the process of repair of DNA damage and V(D)J (variable, V; diversity, D; joining, J) recombination.[1-3] In many respects, V(D)J recombination can be viewed as a type of physiologic DNA repair that is crucial to the development of a diversified repertoire of antigen-processing cells generated in response to, and with specificity for, a variety of antigenic stimuli.[1] The rearrangement of gene sequences encoding the specific components (V, D, J) of T- and B-cell antigen receptors is intrinsic to the normal morphologic and functional differentiation of T and B cells.[1,4] In this regard, both AT and SCID manifest profound defects in both cellular and humoral immunity, striking predisposition to lymphoproliferative malignancies, intrinsic genetic instability, and defective repair of DNA damage that may relate to defects in one or more components that govern V(D)J recombination.[5]

It is becoming increasingly clear that many of the disorders characterized by defective DNA repair processes, including V(D)J recombination, represent a family of diseases, related on the molecular level as well as in terms of cellular behavior and clinical phenotype. On the molecular level, the diseases typically involve the defective expression of genes that encode putative phosphatidylinositol kinases (PIKs). These molecules appear to be intimately involved in cell cycle control, DNA repair, and mitotic recombination events.[6] In one member of this disease family—SCID—the DNA-dependent protein kinase (DNA-PK) is disrupted; although DNA-PK exhibits structural homology to the PIKs, it functionally exhibits serine-threonine kinase activity with no lipid kinase activity detected to date. The exact functions of the other PIKs in this family of diseases are not yet deciphered. Nonetheless, it appears that the loss of such PIK activity could, at least in theory, translate into a clinical constellation typified by radiation hypersensitivity, immunodeficiency, and cancer predisposition. In this regard, the inherited diseases of DNA repair are instructive paradigms, because the mechanisms underlying the genomic instability in such genetic disorders may pertain to diverse types of immune deficiencies, including HIV infection and AIDS.

Ataxia-Telangiectasia: A Classical Disease of Disordered Cell Cycle Checkpoint Controls

AT is an inherited multisystem disorder, arising from mutations in a recessive gene on chromosome 11q23.1.[7] It is characterized on both the cellular and molecular levels by chromosomal fragility and a heightened sensitivity to DNA damage (especially from ionizing radiation).[5] Clinical observations and molecular and cellular biologic studies of this rare and tragic disorder have proved that the AT gene plays a critical role in cell cycle regulation, particularly in response to certain types of DNA damage, and thus is a crucial determinant of cell–environment interactions. People with AT have a striking incidence of lymphoproliferative malignancies (lymphoid leukemias and lymphomas), with a risk that is 70 to 250 times higher than that in the nonaffected population.[8] Overall, roughly 10% to 30% of AT patients develop a malignancy; most are lymphoid, but epithelial cancers also occur involving, for example, breast, ovary, prostate, stomach, and skin.[8]

The unique chromosome instability in AT lymphocytes almost certainly plays a key role in the emergence and perpetuation of aberrant chromosomal translocations.[9,10] The sites of instability occur in the areas of both the immunoglobulin heavy chain genes (14q32) and, of particular note, the various related chains of the T-cell antigen-recognition receptor (alpha and delta, 14q11; beta, 7p14–15; gamma, 7q33–35).[9,11] The instability at these gene loci may intensify the physiologic recombination that normally takes place during T- and B-cell differentiation in a way that permits the emergence and expansion of dysregulated lymphoid clones.[4]

Although full-blown, homozygous AT is rare, affecting between 1 in 40,000 and 1 in 200,000 people worldwide, the heterozygous state may be remarkably common, affecting approximately 1% of the U.S. population.[8,12] Some studies in the United States, England, and Norway have detected a three- to sevenfold increased risk of breast cancer in women who are known AT heterozygotes, suggesting that 4% of all breast cancer cases might occur in AT heterozygotes.[8,12] Nonetheless, these figures are estimates based on selected family studies; they are not yet corroborated by molecularly based population studies. In this regard, the recent isolation of the gene responsible for AT (called *ATM* for "mutated in AT")[7] offers the promise that we will be able to identify clearly those individuals who are AT heterozygotes and to dissect with accuracy the relationship among AT heterozygosity, radiation hypersensitivity, and the potentially heightened cancer risk. Although there is only one gene without multiple complementation groups, *ATM* is very large, with more than 40 mutations detected to date.[7] Still, with *ATM* in hand, it will eventually be possible to identify the intracellular pathways in which *ATM* participates, either as a trigger or as a pivotal intermediary.

The fully functional *ATM* acts to halt the cell cycle at the G_1 checkpoint (the preparatory stopping point before DNA synthesis, or S phase) in the setting of DNA damage and ongoing repair. It does so by up-regulating the cell cycle–regulating p53 tumor suppressor protein. In this regard, *ATM*, p53, the cell cycle inhibitory protein p21$^{WAF1/CIP1}$, and a specific growth arrest DNA damage-inducible (GADD) gene are linked in a molecular pathway for repair of DNA that has been damaged by certain types of ionizing radiation or by cytotoxic agents that mimic the DNA-damaging effects of radiation.[13,14] p21 is involved in cell cycle arrest, but the functional significance of GADD has not yet been determined.[13] *ATM* also exerts checkpoint arrest in G_2 (the resting phase between S phase and the completion of cell division, or mitosis) in response to radiation-induced DNA damage.[15,16] Failure to arrest the cell cycle in G_2 results in the high frequency of chromatid breaks seen in the lymphocytes and fibroblasts of AT homozygotes. Recent studies in yeast with AT-related genetic defects in DNA repair raise the possibility that *ATM* plays a regulatory role in S phase as well, impeding the initiation of DNA synthesis in the face of DNA damage.[17] Thus, it appears that *ATM* may exert a negative regulatory influence during all phases of the cell cycle in the genetically damaged cell, placing *ATM* in a critical position with regard to the cell's ability to repair damaged DNA and to preserve the fidelity of DNA replication.

The ATM protein is a large molecule with multiple domains. Its C-terminal is homologous with several members of the PIK family, in particular the PI3K subtype.[7] PIKs phosphorylate lipids and proteins—as such, they are a multifunctional group with roles in signaling, cytoskeletal, and genomic organization, and in DNA repair.[6,18] This group of conserved, structurally interrelated gene sequences and proteins includes Drosophila *mei-41*[19] and several yeast DNA repair genes, including the *tor* genes, the multifunctional *rad-3*, *mec-1*, and *tel-1*.[7,18,20,21] In particular, *tel-1*, which encodes a 322-kd protein with a PIK motif, shares the greatest structural homology with *ATM*.[20] Functionally, *tel-1* appears to be involved in the maintenance of telomere length (which may, in turn, prevent premature senescence in certain cell types) and in the fidelity of mitotic recombination. In this light, it is germane that AT cells may exhibit defective telomere metabolism, as evinced by telomere shortening and end-to-end fusions.[10,20]

Although our molecular genetic knowledge is accruing rapidly, to date we know little about the specific biochemical functions of this family of interrelated DNA repair genes.[21] The mechanisms by which these PIK-related kinases interact with lipids, proteins, and DNA remain to be uncovered. The full biochemical characterization and mechanistic dissection of members of this PIK-related kinase family should help us to define the relative contributions of the individual genes and gene products to orderly cell cycle progression, repair of DNA damage, replication integrity, and overall cell survival in both simple and complex organisms from yeast to humans.

SCID: Multiple Mechanisms in a Failure of Recombination

SCID involves a fundamental defect of both B- and T-cell development; affected individuals lack both humoral and cellular responses. The clinical constellation of SCID can evolve from a number of distinctive mechanisms. The X-linked SCID variant exemplifies a failure of growth factor–driven lymphoid growth and differentiation, especially (but not exclusively) in the T-cell line.[22] One factor in this failure is an aberrancy in the interleukin (IL)-2 cytokine-receptor interaction. The IL-2 receptor gamma chain is encoded by a gene on chromosome Xq13, the site of mutations in X-linked SCID. Many cell surface growth factor receptors are membrane-spanning molecules composed of extracellular and intracellular domains that require two or more chains to accomplish ligand-receptor binding, receptor activation, and intracellular signal transduction. Some of these chains have the capacity to bind multiple growth factors.[23,24] The IL-2 receptor gamma chain is a case in point. It serves as a common subunit for multiple immune-acting cytokines—namely, IL-4, IL-7, IL-9 and IL-15 (related to IL-2).[22,25] In turn, each of the IL-2 receptor gamma chain–linked cytokines stimulates a distinct stage of T (and, to a lesser degree, B) cell development. In this regard, IL-7 drives V(D)J recombination in T cells, and the absence of IL-7–based signaling leads to a blockade in overall thymic development and to a deficiency in T-cell driven B-cell proliferation and differentiation.[22] Thus, a defect in the structural and functional integrity of the IL-2 receptor gamma chain would be expected to lead to an amplified immune deficiency, due to the inability of the target cells to respond to multiple growth factor signals.

Another formative defect in SCID is the lack of expression of the catalytic subunit of the DNA-dependent protein kinase (DNA-PK$_{CS}$).[26,27] The immune deficits seen in human SCID are closely paralleled in an inbred strain of mice that suffers from combined humoral and cellular immunodeficiency. Studies in the SCID mouse have uncovered the pivotal role of the multicomponent DNA-PK complex in DNA repair. DNA-PK is necessary for a cell to recognize and rejoin the free DNA ends generated by double-strand DNA breaks—both endogenous breaks that culminate in V(D)J recombination and breaks caused by radiation.[27] The loss of DNA-PK activity, in turn, leads to a morphologic and functional blockade of T- and B-cell differentiation. Like *ATM*, the *DNA-PK$_{CS}$* gene contains sequences that encode a PIK; however, unlike the AT-related PIKs, the resultant DNA-PK$_{CS}$ appears to exhibit only serine-threonine kinase activity, with no known lipid kinase activity.[6,26,28] The genetic defect in the SCID mouse localizes to the gene encoding DNA-PK$_{CS}$ which, in turn, colocalizes to human chromosome 8q11.[27] Although the responsible gene and the specific molecular mechanisms in SCID are distinct from those in AT, the net result is that the absence of functional DNA-PK$_{CS}$ in SCID confers a defect in appropriate lymphoid differentiation leading to immunodeficiency and to heightened cancer susceptibility—a clinical phenotype that is similar to AT.

IATROGENIC IMMUNODEFICIENCY: POSTTRANSPLANT LYMPHOPROLIFERATIVE DISORDERS

The etiologic relationship between immunodeficiency and the pathogenesis of certain malignancies is further exemplified by the striking incidence of posttransplant immunodeficiency disorders (PTLDs) that arise in patients receiving immunosuppressive therapy for autoimmune disorders and particularly during organ allotransplantation (both solid organ and bone marrow transplants) to prevent graft rejection and graft versus host disease (GVHD).[29–33] The incidence of PTLDs ranges from roughly 1% to 1.5% following renal transplantation to 5% (and in some reports as high as 10%) following liver, heart, and lung transplantation, in large part related to the intensity of the immunosuppressive regimen.[34–36] Although most immunosuppressive posttransplantation regimens can predispose to PTLDs, the greatest risks and shortest latency periods are seen with the maximally T cell–suppressive regimens incorporating cyclosporine A (especially in combination with azathioprine) or antilymphocyte antibodies such as OKT3[37] and anti-CD5.[29] Some PTLDs can regress upon withdrawal of the underlying immunosuppression,[38] but such regression occurs in less than 25% of cases, especially for high-grade lymphomas. Aggressive combination chemotherapy[39] and immunotherapy with monoclonal antibodies (MoAb) directed against certain B-cell surface antigens,[34] however, have yielded promising results in early clinical testing.

PTLDs can range from nonmalignant, localized, polyclonal B-cell proliferations without genetic alterations to highly aggressive, widely disseminated, monoclonal or multiclonal immunoblastic lymphomas (large cell with plasmablastic features), or multiple myelomas. These tumors may be accompanied by structural and functional alterations in the oncogenes *c-myc* and *N-ras* and/or the tumor suppressor gene *p53*.[31] Approximately 80% of these PTLDs belong to the B-cell lineage and are linked to Epstein-Barr virus (EBV) infection (see Chapter 7).[30,34,36,37] In this situation, EBV may provoke polyclonal B-cell activation that, in the absence of normal T-cell controls, may permit unopposed B-cell expansion with an increased number of cells susceptible to destabilizing genetic events, such as chromosomal breaks and recombinations. The formative role of EBV in these PTLDs is substantiated by the findings that the detection of EBV gene expression can precede the clinical and histologic occurrence of PTLD.[36] Morevoer, posttransplant increases in EBV viral load (measured by the numbers of EBV-infected circulating lymphocytes) and decreases in the production of antibodies directed against EBV nuclear antigens (EBNAs) can predict for the eventual development of PTLD.[40,41]

In addition to PTLDs, immunosuppression also engenders increased risk of development of Kaposi's sarcoma (KS) and of epithelial cancers involving the skin. KS is especially likely in the setting of cyclosporine use, where the risk of KS is increased 200- to 400-fold over that in the general population.[38] This heightened risk of KS in the setting of iatrogenic immunosuppression appears to be linked to a newly discovered herpesvirus, HHV-8. This virus was initially detected in AIDS-related KS; it has now also been found in cases of transplant-associated KS (to be discussed more fully later and in Chapter 8).[42,43] The mechanisms underlying KS pathogenesis in the setting of iatrogenic immunosuppression could parallel the mechanisms by which PTLDs emerge—namely, the activation and proliferation of pathogenic herpesviruses. Intriguingly, cyclosporine A has been found to induce interleukin-6 (IL-6) production by peripheral blood mononuclear cells (PBMCs),[44] which, in turn, may play a pivotal role in the establishment and expansion of malignant clones in both lymphoproliferative disorders and KS.[23,45]

AIDS LYMPHOMAS: A PARADIGM OF LYMPHOMAGENESIS IN THE IMMUNOCOMPROMISED STATE

Soon after AIDS was recognized as a new disease, researchers observed that people with AIDS or at risk of AIDS had a high incidence of non-Hodgkin's lymphomas (NHLs). These NHLs tended to be of B-cell origin, high grade, and to occur in extranodal sites. In a prospective, ongoing study, scientists at the National Cancer Institute (NCI) have followed a group of patients on long-term studies of antiretroviral therapy, including the first patients to receive zidovudine (AZT), zalcitabine (ddC), or didanosine (ddI).[46–49] Eight of 55 patients on protocols of AZT alone or with ddC developed NHL, yielding a rate of 29% after 3 years on therapy,[46] and 4 of 61 patients receiving ddI developed NHL, yielding a rate of 9.5% after 3 years.[47] Additional studies have found that patients with less than 50 CD4 cells/mm^3 are at particularly high risk,[48] and that patients who have high serum levels of IL-6 are also at high risk.[49]

The unique immunologic milieu induced by HIV infection probably has a formative role in the pathogenesis and pathophysiology of AIDS-related lymphomas. This environment is characterized by defects in immune regulation, loss of specific immune-cell subsets, presence of abnormal cytokine levels, changes in the architecture of germinal centers and other lymphoid tissues, and aberrant immune surveillance. Any or all of these factors may contribute in a pivotal way to the high incidence and distinctive characteristics of AIDS-associated lymphoma. The dysregulation may lead to an increase in the rate of generation of transformed lymphocytes and to enhanced capacity of these cells to escape surveillance and thus to cause disease.

In addition to T-cell destruction, HIV infection may also cause an intrinsic impairment in B-cell maturation. Lymphohematopoietic malignancies are characterized by the clonal expansion of cells that have been arrested at a specific developmental stage. The capacity for self-renewal is preserved, but the capacity for terminal differentiation into mature cells is blocked. With HIV infection, this failure of maturation relates in part to a clonal defect in rearrangements of the VH3L subfamily of genes encoding the variable region of the immunoglobulin heavy chain (V$_H$).[50] The clonal defect occurs in B cells within lymph-node germinal centers, and results in a B-cell maturation arrest that, in turn, leads to a deficit in memory B cells. This deficit is accompanied by an increase in circulating levels of IL-6[51] that may provide a chronic proliferative stimulus for the arrested B-cell clone and thereby may drive the clone's expansion. Maturation arrest and chronic IL-6 stimulation (perhaps a compensatory, feedback attempt to override the maturation blockade and to push the arrested clone toward a more differentiated state) may serve as a foundation on which malignant B-cell transformation is built.

Like other retroviruses (see Chapter 11 on HTLV-1), HIV may also play a more direct etiologic role in certain cases of AIDS-related lymphoma.

Although at least 90% of AIDS NHLs are of B-cell origin, the incidence of rare T-cell lymphomas appears to be increasing. Molecular analyses of four such T-cell tumors reveal the presence of monoclonal HIV-long terminal repeat sequences integrated within the human *fur* gene, located just upstream of the tyrosine kinase–encoding *fes* oncogene on chromosome 15.[52] Theoretically, HIV could drive malignant transformation through mechanisms recognized for other retroviruses, such as insertional mutagenesis and up-regulation of oncogene expression, disturbance of normal DNA repair mechanisms, and clonal selection.

AIDS lymphomas can possess a variety of genetic lesions, some of which appear to be specific to particular etiologic agents and/or lymphoma cell types. One classical genetic lesion involves the disruption and translocation of the growth-promoting *c-myc* oncogene on chromosome 8q24 to one of the immunoglobulin gene loci (most commonly the heavy chain locus on chromosome 14q32), with transcriptional activation and constitutive overexpression of *c-myc*.[45,53–55] *c-myc* mutations and/or rearrangements occur in 50% to 70% of all AIDS NHLs.[45,55,56] Mutations of *p53* can be detected in roughly 50% to 70% of AIDS-related Burkitt's lymphomas, often linked to *c-myc* rearrangement and activation. *p53* mutations have also been found in 40% of non-AIDS Burkitt's.[56–58] Losses of one or more segments of the long arm of chromosome 6 (6q21–23 and 6q25–27)— sites of multiple putative tumor suppressors—occur in about 20% of all lymphomas, including those associated with AIDS.[56] Interestingly, *ras* mutations are detectable in about 10% to 15% of AIDS-related Burkitt's lymphomas but are absent in non-HIV lymphomas.[56] Rearrangements of *bcl-6* on chromosome 3q27—a transcription factor–encoding gene that is rearranged in 30% to 40% of diffuse large-cell lymphomas (DLCLs) arising in nonimmunosuppressed hosts—are evident in roughly 20% of AIDS-related DLCLs (both large noncleaved and immunoblastic variants) but not in small noncleaved cell lymphomas.[59] The *bcl-6* lesions are independent of the presence or absence of EBV and are not accompanied by alterations in *c-myc* and *p53*. Continued elucidation of the multiple factors and genetic alterations that may contribute to the HIV-infected state should provide a scientific scaffold for design of molecularly targeted therapies, definition of individual risk, and design of prevention strategies.

Epstein-Barr Virus: Mechanisms for Malignant Transformation

The role of EBV in B-cell lymphomagenesis has been established for endemic (African) Burkitt's lymphoma and has been postulated for many of the non-Burkitt's B-cell malignancies that arise in the setting of chronic immunosuppression, including HIV infection (see Chapter 7). One mechanism by which EBV may accomplish such B-cell growth dysregulation is through the activation of EBV latent genes encoding at least six transcriptionally active viral nuclear antigens (EBNAs) and two or more signal-transducing latent membrane proteins (LMPs). These proteins enhance the survival and self-renewal capacity of both EBV-infected host cells and the viral genome.[60] Their actions with respect to B cells—that is, blocking one form of programmed cell death known as apoptosis and extending B-cell longevity—may mimic that of *bcl-2*, an antiapoptosis oncogene that is overexpressed in diverse leukemias, lymphomas, and epithelial malignancies.[61] Of particular relevance in this context is the demonstration that EBNA-2, and especially LMP, can induce the expression of *bcl-2* in Burkitt's lymphoma cell lines, where *bcl-2* is not commonly detected in vivo.[62,63] This finding supports the notion that EBV may immortalize and/or enhance the survival of B cells through *bcl-2* up-regulation and abrogation of apoptosis. Along these lines, the EBV gene *BHRF1*, a homologue of *bcl-2*, appears to be transcribed in certain EBV-infected malignant B cells.[64] In the setting of PTLDs, however, *bcl-2* expression is not coupled to BHRF1 but rather appears to be linked to LMP1.[65] Thus, EBV infection can culminate in prolonged B-cell survival in vivo by at least two distinctive, noncompetitive mechanisms operating in concert or independently: (1) by the direct activity of a *bcl-2*-like viral gene and (2) by the viral induction of host *bcl-2* expression.

EBV gene products may also subvert host-cell machinery by inducing expression of B-cell surface antigens that enhance both viral and B-cell activation. Two such antigens have been reported: CD21, a receptor for EBV that is involved in EBV internalization, B-cell activation, and possibly EBV-induced autostimulation; and CD23, the low-affinity IgE receptor also known as B-cell activating factor.[66] EBV has also been reported to influence expression of lymphocyte adhesion molecules involved in immune responses that require cell-to-cell contact, including cytotoxic T-cell recognition.[67] Another posited mechanism of EBV-induced B-cell stimulation operates through BCRF-1, an EBV-encoded protein that shares structural and functional homology with IL-10.[68] This mechanism is discussed later in the context of AIDS-related lymphomagenesis.

EBV-linked lymphoproliferative malignancies that arise in the setting of chronic, profound immunosuppression are often characterized by the presence of multiple neoplastic clones and by an immunoblastic large-cell morphology with plasmacytoid features.[29–33,69] In this situation, the virus may provoke polyclonal B-cell activation, permitting unopposed B-cell expansion in the absence of normal T-cell controls. The result is increased numbers of cells susceptible to destabilizing genetic events such as chromosomal breaks and recombinations. Researchers have demonstrated the etiologic effects of EBV by inducing lymphomas in SCID mice that have been reconstituted with EBV-negative human peripheral or nodal lymphocytes (SCID/hu chimeric mice) and subsequently infected with EBV[70] or with peripheral blood lymphocytes from EBV-seropositive donors.[71] Of note, in the resulting tumors, *c-myc* and *bcl-2* translocations or rearrangements are absent. This tumor model parallels the large-cell immunoblastic B lymphomas that occur in people with severe immunodeficiency, such as that seen after organ transplantation[29-33] or the AIDS-related primary central nervous system (CNS) lymphomas.[69,72,73] In humans, as in the SCID/hu mouse, the EBV genome is present in tumor cells that arise from a background of polyclonal B cells activated by the infection.

Several investigators have demonstrated the particularly close relationship between primary CNS lymphomas and EBV infection.[69,72,74-76] EBV gene sequences and EBV-encoded RNAs (EBER) are detectable in virtually 100% of these tumors, and LMP can be found in roughly 40% to 60% of them.[75,76] In contrast, EBV DNA and EBER have been detected in only 50% (as high as 80% in some series) of non-CNS systemic AIDS lymphomas.[69,72,74,77] Viral protein expression differs in CNS compared to systemic HIV-related NHLs Along these lines, Camilleri-Broet and colleagues[74] detected the expression of both LMP1 and bcl-2 in 10 of 11 EBV-positive primary CNS lymphomas. In contrast, although 46 of 57 (80%) of the systemic NHLs examined in this series were linked to EBV, only 21 (46%) of the EBV-positive tumors expressed LMP1; a mere three systemic tumors, all extranodal, expressed bcl-2.[87]

EBV gene expression also differs in polyclonal compared to monoclonal tumors. In a series from Shiramizu and associates in San Francisco,[72] roughly 40% of all AIDS-related B-cell NHLs contained EBV gene sequences; EBV sequences were particularly prevalent in monoclonal tumors. When the data were stratified by tumor locations, however, *all* CNS tumors were EBV positive, whereas only one third of the systemic NHLs contained detectable EBV genomic material. In this population, *c-myc* rearrangements were linked exclusively to monoclonal NHLs. Overall, the most common lymphoma in this patient group was a polyclonal, high-grade systemic B-cell NHL without detectable EBV infection or *c-myc* rearrangements.[78] The polyclonal NHLs occurred in the setting of a higher CD4 count. In response to chemotherapy, patients with polyclonal disease—especially those with CD4 counts of $200/mm^3$ or more—enjoyed a longer survival (more than 50% were alive at 26^+ to 65^+ months) relative to those who had monoclonal tumors and CD4 counts less than $200/mm^3$ (median survival 3.5 months). The presence of EBV conferred a strikingly poor prognosis, independent of clonality status, with overall median survival of 3.2 months for those with EBV-positive disease versus 9 months for those with EBV-negative tumors.

Although EBV is often accompanied by alterations and deregulation of *c-myc*, the two are not linked inextricably.[69,79] Primary CNS lymphomas may contain the EBV genome without accompanying *c-myc* gene rearrangements.[69] More commonly, however, when there is dissociation between EBV and *c-myc*, the *c-myc* alterations occur in the absence of detectable EBV.[79] The majority of these EBV-negative, non-Burkitt's NHLs have *c-myc* rearrangements and 14q32 switch region breaks that mimic the mutations seen in "sporadic" Burkitt's type lymphomas. In a minority (approximately 25%) of EBV-negative, non-Burkitt's NHLs, breakpoints in both *c-myc* and 14q32 parallel those of "endemic" Burkitt's lymphomas; these changes are accompanied by point mutations in the first *myc* exon.[55] The net result of *c-myc* translocation to the immunoglobulin gene locus for either the endemic or the sporadic type of Burkitt's lymphoma is the abrogation of the effects of negative regulatory elements on *c-myc* transcription. More than transcriptional activation or amplification of *c-myc* per se, these gene rearrangements result in constitutive C-myc expression. This failure of the normal control mechanisms, in turn, leads to a net overexpression of the *c-myc* mRNA and DNA binding phosphoprotein.[53,54] Whatever the specific breakpoints and mechanisms of deregulation, the prevalence of abnormalities in *c-myc* structure and function is consistent with the notion that *c-myc* has a central role in the malignant transformation and clonal expansion of B-cell lymphomas in AIDS.

Interleukins in the Pathogenesis and Treatment of AIDS Lymphomas

The production of hematopoietic and immunomodulatory cytokines in response to infection may contribute to the development of lymphomas, particularly in HIV-infected hosts. The major cellular sources of cytokine production are T cells, monocytes, and bone marrow stromal cells, all of which can be infected by HIV and can perturb net cytokine production.[80] In this regard, HIV-related changes in IL-6 production may be especially relevant both to "premalignant" polyclonal B-cell expansion and to eventual malignant transformation in AIDS (and non-AIDS) lymphomas.

IL-6 affects proliferation, differentiation, and net expression of multiple arms of the immune system, including B cells and cytotoxic T cells.[23] The increase in serum IL-6 levels that accompanies the clonal VH3L defect in B-cell maturation occurs early in HIV infection, even before there is evidence of cellular immune impairment.[50] Thus, IL-6 may drive B-cell proliferation over a long period of time. Furthermore, IL-6 may augment HIV replication and infection progression in an autocrine fashion by enhancing T-cell and monocyte growth.[80] The production of IL-6 by HIV-infected monocytes also promotes the proliferation of activated B cells (for example, by EBV), thereby driving immunoglobulin synthesis and causing the nonspecific hyperglobulinemia commonly seen in early HIV infection.[80,81]

Based on these data, IL-6 is considered a likely promotor of malignant transformation in B-cell precursors. It is provocative that among the AZT-treated AIDS patients followed by the National Cancer Institute, those who eventually developed B-cell NHL had relatively elevated serum IL-6 levels at the time of study entry compared to those who did not develop NHL; they also manifested continued IL-6 increases over time.[49] The hypothetical linkage between IL-6 and B-cell dyscrasias is further supported by data suggesting that IL-6 is implicated in the pathogenesis of multiple myeloma through its activity as an autocrine growth factor for malignant plasma cells.[23] Along these lines, Emilie and coworkers,[82] examining high-grade B-cell NHLs, found striking expression of both IL-6 and IL-6 receptors predominantly in the non-Burkitt's, immunoblastic subset (which has a prominent plasmacytoid phenotype), independent of HIV and/or EBV positivity.

Because IL-6 and its receptor may be pivotal effectors in the genesis and clonal expansion of AIDS lymphomas, investigators are testing several novel anti–IL-6 strategies for lymphoma treatment. Kreitman and colleagues[83] have developed an immunotoxin by coupling IL-6 to a mutant *Pseudomonas* exotoxin (IL-6-PE^{4E}) that is cytotoxic to approximately 50% of fresh myeloma cell populations, as well as to other malignant cells that express the IL-6 receptor (namely, prostate and hepatocellular cancers). In human studies of IL-6–directed therapy, 50% of patients with advanced myeloma treated with a murine anti–IL-6 monoclonal antibody demonstrated marked inhibition of myeloma cell proliferation and overall IL-6 production.[84] A different murine anti–IL-6 monoclonal antibody tested in a small series of patients with AIDS-related NHLs stabilized disease and led to clinical improvement of 2 to 7 months' duration in about 50% of the treated subjects.[85] These or related monoclonal antibody–based constructs could furnish a molecularly targeted approach to AIDS lymphomas, non-AIDS lymphomas, and other IL-6–driven malignancies in which the malignant clone expresses both IL-6 and the IL-6 receptor.

In addition to IL-6, IL-10 also may be an important cytokine in AIDS lymphoma pathogenesis.[45,86,87] IL-10, which shares significant homology with the EBV protein BCRF-1, impairs the ability of the T_H1 subset of CD4+ helper T cells to synthesize interferon gamma and IL-2. Both of these cytokines exert antiviral activity against EBV and are crucial to the generation of cytotoxic CD8+ T cells.[68,88] EBV-positive Burkitt's lymphoma cell lines—particularly those derived from AIDS patients—are capable of producing IL-10 in a constitutive fashion.[86] Moreover, if the SCID/hu chimeric mouse model is repopulated with peripheral blood lymphocytes from EBV-infected individuals, the resultant EBV-positive human tumor cells produce both IL-10 and the IL-10 receptor. Autocrine growth stimulation of B cells results from this stimulation, as does concomitant IL-10–induced abrogation of apoptosis.[89] Intriguingly, IL-10–producing cell lines also secrete IL-6, providing yet another mechanism by which IL-10 may promote B-cell proliferation and immortalization.[87] The potential central role of IL-10 in AIDS-related lymphomagenesis suggests that IL-10 could be an important molecular target for inhibition by drugs designed to block IL-10's interactions with other cytokine-producing cells—namely, T_H1 cells and monocytes.

The SCID mouse repopulated with peripheral blood lymphocytes from EBV-infected hosts provides an elegant model of IL-2–based immunotherapy for EBV-induced, B-cell lymphoproliferative tumors. This model has served as the foundation for an innovative clinical approach in AIDS-related NHLs.[90,91] Human NHL cells generate copious amounts of IL-6 and IL-10, both of which are down-regulated by IL-2.[89] In the SCID/hu chimera, low-dose IL-2 has prevented the establishment of fatal EBV-positive lymphomatous disease, an effect that is mediated by NK and CD8+ T cells.[90,91] In human studies of HIV-related NHLs, administration of low-dose IL-2 following chemotherapy induced partial or complete remission in a majority of patients and prevented or forestalled relapse or disease progression for up to 1 year, even when CD4 counts were less than 100/ mm^3.[91] These exciting observations have formed the basis for a confirmatory national trial to define the influence of daily, postchemotherapy, low-dose IL-2 given as maintenance immunotherapy based on duration of response, viral load and replication activity, cellular and humoral immunologic parameters, and infectious complications.

A New Herpesvirus with Possible Etiologic Links to Kaposi's Sarcoma and Lymphoma

Kaposi's sarcoma (KS) is a malignancy that in the United States predominantly strikes patients with HIV infection or other immunodeficiency states. Its etiology, pathogenesis, and pathophysiology are incompletely understood. There are several variants of the disease, some of which are linked to iatrogenic immunodeficiency and, most strikingly, to AIDS.[73,92] A new inroad into understanding the pathogenesis of KS was made with the discovery of specific DNA sequences from a putative new herpesvirus, HHV-8, in tumor tissue (see Chapter 8). HHV-8 sequences were similarly observed in body-cavity lymphomas.[42,43,93] These unique sequences (called KS330$_{233}$) bear significant homology to genes encoding the minor capsid and tegument proteins of two Gammaherpesviriae with oncogenic activity: EBV and herpesvirus saimiri (HVS).[42,43] As described above and in Chapter 7, EBV is pathogenically linked to a diversity of malignancies, including lymphomas, nasopharyngeal carcinomas, and smooth muscle tumors arising in HIV-infected children and immunocompromised organ transplant recipients.[45,73,94,95] HVS induces a fatal polyclonal T-cell lymphoproliferative disease in nonimmune primates, in much the same manner that EBV causes B-cell lymphoproliferative disorders in humans.[96] Of particular interest is the presence of a gene in HVS that has homology with an oncogene, bcl-1, that encodes the cell cycle–promoting protein cyclin D$_1$.[97] Cyclin D$_1$ is often overexpressed in intermediate lymphomas and is amplified in certain epithelial cancers (esophageal, breast, bladder and non–small-cell lung cancers).[98]

The initial reports of HHV-8 in tumor tissue have been bolstered by the findings that 95% of KS lesions from AIDS patients, as well as of lesions from patients with "classic" (Mediterranean) KS and from HIV-negative homosexual men with KS, contain the sequences.[43,99] In addition, roughly 20% of clinically uninvolved skin lesions from all KS subgroups contained HHV-8.[42,43] However, some studies have called into question the specific etiologic role of this virus in KS, as HHV-8 sequences have been detected in both benign and malignant posttransplant skin lesions[100] and in sperm samples[101] in the absence of both HIV and KS. Nonetheless, Whitby and associates[102] have detected HHV-8 sequences in the PBMCs in more than 50% of the KS patients examined, but in only 8% of HIV-infected patients without KS. Further, HHV-8 was detectable prior to the clinical develop-ment of KS and was predictive for the eventual emergence of KS. Taken together, these findings add credence to the notion that HHV-8 may be important in KS etiology.

The emerging story of HHV-8 becomes even more complex with the finding of a specific linkage between HHV-8 and AIDS-related NHLs of the pleura, pericardium, and peritoneum.[93] These body-cavity NHLs are immunoblastic with a mature B-cell phenotype and EBV sequences but without accompanying *c-myc* rearrangements. HHV-8 has also been de-tected in the peripheral blood and lymph nodes of patients with multi-centric Castleman's disease, a polyclonal lymphoproliferative disorder ac-companied by vascular hyperplasia that can arise in the setting of HIV infection and can be associated with the development of KS and NHLs.[103,104] This finding and the independent detection of additional cases of HHV-8 in HIV-related body cavity NHLs (again, with clonal EBV DNA sequences and immunoglobulin gene rearrangements without accompanying *c-myc* alterations)[105] further substantiate the postulated etiologic role of HHV-8 in both vascular and lymphoid neoplasias.

FUTURE DIRECTIONS

The most effective strategies for addressing malignancy are those targeted to prevention. This assertion is as true for malignancies arising in the setting of profound immunodeficiency—be it genetic, iatrogenic, or in-fectious in its foundations—as for other tumors. Yet, we still need a much better understanding of the factors that instigate emergence and perpetu-ation of malignant cells. The study of DNA repair mechanisms, illumi-nated to a large degree by the dissection of certain genetic immunodefi-ciencies and other familial cancer-prone syndromes, has direct bearing on the means by which infectious agents—especially HTLV-1 and HIV—sub-vert the host cellular response and thereby initiate and propagate genet-ically aberrant clones. The current and prospective approaches listed in Table 5.2 aim to exploit certain molecular components that contribute to the etiology, pathogenesis, and pathophysiology of malignancies arising on a background of immune aberration. Many of these modalities— which, in some cases, are already in the clinical testing arena—have appli-cations for both treatment and prevention. Those aimed at reversing the underlying causes and formative consequences of immunosuppression ap-pear to hold particular promise.

AIDS-related malignancies exemplify the complexity of mechanisms and the multiple factors that interdigitate to engender and sustain tumor-igenesis. Early in the course of active HIV infection, interventions that interfere with factors that promulgate hyperproliferation and clonal ex-pansion (for example, growth factors such as IL-6 and IL-10, or concomi-tant viral infections such as EBV and HHV-8) might decrease the occur-

Table 5.2 Exploiting molecular pathogenesis for therapy and prevention of lymphoproliferative malignancies

---

Cytotoxic therapies
  New mechanisms (e.g., paclitaxel and other tubulin-directed agents, camptothecins)
  Mechanisms to overcome drug resistance

Cytokine-based (biomodulatory) therapies
  IL-2, IL-12, interferon
  Anti–IL-6, anti–IL-10, anti–tumor necrosis factor

Immune-based therapies
  Monoclonal antibodies, including immunotoxins and radioimmunoconjugates
  Vaccines (anti-idiotype, antiviral)

Immunorestorative approaches
  Bone marrow transplantation
  Stem cell reconstitution (gene-altered)
  Adoptive immunotherapy (HIV, EBV, CMV)
  Immunopotentiating hormones

Gene-targeted approaches
  Antisense (host and viral genomes)
  Ribozymes

Antiviral strategies
  New virocidal agents (including anti-KSHV)
  Antiviral immunity
    Adoptive immunotherapy, immunomodulation, vaccines
  Modulation of EBNA gene expression (alteration of gene methylation)
  Antiretroviral targets
    Reverse transcriptase, protease, nucleocapsid protein, integrase

---

rence or prolong the time to development of AIDS-related malignancies. Ultimately, however, the key strategies will be those directed toward maintaining cellular immunity at a level that prevents the establishment and perpetuation of transformed clones. In this regard, the potential to restore some immune responsiveness through adoptive transfer technologies or cytokine-based immunomodulatory therapies is provocative, particularly if implemented before irrevocable immune-cell depletion ensues. Such approaches stand to serve patients at risk for diverse malignancies arising in the setting of immunodeficiency, in particular those malignancies in which viral and other infectious cofactors may play a formative pathogenic role.

REFERENCES

1. Lieber MR. The mechanism of V(D)J recombination: a balance of diversity, specificity, and stability. Cell 1992;70:873–876.

2. Taccioli GE, Rathbun G, Oltz E, Stamoto T, Jeggo PA, Alt FW. Impairment of V(D)J recombination in double-strand break repair mutants. Science 1993; 260:207–210.

3. Waldmann TA. The arrangement of immunoglobulin and T-cell receptor genes in human lymphoproliferative disorders. Adv Immunol 1987;40:247–321.

4. Waldmann TA, Korsmeyer SJ, Bakhshi A, Arnold A, Kirsch IR. Molecular genetic analysis of human lymphoid neoplasms. Immunoglobulin genes and the *c-myc* oncogene. Ann Intern Med 1985;102:497–510.

5. Waldmann TA, Misiti J, Nelson DL, Kraemer CH. Ataxia-telangiectasia: a multisystem hereditary disease with immunodeficiency, impaired organ maturation, X-ray hypersensitivity, and a high incidence of neoplasia. Ann Intern Med 1983;99:367–379.

6. Keith CT, Schreiber SL. PIK-related kinases: DNA repair, recombination, and cell cycle checkpoints. Science 1995;210:50–51.

7. Savitsky K, Bar-Shira A, Gilad S, et al. A single ataxia telangiectasia gene with a product similar to PI-3 kinase. Science 1995;268:1749–1753.

8. Gatti RA, McConville CM, Taylor AMR. Sixth international workshop on ataxia telangiectasia (meeting report). Cancer Res 1994;54:6007–6010.

9. Hecht F, Hecht BKM. Chromosome changes connect immunodeficiency and cancer in ataxia-telangiectasia. Am Pediatr Hematol Oncol 1987;9:185.

10. Taylor AMR, Metcalfe JA, McConville C. Increased radiosensitivity and the basic defect in ataxia telangiectasia. Int J Radiat Biol 1989;56:677–684.

11. Lipkowitz S, Stern M-H, Kirsch IR. Hybrid T cell receptor genes formed by interlocus recombination in normal and ataxia-telangiectasia lymphocytes. J Exp Med 1990;172:409–418.

12. Swift M, Morrell D, Massey RB, Chase CL. Incidence of cancer in 161 families affected by ataxia-telangiectasia. N Engl J Med 1991;325:1831–1836.

13. Canman C, Wolff A, Chen C, et al. The p53–dependent G1 cell cycle checkpoint pathway and ataxia-telangiectasia. Cancer Res 1994;54:5054–5058.

14. Kastan MB, Zhan Q, El-Deiry WS, et al. A mammalian cell cycle checkpoint pathway utilizing p53 and GADD 45 is defective in ataxia-telangiectasia. Cell 1992;71:587–597.

15. Lavin MF, Le Poidevin P, Bates P. Enhanced levels of radiation-induced G2 phase delay in ataxia-telangiectasia heterozygotes. Cancer Genet Cytogenet 1992;60:183–187.

16. Sanford KK, Parshad R, Price FM, et al. Enhanced chromatid damage in blood lymphocytes after G2 phase x irradiation, a marker of the ataxia-telangiectasia gene. J Natl Cancer Inst 1990;82:1050–1054.

17. Paulovich AG, Hartwell LH. A checkpoint regulates the rate of progression through S phase in S. cerevisiae in response to DNA damage. Cell 1995;82: 841–847.

18. Zakian VA. ATM-related genes: what do they tell us about functions of the human gene? Cell 1995;82:685–687.

19. Hari KL, Santerre A, Sekelsky JJ, McKim KS, Boyd JB, Hawley RS. The mei-41 gene of D. melanogaster is a structural and functional homolog of the human ataxia telangiectasia gene. Cell 1995;82:815–821.

20. Greenwell PW, Kronmal SL, Porter SE, Gassenhuber J, Obermaier B, Petes TD. *Tel1*, a gene involved in controlling telomere length in S. cerevisiase, is homologous to the human ataxia telangiectasia gene. Cell 1995;82:823–829.

21. Morrow DM, Tagle DA, Shiloh Y, Collins FS, Hieter P. *Tel1*, an S. cerevisiae homolog of the human gene mutated in ataxia telangiectasia, is functionally related to the yeast checkpoint gene *mec1*. Cell 1995;82:831–840.

22. Voss SD, Hong R, Sondel PM. Severe combined immunodeficiency, interleukin-2 (IL-2), and the IL-2 receptor: experiments of nature continue to point the way. Blood 1994;83:626–635.

23. Kishimoto T, Akira S, Narazaki M, Taga T. Interleukin-6 family of cytokines and gp130. Blood 1995;86:1243–1254.

24. Waldmann TA, Pastan IH, Gansow OA, Junghans RP. The multichain interleukin-2 receptor: a target for immunotherapy. Ann Intern Med 1992;116: 148–160.

25. Matthews DJ, Clark PA, Herbert J, et al. Function of the interleukin-2 (IL-2) receptor gamma chain in the biologic responses of X-linked severe combined immunodeficient B cells to IL-2, IL-4, IL-13, and IL-15. Blood 1995;85: 38–42.

26. Blunt T, Finnie NJ, Taccioli GE, et al. Defective DNA-dependent protein kinase activity is linked to V(D)J recombination and DNA repair defects associated with the murine *scid* mutation. Cell 1995;80:813–823.

27. Kirchgessner CU, Patil CK, Evans JW, et al. DNA-dependent kinase (p350) as a candidate gene for the murine SCID defect. Science 1995;267:1178–1183.

28. Hartley KO, Gell D, Smith GCM, et al. DNA-dependent protein kinase catalytic subunit: a relative of phosphatidylinositol 3–kinase and the ataxia telangiectasia gene product. Cell 1995;82:849–856.

29. Antin JH, Bierer BE, Smith BR, et al. Selective depletion of bone marrow T lymphocytes with anti-CD5 monoclonal antibodies: effective prophylaxis for graft-versus-host disease in patients with hematologic malignancies. Blood 1991;78:2139–2149.

30. Hanto DW, Frizzera G, Gajl-Peczalska KJ, et al. Epstein-Barr virus-induced B-cell lymphoma after renal transplantation. N Engl J Med 1982;306:913–918.

31. Knowles DM, Cesarman E, Chadburn A, et al. Correlative, morphologic and molecular genetic analysis demonstrates three distinct categories of posttransplantation lymphoproliferative disorders. Blood 1995;85:552–565.

32. Penn I. Tumors arising in organ transplant recipients. Adv Cancer Res 1978;28:31–61.

33. Shearer WT, Ritz J, Finegold MJ, et al. Epstein-Barr virus-associated B-cell proliferations of diverse clonal origins after bone marrow transplantation in a 12-year-old patient with severe combined immunodeficiency. N Engl J Med 198;312:1151–1159.

34. Lebland V, Sutton L, Dorent R, et al. Lymphoproliferative disorders after organ transplantation: a report of 24 cases observed in a single center. J Clin Oncol 1995;13:961–968.

35. Opelz G, Henderson R, for the Collaborative Transplant Group. Incidence of non-Hodgkin lymphoma in kidney and heart transplant recipients. Lancet 1993;342:1514–1516.

36. Randhawa PS, Jaffe R, Demetris AJ, et al. Expression of Epstein-Barr virus-encoded small RNA (by the EBER-1 gene) in liver specimens from transplant recipients with post-transplantation lymphoproliferative disease. N Engl J Med 1992;327:1710–1714.

37. Swinnen LJ, Costanzo-Nordin MR, Fisher SG, et al. Increased incidence of

lymphoproliferative disorder after immunosuppression with the monoclonal antibody OKT3 in cardiac transplant recipients. N Engl J Med 1990;323: 1723–1728.

38. Cockburn ITR, Krupp P. The risk of neoplasms in patients treated with cyclosporine A. J Autoimmun 1989;2:723–731.

39. Swinnen LJ, Mullen GM, Carr TJ, Costanzo MR, Fisher RI. Aggressive treatment for postcardiac transplant lymphoproliferation. Blood 1995;86:3333–3340.

40. Riddler SA, Breinig MC, McKnight JLC. Increased levels of circulating Epstein-Barr virus (EBV)-infected lymphocytes and decreased EBV nuclear antigen antibody responses are associated with the development of posttransplant lymphoproliferative disease in solid-organ transplant recipients. Blood 1994;84:972–984.

41. Savoie A, Perpete C, Carpentier L, Joncas J, Alfieri C. Direct correlation between the load of Epstein-Barr virus-infected lymphocytes in the peripheral blood of pediatric transplant patents and risk of lymphoproliferative disease. Blood 1994;83:2715–2722.

42. Chang Y, Cesarman E, Pessin MS, et al. Identification of herpesvirus-like DNA sequences in AIDS-associated Kaposi's sarcoma. Science 1994;266:1865.

43. Moore P, Chang Y. Detection of herpesvirus-like DNA sequences in Kaposi's sarcoma in patients with and without HIV infection. N Engl J Med 1995;332: 1181.

44. Tanner JE, Menezes J. Interleukin-6 and Epstein-Barr virus induction by cyclosporine A: potential role in lymphoproliferative disease. Blood 1994;84: 3956–3964.

45. Karp JE, Broder S. Acquired immunodeficiency syndrome and non-Hodgkin's lymphomas. Cancer Res 1992;51:4743–4756.

46. Pluda JM, Yarchoan R, Jaffe ES, et al. Development of non-Hodgkin's lymphoma in a cohort of patients with severe immunodeficiency virus (HIV) infection on long-term antiretroviral therapy. Ann Intern Med 1990;113:276–282.

47. Nguyen B-Y, Yarchoan R, Wyvill KM, et al. Five-year follow-up of a phase I study of didanosine in patients with advanced human immunodeficiency virus infection. J Infect Dis 1995;171:1180–1189.

48. Yarchoan R, Venzon DJ, Pluda JM, et al. CD4 count as a mortality risk indicator in human immunodeficiency virus (HIV)-infected patients receiving antiretroviral therapy: experience in a research hospital. Ann Intern Med 1991; 115:184–189.

49. Pluda JM, Venzon DJ, Tosato G, et al. Parameters affecting the development of non-Hodgkin's lymphoma in patients with severe human immunodeficiency virus infection receiving antiretroviral therapy. J Clin Oncol 1993;11: 1099–1107.

50. Berberian L, Valles-Ayoub Y, Sun N, Martinez-Maza O, Braun J. A VH clonal deficit in human immunodeficiency virus-positive individuals reflects a B-cell maturational arrest. Blood 1991;78:175–179.

51. Breen EC, Rezai AR, Nakajima K, et al. Infection with HIV is associated with elevated IL-6 levels and production. J Immunol 1990;144:480–484.

52. Shiramizu B, Herndier BG, McGrath MS. Identification of a common clonal human immunodeficiency virus integration site in human immunodeficiency virus-associated lymphomas. Cancer Res 1994;54:2069–2072.

53. Croce CM, Nowell PC. Molecular basis of human B cell neoplasia. Blood 1985;65:1–7.

54. Dalla-Favera R, Bregni M, Erikson J, Patterson D, Gallo RC, Croce CM. Human c-myc oncogene is located on the region of chromosome 8 that is translocated in Burkitt lymphoma cells. Proc Natl Acad Sci USA 1982;79:7824–7827.

55. Ladanyi M, Offitt K, Jhanwar SC, Filippa DA, Chaganti RSK. MYC rearrangement and translocations involving band 8q24 in diffuse large cell lymphomas. Blood 1991;7:1057–1063.

56. Ballerini P, Gaidano G, Gong JZ, et al. Multiple genetic lesions in acquired immunodeficiency syndrome-related non-Hodgkin's lymphoma. Blood 1993; 81:1166–1176.

57. De Re V, Carbone A, De Vita S, et al. p53 protein over-expression and p53 gene abnormalities in HIV-1 related non-Hodgkin's lymphomas. Int J Cancer 1994;56:662–667.

58. Edwards RH, Raab-Traub N. Alterations of the p53 gene in Epstein-Barr virus-associated immunodeficiency-related lymphomas. J Virol 1994;68:1309–1315.

59. Gaidano G, Lo Coco F, Ye BH, Shibata D, Levine AM, Knowles DM, Dalla-Favera R. Rearrangements of the BCL6 gene in acquired immunodeficiency syndrome-associated non-Hodgkin's lymphoma: association with diffuse large-cell subtype. Blood 1994;84:397–402.

60. Gregory CD, Dive C, Henderson S, et al. Activation of Epstein-Barr virus latent genes protects human B cells from death by apoptosis. Nature 1991;349: 612–614.

61. Korsmeyer SJ. Bcl-2 initiates a new category of oncogenes: regulators of cell death. Blood 1992;80:879–886.

62. Finke J, Fritzen R, Ternes P, et al. Expression of bcl-2 in Burkitt's lymphoma cell lines: induction by latent Epstein-Barr virus genes. Blood 1992;80:459–469.

63. Henderson S, Rowe M, Gregory C, et al. Induction of bcl-2 expression by Epstein-Barr virus latent membrane protein 1 protects infected B cells from programmed cell death. Cell 1991;65:1107–1115.

64. Oudejans JJ, van den Brule AJC, Jiwa NM, et al. BHRF1, the Epstein Barr virus (EBV) homologue of the BCL-2 proto-oncogene, is transcribed in EBV-associated B-cell lymphomas and in reactive lymphocytes. Blood 1995;86: 1893–1902.

65. Murray PG, Swinnen LJ, Constandinou CM, et al. BCL-2 but not its Epstein-Barr virus-encoded homologue, BHRF1, is commonly expressed in post-transplantation lymphoproliferative disorders. Blood 1995;87:706–711.

66. Calender A, Cordier M, Billaud M, Lenoir GM. Modulation of cellular gene expression in B lymphoma cells following in vitro infection by Epstein-Barr virus (EBV). Int J Cancer 1990;46:658–663.

67. Inghirami G, Grignani F, Sternas L, Lombardi L, Knowles DM, Dalla-Favera R. Down-regulation of LFA-1 adhesion receptors by C-myc oncogene in human B lymphoblastoid cells. Science 1990;250:682–686.

68. Moore KW, Vieira P, Fiorentino DF, Trounstine ML, Khan TA, Mosmann TR. Homology of cytokine synthesis inhibitory factor (IL-10) to the Epstein-Barr virus gene BCRF1. Science 1990;248:1230–1234.

69. Meeker TC, Shiramizu B, Kaplan L, et al. Evidence for molecular subtypes of

HIV-associated lymphoma: division into peripheral monoclonal, polyclonal and central nervous system lymphoma. AIDS 1991;5:669–674.

70. Cannon MJ, Pisa P, Fox RI, Cooper NR. Epstein-Barr virus induces aggressive lymphoproliferative disorders of human B cell origin in SCID/hu chimeric mice. J Clin Invest 1990;85:1333–1337.

71. Rowe M, Young LS, Crocker J, Stokes H, Henderson S, Rickinson AB. Epstein-Barr virus (EBV)-associated lymphoproliferative disease in the SCID mouse model: implications for the pathogenesis of EBV-positive lymphomas in man. J Exp Med 1991;173:147–158.

72. Shiramizu B, Herndier B, Meeker T, Kaplan L, McGrath M. Molecular and immunophenotypic characterization of AIDS-associated Epstein-Barr virus-negative, polyclonal lymphoma. J Clin Oncol 1992;10:383–389.

73. Levine AM. AIDS-related malignancies: the emerging epidemic. J Natl Cancer Inst 1993;85:1382–1396.

74. Camilleri-Broet S, Davi F, Feuillard J, et al. High expression of latent membrane protein 1 of Epstein Barr virus and BCL-2 oncoprotein in acquired immunodeficiency syndrome-related primary brain lymphomas. Blood 1995; 86:432–435.

75. Hamilton-Dutoit SJ, Raphael M, Audouin J, et al. In situ demonstration of Epstein-Barr virus small RNAs (EBER-1) in acquired immunodeficiency syndrome-related lymphomas: correlation with tumor morphology and primary site. Blood 1993;82:619–624.

76. MacMahon EME, Glass JD, Hayward D, et al. Epstein-Barr virus in AIDS-related primary central nervous system lymphoma. Lancet 1991;338:969–973.

77. Shibata D, Weiss LM, Hernandez AM, Nathwani BN, Bernstein L, Levine AM. Epstein-Barr virus-associated non-Hodgkin's lymphoma in patients infected with the human immunodeficiency virus. Blood 1993;81:2102–2109.

78. Kaplan LD, Shiramizu B, Herndier B, et al. Influence of molecular characteristics on clinical outcome in human immunodeficiency virus-associated non-Hodgkin's lymphoma: identification of a subgroup with favorable clinical outcome. Blood 1995;85:1727–1735.

79. Subar M, Neri A, Inghirami G, Knowles DM, Dalla-Favera R. Frequent c-myc oncogene activation and infrequent presence of Epstein-Barr virus genome in AIDS-associated lymphoma. Blood 1988;72:667–671.

80. Birx DL, Redfield RR, Tencer K, Fowler A, Burke DS, Tosato G. Induction of interleukin-6 during human immunodeficiency virus infection. Blood 1990; 76:2303–2310.

81. Yarchoan R, Redfield RR, Broder S. Mechanisms of B cell activation in patients with acquired immunodeficiency syndrome and related disorders. J Clin Invest 1986;78:439–447.

82. Emilie D, Coumbaras J, Raphael M, et al. Interleukin-6 production in high grade B lymphomas: correlation with the presence of malignant immunoblasts in acquired immunodeficiency syndrome and in human immunodeficiency syndrome virus-seronegative patients. Blood 1992;80:498–504.

83. Kreitman RJ, Siegall CB, FitzGerald DJP, Epstein J, Barlogie B, Pastan I. Interleukin-6 fused to a mutant form of *Pseudomonas* exotoxin kills malignant cells from patients with multiple myeloma. Blood 1992;79:1775–1780.

84. Bataille R, Barlogie B, Lu ZY, et al. Biologic effects of anti-interleukin-6 murine monoclonal antibody in advanced multiple myeloma. Blood 1995;86:685.

85. Emilie D, Wijdenes J, Gisselbrecht C, et al. Administration of an anti-inter-
    leukin-6 monoclonal antibody to patients with acquired immunodeficiency
    syndrome and lymphoma: effect on lymphoma growth and on B clinical
    symptoms. Blood 1994;84: 2472–2479.
86. Benjamin D, Knobloch TJ, Dayton MA. Human B-cell interleukin-10: B-cell
    lines derived from patients with acquired immunodeficiency syndrome and
    Burkitt's lymphoma constitutively secrete large quantities of interleukin-10.
    Blood 1992;80:1289–1298.
87. Masood R, Zhang Y, Bond MW, et al. Interleukin-10 is an autocrine growth
    factor for acquired immunodeficiency syndrome-related B-cell lymphoma.
    Blood 1995;85:3423–3430.
88. Fiorentino DF, Zlotnik A, Vieira P, et al. IL-10 acts on the antigen-presenting
    cell to inhibit cytokine production by Th1 cells. J Immunol 1991;146:3444–
    3451.
89. Baiocchi RA, Ross ME, Tan JC, et al. Lymphomagenesis in the SCID-hu
    mouse involves abundant production of human interleukin-10. Blood 1995;
    85:1063–1074.
90. Baiocchi RA, Caligiuri MA. Low-dose interleukin 2 prevents the development
    of Epstein-Barr virus (EBV)-associated lymphoproliferative disease in *scid/scid*
    mice reconstituted i.p. with EBV-seropositive human peripheral blood lym-
    phocytes. Proc Natl Acad Sci USA 1994;91:5577–5581.
91. Bernstein ZP, Porter MM, Gould M, et al. Prolonged administration of low-
    dose interleukin-2 in human immunodeficiency virus-associated malignancy
    results in selective expansion of innate immune effectors without significant
    clinical toxicity. Blood 1995;86:3287–3294.
92. Rabkin CS, Biggar RJ, Horm JW. Increasing incidence of cancers associated
    with the human immunodeficiency virus epidemic. Int J Cancer 1991;47:
    692–696.
93. Cesarman E, Chang Y, Moore PS, et al. Kaposi's sarcoma-associated her-
    pesvirus-like DNA sequences in AIDS-related body-cavity-based lymphomas. N
    Engl J Med 1995;332:1186–1191.
94. Lee ES, Locker J, Nalesnik M, et al. The association of Epstein-Barr virus with
    smooth muscle tumors occurring after organ transplantation. N Engl J Med
    1995;332:19–25.
95. McClain KL, Leach CT, Jenson HB, et al. Association of Epstein-Barr virus
    with leiomyosarcomas in young people with AIDS. N Engl J Med 1995;332:
    12–18.
96. Chu EW, Rabson AS. Chimerism in lymphoid cell culture lines derived from
    lymph node of marmoset infected with Herpesvirus saimiri. J Natl Cancer
    Inst 1972;48:771–775.
97. Nicholas J, Cameron KR, Honess RW. Herpesvirus saimiri encodes homo-
    logues of G protein-coupled receptors and cyclins. Nature 1992;355:362–365.
98. Motokura T, Arnold A. Cyclin D and oncogenesis. Curr Opin Genet Devel
    1993;3:5–10.
99. Schalling M, Ekman M, Kaaya EE, et al. A role for a new herpes virus (KSHV)
    in different forms of Kaposi's sarcoma. Nature Med 1995;1:707–708.
100. Rady PL, Yen A, Rollefson JL. Herpesvirus-like DNA sequences in non-
     Kaposi's sarcoma skin lesions of transplant patients. Lancet 1995;345:1339–
     1340.
101. de Lillis L, Fabris M, Cassai E, et al. Kaposi's sarcoma herpesvirus (KSHV-8)

DNA sequences in the uro-genital tract, prostate and human sperm. AIDS Res Hum Retroviruses 1995;11 (Suppl 1):S98.

102. Whitby D, Howard MR, Tenant-Flowers M, et al. Detection of Kaposi's sarcoma associated herpesvirus in peripheral blood of HIV-infected individuals and progression to Kaposi's sarcoma. Lancet 1995;346:799–802.

103. Dupin N, Gorin I, Deleuze J, et al. Letter to the Editor: Herpes-like DNA sequences, AIDS-related tumors, and Castleman's disease. N Engl J Med 1995;333:798.

104. Soulier J, Grollet L, Oksenhendler E, et al. Kaposi's sarcoma-associated herpesvirus-like DNA sequences in multicentric Castleman's disease. Blood 1995;86:1276–1280.

105. Karcher DS, Alkan S. Letter to the Editor: Herpes-like DNA sequences, AIDS-related tumors, and Castleman's disease. N Engl J Med 1995;333:797.

II
INFECTIONS
AND CANCER:
VIRUSES

6

Human Papillomaviruses
and Squamous Cell Carcinomas

PETER M. HOWLEY AND KARL MÜNGER

Papillomaviruses are small, nonenveloped DNA viruses with a closed, circular double-stranded genome. Papillomaviruses have been described in many higher vertebrate species ranging from bird to human. They are highly restrictive and do not appear to cross from one species to another. They are also highly tissue specific and productively infect only squamous epithelial cells, causing benign hyperplastic epithelial lesions (warts or papillomas). A viral etiology of common warts in humans was established almost 100 years ago by transmission studies with cell-free filtrates.[1] Despite this long history, the causative viruses remained poorly understood because of an inability to propagate them in standard laboratory tissue culture systems. Although there have been advances in replicating some papillomaviruses in organotypic cultures of squamous epithelial cells, our current knowledge of the papillomaviruses has been derived largely by reverse genetics and through the application of recombinant technology. The molecular cloning and sequencing of the genomes of many of the papillomaviruses has provided the molecular platform to perform systematic mutational analyses, which led to the definition of the biological and biochemical activities of the genes encoded by these viruses. Although the bovine papillomavirus (BPV) has served as the prototype for many of these studies, the association of certain human papillomaviruses (HPVs) with cancer has motivated research on the transformation properties of this family of viruses.

More than 70 different HPV types have been described, and many of their genomes have been sequenced completely or in part. Because standardized type-specific antisera are not yet available, it has not been possible to type the papillomaviruses by serologic methods. Currently, the DNA sequence of a portion of the L1 open reading frame (ORF) is used to define new HPV types. A list of 77 HPVs, with the clinical syndromes with which they are associated or from which they have been isolated, is presented in Table 6.1.

The HPV genomes that have been sequenced to date all consist of a double-stranded DNA circle of approximately 8000 base pairs in size that have similar genomic organization. RNA-expression studies have indicated that only one DNA strand is transcribed. A detailed description of the general molecular biology of the papillomaviruses can be found in the third edition of *Field's Virology*.[2]

Papillomavirus genomes can be divided into three distinct regions: (1) the early (E) region, which encodes the viral proteins that are primarily involved in viral DNA replication, transcriptional regulation, and cellular transformation, (2) a late (L) region, which encodes the two viral capsid proteins, and (3) a long control region, or LCR, with no apparent coding potential, which contains the important cis elements of the viral genome required for viral DNA replication and for gene expression. For instance, the viral DNA replication origin as well as keratinocyte-specific enhancer elements are located in the LCR. A schematic map of a typical papillomavirus genome is shown for HPV 16 in Figure 6.1. Genes located in the early region of the genome are designated with the prefix "E." The genes located in the late region of the genome are designated L1 and L2. The HPV E4 gene, despite its location within the early region of the genome, actually encodes a late function that is expressed only when the viral particles are produced.[3] A listing of the functions assigned to the HPV-16 ORFs is provided in Table 6.2.

As noted, the papillomaviruses have a specific tropism for squamous epithelial cells, and their full replicative cycle is limited to these cells. Moreover, stages of HPV replicative cycle depend on the differentiation state of the host cell. In a stratified squamous epithelium, normally only the basal cells are capable of supporting cellular DNA synthesis and of undergoing cellular division. Once a squamous epithelial cell exits the basal layer, it leaves the cell cycle and enters a program of differentiation. Therefore, to induce a persistent infection, papillomaviruses must infect the cells of the basal layer. Consistent with this model, *in situ* hybridization experiments have demonstrated the presence of papillomavirus DNA within the basal cell layer.[4] The "late" viral replication functions, such as vegetative viral DNA synthesis, the production of viral capsid proteins, and the assembly of virion particles, are restricted to the most superficial layers containing terminally differentiated keratinocytes.

During a productive infection, when viral particles are produced, messenger RNAs derived from both the early and the late regions of the genome are transcribed.[5] During a nonproductive infection of host cells (as seen in the lower cells of the epithelium in a wart or in HPV-associated cancers) viral gene expression is restricted to mRNAs derived from the early region of the genome. This regulation of viral gene transcription is at the levels of the initiation of RNA synthesis, RNA stability, and of transcriptional termination.

EPIDEMIOLOGY OF HUMAN PAPILLOMAVIRUS

HPVs cause infection of the squamous epithelium in the genital tract, skin, and upper respiratory tract. Although warts may be evident in these sites, the majority of HPV infections are clinically silent. HPVs appear to be very common worldwide. Most studies that have investigated disease incidence and prevalence have focused on the genital tract. In asymptomatic women with normal Pap smears, HPV has been detected at prevalences ranging from 4% in the Netherlands to 48% in Tanzania.[6] Prevalence of infection has been generally higher in younger than in older women. For example, in the United States, HPV has been found in 30% to 40% of young women visiting university health clinics wheras prevalence was considerably lower (17%) in somewhat older women visiting health maintenance organization clinics.[6] Prevalence of genital HPV is higher among women infected with human immunodeficiency virus (HIV) infection than among HIV uninfected hosts. Moreover, in HIV-infected women, HPV infection often becomes chronic, particularly as CD4+ counts decline; in HIV-uninfected women, HPV infection resolves over time.[7] Less information is available on genital HPV prevalence in men. The little information from urethral swabs that has been obtained, however, suggests that asymptomatic HPV prevalence is similar in men and women of comparable age.[6] Rates of infection may be substantially higher, however, among men attending sexually transmitted disease clinics.

Skin warts caused by papillomavirus occur in up to 2% to 20% of young adults and schoolchildren; this prevalence declines with increasing age. For unknown reasons, meat handlers appear to be at particularly high risk for skin warts.[8,9] No data are available on the prevalence of respiratory papillomatosis. In one study conducted among all U.S. registered otolaryngologists, however, the annual incidence of respiratory papillomatosis was predicted to be 1.8 per 100,000 in adults and 4.3 per 100,000 in children.[10]

Transmission of papillomavirus-associated lesions of the anogenital tract is characteristic of a venereal transmitted disease with a high prevalence in populations with high sexual promiscuity.[11,12] HPV is rarely found in sexually inexperienced women; the prevalence increases in parallel with the number of recent sexual partners.[6] The higher than expected concordance of infection in married couples also supports sexual transmission. Because HPV often involves other genital areas, including the base of the penis, condoms may not protect against sexual transmission.[6] Respiratory papillomatosis in infants is presumed to be acquired vertically, probably at the time of delivery.

CANCERS ASSOCIATED WITH
PAPILLOMAVIRUS INFECTIONS

Most hyperplasias that are caused by papillomaviruses are benign. This chapter specifically focuses on human cancers and HPVs, yet it was the

Table 6.1 The Human papillomaviruses[a]

HPV Type	Location	Associated diseases
1	Cutaneous	Plantar warts
2	Cutaneous	Common warts
3	Cutaneous	Flat warts
4	Cutaneous	Common and plantar warts
5	Cutaneous	Macular lesions in EV[b] and cancers
6	Genital tract, other mucosal sites	Genital warts, laryngeal papillomatosis
7	Genital tract, other mucosal sites	"Butcher's" warts
8	Cutaneous	Macular lesions (EV) and cancers
9	Cutaneous	Macular lesions (EV)
10	Cutaneous	Flat warts
11	Genital tract, other mucosal sites	Genital warts, laryngeal papillomas
12	Cutaneous	Macular lesions (EV)
13	Oral	Oral focal epithelial hyperplasia
14	Cutaneous	Macular lesions (EV) and cancers
15	Cutaneous	Macular lesions (EV)
16	Genital tract, other mucosal sites	Intraepithelial neoplasias and cancers
17	Cutaneous	Macular lesions (EV) and cancers
18	Genital tract, other mucosal sites	Intraepithelial neoplasias and cancers
19	Cutaneous	Macular lesions (EV)
20	Cutaneous	Macular lesions (EV) and cancers
21	Cutaneous	Macular lesions (EV)
22	Cutaneous	Macular lesions (EV)
23	Cutaneous	Macular lesions (EV)
24	Cutaneous	Macular lesions (EV)
25	Cutaneous	Macular lesions (EV)
26	Cutaneous	Common warts
27	Cutaneous	Common warts
28	Cutaneous	Flat warts
29	Cutaneous	Common warts
30	Genital tract, other mucosal sites	Intraepithelial neoplasias and cancers
31	Genital tract, other mucosal sites	Intraepithelial neoplasias and cancers
32	Cutaneous	Oral focal epithelial hyperplasia, oral papillomas
33	Genital tract, other mucosal sites	Intraepithelial neoplasias and cancers
34	Genital tract, other mucosal sites	Intraepithelial neoplasias
35	Genital tract, other mucosal sites	Intraepithelial neoplasias and cancers
36	Cutaneous	Actinic keratosis, EV lesions
37	Cutaneous	Not yet known, isolated from a keratoacanthoma
38	Cutaneous	Not yet known, isolated from a melanoma
39	Genital tract, other mucosal sites	Intraepithelial neoplasias and cancers
40	Genital tract, other mucosal sites	Intraepithelial neoplasias
41	Cutaneous	Flat warts
42	Genital tract, other mucosal sites	Intraepithelial neoplasias

(continued)

discovery of malignant papillomatous tumors in cottontail rabbits that began the modern era of viral oncology. The Shope papillomavirus (also
known as the cottontail rabbit papillomavirus, CRPV), the best-studied of
the oncogenic animal papillomaviruses, was identified by Richard Shope
in 1933.[13] Treatment of these virus-induced papillomas with coal tar or

Table 6.1 (Continued)

HPV Type	Location	Associated diseases
43	Genital tract, other mucosal sites	Intraepithelial neoplasias
44	Genital tract, other mucosal sites	Intraepithelial neoplasias
45	Genital tract, other mucosal sites	Intraepithelial neoplasias and cancers
46	Cutaneous	Macular lesions (EV)
47	Cutaneous	Macular lesions (EV)
48	Cutaneous	Cutaneous squamous cell carcinoma (transplant patient)
49	Cutaneous	Flat wart (immunocompromised patient)
50	Cutaneous	Macular lesions (EV)
51	Genital tract, other mucosal sites	Intraepithelial neoplasias and cancers
52	Genital tract, other mucosal sites	Intraepithelial neoplasias and cancers
53	Genital tract, other mucosal sites	Intraepithelial neoplasias
54	Genital tract, other mucosal sites	Intraepithelial neoplasias
55	Genital tract, other mucosal sites	Intraepithelial neoplasias
56	Genital tract, other mucosal sites	Intraepithelial neoplasias and cancers
57	Oral, genital tract, other mucosal sites	Oral papillomas and inverted maxillary sinus papilloma
58	Genital tract, other mucosal sites	Intraepithelial neoplasias and cancers
59	Genital tract, other mucosal sites	Anogenital intraeipithelial neoplasias
60	Cutaneous	Epidermoid cysts, plantar warts
61	Genital tract, other mucosal sites	Intraepithelial neoplasias
62	Genital tract, other mucosal sites	Intraepithelial neoplasias
63	Cutaneous	Isolated from a plantar wart
64	Genital tract, other mucosal sites	Intraepithelial neoplasias
65	Cutaneous	Isolated from a pigmented wart
66	Genital tract, other mucosal sites	Intraepithelial neoplasias and cancers
67	Genital tract, other mucosal sites	Isolated from an intraepithelial neoplasia
68	Genital tract, other mucosal sites	Isolated from an intraepithelial neoplasia
69	Genital tract, other mucosal sites	Intraepithelial neoplasias and cancers
70	Genital tract, other mucosal sites	Isolated from a vulvar papilloma
71	Genital tract, other mucosal sites	Isolated from an intraepithelial neoplasia
72	Oral	Isolated from an oral papilloma (HIV)
73	Oral	Isolated from an oral papilloma (HIV)
74	Genital tract, other mucosal sites	Isolated from an intraepithelial neoplasia
75	Cutaneous	Isolated from a common wart in organ allograft recipient
79	Cutaneous	Isolated from a common wart in organ allograft recipient
77	Cutaneous	isolated from a common wart in organ allograft recipient

ᵃFrom references 48, 113, 114.
ᵇEV = Epidermodysplasia verruciformis.

other carcinogens leads to the formation of carcinomas at a high frequency. CRPV has served as a valuable model for papillomavirus-associated multistep carcinogenesis.[14-16] The synergy of the viral infection with cocarcinogens in tumor progression has proved to be a hallmark of papillomavirus-associated carcinogenesis. These CRPV-associated carcinomas

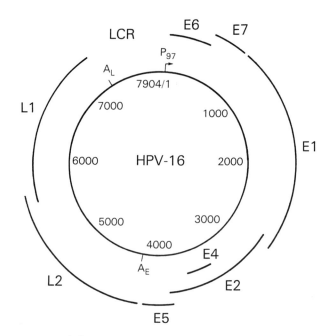

Figure 6.1. Map of the 7.9-kb HPV-16 genome. The nucleotide numbers are indicated within the circular map. Transcription proceeds in a clockwise direction, and the major open reading frames (E1 to E7, L1, and L2) are indicated. The transcriptional promoter that directs the expression of E6 and E7 is designated (P₉₇). A_E and A_L represent the polyadenylation signals for the early and late transcripts, respectively. The major functions of the genes encoded by HPV-16 are indicated in Table 6.2.

Table 6.2 HPV-16 Gene functions

ORF	Function
L1	L1 protein, major capsid protein
L2	L2 protein, minor capsid protein
E1	Initiation of viral DNA replication, helicase, ATPase, ori binding, complex E2
E2	Transcriptional regulatory protein, auxiliary role in viral DNA replication, complex E1
E4	Late protein; disrupts cytokeratins
E5	Membrane transforming protein; interacts with growth factor receptors (BPV)
E6	Oncoprotein; binds E6AP to ubiquitinate p53; activates telomerase; binds paxillin
E7	Oncoprotein; binds to pRB and other "pocket proteins"; complexes p21CIP1

ORF = open reading frame.

162

contain copies of the viral DNA that are transcriptionally active, consistent with the hypothesis that CRPV plays an active and ongoing role in the cancers that develop. Because it is now possible to induce skin papillomas by delivering CRPV DNA directly into the skin of rabbits, the functions of the individual CRPV genes in viral pathogenesis and carcinogenesis can be studied.

Epidermodysplasia Verruciformis and HPV

The first studies to implicate an HPV in human cancer were of patients who had a rare skin disease called epidermodysplasia verruciformis (reviewed in reference 17). This life-long disease usually begins in infancy or early childhood. It is characterized by disseminated polymorphic cutaneous lesions that resemble flat warts, and by reddish macules sometimes referred to as pityriasis-like lesions.[18] More than 20 different HPV types have been demonstrated in individual lesions in patients with this disease (see Table 6.1). Approximately 50% of EV patients develop multiple skin cancers, usually during the third of fourth decade of life. These cancers can be bowenoid carcinomas, *in situ* carcinomas, or invasive squamous cell carcinomas. Only a subset of the EV-associated HPVs—most notably HPV-5 and HPV-8—has been linked to malignant progression. A mechanistic role of these specific HPVs in EV-derived cancers is suggested by the presence of transcriptionally active viral DNA in the carcinomas.[19] The carcinomas that develop in these patients typically arise in sun-exposed areas, therefore, it has been postulated that ultraviolet radiation plays a cocarcinogenic role with the virus in the etiology of these cancers.

The underlying genetic defect that predisposes EV patients to HPV infections and to carcinogenic progression has not yet been determined. Genetic studies, however, have suggested that EV is linked to a recessive, abnormal allele of an X-linked gene. The majority of the EV patients have an impaired cell-mediated immunity (EV-like lesions have also been observed in immunosuppressed patients following organ transplantation[11] and in HIV-positive individuals[20]). This immunologic impairment may be responsible for the sustained, lifelong infection these patients suffer with these specific papillomaviruses; regression of these cutaneous HPV lesions is rare. Of interest. however, there does not appear to be an increased sensitivity to anogenital HPV infections in EV patients.

The skin cancers in EV patients provide an excellent example of multifactorial malignancies arising from a mixture of genetic, infectious (HPV), and environmental factors (UV light). Moreover, what has been learned from EV and HPV may be germane to other forms of cutaneous tumors. HPVs similar to those associated with EV have also been detected in nonmelanoma skin cancers in both immunosuppressed and immunocompetent patients.[21,22]

Association of HPVs with Oral and Upper Airway Cancers

Conceivably, any carcinoma of a squamous epithelium, or of an epithelium that can undergo squamous metaplasia, could have the potential to be HPV-associated. Thus, a variety of human cancers have been screened for HPV sequences. Some oral and upper airway carcinomas contain HPV-positive carcinomas, although the exact proportion that has HPV is unknown.[23-25] Specific HPVs also have been detected in benign oral papillomas,[26-29] and in oral focal epithelial hyperplasia.[30,31] HPV-11 has been detected in one squamous cell carcinoma of the lung arising in a young adult with a history of laryngotracheobronchial papillomatosis. The viral genome was transcriptionally active consistent with the notion that expression of the virus may have contributed to carcinogenic progression.[32] In this case, metastases to the liver and lymph nodes were also HPV-11 positive. HPV-16 sequences have been detected in a verrucous carcinoma of the larynx. The esophagus is lined by a squamous epithelium and squamous cell papillomas of the esophagus have been described in humans.[33] There is no convincing evidence, however, that a significant portion of human esophageal carcinomas are associated with an HPV infection.

HPVs and Cancers of the Anogenital Tract

Cancers of the anogenital tract include cancers of the cervix, vulva, anus, and penis. Of these, cervical cancer is by far the most common; it is the second leading cause of cancer among women worldwide. Annually, there are 500,000 new cases of cervical cancer; of these, 13,500 new cases are in the United States causing approximately 5000 deaths. An increase in the incidence of anal cancer in men may be due to a high prevalence of anal HPV infection in HIV-seropositive homosexual men.

Epidemiological studies have long indicated that cervical carcinoma is associated with the venereal transmission of an infectious carcinogenic agent that has a long latency period.[34,35] Sexual promiscuity and an early age of onset of sexual activity are two of the risk factors for cervical carcinoma. In many parts of the world, there is also an excellent correlation between the rates of incidence rates of cervical and penile carcinoma. Although the incidence rates for penile carcinoma are 20-fold lower than those of cervical carcinoma, the similar ratio of incidence between cervical carcinoma and penile carcinoma is maintained in areas of high, medium, and low prevalence. These observations suggest that etiologic factors for penile and cervical carcinoma may be shared. As further evidence for this model, monogamous women whose spouses have multiple sexual partners are at a higher risk for cervical carcinoma than women whose spouses are also monogamous.

These epidemiological data prompted a variety of different studies evaluating infectious genital pathogens as potential causative agents in the etiology of cervical carcinoma. A viral etiology for cervical carcinoma was suggested in the late 1960s and early 1970s when several studies indicated a link with genital infections by herpes simplex virus (HSV) type 2.[36,37] This notion was further strengthened by laboratory studies that showed that HSV can transform certain rodent cells in vitro. In addition, HSV-2 specific antibodies were found more frequently in patients who had cervical cancer than in control populations. However, this association fell apart at the molecular level when investigators were unable to find evidence of HSV DNA or mRNA in cervical cancer tissues, effectively ruling out HSV-2 as the principal etiologic agent responsible for the malignancy.[38] At the same time, a larger, well-controlled seroepidemiologic study carried out by Vonka failed to support the involvement of genital herpesvirus infections in cervical cancer.[39,40] In the mid-1970s, zur Hausen postulated that HPV infections might be associated with genital cancers[41] Support for this hypothesis came from the observations of pathologists who recognized that a particular abnormal cell, the koilocyte, was characteristically present in Papanicolaou smears and in cervical biopsies of patients with cervical dysplasia.[42] Electron microscopy studies demonstrated papillomavirus particles in these cells, thereby linking infections with HPV directly with the koilocytotic changes and cervical dysplasia—a precursor lesion to cervical cancer.[43-45] The viral etiology of cervical dysplasia was then confirmed by numerous investigators through the detection of papillomavirus-specific capsid antigens and specific HPV DNA within the lesions of cervical dysplasia.

The nature of cervical dysplasia (also referred to as cervical intraepithelial neoplasia [CIN] and sqamous intraepithelial lesion [SIL]) as a precursor to carcinoma in situ and to invasive squamous cell carcinoma of the cervix prompted the screening of cervical cancers for specific HPV sequences. Using HPV-11 DNA as a low-stringency hybridization probe, zur Hausen and his colleagues identified and cloned two new papillomavirus DNAs (HPV-16 and HPV-18) from human cervical carcinomas.[46,47] In subsequent studies, HPV-16 and HPV-18 were detected in approximately 70% of cervical carcinomas.[48] Screening of genital tract lesions by low-stringency hybridization and, more recently by PCR with degenerate primers has led to the identification of approximately 20 additional HPVs (see Table 6.1). Several other human carcinomas of the anogenital tract—including penile, vulvar, and perianal carcinomas—also contain HPVs. Bowenoid papulosis of the penis (also referred to as penile intraepithelial neoplasia [PIN]) is associated with HPV-16 and is the male counterpart of CIN in the female.[49,50]

Two types of HPV-associated anogenital lesions can be differentiated by their clinical appearance and histology: condyloma acuminata (or venereal warts) and squamous intraepithelial lesions (SIL). Condyloma acuminata can be found on the penis, the vulva, the perineum, the anus, and, rarely, the uterine cervix. Electron microscopy studies have revealed papillomavirus particles in nuclei in these lesions[51,52] and the genomes of specific HPV types (HPV-6 and HPV-11) have been directly cloned from them. Molecular epidemiological studies have shown that most (>90%) of condyloma acuminata contain DNA from HPV-6, HPV-11, or closely related HPV types. The rate of malignant conversion of these lesions to squamous cell carcinoma is very low, with the giant condyloma described by Buschke and Löwenstein as the exceptions; these giant lesions are associated with HPV-6 and HPV-11 but have characteristics similar to locally invasive squamous cell carcinoma.[53] The vast majority of carcinomas of the anogenital tract, however, are not associated with HPV-6 and HPV-11. Due to their association with clinical lesions that are at a low risk for malignant progression, HPV-6 and HPV-11 are classified as "low-risk" HPV types.

HPV types that are associated with anogenital tract lesions that are at a significant risk for malignant progression are referred to as the "high-risk" HPVs. The prototypical high-risk HPVs are HPV-16 and HPV-18. Other high-risk HPVs are HPV-31, HPV-33, HPV-35, HPV-39, HPV-45, HPV-51, HPV-52, and HPV-56; each is detected in a small percentage of cervical carcinomas (see Table 6.1). It is estimated that high-risk HPV DNA can be detected in approximately 90% to 95% of the cervical carcinomas.

PATHOGENIC MECHANISMS OF HPV-ASSOCIATED CANCER

Although the HPV-16 and HPV-18 viral genomes are generally maintained as episomes in benign precancerous lesions, carcinogenic progression of these lesions is almost always accompanied by integration of the viral genome into the genome of the host human cell. Rarely, the viral DNA remains extrachromosomal. The viral DNA does not preferentially integrate at specific sites in the host genome, although in some cell lines the integration event has occurred in the vicinity of known oncogenes. For instance, in the HPV-18–positive human cervical carcinoma cell line HeLa, the viral integration site has been mapped to chromosome 8, within approximately 50 kilobases of the *c-myc* locus.[54] The clonal integration pattern of the HPV genome that is detected in HPV-positive cervical cancers and the derived cell lines indicates that integration of the viral genome preceded the clonal outgrowth of the tumor—an observation that supports a mechanistic role for the virus as a step in the malignant progression to cervical cancer.

Integration of the viral genome into the host genome during malignant progression selectively retains the integrity of the viral regulatory region and of the coding region for the E6 and E7 genes. Furthermore, high level expression of the E6 and E7 genes is regularly detected in HPV-positive cervical cancers; expression of the viral E2 and E1 is typically lost.[55–58] An example of the integrated HPV-16 genome in the SiHa cell line, derived from a human cervical carcinoma, is shown in Figure 6.2. The HPV E2 ORF encodes an important viral regulatory factor that can negatively regulate the promoter that controls transcription of the E6 and E7 genes.[59,60] The disruption of the E2 gene by the integration abrogates this negative

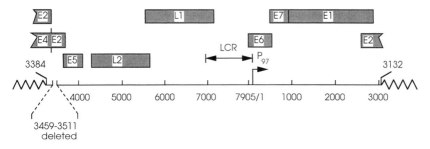

Figure 6.2. Structure of the single copy of the HPV-16 DNA integrated into the host chromosome in the SiHa cell line derived from a cervical carcinoma.[56] The jagged line represents human chromosomal DNA. The early and late HPV open reading frames (ORFs) are indicated. Integration has occurred in the E2 ORF and a portion of the E2 ORF has been deleted. The deregulated transcription of E6 and E7 is from the P97 promoter.

regulatory circuit and results in the increased expression of the E6 and E7 genes. Consistent with this model, disruption of the E1 or E2 regulatory genes of HPV-16 results in an increase in the immortalization capacity of the viral genome.[61] E2 expression in cervical cancer cell lines, on the other hand, inhibits the growth of these cells.[59,62,63]

An important step in establishing an etiologic role for the high-risk HPVs in the HPV-associated cancers was the demonstration that the genomic DNA of the high-risk HPVs can extend the life span and lead to the immortalization of primary human genital keratinocytes (the normal host cell for the HPVs) in cell culture, whereas the genomic DNA of the low-risk types does not.[56,64,65] Genetic studies revealed that the E6 and E7 genes were necessary and sufficient for this activity.[66–68] When high-risk HPV E6–E7 expressing keratinocytes are grown under conditions that allow the formation of stratified epithelial-like structures, they form abnormal structures that histologically resemble high-grade SILs. In transgenic animals, expression of the E6 and E7 genes by epithelial-specific promoters induces skin hyperplasias that can progress to carcinomas.[69–71] Such studies have been immensely useful in elucidating cellular targets of the high-risk HPV E6 and E7 oncoproteins, and in pinpointing biochemical differences between the E6 and E7 proteins of the high- and the low-risk HPVs.

Functions of the HPV E6 Proteins

The high-risk HPV E6 and E7 proteins together contribute to the immortalization of primary human cells.[66–68] E6, by itself, is sufficient for the immortalization of primary human mammary epithelial cells and can cooperate with the *ras* oncogene to transform primary mouse embryo fibroblasts.[72,73] A biochemical mechanism that accounts for some of the transformation activities of E6 is the ability of the E6 proteins of the high-risk, but not of the low-risk, HPVs to form complexes with the tumor suppressor protein p53.[74] The ability of HPV16 and HPV18 E6 to enter complexes with p53 is shared with the large tumor antigen of SV40 (SV40TAg) and with the 55 kd form of the adenovirus E1B (AdE1B) protein (see Figure 6.3).[72,75–77] The biochemical consequences of the interaction between E6 and p53 are unique, however. Whereas interaction of SV40 TAg and Ad E1B (55 kD) results in the metabolic stabilization of p53, E6 decreases the steady state levels of p53. High-risk HPV-expressing cell lines contain low levels of the wild-type p53, and the metabolic half-life of p53 in high-risk E6-expressing cells is reduced compared to in normal squamous epithelial cells.[78,79]

The interaction of E6 with p53 is not direct but rather is mediated by a cellular protein, called the E6-associated protein (E6AP).[80] E6AP is a ubiquitin protein ligase and, in the presence of E6, directly participates in

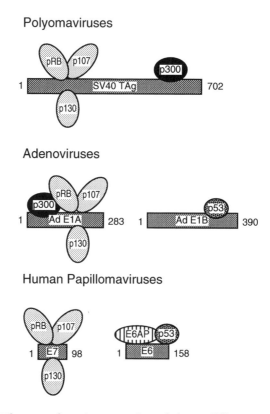

Figure 6.3. The transforming proteins of three different groups of DNA tumor viruses target similar cellular proteins. The binding of HPV-16 E6 to p53 is not direct but rather is mediated by a cellular protein called E6AP.

the ubiquitination of p53.[81] Multi-ubiquitinated p53 is then recognized by and degraded by the 26S proteasome. Through its ubiquitination of p53, HPV 16 E6 has also been shown to abrogate the transcriptional activation and repression properties of p53[82,83] and to disrupt the ability of wild-type p53 to mediate cell cycle arrest in response to DNA damage.[84] One of the functions of p53 is to sense DNA damage and, by then arresting the cell cycle, to prevent the replication of a mutated cell. Thus, the functional abrogation of p53 by the high-risk HPV E6 protein results in decreased genomic stability and in accumulation of DNA abnormalities in high-risk HPV E6 expressing cells. Hence, E6 can be directly implicated in the establishment and propagation of genomic instability—a hallmark in the pathology of malignant progression of cervical lesions.[85]

The high-risk HPV E6 proteins also have other activities that are not linked to their ability to target p53. For instance, investigators have shown that expression of the HPV E6 oncoprotein results in the activation of telomerase activity in infected cells, potentially preventing cell senescence.[86] Furthermore, E6 can interact with several additional cellular proteins, including a putative calcium-binding protein referred to as the E6 binding protein, although the physiologic significance of this interaction has yet to be established.[87] Recently, researchers have also shown that the high-risk HPV E6 proteins can complex with paxillin, a cellular focal adhesion protein that may serve as an adaptor in transmitting signals from integrin molecules to the actin cytoskeleton.[88] Additional targets of the HPV E6 proteins have been identified, but the interaction with p53 appears to have the most relevance for the role of the HPVs in carcinogenesis.

Functions of the HPV E7 Proteins

The high-risk HPV E7 proteins have transforming activities in several assays, including focus formation in rodent fibroblast cell lines, cooperation with ras in the transformation of primary baby rat kidney cells and, with E6, immortalization of primary human fibroblasts and keratinocytes. The HPV E7 proteins encode low-molecular-weight phosphoproteins, which share functional and structural similarities with other transforming proteins encoded by small DNA tumor viruses, including SV40 TAg and the adenovirus E1A (AdE1A) oncoprotein (see Figure 6.3). These conserved sequences are critical for the transforming activities in all three viral oncoproteins and have been shown to participate in the binding of a number of important cellular regulatory proteins, including the product of the retinoblastoma tumor suppressor gene (pRB), and the related pocket proteins, p107 and p130.[89–91] Interaction of HPV E7 with the pocket proteins leads to their destabilization.[92,93]

Members of the E2F family of transcription factors are involved in mediating the functions of the pocket proteins. The transcriptional activity of E2F is modulated by pRB; when bound to the G_0/G_1-specific hypophosphorylated form of pRB, E2F functions as a transcriptional repressor. When pRB is phosphorylated by cyclin-dependent kinase complexes near the G_1-to-S boundary, the pRB–E2F complex dissociates and E2F can act as a transcriptional activator. The regulated conversion of the transcriptional activity of E2F between repressor and activator contributes to the regulation of G_1/S progression. Consistent with this model, it has been shown that overexpression of E2F results in cell cycle progression and can induce morphological changes in cultured cells that are characteristic of cellular transformation. Most of the experimental evidence is consistent with a model in which the high-risk HPV E7 protein contributes to carcinogenic progression, at least in part, by disrupting this regulatory network. Although the complex formed between E7 and the pRB family of pocket proteins contributes to carcinogenesis, these interactions do not account for the full immortalization and transforming functions of E7. Thus, there must be additional cellular targets of E7. Jewers and colleagues have reported that E7 can interact with several members of the AP-1 family of transcription factors. This protein–protein interaction requires sequences in the carboxyl terminus of E7 that have been shown to be necessary for the immortalization of primary human foreskin keratinocytes.[94] The carboxyl terminus of E7 also functions as a dimerization domain, but it is not clear whether dimerization is necessary for the biological activities of E7.[95–97]

The HPV E7 protein can also interact with cyclin-dependent kinase inhibitors (CKIs). Scientists have reported that, like the Ad E1A protein,[98] HPV-16 interacts with and abrogates the inhibitory activity of $p27^{kip1}$.[99] Because $p27^{kip1}$ is involved in mediating cellular growth inhibition by TGF-β,[100] this interaction may contribute to the ability of HPV-16 E7 and Ad E1A to overcome transforming growth factor β associated growth arrest.[101] The HPV-16 E7 protein can also interact with the CKI $p21^{cip1}$ and can abrogate $p21^{cip1}$-mediated inhibition of cyclin-dependent kinase activity as well as inhibition of PCNA-dependent DNA replication (see Figure 6.4).[102,103] The CKI $p21^{cip1}$ is induced during keratinocyte differentiation through a p53-independent pathway.[104] Viral DNA replication is dependent on the activity of the cellular replication machinery, so it is necessary for HPVs to uncouple cellular differentiation and proliferation in the infected epithelial cells. Previous studies have shown that the HPV E7 protein is able to uncouple these processes.[105,106] Thus, the interaction of E7 and $p21^{cip1}$ may be critical to induce or maintain cellular DNA-replication in terminally differentiated keratinocytes.

An amino terminal domain in E7 that shares sequence similarity to the conserved region 1 in the AdE1A protein and to the conserved sequence in SV40 TAg also contributes to cellular transformation. This sequence does not contribute directly to pocket protein binding by E7, but it is necessary for E7-mediated destabilization of pRB.[93]

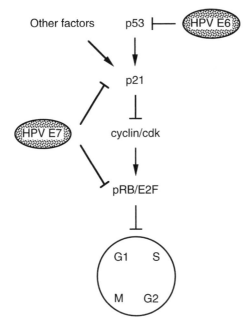

Figure 6.4. The HPV-16 E6 and E7 oncoproteins target and inactivate cellular proteins involved in regulating the cell cycle. E6 targets the inactivation of p53 by causing its ubiquitination and degradation. E7 complexes with pRB (and the other pocket proteins p107 and p130) freeing up E2F, promoting cell cycle progression from G_1 to S. E7 also can complex and functionally inactivate the cyclin dependent kinase inhibitor p21.

Additional Factors Involved in Carcinogenic Progression in HPV-Associated Malignancies

Cancer is a rare outcome of infection, even with a high-risk HPV, such as HPV 16 or HPV 18. It is estimated, for example, that a woman infected with a high-risk HPV has approximately a 1-in-30 lifetime risk of developing cervical cancer. Moreover, the time period between HPV infection and the development of invasive cancer can be several decades. Thus, infection with a high-risk HPV constitutes only one step in carcinogenesis, and the genetic information carried by the virus per se is not sufficient to cause cancer. Other factors must be involved in the progression of viral-associated lesions to these genital-tract cancers, and there is a clear requirement for an infected cell to sustain additional genetic mutations for a cancer to arise. The deregulated expression of the viral E6 and E7 proteins in these lesions, however, does contribute mechanistically to the loss of genomic stability and to the accumulation of host cellular mutations.[85]

Specific chromosomal abnormalities have been detected in cervical cancer. Loss of heterozygosity on the short arm of chromosome 3 (3p21) has been detected in many cervical cancers, suggesting loss of tumor suppressor gene at the site.[107] This locus contains the recently described FHIT gene, which has been implicated in tumor suppression in a variety of human cancers.[108] Recessive host cell mutations have also been described in the somatic cell hybrid work of Stanbridge.[109] A gene on human chromosome 11 can suppress the tumorigenicity of HPV-positive cervical carcinoma cells. Zur Hausen has proposed a model in which this gene modulates the expression of the cellular factor [termed cellular interfering factor [CIF]) that negatively regulates HPV expression.[48] He has postulated that the disruption of this locus results in a further dysregulation of HPV oncogene expression. This model is consistent with experimental evidence that shows that fibroblasts with a deletion in the short arm of chromosome 11 can be immortalized by HPV-16 more efficiently than can normal fibroblasts.[110] A candidate gene on chromosome 11 has not yet been identified and the molecular mechanisms of CIF-action remain to be defined. Tumor progression is a complex process that is likely to involve many additional loci. For instance, cellular mutations may also be involved in down-regulating the ability of an HPV-positive cancer cell to be recognized by the host cellular immune response.

CONTROL AND IMPLICATIONS FOR CLINICAL MANAGEMENT

Currently, there is no specific treatment for HPV infection. Destruction or excision can be used to manage warts and dysplastic lesions; however, these do not necessarily remove the infection. Although not discussed in this chapter, the replication of the viral DNA is dependent on two viral gene products, E1 and E2, that bind together at the origin of DNA replication within the viral genome to initiate DNA replication.[2] The E1 and E2 proteins therefore provide reasonable targets for the development of specific antiviral therapies. In advanced stage cervical cancers, the expression of the HPV E6 and E7 oncoprotein is maintained. Studies with cervical cancer cell lines that have sustained myriad cellular mutations have shown clearly that expression of E6 and E7 is necessary for the maintenance of the transformed phenotype. The high-risk HPV E6 and E7 proteins, and the factors that control their expression, therefore provide promising targets for the development of therapies that may prevent or cure HPV-associated cancers and the relevant precursors.

Significant advances have been made recently in the development of vaccines against papillomavirus infections. The expression of the major capsid protein in yeast and in insect cells leads to the assembly of viruslike particles (VLPs) that are morphologically identical to native virion particles.[111,112] Further, these VLPs present the conformational epitopes that are necessary for the development of a high-titer neutralizing antisera. Such VLPs are now being employed in clinical trials in humans.

Until vaccines and antiviral agents become available, the best hope for controlling HPVs rests in prevention. Prevention strategies include (1) primary prevention by instructing teenagers and adults on the health hazards of both protected and unprotected sex, (2) secondary prevention by conducting regular physical examinations of the skin and genitalia and removing suspicious lesions, and (3) tertiary prevention by Pap smear surveillance and removal of early tumors before they become untreatable. These activities have succeeded in rapidly diminishing the mortality from cervical and penile cancers in developed countries. Vigorous implementation of these strategies worldwide would further diminish the long-term consequences of HPV infection until such time as specfic interventions against the virus become available.

REFERENCES

1. Ciuffo G. Imnfesto positivo con filtrato di verruca volgare. Giorn Ital Mal Venereol 1907;48:12–17.
2. Howley PM. Papillomavirinae: the viruses and their replication. In: Bernard N. Fields, David M. Knipe, Peter M. Howley, eds. Fields Virology. Vol. 2. Philadelphia: Lipppincott-Raven; 1996:2045–2076.
3. Doorbar J, Campbell D, Grand RJA, Gallimore PH. Identification of the human papillomavirus-1a E4 gene products. EMBO J 1986;5:355–362.
4. Schneider A, Oltersdorf T, Schneider V, Gissmann L. Distribution of human papillomavirus 16 genome in cervical neoplasia by molecular in situ hybridization of tissue sections. Int J Cancer 1987;39:717–721.
5. Baker CC, Howley PM. Differential promoter utilization by the papillomavirus in transformed cells and productively infected wart tissues. EMBO 1987; 6:1027–1035.
6. IARC Working Group on the Evaluation of Carcinogenic Risks to Humans. Human papillomaviruses. Lyon: International Agency for Research on Cancer;1995:58–65.
7. Sun X-W, Kuhn L, Ellerbrock TV, Chiasson MA, Bush TJ, Wright TC. Human papillomavirus infection in women infected with the human immunodeficiency virus. N Engl J Med 1997;337:1343–1349.
8. Kilkenny M, Marks R. The descriptive epidemiology of warts in the community. Australas J Dermatol 1996;37:80–86.
9. Keefe M, al-Ghamdi A, Coggon D, Maitland NJ, Egger P, Keefe CJ, Carey A, Sanders CM. Cutaneous warts in butchers. Br J Dermatol 1994;130:9–14.
10. Derkay CS. Task force on recurrent respiratory papillomas: a preliminary report. Arch Otolaryngol 1995;121:1386–1391.
11. Underwood PB, Hester L. Diagnosis and treatment of premalignant lesions of the vulva. Am J Obstet Gynecol 1971;110:849–857.
12. Waugh M. Condylomata acuminata. Br Med J 1972;2:527–528.
13. Shope RE, Hurst EW. Infectious papillomatosis of rabbits; with a note on the histopathology. J Exp Med 1933;58:607–624.

14. Rous P, Beard JW. Carcinomatous changes in virus-induced papillomas of rabbits. Proc Soc Exp Bio Med 1935;32:578–580.

15. Rous P, Kidd JG. The carcinogenic effect of a virus upon tarred skin. Science 1936;83:468–469.

16. Rous P, Kidd JG, Smith WE. Experiments on the cause of the rabbit carcinomas derived from virus-induced papillomas. J Exp Med 1953;96:159–174.

17. Jablonska S, Majewski S. Epidermoplasia verruciformis: immunological and clinical aspects. Curr Top Microbiol Immunol 1994;186:157–175.

18. Lutzner M. An autosomal recessive disease characterized by viral warts and skin cancer: a model for viral oncogenesis. Bull Cancer 1978;65:169–182.

19. Yutsudo M, Hakura A. Human papillomavirus type 17 transcripts expressed in skin carcinoma tissue of a patient with epidermodysplasia verruciformis. Int J Cancer 1987;39:586–589.

20. Prose N, von Knebel Doeberitz C, Miller S, Milburn PB, Heilman E. Widespread flat warts associated with human papillomavirus type 5: a cutaneous manifestation of human immunodeficiency virus infection. J Am Acad Dermatol 1990;23:978–981.

21. Berkhout RJM, Tieben LM, Smits HL, Bouwes Bavinck JN, Vermeer BJ, ter Schegget J. Nested PCR approach for detection and typing of epidermoplasia verruciformis-associated human papillomavirus types in cutaneous cancers from renal transplant recipients. J Clin Microbiol 1995;33:690–695.

22. Shamanin V, Glover M, Rausch C, et al. Specific types of human papillomavirus found in benign proliferations and carcinomas of the skin in immunosuppressed patients. Cancer Res 1994;54:4610–4613.

23. Kahn T, Schwarz E, zur Hausen H. Molecular cloning and characterization of the DNA of a new human papillomavirus from a laryngeal carcinoma. Int J Cancer 1986;37:61–65.

24. Loning T, Ikenberg H, Becker J, Gissmann L, Hoepfer I, zur Hausen H. Analysis of oral papillomas, leukoplakias, and invasive carcinomas for human papillomavirus type related DNA. J Invest Dermatol 1985;84:417–420.

25. Brandsma JL, Steinberg BM, Abromson AL, Winkler B. Presence of human papillomavirus type 16 related sequences in verrucous carcinoma of the larynx. Cancer Res 1986;46:2185–2188.

26. Jenson AB, Lancaster WD, Hartmann DP, Shaffer EL. Frequency and distribution of papillomavirus structural antigens in verrucae, multiple papillomas, and condylomata of the oral cavity. Am J Pathol 1982;107:212–218.

27. Lind PO, Syrjanen SM, Syrjanen KJ, Koppang HS, Aas E. Local immunoreactivity and human papillomavirus (HPV) in oral precancer and cancer lesions. Scand J Dent Res 1986;94:419–426.

28. DeVilliers EM, Neumann C, Le JY, Weidauer H, zur Hausen H. Infection of the oral mucosa with defined types of human papillomaviruses. Med Microbiol Immunol (Berl) 1986;174:287–294.

29. Naghasfar Z, Sawada E, Kutcher MK, et al. Identification of genital tract papillomaviruses HPV-6 and HPV-16 in warts of the oral cavity. J Virol 1985;62:660–667.

30. Pfister H, Hettich I, Runne U, Gissman L, Chilf GN. Characterization of human papillomavirus type 13 from lesions of focal epithelial hyperplasia Heck. J Virol 1983;47:363–366.

31. Beaudenon S, Praetorius F, Kremsdorf D, et al. A new type of human papil-

lomavirus associated with oral focal epithelial hyperplasia. J Invest Derm 1987;88:130–135.

32. Byrne JC, Tsao MS, Fraser RS, Howley PM. Human papillomavirus-11 DNA in a patient with chronic laryngotracheobronchial papillomatosis and metastatic squamous-cell carcinoma of the lung. N Engl J Med 1987;317:873–878.

33. Winkler B, Capo V, Reumann W, et al. Human papillomavirus infection of the esophagus. Cancer 1985;55:149–155.

34. Kessler IL. Human cervical cancer as a venereal disease. Cancer Res 1976;36: 783–791.

35. zur Hausen H. Human papillomaviruses and their possible role in squamous cell carcinomas. Curr Top Microbiol Immunol 1977;78:1–30.

36. Rawls WE, Tompkins WAF, Figueroa ME, Melnick JL. Herpes simplex virus type 2: Association with carcinoma of the cervix. Science 1968;161:1255–1256.

37. Nahmias AJ, Josey WE, Naib ZM, Luce CF, Guest BA. Antibodies to herpes virus hominus types 1 and 2 in humans. II. Women with cervical cancer. Am J Epidemiol 1970;91:547–552.

38. zur Hausen H. Herpes simplex virus in human genital cancer. Int Rev Exp Pathol 1983;25:307–326.

39. Vonka V, Kanda J, Hirsch I, et al. Prospective study on the relationship between cervical neoplasia and herpes simplex type-2 virus. II. Herpes simplex type-2 antibody presence in sera taken at enrollment. Int J Cancer 1984;33: 61–66.

40. Vonka V, Kanda J, Jelinek J, et al. Prospective study on the relationship between cervical neoplasia and herpes simplex type-2 virus. I. Epidemiological Characteristics. Int J Cancer 1984;33:49–60.

41. zur Hausen H. Condylomata acuminata and human genital cancer. Cancer Res. 1976;36:530.

42. Koss LG, Durfee GR. Unusual patterns of squamous epithelium of the uterine cervix: Cytologic and pathologic study of koilocytotic atypia. Ann NY Acad Sci 1956;63:1245–1261.

43. Meisels A, Fortin R. Condylomatous lesions of the cervix and vagina. I. Cytologic patterns. Acta Cytol 1976;20:505–509.

44. Purola E, Savia E. Cytology of gynecologic condyloma acuminatum. Acta Cytol 1977;21:26–31.

45. Laverty CR, Russell P, Hills E, Booth N. The significance of noncondylomatous wart virus infection of the cervical transformation zone. Acta Cytol 1978;22:195–201.

46. Durst M, Gissmann L, Idenburg H, zur Hausen H. A papillomavirus DNA from a cervical carcinoma and its prevalence in cancer biopsy samples from different geographic regions. Proc Natl Acad Sci USA 1983;80:3812–3815.

47. Boshart M, Gissman L, Ikenberg H, Kleinheinz A, Scheurlen W, zur Hausen H. A new type of papillomavirus DNA, its presence in genital cancer biopsies and in cell lines derived from cervical cancer. EMBO J 1984;3:1151–1157.

48. zur Hausen H. Papillomavirus infections—a major cause of human cancers. Biochim Biophys Acta 1996;1288:55–78.

49. Ikenberg H, Gissmann L, Gross G, Grussendorf, Conen E, zur Hausen H. Human papillomavirus type-16-related DNA in genital Bowen's disease and in Bowenoid papulosis. Int J Cancer 1983;32:563–565.

50. Gross G, Hagedorn M, Ikenberg H, et al. Bowenoid papulosis. Presence of human papillomavirus (HPV) structural antigens and of HPV-16 related DNA sequences. Arch Dermatol 1985;121:858–863.

51. Dunn AE, Ogilvie MM. Intranuclear virus particles in human genital wart tissue: Observation on the ultrastructure of epidermal layer. J Ultrastruct Res 1968;22:282–295.

52. Oriel JD, Almeida JD. Demonstration of virus particles in human genital warts. Br J Vener Dis 1970;46:37–42.

53. Boshart M, zur Hausen H. Human papillomaviruses in Buschke-Lowenstein tumors: Physical state of the DNA and identification of a tandem duplication in the noncoding region of a human papillomavirus 6 subtype. J Virol 1986; 58:963–966.

54. Durst M, Croce C, Gissmann L, Schwarz E, Huebner K. Papillomavirus sequences integrate near cellular oncogenes in some cervical carcinomas. Proc Natl Acad Sci USA 1987;84:1070–1074.

55. Schwarz E, Freese UK, Gissman L, et al. Structure and transcription of human papillomavirus sequences in cervical carcinoma cells. Nature 1985;314: 111–114.

56. Baker CC, Phelps WC, Lindgren V, Braun MJ, Gonda MA, Howley PM. Structural and transcriptional analysis of human papillomavirus type 16 sequences in cervical carcinoma cell lines. J Virol 1987;61:962–971.

57. Durst M, Dzarlieva PR, Boukamp P, Fusenig NE, Gissmann L. Molecular and cytogenetic analysis of immortalized human primary keratinocytes obtained after transfection with human papillomavirus type 16 DNA. Oncogene 1987; 1:251–256.

58. Jeon S, Lambert PF. Integration of HPV16 DNA into the human genome leads to increased stability of E6/E7 mRNAs: implications for cervical carcinogenesis. Proc Natl Acad Sci USA 1995;92:1654–1658.

59. Thierry F, Yaniv M. The BPV1 E2 trans-acting protein can be either an activator or a repressor of the HPV18 regulatory region. EMBO J 1987;6:3391–3397.

60. Romanczuk H, Thierry F, Howley PM. Mutational analysis of cis-elements involved in E2 modulation of human papillomavirus type 16 P97 and Type 18 P105 promoters. J Virol 1990;64:2849–2859.

61. Romanczuk H, Howley PM. Disruption of either the E1 or the E2 regulatory gene of human papillomavirus type 16 increases viral immortalization capacity. Proc Natl Acad Sci USA 1992;89:3159–3163.

62. Dowhanick JJ, McBride AA, Howley PM. Suppression of cellular proliferation by the papillomavirus E2 protein. J Virol 1995;69:7791–7799.

63. Hwang ES, Riese DJ, Settleman J, et al. Inhibition of cervical carcinoma cell line proliferation by the introduction of a bovine papillomavirus regulatory gene. J Virol 1993;67:3720–3729.

64. Schlegel R, Phelps WC, Zhang YL, Barbosa M. Quantitative keratinocyte assay detects two biological activities of human papillomavirus DNA and identifies viral types associated with cervical carcinoma. EMBO J 1988;7:3181–3187.

65. Woodworth CD, Bowden PE, Doninger J, et al. Characterization of normal human exocervical epithelial cells immortalized in vitro by papillomavirus types 16 and 18 DNA. Cancer Res 1988;48:4620–4628.

66. Hawley-Nelson P, Vousden KH, Hubbert NL, Lowy DR, Schiller JT. HPV16 E6 and E7 proteins cooperate to immortalize human foreskin keratinocytes. EMBO J 1989;8:3905–3910.

67. Münger K, Phelps WC, Bubb V, Howley PM, Schlegel R. The E6 and E7 genes of the human papillomavirus type 16 together are necessary and sufficient for transformation of primary human keratinocytes. J Virol 1989;63: 4417–4421.

68. Hudson JB, Bedell MA, McCance DJ, Laimins LA. Immortalization and altered differentiation of human keratinocytes in vitro by the E6 and E7 open reading frames of human papillomavirus type 18. J Virol 1990;64:519–526.

69. Arbeit JM, Munger K, Howley PM, Hanahan D. Progressive squamous epithelial neoplasia in K14–HPV16 transgenic mice. J Virol 1994;68:4358–4368.

70. Arbeit JM, Howley PM, Hanahan D. Chronic estrogen-induced cervical and vaginal squamous carcinogenesis in human papillomavirus type 16 transgenic mice. Proc Natl Acad Sci USA 1996;93:2930–2935.

71. Herber R, Liem A, Pitot H, Lambert PF. Squamous epithelial hyperplasia and carcinoma in mice transgenic for the human papillomavirus type 16 E7 oncogene. J Virol 1996;70:1873–1881.

72. Band V, DeCaprio JA, Delmolino L, Kulesa V, Sager R. Loss of p53 protein in human papillomavirus type 16 E6-immortalized human mammary epithelial cells. J Virol 1991;65:6671–6676.

73. Matlashewski G, Schneider J, Banks L, Jones N, Murray A, Crawford L. Human papillomavirus type 16 DNA cooperates with activated ras in transforming primary cells. EMBO J 1987;6:1741–1746.

74. Werness BA, Levine AJ, Howley PM. Association of human papillomavirus types 16 and 18 E6 proteins with p53. Science 1990;248:76–79.

75. Lane DP, Crawford LV. T antigen is bound to a host protein in SV40–transformed cells. Nature 1979;278:261–263.

76. Linzer D, Levine AJ. Characterization of a 54K dalton cellular SV40 tumor antigen present in SV40–transformed cells and uninfected embryonal carcinoma cells. Cell 1979;17:43–52.

77. Sarnow P, Ho YS, Williams J, Levine AJ. Adenovirus E1b-58kd tumor antigen and SV40 large tumor antigen are physically associated with the same 54 kd cellular protein in transformed cells. Cell 1982;28:387–394.

78. Hubbert NL, Sedman SA, Schiller JT. Human papillomavirus type 16 E6 increases the degradation rate of p53 in human keratinocytes. J Virol 1992;66: 6237–6241.

79. Scheffner M, Munger K, Byrne JC, Howley PM. The state of the p53 and retinoblastoma genes in human cervical carcinoma cell lines. Proc Natl Acad Sci USA 1991;88:5523–5527.

80. Huibregtse JM, Scheffner M, Howley PM. A cellular protein mediates association of p53 with the E6 oncoprotein of human papillomavirus types 16 or 18. EMBO J 1991;10:4129–4135.

81. Scheffner M, Huibregtse JM, Vierstra RD, Howley PM. The HPV-16 E6 and E6-AP complex functions as a ubiquitin-protein ligase in the ubiquination of p53. Cell 1993;75:495–505.

82. Mietz JA, Unger T, Huibregtse JM, Howley PM. The transcriptional transactivation function of wild-type p53 is inhibited by SV40 large T-antigen and by HPV-16 oncoprotein. EMBO J 1992;11:5013–5020.

83. Lechner MS, Mack DH, Finicle AB, Crook T, Vousden KH, Laimins LA. Human papillomavirus E6 proteins bind p53 in vivo and abrogate p53-mediated repression of transcription. EMBO J 1992;11:3045–3052.

84. Kessis TD, Slebos RJ, Nelson WG, et al. Human papillomavirus 16 E6 expres-

sion disrupts the p53-mediated cellular response to DNA damage. Proc Natl Acad Sci USA 1993;90:3988–3992.

85. White A, Livanos EM, Tlsty TD. Differential disruption of genomic integrity and cell cycle regulation in normal human fibroblasts by the HPV oncoproteins. Genes Dev 1994;8:666–677.

86. Klingelhutz AJ, Foster SA, Mcdougall JK. Telomerase activation by the E6 gene product of human papillomavirus type 16. Nature 1996;380:79–81.

87. Chen JJ, Reid CE, Band V, Androphy EJ. Interaction of papillomavirus E6 oncoproteins with a putative calcium-binding protein. Science 1995;269:529–531.

88. Tong X, Howley PM. The bovine papillomavirus E6 oncoprotein interacts with paxillin and disrupts the actin cytoskeleton. Proc Natl Acad Sci USA 1997;94:4412–4417.

89. DeCaprio JA, Ludlow JW, Lynch D, et al. The product of the retinoblastoma susceptibility gene has properties of a cell cycle regulatory element. Cell 1989;58:1085–1095.

90. Whyte P, Williamson NM, Harlow E. Cellular targets for transformation by the adenovirus E1A proteins. Cell 1989;56:67–75.

91. Münger K, Werness BA, Dyson N, Phelps WC, Howley PM. Complex formation of human papillomavirus E7 proteins with the retinoblastoma tumor suppressor gene product. EMBO J 1989;8:4099–4105.

92. Boyer SN, Wazer DE, Band V. E7 protein of human papilloma virus-16 induces degradation of retinoblastoma protein through the ubiquitin-proteasome pathway. Cancer Res 1996;56:4620–4624.

93. Jones DL, Münger K. Analysis of the p53- mediated G1 growth arrest pathway in cells expressing the human papillomavirus type 16 E7 oncoprotein. J Virol 1997;71:2905–2912.

94. Jewers RJ, Hildebrandt P, Ludlow JW, Kell B, McCance DJ. Regions of human papillomavirus type 16 E7 oncoprotein required for immortalization of human keratinocytes. J Virol 1992;66:1329–1335.

95. McIntyre MC, Frattini MG, Grossman SR, Laimins LA. Human papillomavirus type 18 E7 protein requires intact Cys-X-X-Cys motifs for zinc binding, dimerization, and transformation but not for Rb binding. J Virol 1993;67:3142–3150.

96. Clemens KE, Brent R, Gyuris J, Munger K. Dimerization of the human papillomavirus E7 oncoprotein in vivo. Virology 1995;214:289–293.

97. Zwerschke W, Joswig S, Jansen Durr P. Identification of domains required for transcriptional activation and protein dimerization in the human papillomavirus type-16 E7 protein. Oncogene 1996;12:213–220.

98. Mal A, Poon RYC, Howe PH, Toyoshima H, Hunter T, Harter ML. Inactivation of p27Kip1 by the viral E1A oncoprotein in TGFβ-treated cells. Nature 1996;380:262–265.

99. Zerfass-Thome K, Zwerschke W, Mannhardt B, Tindle R, Botz JW, Jansen-Durr P. Inactivation of the cdk inhibitor p27KIP1 by the human papillomavirus type 16 E7 oncoprotein. Oncogene 1996;13:2323–2330.

100. Polyak K, Kato JY, Solomon MJ, et al. p27(kip1), a cyclin-cdk inhibitor, links transforming growth factor-beta and contact inhibition to cell cycle arrest. Genes Dev 1994;8:9–22.

101. Pietenpol JA, Holt JT, Stein RW, Moses HL. Transforming growth factor β1 suppression of c-myc gene transcription: Role in inhibition of keratinocyte proliferation. Proc Natl Acad Sci USA 1990;87:3758–3762.

102. Funk JO, Waga S, Harry JB, Espling E, Stillman B, Galloway DA. Inhibition of CDK activity and PCNA-dependent DNA replication by p21 is blocked interaction with the HPV–16 E7 oncoprotein. Genes Dev 1997;11:2090–2100.

103. Jones DL, Alani RM, Münger K. The human papillomavirus E7 oncoprotein can uncouple cellular differentiation and proliferation in human keratinocytes by abrogating p21cip1-mediated inhibition of cdk2. Genes Dev 1997;11: 2101–2111.

104. Missero C, Calautti E, Eckner R, et al. Involvement of the cell-cycle inhibitor Cip1/WAF1 and the E1A-associated p300 protein in terminal differentiation. Proc Natl Acad Sci USA 1995;92:5451–5455.

105. Blanton RA, Coltrera MD, Gown AM, Halbert CL, McDougall JK. Expression of the HPV16 E7 gene generates proliferation in stratified squamous cell cultures which is independent of endogenous p53 levels. Cell Growth Differ 1992;3:791–802.

106. Cheng S, Schmidt-Grimminger DC, Murant T, Broker TR, Chow LT. Differentiation-dependent up-regulation of the human papillomavirus E7 gene reactivates cellular DNA replication in suprabasal differentiated keratinocytes. Genes Dev 1995;9:2335–2349.

107. Yokota J, Tsukada Y, Najajima T, et al. Loss of heterozygosity on the short arm of chromosome 3 in carcinoma of the uterine cervix. Cancer Res 1989;49: 3598–3601.

108. Ohta M, Inoue H, Cotticelli MG, et al. The FHIT gene, spanning the chromosome 3p14.2 fragile site and renal carcinoma-associated t(3;8) breakpoint, is abnormal in digestive tract cancers. Cell 1996;84:587–597.

109. Stanbridge EJ. Suppression of malignancy in human cells. Nature 1976;260: 17–20.

110. Smits HL, Raadsmeer E, Rood I, et al. Induction of anchorage independent growth of human fibroblasts with a deletion in the short arm of chromosome 11 by human papillomavirus 16 DNA. J Virol 1988;62:4538–4543.

111. Kirnbauer R, Taub J, Greenstone H, et al. Efficient self-assembly of human papillomavirus type 16 L1 and L1-L2 into virus-like particles. J Virol 1993;67: 6929–36.

112. Zhou J, Stenzel DJ, Sun XY, Frazer IH. Synthesis and assembly of infectious bovine papillomavirus particles in vitro. J Gen Virol 1993;74:763–8.

113. DeVilliers EM. Heterogeneity of the human papillomavirus group. J Virol 1989;63:4898–4903.

114. DeVilliers E-M. Human pathogenic papillomaviruses: an update. Curr Top Microbiol Immunol 1994;86:1–12.

7

Epstein-Barr Virus, Lymphoproliferative Diseases, and Nasopharyngeal Carcinoma

NANCY RAAB-TRAUB

The Epstein-Barr virus (EBV) is a ubiquitous human herpesvirus that infects greater than 90% of the world's population. It is the prototype member of the Herpesvirus subfamily, Gammaherpesviridae, and, like other herpesviruses, EBV establishes a latent infection with life-long persistence in the infected host.[1,2] EBV is transmitted by salivary exchange and is believed initially to infect the epithelial cells of the oropharynx and posterior nasopharynx, as well as the parotid gland and duct.[2,3] The virus subsequently infects B cells. The infected B cells usually do not produce virus and the virus is thought to establish a permanent latent infection in B cells in bone marrow and peripheral blood.[2,4]

Asymptomatic primary infection usually occurs in childhood; in relatively developed countries, however, infection may be delayed until after adolescence. This delayed primary infection may result in the clinical syndrome infectious mononucleosis (IM), a fact discovered serendipitously.[2] While conducting early seroepidemiologic studies of EBV infection, a laboratory worker performing the studies was the control seronegative. Her seroconversion during an episode of IM prompted the retrospective study of serum repositories at Yale University containing pre- and post-IM serum samples. These studies unequivocally established that IM occurred as a result of primary EBV infection.[5,6]

Following acute infection, virus can be detected in saliva and is sporadically secreted into saliva for years.[6,7] Hybridization *in situ* has detected evidence of EBV DNA in epithelial cells lining the parotid duct, and EBV DNA and replicative mRNAs have been detected in sloughed oropharyngeal and cervical epithelial cells. This suggested that these epithelial cells are permissively infected and may be the source of oropharyngeal virus shedding.[3,8,9]

In addition, a subset of peripheral blood lymphocytes persistently contains EBV. These cells can be established as permanent cell lines after explantation into culture in vitro.[2] The majority of the infected cells in the cell lines do not produce virus, but instead maintain the EBV genome as a multicopy episome.[10] An occasional cell in some cell lines may reactivate into viral replication. The infectious virus produced by such cells, or virus that is present in throat washings, will infect primary B cells, establish a latent infection, and induce growth transformation.[2]

Growth transformation is induced by the coordinate expression of multiple viral gene products.[1,2] It is thought that reactivation and expression of the growth-inducing viral functions also occurs *in vivo*. *In vivo*, the overgrowth of the transformed cells is controlled by viral-specific cytotoxic T cells that can be detected continuously in the peripheral blood of infected individuals.[11-14] This continued surveillance and protection from proliferating EBV-infected cells by cytotoxic T cells is a critical component in the control of EBV infection because EBV-infected lymphomas occur with high frequency in allograft recipients with T-cell immunosuppression.[15]

BIOCHEMICAL AND MOLECULAR CHARACTERISTICS

Like other herpesviruses, the virion of EBV consists of a core wrapped with DNA that is contained within an icosadeltahedral capsid. The virus has a membranous envelope with glycoprotein spikes. The pleomorphic envelope is separated from the capsid by an amorphous substance called the tegument that contains many virally encoded proteins.[1]

The EBV genome that is encapsidated in the virion is a 172-kb double-stranded, linear DNA molecule. The linear DNA has homologous direct tandem repeats (TR) of approximately 500 bp at each terminus and a large 3.0-kb internal repeat (IR1) that separates the genome into two regions of unique DNA.[1] The IR1 sequence is cut once by the enzyme BamHI. There are 5 to 10 copies of IR1 per viral genome, so this digestion produces a supermolar 3.0-kb DNA fragment, BamHI W, that can be detected with great sensitivity on Southern blots and has thus been useful for diagnostic studies.[16]

Identification of the terminal fragments is also useful diagnostically. The ends of the linear genome have multiple copies of the TR sequences.[17] The terminal restriction enzyme fragments are heterogeneous in size because of the variable numbers of the terminal repeat elements. Hybridization with a probe that identifies the terminal restriction enzyme fragments on Southern blots of virion DNA will detect ladder arrays of fragments that have differing numbers of repeat elements (Figure 7.1). After entry into the cell, the linear form circularizes through the TR to

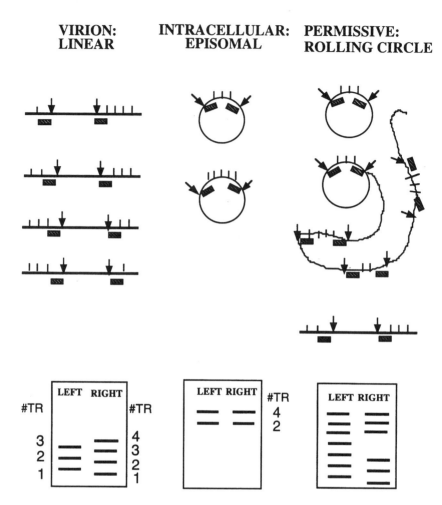

VIRION: LINEAR   **INTRACELLULAR: EPISOMAL**   **PERMISSIVE: ROLLING CIRCLE**

Figure 7.1. Structure of the EBV termini in Virus, latent, and permissive infection. The linear form of EBV DNA that is present in the virion has multiple copies at both termini of a 500-base-pair direct repeat (TR), indicated by small cross lines. When virion DNA is cleaved with a restriction enzyme that cuts in the unique DNA adjacent to the TRs, heterogeneous fragments are produced that differ in the number of repeat elements. Hybridization with DNA probes (hatched bars) representing unique DNA from either the left or right ends of the linear viral genome will identify the left or right terminal fragments.

The intracellular episomal form of DNA is formed through joining of the TR. This generates a fused terminal fragment that is identified on Southern blots by both the left and right end DNA probes. These fused fragments can be quite heterogeneous, thus the identification of a single fragment or clonal EBV episomes suggests cellular clonality.[18]

In permissive infections, episomal DNA, linear DNA, and replicative intermediates may all be present. Thus ladder arrays of fragments that do not align and represent linear DNA will be detected as well as multiple fused fragments that represent episomal and concatameric DNA.

182

form viral episomal DNA. The restriction enzyme fragment representing the fused termini of the episomal form of EBV can be distinguished from the restriction fragments of the linear genomes, because the fused fragments are larger and contain the unique DNA sequences adjacent to the terminal repeats. Therefore, these fragments will hybridize to DNA probes from both ends of the linear genome.[18]

This assay has significant diagnostic value because it permits discrimination between viral replicative and latent states; also, it is a predictor of the clonality of the genome.[18,19] In the initial studies, a single band representing the EBV-fused termini was detected in nasopharyngeal carcinoma (NPC) and in monoclonal lymphomas.[18] The identification of a single band indicated that all the EBV episomes were identical to one another with regard to the number of TR. This homogeneity indicated a clonal population of EBV genomes and by extension suggested cellular monoclonality. This study provided the first evidence that NPC, like Burkitt's lymphoma (BL), is a monoclonal proliferation and it revealed that the malignancy had developed from a single EBV-infected cell.[18]

Similar analyses of cell lines cloned in vitro identified clonal or oligoclonal fused terminal fragments and ladder arrays representing linear DNAs, revealing viral replication in some lines.[19] Arrays of terminal fragments have also been detected in DNA from many types of EBV-infected lymphoproliferations, some of which developed in patients who had AIDS or were organ-transplant recipients.[20] Scientists believe that during viral replication, rolling circle replicative intermediates are formed that have varying numbers of TR from the parental episome. The cleavage of replicative intermediates by restriction enzymes generates multiple fragments that hybridize to both probes even though they do not represent episomal DNA (Figure 7.1). Thus, is it difficult to assess clonality accurately when there is evidence of replication. Usually, however, in both cell lines in vitro and in lymphoproliferations in vivo, predominant fused terminal bands are detected, suggesting that most proliferations are monoclonal or oligoclonal.[20] An example of a clonal posttransplant lymphoma (PTL) with evidence of linear, virion DNA, and an example of a biclonal PTL, are shown in Figure 7.2. The detection of clonal EBV episomes and of the EBV-encoded small RNAs (EBER) within the malignant cells are the main diagnostic indicators of the association of EBV with a specific cancer.

SIGNIFICANCE OF EBV FOR WORLD HEALTH

The ability of EBV to transform B cells efficiently in culture to immortalized, transformed cells undoubtedly underlies its connection to human cancers. EBV is linked to at least five distinct major malignancies of lymphoid and epithelial cellular origin, and has been detected in a subset of many other cancers. The most consistent and significant associations include immunodeficiency-associated malignancies, Burkitt's lymphoma

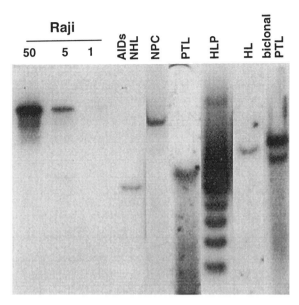

Figure 7.2. Identification of the EBV termini in EBV-associated disease. A Southern blot hybridized to the XhoI a fragment, which represents unique sequences from the right end of the linear EBV genome. The prototype Burkitt lymphoma, Raji, cell line and dilutions of Raji DNA are included for copy number comparisons (50, 5, 1 copy/cell). The samples include a monoclonal, non-Hodgkin's AIDS associated lymphoma (AIDS NHL), an NPC, a PTL with evidence of viral replication, a hairy leukoplakia (HLP) with abundant ladder arrays, a Hodgkin's lymphoma (HL), and a biclonal PTL.

(BL), Hodgkin's disease (HD), T-cell lymphoma, and nasopharyngeal carcinoma (NPC).[16,21-25] EBV infection is clearly etiologic to the development of lymphoma in organ transplant recipients, a disease of increasing worldwide significance; there were more than 50,000 transplantations in the United States in 1995.[16] EBV also contributes to the development of approximately one half of AIDS-associated lymphoproliferations.[26] As fewer AIDS patients succumb to opportunistic infections, such as *Pneumocystis carinii*, an increasing number of them develop cancer, with a projected 5000 lymphoma cases expected annually in the United States.[27] EBV is also linked to a significant proportion of HD, the most frequently occurring lymphoma in young adults.[28] HD has an incidence of $5.5/10^5$ in the 20- to 24-year-old age group.[29] Burkitt's lymphoma, although relatively rare in Western countries, is the most common childhood malignancy in equatorial Africa.[30] Finally, in terms of world health significance, nasopharyngeal carcinoma is one of the most significant virus-associated tumors.[30]

Virologic studies have characterized the viral infection in each of these malignancies and have identified the viral genes that are expressed. These studies have revealed that EBV expression is distinct in PTL, BL, HD, and

NPC, suggesting that the contribution of EBV to the etiology of these individual diseases may differ.[31–35] The extraordinarily elevated incidence of some of the EBV-associated malignancies—such as BL and NPC—in distinct populations has promoted intensive epidemiological investigations to identify contributing environmental and genetic elements. The relationship of a ubiquitous infectious agent to these diseases could reflect unique viral–cellular interactions, perhaps due to unique genetic and environmental components.

HISTORY AND EPIDEMIOLOGICAL ASSOCIATIONS

EBV has been linked to malignancies of both lymphoid and epithelial origin. Because of its ubiquity in normal hosts, however, these associations have been difficult to prove. Despite these difficulties, it is now widely accepted that EBV plays a role in the development of Burkitt's lymphoma, nasopharyngeal carcinoma, and lymphomas in immunocompromised patients. Other tumor associations are less consistent.

Burkitt's Lymphoma

EBV was first detected in cell lines established from the unusual childhood malignancy Burkitt's lymphoma (BL).[36] BL was first recognized by a British missionary surgeon, Denis Burkitt, working in East Africa. He described the clinical and epidemiological features of this tumor and discovered that the tumor occurred with high incidence in an endemic geographic region that was coincident with the endemic malarial belt of Central and East Africa.[21] Fresh tumor biopsies were sent to Dr. Anthony Epstein in London, where Drs. Epstein and Barr succeeded in establishing cell lines. In some lines, herpesvirus particles were detected by electron microscopy.[36] This virus was later shown to be distinct from other known human herpesviruses and subsequent seroepidemiologic studies revealed that EBV infection was widespread in all populations worldwide, with the majority of adults having antibodies to the virus.[37]

In endemic areas, BL occurs with the unusually high incidence of approximately 10 per 100,000 population per year for the first 15 years of life.[30] Early seroepidemiologic studies in endemic regions provided evidence that EBV was associated with the cancer. Children become infected with EBV during the first 2 years of life, and endemic BL patients have significantly elevated titers of antibody to viral antigens, including the viral capsid antigen (VCA) and early replicative functions (early antigen, EA).[37] Prospective epidemiological studies in Uganda indicated that high EBV VCA antibodies preceded the development of the tumor by months or years.[30] The high incidence of BL is coincident with high malarial infection both in equatorial Africa and in coastal New Guinea, suggesting that malarial infection may be a contributing factor to the development of this cancer.[22,38]

All of the tumors from the endemic areas contain EBV in all of the malignant cells, and each tumor contains a clonal form of the EBV episome, indicating that the tumor developed from a single EBV-infected cell.[18] The Raji cell line, a prototype latently infected BL cell line that contains clonal EBV episomes, is shown in Figure 7.2. BL was one of the first tumors shown to have a characteristic chromosomal translocation. The reciprocal translocations involve chromosome 8 near the location of the c-*myc* oncogene and either the immunoglobulin heavy chain locus on chromosome 14 or the light chain loci on chromosomes 2 and 22.[39]

In Western countries, rare childhood lymphomas were subsequently shown to resemble BL histologically.[40] These sporadic tumors occur 100-fold less frequently than the endemic form, but also are marked by the characterisitic translocations between c-*myc* and the immunoglobulin loci. It is intriguing that the sporadic and endemic forms of BL have different breakpoints with regard to c-*myc*. The endemic form has breakpoints several thousand base pairs upstream to the c-*myc* gene, whereas the breakpoint in the sporadic form usually occurs in the first exon or intron of the c-*myc* gene itself.[41]

In recent years, due to the epidemic of human immunodeficiency virus (HIV) infection, the incidence of sporadic BL has increased greatly. Although, in HIV infection, many types of lymphoid malignancies may develop, BL tends to arise early in the course of AIDS progression.[26] The tumors resemble classic BL histologically and also possess the characteristic translocations, with the chromosomal breakpoints similar to those in the sporadic BL. The association of EBV with sporadic BL is much less consistent than that with endemic BL, yet approximately 20% of the tumors of the childhood form contain EBV, and approximately 50% of those of the AIDS-associated form are EBV positive.[26]

Nasopharyngeal Carcinoma

Nasopharyngeal carcinoma (NPC) is an epithelial tumor that, like BL, is characterized by marked geographic and population differences in incidence.[2,30] It is common in southern China and southeast Asia, where it may represent 20% of all cancer cases, occurring at a rate of 30 to 100 per 100,000 population per year.[30,42] The tumor also frequently develops in Eskimo populations and occurs with elevated incidence in Mediterranean Africa.[43]

Early seroepidemiologic studies revealed that, like patients with BL, patients with NPC had elevated antibody titers to VCA and EA. Only NPC patients, however, had elevated IgA antibodies to these antigens.[44] Detection of IgA antibodies to EBV predated the development of NPC by several years and also correlated with tumor burden and recurrence. Subsequent studies revealed that viral DNA and the EBV nuclear antigen,

EBNA, were detected in the malignant epithelial cells rather than in the abundant infiltrating lymphoid cells.[45] This was the first detection of EBV within epithelial cells.

The incidence of NPC is low in Western populations, where it accounts for only 0.25% of all cancers and occurs at a rate of 0.1 per 100,000 population per year. In contrast to the relationship of EBV to BL, however, EBV is consistently detected in NPC, regardless of geographic location or the racial background of the patient.[16,46] The consistent association with a ubiquitous herpesvirus and the remarkable patterns of incidence suggest that other cofactors contribute to the development of this cancer.[47]

Comparisons of EBV infection among Indian and Chinese people living in Singapore revealed that both populations were infected with EBV early in life, usually between the ages of 6 and 9 years. Although the two ethnic groups were living in the same general area of Singapore, the NPC incidence was high only in the Chinese population. Elevated incidence is also retained by second-generation Chinese people in other nonendemic regions. This continued elevated incidence suggested that environmental contaminants are not likely to be a cofactor; rather, genetic or cultural and dietary differences probably contribute to the development of this disease.[47] One suggested dietary component is exposure to salted fish at an early age.[48] Tumor-promoting compounds have also been identified in food products in other populations that have elevated incidence of NPC.[49]

NPC presents with varying degrees of differentiation and has been classified by the World Health Organization into three categories.[50] Squamous cell carcinomas, WHO1 tumors, are highly differentiated, with characteristic epithelial growth patterns and keratin filaments. Nonkeratinizing WHO2 carcinomas retain epithelial cell shape and growth patterns. Undifferentiated carcinomas, WHO3, do not produce keratin and lack a distinctive growth pattern. In addition, many tumors have mixed degrees of differentiation or may present as WHO3 at the primary site with increased differentiation in metastatic lymph nodes.[50] The WHO2 and WHO3 tumors have elevated IgG and IgA titers to VCA and EA, whereas the WHO1 tumors have EBV serologic profiles similar to those of control populations.[51] The similarity in EBV serology between WHO1 cases and controls initially suggested that EBV was associated with only the WHO2 and WHO3 types. This remains controversial. Two subsequent studies consistently detected EBV in WHO1 tumors from both Asia and the United States[16,52]; in one other study, however, EBV was not detected in WHO1 NPC from certain areas.[53]

Of note, all forms of NPC contain clonal EBV episomes (Figure 7.2), suggesting that the tumor developed from a single EBV infected cell. This fact, and the consistent detection of EBV in most NPC, suggests that EBV is an essential cofactor in the development of this tumor.[42]

A recent study identified examples of dysplasia and isolated carcinoma *in situ* (CIS), collected at the Tumor Institute in Guangzhou, China, and the University of Malaya, Kuala Lumpur, Malaysia.[54] These isolated lesions were extremely rare (11 [0.6%] of 1798 NPCs) although examples of na-sopharyngeal intraepithelial neoplasia coexistent with invasive cancer were detected more frequently (58 [3%] of 1798 NPCs). The extreme rarity of lesions without concomitant carcinoma, the more frequent detection of dysplasia with invasive carcinoma, and the development of invasive carcinoma within 1 year of follow-up suggest a rapid progression of the initiated cell through the sequence of dysplasia, CIS, and invasive cancer. Thus, the biologic behavior of NPC is distinct from that observed in the malignant progression of mammary carcinoma or cervical cancer, where intraductal cancer of the breast or CIS of the cervix may persist for years.[55]

In the Tumor Institute–University of Malaya study, EBV was found in all the examples of dysplasia and CIS, with detection of EBER by *in situ* hybridization and latent membrane protein 1 (LMP1) by immunohistochemistry. In all samples, LMP1 was detected in all cells, indicating that the lesions were homogeneously infected. In Figure 7.3, LMP1 staining is shown in an example of severe dysplasia. Interestingly, in the surface epithelial cells that show evidence of differentiation, the detection of LMP1 is more intense, suggesting that LMP1's expression increases dur-

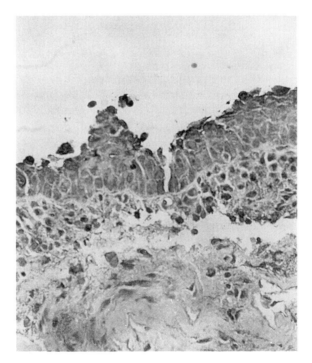

Figure 7.3. Detection of LMP1 in CIS. Expression of LMP1 is detected throughout the epithelial layer of this example of CIS. The entire affected epithelial layer stains positively for LMP1 as evidenced by the darker gray staining. LMP1 was detected with a cocktail of monoclonal antibodies (CS1-4) with a standard immunoperoxidase staining procedure.[54]

ing differentiation. In these samples, clonal EBV episomes were detected without detectable linear forms of the genome, revealing that the neoplasias were a predominantly latent infection.[54] The presence of a single clonal form of EBV implies that the hyperplasia or dysplasia represents a focus of EBV-induced cellular proliferation. Such lesions might spontaneously regress; however, their rarity and the more frequent detection of CIS concomitant with invasive cancer suggests that this clonal proliferation progresses rapidly to malignancy.

During primary and reactivated infection, oropharyngeal epithelial cells with evidence of viral replication have been detected and are thought to be the source for viral shedding.[3] The high titers of IgA to EBV replicative antigens (particularly VCA) that precede the development of NPC probably reflect increased antigenic stimulation. It has been shown that secretory IgA facilitates viral entry into epithelial cells.[56] This finding suggests that the elevated IgA titers may actually contribute to the development of NPC by enhancing epithelial infection.[56]

In the development of NPC, increased viral replication, perhaps at lymphoid–mucosal epithelial interfaces, increases the likelihood of the establishment of a latent, transforming infection of an epithelial cell. When a latent, transforming infection occurs, the infected cell begins to proliferate, creating the state of infection in the preinvasive lesion. The establishment of latent infection and expression of viral transforming functions in epithelial cells probably are critical events that lead to the development of NPC. This process could be influenced by genetic or environmental factors. Expression of the viral transforming functions, however, may be all that is needed to induce growth such that the dysplasia is rapidly invasive. Additional genetic changes—such as p53 mutation, Rb alterations, or ras mutations—would not be required and have not been detected in NPC.[57–59] However, these genetic changes could subsequently develop during tumor growth and contribute to tumor progression and metastasis.

Hodgkin's Disease

Hodgkin's disease (HD) or Hodgkin's lymphoma is a common malignant lymphoma characterized by the loss of lymph-node architecture, with the majority of infiltrating cells of a nonmalignant phenotype. The malignant cells are the unusual Hodgkin and Reed-Sternberg (RS) cells; these constitute about 2% of the tumor mass. Depending on the proportion of RS cells and the type of infiltrate, HD is histologically distinguished as lymphocyte predominant, nodular sclerosing, or lymphocyte depleted.[60]

HD occurs worldwide but is particularly frequent in higher socioeconomic groups in Western populations, where it occurs with two peaks of incidence at ages 25 to 30 years and at later than age 45 years.[29] Researchers observed years ago that the profile of the early-age–onset group was similar to that of patients who developed IM—the pathologic manifestation of primary EBV that occurs in post-adolescent infection.[61] A history of IM was associated with a two to four-fold increased risk of HD. Retrospective analyses of the serum repository at Yale revealed that elevated EBV titers preceded the development of HD by 2 to 3 years.[61]

The key finding supporting an etiologic association of EBV with HD was the detection of the viral genome and virally encoded proteins in the RS cells. Again, the analysis of the EBV genome revealed that HD had clonal EBV episomes (Figure 7.2).[62] This clonality indicated that HD develops from a single EBV-infected cell. Immunoglobulin gene rearrangements and, in some cases, T-cell receptor rearrangements also exhibit monoclonality.

HD tumors also have variable expression of B- or T-cell markers in some cases.[63] This variation in phenotype may indicate that the tumor developed following EBV infection of an immature cell that was not yet committed to either lymphocyte lineage.

Immunodeficiency-Associated Lymphomas

The ability of EBV to cause cancer is most clearly indicated by the development of B-cell lymphoproliferations in patients who are immunocompromised (see Chapter 5). In genetically affected families with X-linked lymphoproliferative syndrome, the majority of affected males die of fatal infectious mononucleosis or lymphomas that develop almost immediately after primary infection.[64] The cells are lymphoblastoid in appearance, and multiple clones of proliferating cells are found infiltrating various organs.

EBV lymphoproliferations and lymphomas also develop in patients who are immunosuppressed following allograft transplantation and in patients with AIDS.[15,20,21,65] All cases of posttransplant lymphoma (PTL) are EBV positive and may be polyclonal, oligoclonal, or monoclonal at diagnosis (Figure 7.2). Depending on the degree of or regimen for immunosuppression, PTL develops in 5% to 15% of cardiac transplants, 10% of heart-–lung transplants, 1% to 3% of renal transplants, and approximately 1% to 2% of bone-marrow transplants.[15] In some cases, the disease may regress after reduction in immunosuppressive therapy, indicating that the cells are still susceptible to EBV-specific cytotoxic T cells. Adoptive immunotherapy has been applied successfully in some cases.[66,67] However, the majority of EBV-positive lymphomas develop in patients who acquire the virus from the transplanted organ or subsequent transfusions and therefore lack EBV antibodies and EBV-specific CTLs.

Lymphomas develop in approximately 3% of AIDS patients. BL may develop early in AIDS progression and, as mentioned previously, approximately 25% are EBV positive with c-*myc* translocations similar to other sporadic BL.[26,68] Other B-cell malignancies also occur at high incidence in AIDS; approximately 50% of these are EBV-associated. Central nervous system lymphoma is extremely rare in the general population, but occurs in 0.5% of patients with AIDS.[69] All the CNS lymphomas are EBV positive. Possible epidemiologic factors that contribute to the development of EBV-positive lymphoma or CNS lymphoma have not yet been identified.

T-Cell Lymphomas

Although long believed to be B-cell trophic, EBV has been detected in an occasional T-cell lymphoma. A particular type of T-cell lymphoma that usually presents in the nasal cavity, also referred to as midline granuloma, is a common tumor in Southeast Asians. EBV was first linked to midline granuloma when five tumors in Japanese patients were all found to be EBV positive. These tumors had various T- or NK-cell markers, suggesting EBV infection of a peculiar undifferentiated cell type.[70]

Peripheral T-cell lymphomas that are EBV positive have also been described in Taiwanese and Japanese populations.[24] In some cases, EBV was detected only in some cells, suggesting that the virus infected the tumor secondarily. However, the proportion of EBV-infected cells seems to increase over time, with emergence of a clonal EBV-infected population, indicating that the virally infected cells have some growth advantage and that the fastest growing clone will eventually predominate.[25] The occurrence of T-cell lymphomas is also increasing in AIDS patients; all such tumors are EBV-positive.

Other Tumors Linked to EBV

Undifferentiated carcinomas of other tissues also have been associated with EBV. Clonal EBV episomes have been detected in all examined samples of undifferentiated carcinoma of the parotid gland.[60] Although the parotid gland is a site of viral shedding, carcinoma of the parotid gland involves a clonal proliferation of nonpermissively infected epithelial cells. Undifferentiated carcinoma of the parotid gland is an extremely rare cancer that has been detected most often in Eskimo populations that also have a high incidence of NPC.[43] EBV infection has also been detected in a rare form of undifferentiated gastric carcinoma seen in both Asian and white populations[71]. These findings indicate that EBV may gain access to epithelial cells outside the naso-oropharynx, and that in some of these instances, it leads to the development of carcinoma.

PATHOGENETIC MECHANISMS AND CARCINOGENESIS

EBV has been extensively studied and the functions of many of its genes and proteins are known. Much is yet to be learned, however, about how these elements converge with host factors to cause carcinogenesis.

Expression in Latent Infection

In B-lymphoid cell lines established from the peripheral blood or after infection of B cells *in vitro*, the majority of cells harbor EBV in a latent state with reactivation of viral replication in an occasional cell. In latently infected lymphocytes, the viral DNA is maintained as an episome with expression of multiple viral genes.[1] These genes include six EBNAs and two integral membrane proteins—latent membrane protein 1 (LMP1) and latent membrane protein 2 (LMP2). Potential functions have been identified for some of these proteins.

The EBNA1 protein is essential for maintenance and replication of the viral episome. EBNA1 binds to the origin of replication for the plasmid form of the viral genome and is essential for plasmid replication.[72] The EBNA2 protein is essential for growth transformation of lymphocytes and is also a transcriptional transactivator.[73] It interacts with several cellular proteins and regulates the viral promoters for LMP1, LMP2, CD23 (the B-cell activation marker), and CD21 (the receptor for complement that is also the EBV receptor).[1,74] Two types of EBNA2 have been identified; they are encoded by divergent sequences.[75] The type of EBNA2 gene, EBNA2A or 2B, has been used to define two types of EBV: EBV1 or 2. EBV1 is more prevalent than EBV2 in Western populations; EBV2 infection is more prevalent in central Africa, in New Guinea, and among Alaskan Eskimos.[76,77] Coinfection with both EBV types is detected frequently in HIV-infected patitents and also is seen in immunocompetent hosts.[78,79]

The EBNA3 genes have two forms encoded by distinct sequences that cosegregate with the EBNA2 type[75,80] and help determine the EBV type. The EBNA3 proteins interact with cellular proteins and modulate transactivation of the LMP1 promoter by the EBNA2 protein.[1] The EBNA3C protein also up-regulates expression of CD21.[1]

The LMP1 and LMP2 proteins are located in the cytoplasmic membrane of latently infected cells.[1] LMP1 is a hydrophobic protein with six domains that wind through the cell membrane (Figure 7.4). LMP1 is the only EBV gene product that has transforming ability in rodent fibroblasts and is essential for EBV transformation of lymphocytes.[81,82] Expression of LMP1 at levels comparable to those observed in infected lymphocytes alters the phenotype of lymphoid cells and transforms Rat-1 cells *in vitro* to anchorage-independent growth and tumorgenicity in nude mice.[81] Expression of LMP1 alters expression of B-cell activation antigens, adhesion molecules, transferrin receptor, and sensitivity to transforming growth factor β, and induces expression of the *bcl-2* oncogene.[1,83] The induction of Bcl-2 is thought to be responsible for the inhibition of apoptosis in lymphocytes by LMP1.[26] In epithelial cells, LMP1 activates expression of the epidermal growth factor receptor and of an antiapoptotic factor called A20.[84]

The second membrane protein, LMP2, colocalizes with LMP1 in the cytoplasmic membrane of lymphocytes and is phosphorylated by an associated tyrosine kinase.[85] LMP2 blocks activation of B cells through the immunoglobulin receptor and is thought to prevent reactivation and viral replication, thereby maintaining a latent infection.[1]

In EBV-infected cells, two small nonpolyadenylated RNA molecules designated EBER 1 and EBER 2 are transcribed by RNA polymerase III.[86]

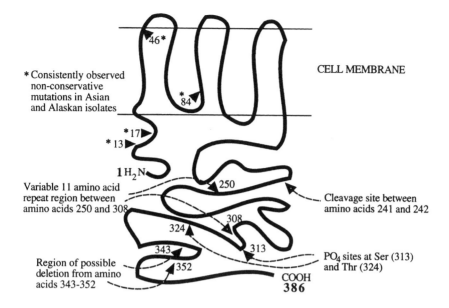

* Consistently observed
non-conservative
mutations in Asian
and Alaskan isolates

CELL MEMBRANE

46
*84
*17
*13
1 H₂N
Variable 11 amino acid
repeat region between
amino acids 250 and 308
250
Cleavage site between
amino acids 241 and 242
308
324
343
313
Region of possible
deletion from amino
acids 343-352
352
PO₄ sites at Ser (313)
and Thr (324)
COOH
386

Figure 7.4. Structure of LMP1 The positions of the nonconservative amino acid changes that are consistently detected in the Alaskan and Chinese EBV strains are marked by asterisks. The presence of the variable repeat element in the carboxy terminus between amino acids 250 and 308 is indicated as well as the region of possible deletion between amino acids 343 and 352. Potential serine and threonine phosphorylations sites are denoted. (Reprinted with permission from reference 99.)

These 170-bp RNAs are encoded by adjacent sequences that have considerable homology. The EBERs exist as ribonucleoprotein complexes and are the most abundantly expressed viral transcript, with 10^5 or 10^6 copies per infected cell. Genetic studies indicate that EBER expression is not essential for lymphocyte transformation and the EBERs' function remains obscure.[87]

In patients with HIV and in occasional transplant recipients, an unusual lesion may develop on the lateral borders of the tongue. This condition, oral hairy leukoplakia (OHL), is the first pathologic manifestation of a permissive EBV infection, and abundant arrays of fragments indicative of virion DNA are detected by the termini assay (Figure 7.2).[88] Viral particles, replicative gene products, and linear viral DNA all confirm that OHL is a site of EBV replication. Of interest, although LMP1 and other viral gene products are detected, OHL lacks episomal EBV DNA and expression of the EBERs.[89] This finding reveals that OHL is not a site of reactivation of replication from latency but rather a *de novo* permissive infection, and that EBER expression is a marker of latent EBV infection. This fact and the extraordinary abundance and stability of the EBER ribonucleoprotein complexes makes *in situ* detection of EBER expression one of the most useful diagnostic tools for identification of latently infected cells.

Replicative Gene Functions

Permissive and latent EBV infection can be distinguished in several ways. Permissively infected cells contain linear forms of DNA detected as ladder arrays in the EBV termini assay (Figures 7.1 and 7.2) and, in OHL, lack EBER expression. A single viral gene is responsible for the induction of viral replication. The EBV replication activator gene (ZEBRA) is encoded by the BamHI Z fragment.[90] ZEBRA regulates the expression of other viral genes and induces the expression of the viral DNA polymerase. Replication by the viral DNA polymerase produces the linear form of the genome that is present in virions.[1] Thus, expression of ZEBRA and detection of linear DNA indicates permissive infection. Although the malignancies associated with EBV represent latently infected transformed cells, the decline in the ability of cytotoxic T cells to recognize and eliminate permissively infected cells could also influence the development of lymphoma. Infectious virus produced by peripheral blood lymphocytes could transform additional cells, increasing the pool of cells at risk for developing lymphoma. Free virus also could be a direct factor in the development of CNS lymphoma.

Clonality and Expression in Vivo

The pattern of EBV expression in transformed lymphoid cell lines is distinct from that detected in the EBV-associated malignancies. In BL and in cells freshly explanted from BL, only the EBNA1 gene is thought to be expressed (type 1 latency).[91] The cells do not form clumps or express the activation antigens associated with EBV infection in transformed lymphoid cell lines. In NPC and in HD, only EBNA1, LMP1, and LMP2 are expressed (type 2 latency).[33,34,92] In the immunoblastic lymphomas, all of the known viral latent proteins, EBNAs and LMPs, are detected (type 3 latency).[32] This pattern of expression is identical to that in transformed cell lines maintained *in vitro*. The patterns of expression found in the three types of latent infection have important implications for control of EBV growth transformed lymphocytes.[14]

HLA class I–restricted cytotoxic T-lymphocytes (CTLs) are important in control of growth of EBV-transformed lymphocytes. EBV infection induces a long-lasting CTL response against one or another of the latent viral proteins presented in the context of a particular HLA class I restriction. The HLA genotype determines the target antigen choice and possibly the strength of the cytotoxic response, with particularly strong CTL responses associated with certain HLA alleles.[11-13]

The most frequently detected and possibly immunodominant target antigens are the EBNA 3A, 3B, and 3C proteins.[12,93] These proteins are detected in the immunoblastic lymphomas that develop in transplant recipients.[32] These lymphomas remain sensitive to virus-specific CTL and respond to reductions in immunosuppression. In contrast, in type 1 and 2 latency detected in BL, NPC, and HD, the CTL response to the viral genes that are expressed (EBNA1, LMP1, and LMP2) is thought to be a minor component of the cellular immune response.[14,94] This variation in expression and immune response raises the possibility of enhancing, for therapeutic purposes, a specific CTL response to the specific viral genes that are expressed in malignancies. One study revealed that a specific polymorphism in the EBV strain prevalent in New Guinea altered the EBNA4 epitope presented by A11, the predominant HLA in New Guinea, and abrogated CTL recognition.[95] This observation suggested that the viral strain had evolved due to immune pressure. A similar finding has been described in CTL responses to HIV. The predominant CTL response in HIV is directed against the gag protein. In studies in HIV-positive donors, genetic variation in HIV gag CTL epitopes led to loss of CTL recognition.[96]

Taken together, these observations indicate that control of EBV-infected B cells and lymphomas is a complex interplay of multiple components. Factors that could influence lymphoma development include the strength of specific CTL responses, which may be governed by HLA type; differences in expression of the immunodominant viral proteins in the malignancy; and potential strain variation in CTL recognition sequences.

LMP1: the EBV Oncogene

A key factor in cell transformation appears to be LMP1, known as the EBV oncogene. This protein's carcinogenic effects may depend somewhat on its genetic sequence, which varies from strain to strain.

Strain Variation

One explanation for the elevated incidence of EBV-associated malignancies in specific populations is variation in strains of EBV. In other words, the prevalence of specific strains with distinct biologic properties within localized populations could contribute to these differences in disease incidence. Analyses of strain variation based on restriction enzyme polymorphisms have identified a predominant strain in NPC from southern China.[77,97] One of the polymorphisms observed in this strain was the loss of an XhoI restriction enzyme polymorphism within the LMP1 gene.[77,98] This polymorphism was also present in all NPC samples from Alaska and in some of the NPC samples from white Americans, but was not seen in samples of NPC from Mediterranean Europe and Africa. Analysis of the EBV type in the NPC samples indicated that Chinese strain was EBV type, 1 based on the EBNA2 sequence; the Alaskan samples were EBV type 2.[77]

Further studies of NPC cases revealed consistent, distinct sequence variation in the amino terminus of LMP1 in both the prevalent EBV type 1 Chinese strain and the EBV type 2 Alaskan Eskimo strain (Figure 7.3).[99]

This finding indicates that the strain variation detected in LMP1 is independent of the EBV type. Moreover, the detection of identical amino acid changes in the amino terminus of LMP1 in Chinese EBV type 1 and in Alaskan EBV type 2 suggests that mutation of these amino acids imparts some advantage to a virus encoding these changes.

The elevated incidence of NPC and BL in restricted populations, such as Alaskan Eskimos and Cantonese from southeastern China, also may reflect a predominance of a specific MHC type. The high incidence of a specific MHC haplotype in these populations could provide an immune selection for viruses with mutations in putative CTL recognition sequences in LMP1. The prevalence of a viral strain with such mutations may allow expression of LMP1 in infected cells to go undetected by virtue of the inability of MHC molecules to process and present mutated LMP1 peptides properly to circulating cytotoxic T cells. Such a mechanism would allow the variant virus to resist immune recognition and might contribute to the prevalence of NPC tumors in specific ethnic groups.

EBV strains can also be distinguished by sequence variation in the LMP1 carboxy terminus; three types of sequence variation have been detected (Figure 7.4). In one type of carboxy sequence variation, the LMP1 sequences differ in the number of 11 amino acid (aa) repeat elements. However, variation in the number of repeat elements may change due to recombination during replication and, therefore, the number of repeat elements does not distinguish EBV strains. In the permissive infection OHL, the LMP1 coding sequence from a single strain has been shown to contain multiple, differing numbers of repeats. A second difference has been identified in the prototype type 1 B95–8 sequence and in the type 1 RAJI and type 2 HR-1 strains, where the third repeat element contains an insertion of five amino acids. The third variation is a deletion of amino acids 343–352 of the B95–8 LMP-1. This deletion is present in the type 1 Chinese strains, but is not seen in the type 2 Alaskan strains, although the Chinese and Alaskan strains have nearly identical amino acid changes in the amino terminus. Strains with or without the deletion have been detected in approximately equal proportions in the various EBV-associated diseases.[99] However, several studies have suggested that LMP1 with the 343–352 deletion has enhanced transforming potential *in vitro* and may be present in more aggressive forms of disease.[100-102]

Biologic and Biochemical Properties

Genetic studies have revealed that the EBV latent membrane protein, LMP1, is essential for transformation of B cells in vitro.[82] Expression of LMP1 affects different cellular genes in lymphocytes and epithelial cells.[84] In both cell types, NF-$\varkappa$B transcription factors are activated, although different forms of NF-$\varkappa$B are activated in the two cell types.[103] Activation of NF-$\varkappa$B increases expression of B-cell activation markers in lymphoid cells, and expression of the A20 gene in both lymphoid and epithelial cells. In epithelial cells only, LMP1 activates transcription of the epidermal growth factor receptor, which is also detected at high levels in NPC.[84]

The biochemical properties of LMP1 that are responsible for these effects on cellular expression probably are due to LMP1's abilities to activate the NF-κB transcription factors and to interact with cellular molecules that mediate signals from the tumor necrosis factor (TNF) family of receptors.[104] The TNF receptor–associated factors (TRAFs) form heteromeric complexes that transduce signals that depending on the receptor may activate NF-κB, induce cellular growth, or induce apoptosis. Thus the activation of the TRAF pathway is likely the key property of LMP1 that mediates its effects on cellular growth regulation.

Contributing Genetic Factors in Carcinogenesis

The development of cancer is thought to be a multistage process that involves alteration of multiple genes. Aberrant activation of oncogenes that stimulate growth, and inactivation of cellular suppressor genes that control cellular proliferation, are frequent steps in the development of cancer. The contribution of cellular oncogenes to the development of many human cancers has been suggested by consistent chromosomal rearrangements that alter cellular gene expression or function. The chromosomal translocation characteristic of BL has been shown to involve the c-*myc* oncogene. Deregulated c-*myc* expression is found in both sporadic and endemic forms of BL, suggesting that this step is an essential one in the development of this lymphoma. As the translocations involve the immunoglobulin loci, it is possible that they occur during variable gene rearrangement or class switching. The cell-surface markers that are characteristic of BL—CD10 and CD77—suggest that BL cells may represent a germinal center B cell. Germinal centers are greatly expanded in chronic malarial infection and in HIV infection. This increase in germinal B cell number could be a contributing factor to the increased risk of development of BL in these conditions.

In contrast with what is observed in BL, c-*myc* is not rearranged in NPC or in PTL. Given that multiple additional viral genes are expressed in these cancers, it is possible that the virus induces cell growth by affecting other pathways, or that it indirectly activates c-*myc* expression.

Mutations of the p53 tumor suppressor gene are among the most common genetic alterations found in human malignancies, including those of the colon, lung, and breast.[105] Alterations in the wild-type p53 lead to loss of the suppressor function and thus contribute to tumorigenesis. In BL and lymphomas in patients with AIDS and Wiskott-Aldrich syndrome, p53 mutation was detected frequently but not in lymphomas that arose in transplant recipients or in NPC.[57,106,107] This suggests that EBV viral gene expression may influence the selection for p53 mutations. In support of this hypothesis, recent studies indicate that LMP1 interferes with p53-mediated apoptosis.

Other studies have shown that other identified suppressor genes—including the retinoblastoma gene, p21, and p16—are not mutated in

NPC.[58,59] The expression or function of these genes may be indirectly affected, however, by the viral transforming genes.

PREVENTION AND CONTROL

As new diagnostic methods are developed, it is evident that the number of cases of disease that can be linked to EBV is increasing, especially in immunocompromised patients. The medical significance of EBV infection underscores the importance of developing a vaccine that could either protect against infection or eliminate specific pathologic consequences. The malignancies associated with EBV represent latent infections in which the viral genome is maintained by the host cell DNA polymerase. These diseases are therefore not susceptible to most antiviral therapies, which target the viral DNA polymerase. Therefore, to control the virus-associated malignancies, we must develop novel immune or molecular therapies.

Vaccination

To prevent viral infection, we may need to neutralize EBV at mucosal surfaces completely; doing so probably would require efficient induction of IgA antibodies. That could theoretically be accomplished with a transformation-defective EBV that would replicate at mucosal surfaces. Several studies indicate that there are naturally occuring EBV strains that lack the EBNA2 gene and do not transform cells. A genetically engineered strain of EBV that lacked essential transforming proteins yet replicated efficiently at mucosal surfaces might be useful as an attenuated vaccine.

An alternate approach would be a subunit vaccine; two possible approaches to developing such a vaccine have been attempted. One approach utilizes the most abundant viral glycoprotein, gp350—a protein essential for viral binding to and infection of host cells.[1] The protective efficacy of gp350 vaccination has been tested in cottontop marmosets challenged with a parenteral inoculation of a lymphoma-inducing dose of EBV.[108] Some protection was provided that seemed to be cell-mediated rather than antibody-mediated. It is possible that gp350 vaccination could produce sufficient antibody and cell-mediated response to prohibit infection of lymphocytes at mucosal epithelial or lymphoid sites. A different gp350 vaccine, a GP350/ vaccinia recombinant, has been tested in China in a small number of seronegative children. After 1 year, all 10 of the control group had seroconverted and had antibodies to VCA, indicating wild-type EBV infection; in the comparison test group, only three of nine had seroconverted.[109] These results may indicate some degree of protection against wild-type infection. The completeness and the durability of this immunity need to be further evaluated. However, posttransplant lymphoma in solid organ transplant recipients usually develops in seronegative recipients. In these patients, the virus is acquired from the donor organ. Thus, the neutralizing antibodies produced to recombinant gp350 and present in serum could provide effective protection against PTL. In addition, whether an infected individual manifests IM may depend on the degree or severity of initial EBV exposure; thus, although the presence of neutralizing antibodies might not provide complete protection from infection, it could reduce the initial viral burden and effectively eliminate the syndrome of IM.

Another subunit approach to vaccination would induce CTL recognition using synthetic peptides. These peptides would represent the predominant CTL epitopes that are presented by the MHC class I type prevalent in a given population. A recent study showed that a cocktail of EBV epitopes expressed in vaccinia virus was processed correctly for the individual HLA classes, and that the virus could activate the correct EBV epitope–specific CTLs in vitro.[110] Many EBV CTL epitopes have been identified, and it is possible that an appropriate cocktail could be selected to protect the majority of individuals.

Immune Therapy

The immunoblastic lymphomas that develop in transplant recipients seem to remain susceptible to T-cell control and may regress with reduced immunosuppression. Through expansion of EBV-specific CTLs *in vitro*, it has been possible to suppress the development of these lymphomas prophylactically.[66,67,111] This approach is currently being tested for Hodgkin's lymphoma.

It may also be possible to enhance a specific CTL response. In NPC and Hodgkins's disease, the viral proteins that induce the immunodominant CTL response are not expressed. It is possible that the viral expression could be manipulated, perhaps through the use of demethylating agents such as azcytidine. This treatment has been shown to induce expression of the EBNA viral proteins that normally are not expressed in NPC, HD, or T-cell lymphomas and theoretically would make the cells susceptible to CTL killing. Alternatively, the CTL response to weaker immunogens, such as LMP1 or LMP2, theoretically could be enhanced, enabling immune recognition and control of the tumor.

CONCLUSIONS

There are compelling epidemiological and biological data that indicate that EBV is a potent inducer of human cancer. The abnormal growth may require the consistent expression of multiple viral proteins. This possibility provides an opportunity for both immune-mediated therapy and specific molecular therapy directed toward the viral functions. The continued study of determinants of immune control and of the biochemical properties of the viral genes will, in the long term, enable us to control viral infection or to eliminate the pathogenic consequences of such infection. In addition, the identification of the interactions of viral and cellular proteins will provide a new understanding of critical cellular pathways that are affected in human cancers.

REFERENCES

1. Kieff E, Liebowitz D. 1990. Epstein-Barr Virus and Its Replication. In: Fields B, Knipe D, eds. Virology. 2nd ed Philadelphia: Lippencott-Raven; 1990: 1889–1920.
2. Miller G. Epstein-Barr virus: biology, pathogenesis, and medical aspects. In: Fields B, Knipe D, eds. virology. 2nd ed. 1990: 1921–1958.
3. Sixbey J, Nedrud JG, Raab-Traub N, Hanes RA, Pagano JS. Detection of Epstein-Barr virus DNA and RNA in human pharyngeal epithelial cells. N Engl J Med 1984;310:1225–1230.
4. Gratama JW, Oosterveer MAP, Zwaan FE, Lepooutre J, Klein G, Ernberg I. Eradication of Epstein-Barr virus by allogeneic bone marrow transplantation: implications for sites of viral latency. Proc Natl Acad Sci USA 1988;85:8693–8696.
5. Henle G, Henle W, Diehl V. Relation of Burkitt tumor associated herpes-type virus to infectious mononucleosis. Proc Natl Acad Sci USA 1968; 59:94–101.
6. Niederman JC, McCollulm RW, Henle G, Henle W. Infectious mononucleosis. JAMA 1968;203:139–143.
7. Miller G, Niederman JC, Andrews LL. Prolonged oropharyngeal excretion of Epstein-Barr virus after infectious mononucleosis. N Engl J Med. 1973; 288:229–232.
8. Sixbey J, Lemon SM, Pagano JS. A second site for Epstein-Barr virus shedding: the uterine cervix. Lancet 1986;2:1122–1125.
9. Wolf H, Haus M, Wilmes E. Persistence of Epstein-Barr virus in the parotid gland. J Virol 1984;51:795–798.
10. Nonoyama M, Pagano J. Separation of Epstein-Barr virus DNA from large, chromosomal DNA in non-virus producing cells. Nature 1972;333:41–45.
11. Appolloni A, Moss D, Stumm R, Burrows S, Suhrbier A, Misko I, Schmidt C, Sculley T. Sequence variation of cytotoxic T cell epitopes in different isolates of Epstein-Barr virus. Eur J Immunol 1992;22:183–189.
12. Gavioli R, Kurilla M, de Campos-Lima P-O, Wallace L, Dolcetti R, Murray, Rickinson A, Masucci M. Multiple HLA A11-restricted cytotoxic T-lymphocyte epitopes of different immunogenetics in the Epstein-Barr virus-encoded nuclear antigen 4. J Virol 1993;67:1572–1578.
13. Khanna R, Burrows SR, Kurilla MG, Jacob CA, Misko IS, Sculley TB, Kieff E, Moss DJ. Localization of Epstein-Barr virus cytotoxic T cell epitopes using recombinant vaccinia: implications for vaccine development. J Exp Med 1992;176:169–176.
14. Murray RJ, Kurilla MG, Brooks JM, Thomas WA, Rowe M, Kieff E, Rickinson AB. Identification of target antigens for the human cytotoxic T cell response to Epstein-Barr virus (EBV): implications for the immune control of EBV-positive malignancies. J Exp Med 1992;176:157–168.

15. Cohen J. Epstein-Barr virus lymphoproliferative disease associated with acquired immunodeficiency. Medicine 1991;70:137–160.
16. Raab-Traub N, Flynn K, Pearson G, Huang A, Levine P, Lanier A, Pagano J. The differentiated form of nasopharyngeal carcinoma contains Epstein-Barr virus DNA. Int J Cancer 1987;39:25–29.
17. Given D, Yee D, Griem K, Kieff E. DNA of Epstein-Barr virus. V. Direct repeats at the ends of Epstein-Barr virus DNA. J Virol 1979;30:852–862.
18. Raab-Traub N, Flynn K. The structure of the termini of the Epstein-Barr virus as a marker of clonal cellular proliferation. Cell 1986;47:883–889.
19. Brown NA, Liu C, Wang YF, Garcia C. B-cell lymphoproliferation and lymphomagenesis are associated with clonotypic intracellular terminal regions of the Epstein-Barr virus. J Virol 1988;62:962–969.
20. Katz BZ, Raab-Traub N, Miller G. Latent and replicating forms of Epstein-Barr virus DNA in lymphomas and lymphoproliferative diseases. J Infect Dis 1989;160:589–598.
21. Hanto DW, Gajl-Peczalska KJ, Frizzera G, Arthur DC, Balfour HH, McClain K, Simmons RL, Najerian JS. Epstein-Barr virus (EBV) induced polyclonal and monoclonal B-cell lymphoproliferative disease occurring after renal transplantation: clinical, pathologic, and virologic findings and implications for therapy. Ann Surg 1983;198:356–369.
22. Burkitt D. A children's cancer dependent upon climatic factors. Nature 1962;194:232–234.
23. Cleary ML, Nalesnik MA, Shearere WT, Sklar J. Clonal analysis of transplant-associated lymphoproliferations based on the structure of the termini of the Epstein-Barr virus. Blood 1988;72:349–352.
24. Su IJ, Hsieh HC, Lin KH. Aggressive peripheral T-cell lymphomas containing Epstein-Barr viral DNA: a clinicopathological and molecular analysis. Blood 1991;77:799–808.
25. Chen CL, Sadler R, Walling D, Su IH, Hsieh H-C, and Raab-Traub N. Epstein-Barr virus (EBV) gene expression in EBV-positive peripheral T-cell lymphomas. J Virol 1993;67:6303–6308.
26. Miller G, Raab-Traub N. Pathogenesis of Epstein-Barr virus infection in HIV-1–positive patients. HIV Adv Res Ther 1993;3:23–29.
27. Gail MH, Pluda JM, Rabkin CS. Projections on the incidence of non-Hodgkin's lymphoma related to acquired immunodeficiency syndrome. J Natl Cancer Inst 1991;83:695–700.
28. Cancer Statistics Review 1973–1989. Miller BA, et al, eds. Bethesda: U.S. Dept. of Health and Human Services.
29. Gutensohn NM, Cole P. Epidemiology of Hodgkins's disease. Semin Oncol 1980;7:92–102.
30. de The G. Epidemiology of Epstein-Barr virus and associated diseases. In Roizman B, ed. The Herpesviruses. New York: Plenum Press; 1982: 25–87.
31. Raab-Traub N, Hood R, Yang CS, Henry B, Pagano JS. Epstein-Barr virus transcription in nasopharyngeal carcinoma. J Virol 1983;98:580–590.
32. Young L, Alfieri C, Hennessy K, Evans H, O'Hara C, Anderson K, Ritz J, Shapiro R, Rickinson A, Kieff E, Cohen J. Expression of Epstein-Barr virus transformation-associated genes in tissues of patients with EBV lymphoproliferative disease. N Engl J Med 1989;321:1080–1085.
33. Young L, Dawson C, Clark D, Rupani H, Busson P, Tursz T, Johnson A, Rick-

inson A. Epstein-Barr virus expression in nasopharyngeal carcinoma. J Gen Virol 1988;69:1051–1065.

34. Gilligan K, Sato H, Rajadurai P, Busson P, Young L, Rickinson A, Tursz T, Raab-Traub N. Novel transcription from the Epstein-Barr virus terminal EcoR1 fragment, DIJhet, in a nasopharyngeal carcinoma. J Virol 1990; 64:4948–4956.

35. Pallesen G, Hamilton-Dutoit SJ, Rowe M, Young LS. Expression of Epstein-Barr virus latent gene products in tumor cells of Hodgkin's disease. Lancet 1991;337:320–322.

36. Epstein MA, Achong BG, Barr YM Virus particles in cultured lymphoblasts from Burkitt's malignant lymphoma. Lancet 1964;1:252–253.

37. Henle G, Henle W, Clifford P. Antibodies to EB virus in BL and control groups. J Natl Cancer Inst 1969;43:1147–1157.

38. O'Connor GT. Persistent immunologic stimulation as a factor in oncogenesis, with special reference to Burkitt's tumor. Am J Med 1970;48:279–285.

39. Dalla-Favera R, Bregni M, Erikson J, Patterson D, Gallo RW, Croce C. Human c-myc oncogene is located on the region of chromosome 8 that is translocated in BL cells. Proc Natl Acad Sci USA 1982;79:7824–7827.

40. O'Connor GT, Rappaport H, Smith EB. Childhood lymphoma resembling BL in the United States. Cancer 1965;18:411–417.

41. Neri A, Barriga F, Knowles DM, Magrath IT, Dalla-Favera R. Different regions of the immunoglobulin heavy chain locus are involved in chromosomal translocations in distinct pathogenetic forms of BL. Proc Natl Acad Sci USA 1988;85:2748–2752.

42. Raab-Traub N. Epstein-Barr virus and nasopharyngeal carcinoma. In: Rickinson A, ed.Seminars in Cancer Biology. London-Saunders Scientific Publishers, Academic Press; 1993: 297–303.

43. Saemundsen AK, Albeck H, Hansen JPH. Epstein-Barr virus, nasopharyngeal and salivary gland carcinomas in Greenland Eskimoes. Br J Cancer 1982; 46:721–728.

44. Henle G, Henle W. Epstein-Barr virus-specific IgA serum antibodies as an outstanding feature of nasopharyngeal carcinoma. Int J Cancer 1979;17:1–17.

45. Wolf H, zur Hausen H, Becker Y. EBV viral genomes in epithelial nasopharyngeal carcinoma cells. Nature Biol 1973; 244:245–267.

46. Desgranges C, Wolf H, de The G, et al. Nasopharyngeal carcinoma X. Presence of Epstein-Barr virus genomes in epithelial cells of tumors from high and medium risk areas. Int J Cancer 1975;16:7–15.

47. Ho JHC. Current knowledge of the epidemiology of nasopharyngeal carcinoma. In: Biggs P, de Thé G, Payne L, eds. Oncogenesis and Herpesviruses. Lyon: IARC, 1972: 357–366.

48. Armstrong RW, Armstrong MH, Yu MC, Henderson BE. Salted fish and inhalants as risk factors for carcinoma in Malaysian Chinese. Cancer Res 1983; 43:2967–2970.

49. Poirier S, Ohshima H, de Thé G, Hubert A, Bourgade MC, Bartsch H. Volatile nitrosamine levels in common foods from Tunisia, South China, and Greenland, high risk areas for nasopharyngeal carcinoma (NPC). Int J Cancer 1987;39:292–296.

50. Shanmugaratnam K, Chan SH, de Thé G, Goh JEH, Khor TH, Simon MJ,

Tye TY. Histopathology of nasopharyngeal carcinoma. Cancer 1979;44:1029–1044.

51. Pearson GR, Weiland LH, Neel HB. Application of Epstein-Barr virus (EBV) serology to the diagnosis of North American nasopharyngeal carcinoma. Cancer 1983;51:260–268.

52. Pathmanathan R, Prasad U, Chandrika G, Sadler RH, Flynn K, Raab-Traub N. Undifferentiated, nonkeratinizing, and squamous cell carcinoma of the nasopharynx: variants of Epstein-Barr virus-infected neoplasia. Am J Pathol 1995;146:1355–1367.

53. Niedobitek G, Hansmann ML, Herbst H. Epstein-Barr virus and carcinomas: undifferentiated carcinomas but not squamous cell carcinomas of the nasopharynx are regularly associated with the virus. J Pathol 1991;165:17–24.

54. Pathmanathan R, Prasad U, Sadler RH, Flynn K, Raab-Traub N. Preinvasive neoplasia of the nasopharynx: a clonal proliferation of EBV-infected cells. N Engl J Med 1995;333:695–698.

55. Buckley CH, Butler EB, Fox H. Cervical intraepithelial neoplasia. J Clin Pathol 1983;35:1–13.

56. Sixbey JW, Yao QY. Immunoglobulin A-induced shift of Epstein-Barr virus tissue tropism. Science 1992;255:1578–1580.

57. Effert P, McCoy R, Abdel-Hamid M, Flynn K, Zhang Q, Busson P, Tursz T, Liu E, Raab-Traub N. Alterations of the p53 gene in nasopharyngeal carcinoma. J Virol 1992;66:3768–3775.

58. Sun Y, Hegameyer G, Colburn N. Nasopharyngeal carcinoma shows no detectable retinoblastoma susceptibility gene alterations. Oncogene 1993; 8:791–795.

59. Sun Y, Hildesheim A, Lanier AP, Cao Y, Yao KT, Raab-Traub N, Yang CS. No point mutation but decreased expression of the p16/MTS1 tumor suppressor gene in nasopharyngeal carcinoma. Oncogene 1995;10:785–788.

60. Lukes RJ, Butler JJ. The pathology and nomenclature of Hodgkin's disease. Cancer Res 1966;26:1063–1083.

61. Mueller N, Evans AL, Harris NL. Hodgkin's disease and Epstein Barr virus: altered antibody patterns before diagnosis. N Engl J Med 320:689–695.

62. Weiss LM, Movahed LA, Warnke RA, et al. Detection of Epstein-Barr viral genomes in Reed-Sternberg cells of Hodgkin's disease. N Engl J Med 1989; 320:502–506.

63. Herbst HG, Tippelman G, Anagnostopoulos I. Immunoglobulin and T cell receptor gene rearrangements in Hodgkin's disease and Ki-1 positive anaplastic large cell lymphoma: dissociation between genotype and phenotype. Leuk Res 1989;13:103–116.

64. Purtilo DT. Hypothesis: Pathogenesis and phenotype of an X-linked lymphoproliferative syndrome. Lancet 1976;2:882–885.

65. Hamilton-Dutoit SJ, Raphael M, Audouin J, Diebold J, Lisse I, Pederson C, Oksenhendler E, Marelle L, Pallesen G. In situ demonstration of Epstein-Barr virus small RNAs (EBER 1) in acquired immunodeficiency syndrome-related lymphomas: correlation with tumor morphology and primary site. Blood 1993;82:619–624.

66. Heslop HE, Brenner MK, Rooney C. 1994. Administration of neomycin resistance gene marked EBV-specific cytotoxic T lymphocytes to recipients of mismatched-related or phenotypically similar unrelated donor marrow grafts. Hum Gene Ther 1994;5:381–397.

67. Papdapoulos EB, Ldanyi M, Emanuel D. Infusions of donor leukocytes to treat Epstein-Barr virus associated lymphoproliferative disorders after allogeneic bone marrow transplantation. N Engl J Med 1994;330:1185–1191.

68. Pelicci PG, Knowles DM, Arlin ZA, Wieczorek R, Luciw P, Dina D, Basilico C, Dalla-Favera R. Multiple monoclonal B-cell expansions and c-*myc* oncogene rearrangements in acquired immune deficiency syndrome-related lymphoproliferative disorders: implications for lymphomagenesis. J Exp Med 1986; 164:2049–2058.

69. MacMahon E, Glass JD, Hayward SD, Mann RB, Becker PS, Charache P, McArthur JC, Ambinder RF. Epstein-Barr virus in AIDS-related primary central nervous system lymphoma. Lancet 1991;338:969–973.

70. Harabuchi Y, Yamanaka N, Kataura A. Epstein-Barr virus in nasal T-cell lymphoma in patients with midline granuloma. Lancet 1990;1:128–130.

71. Shibata D, Weiss LM. Epstein-Barr virus associated gastric adenocarcinoma. Amer J Pathol 1992;140:769–774.

72. Yates J, Warren N, Reisman D, Sugden B. A cis-acting element from the Epstein-Barr viral genome that permits stable replication of recombinant plasmids in latently infected cells. Proc Natl Acad Sci USA 1984;81:3806–3810.

73. Cohen J, Wang F, Mannick J, Kieff E. Epstein-Barr virus nuclear protein 2 is a key determinant of lymphocyte transformation. Proc Natl Acad Sci USA 1989;86:9558–9562.

74. Wang F, Tsang SF, Kurilla G, Cohen JI, Kieff E. Epstein-Barr virus nuclear antigen 2 transactivates latent membrane protein LMP1. J Virol 1990; 54: 3407–3416.

75. Sample J, Young L, Martin B, Chatman E, Rickinson A, and Kieff E. Epstein-Barr virus type 1 and type 2 differ in their EBNA-3A, EBNA-3B and EBNA-3C genes. J Virol 1990;64:4084–4092.

76. Young LS, Yao QY, Rooney CM. New type B isolates of Epstein-Barr virus from Burkitt's lmphoma and normal individuals. J Gen Virol 1987;68:2853–2862.

77. Abdel-Hamid M, Chen J-J, Constantine N, Massoud M, Raab-Traub N. EBV strain variation: geographical distribution and relation to disease state. Virology 1992;190:168–175.

78. Walling D, Edmiston SN, Sixbey JW, Abdel-Hamid M, Resnick L, Raab-Traub N. Coinfection with multiple strains of the Epstein-Barr virus in human immunodeficiency virus-associated hairy leukoplakia. Proc Natl Acad Sci USA 1992; 89:6560–6564.

79. Walling, DM, Clark NM, Markovitz DM, Frank T, Braun DK, Eisenberg E, Krutchkoff DJ, Felix DH, Raab-Traub N. Epstein-Barr virus coinfection and recombination in non-HIV associated oral hairy leukoplakia. J Infect Dis. 1995;171:1122–1130.

80. Rowe M, Young L, Cadwallader K, Petti L, Kieff E, Rickinson A. Distinction between Epstein-Barr virus type-A (EBNA-2A) and type-B (EBNA-2B) isolates extends to the EBNA-3 family of nuclear proteins. J Virol 1989;63:1031–1039.

81. Wang D, Liebowitz D, Kieff E. An EBV membrane protein expressed in immortalized lymphocytes transforms established rodent cells. Cell 1985;43:831–840.

82. Kaye K, Izumi K, Kieff E. Epstein-Barr virus latent membrane protein 1 is essential for B-lymphocytes growth transformation. Proc Natl Acad Sci USA 1993;90:9150–9154.

83. Henderson S, Rowe M, Gregory C, Croom-Carter D, Wang F, Longnecker R, Kieff E, Rickinson A. Induction of bcl-2 expression by Epstein-Barr virus latent membrane protein1 protects infected B cells from programmed cell death. Cell 1991;65:1107–1115.
84. Miller WE, Earp HS, Raab-Traub N. The Epstein-Barr virus latent membrane protein 1 induces expression of the epidermal growth factor receptor. J Virol 1995;69:4390–4398.
85. Longnecker R, Kieff E. A second Epstein-Barr virus membrane protein (LMP2) is expressed in latent infection and colocalizes with LMP1. J Virol 1990;64:2319–2326.
86. Arrand JR, Rymo L. Characterization of the major Epstein-Barr virus-specific RNA in Burkitt lymphoma-derived cells. J Virol 1982;41:376–389.
87. Swaminathan S, Tomkinson B, Kieff E. Recombinant Epstein-Barr virus deleted for small RNA (EBER) genes transforms lymphocytes and replicates in vitro. Proc Natl Acad Sci USA 1991;88:1546–1550.
88. Greenspan JS, Greenspan D, Lennette ET, Abrams DI, Conant MA, Petersen V, Freese VK. Replication of Epstein-Barr virus within the epithelial cells of oral "hairy" leukoplakia, and AIDS-associated lesion. N Engl J Med 1985; 313:1564–1571.
89. Gilligan K, Rajadurai P, Resnick L, Raab-Traub N. Epstein-Barr virus small nuclear RNAs are not expressed in permissively infected cells in AIDS-associated leukoplakia. Microbiology 1990;87:8790–8794.
90. Countryman J, Miller G. Activation of expression of latent Epstein-Barr herpesvirus after gene transfer with a small cloned subfragment of heterogeneous DNA. Proc Natl Acad Sci USA 1985;82:4085–4089.
91. Rowe M, Rowe DT, Gregory CD, Young LS, Farrell PJ, Rupani H, Rickinson AB. Differences in B cell growth phenotype reflect novel patterns of Epstein-Barr virus latent gene expression in BL cells. EMBO J 1987;6:2743–2751.
92. Fahraeus R, Fu JL, Ernberg I, Finke I, Rowe M, Klein G, Falk K, Nilsson E, Yadav M, Busson P, Tursz T, Kallin B. Expression of Epstein-Barr virus-encoded proteins in nasopharyngeal carcinoma. Int J Cancer 1988; 42: 329–338.
93. Brooks JM, Murray RJ, Thomas WA, Kurilla MG, Rickinson AB. Different HLA-B27 subtypes present the same immunodominant Epstein-Barr virus peptide. J Exp Med 1993;178:879–887.
94. Lee SP, Thomas WA, Murray RJ, Khanim F, Kaur S, Young LS, Rowe M, Kurilla M, Rickinson B. HLA A2.1-Restricted cytotoxic T cells recognizing a range of Epstein-Barr virus isolates through a defined epitope in latent membrane protein LMP2. J Virol 1993;67:7428–7435.
95. de Campos-Lima PO, Gavioli R, Zhang Q, Wallace Q, Dolcetti R, Rowe M, Rickinson A, Masucci M. HLA-A11 epitope loss isolates of Epstein-Barr virus from a highly A11+ population. Science 1993;260:98–100.
96. Phillips RE, Rowland-Jones S, Nixon DF, Gotch FM, Edwards JP, Ogunlesi A, Elvin JG, Rothbard JA, Bangham C, Rizza C, McMichael AJ. Human immunodeficiency virus genetic variation that can escape cytotoxic T cell recognition. Nature 1991;354:453–459.
97. Lung M, Chang R, Huanf M, Guo H-Y, Choy D, Sham J, Tsao S, Cheng P, Ng M. Epstein-Barr virus genotypes associated with nasopharyngeal carcinoma in southern China. Virology 1990;177:44–53.
98. Hu LF, Zabarovsky ER, Chen F, Cao SL, Ernberg I, Klein G, Winberg G.

Isolation and sequencing of the Epstein-Barr virus BNLF-1 (LMP1) from a Chinese nasopharyngeal carcinoma. J Gen Virol 1991;72:2399–2409.

99. Miller WE, Edwards RH, Walling DM, Raab-Traub N. 1993. Sequence variation in the Epstein-Barr virus latent membrane protein 1. J Gen Virol 1994;75:2729–2740.

100. Li SN, Chang YS, Liu ST. Effect of a 10 amino acid deletion on the oncogenic activity of latent membrane protein 1 of Epstein-Barr virus. Oncogene 1996;12:2129–2135.

101. Knecht H, Bachmann E, Brousset P, Sandjev K, Nadal D, Bachman F, Odermatt BF, Delsol G, Pallesen G. Deletions within the LMP1 oncogene of Epstein-Barr virus are clustered in Hodgkin's disease and identical to those observed in nasopharyngeal carcinoma. Blood 1993;82:2937–2942.

102. Hu LF, Chen F, Zheng X, Ernberg I, Cao SL, Christensson B, Klein G, Winberg G. Clonability and tumorigenicity of human epithelial cells expressing the EBV encoded membrane protein LMP1. Oncogene 1993;8:1575–1585.

103. Paine E, Scheinman RI, Baldwin Jr AS, Raab-Traub N. Expression of LMP1 in epithelial cells leads to the activation of a select subset of NF-κB/Rel family proteins. J Virol 1995;69(7):4572–4576.

104. Mosialos G, Birkenbach M, Yalamanchili R, VanArsdale T, Ware C, Kieff E. The Epstein-Barr virus transforming protein LMP1 engages signaling proteins for the tumor necrosis factor receptor family. Cell 1995;80:389–399.

105. Nigro JM, Baker SJ, Preisinger AC, Jessup JM, Hostetter R, Cleary K, Bigner SH, Davidson N, Baylin S, Devilee P, Glover T, Collins FS, Weston A, Modalli R, Harris CC, Vogelstein B. Mutations in the p53 gene occur in diverse human tumour types. Nature 1989; 342:705–708.

106. Edwards RH, Raab-Traub N. Alterations of the p53 gene in Epstein-Barr virus-associated immunodeficiency-related lymphomas. J Virol 1993;68:1309–1315.

107. Farrell PJ, Allan GJ, Shanahan F, Vousden KH, Crook T. p53 is frequently mutated in BL cell lines. EMBO J 1991;10:2879–2887.

108. Finerty S, Tarlton J, Mackett M, Morgan A. Protective immunization of cottontop tamarins against Epstein-Barr virus induced disease using the envelope glycoprotein gp340 introduced from a bovine papilloma expression vector. J Gen Virol 1991;73:449–453.

109. Gu SY, Huang TM, Ruan L, Miao YH, Lu H, Chu CM, Motz M, Wolf H. First EBV vaccine trial in humans using recombinant vaccinia virus expressing the major membrane antigen. Dev Biol Stand 1995;84:171–177.

110. Thomson SA, Khanna R, Gardner J, Burrows SR, Coupar B, Moss DJ, Suhrbier A. Minimal epitope expression in a recombinant polypeptide protein are processed and presented to CD8+ cytotoxic T cells: implications for vaccine development. Proc Natl Acad Sci USA 1995;92:5845–5849.

111. Rooney CM, Smith CA, Brenner MK, Heslop HE. Prophylaxis and treatment of Epstein-Barr virus lymphoproliferative disease using genetically modified cytotoxic T lymphocytes. Lancet 1995;345:9–13.

8

KSHV, Kaposi's Sarcoma, and Related Lymphoproliferative Disorders

YUAN CHANG

Kaposi's sarcoma–associated herpesvirus (KSHV), formally designated human herpesvirus 8 (HHV8), is a gamma-2 herpesvirus and is the first known member of this genus of herpesviruses to be associated with clinical disease in humans. Since its identification by representational difference analysis in an AIDS Kaposi's sarcoma (KS) skin lesion,[1] KSHV has been found in all forms of KS[2-5] as well as in related lymphoproliferative disorders, including a rare subtype of B-cell lymphoma referred to as primary effusion (body cavity–based) lymphomas[6,7] and some cases of multicentric Castleman's disease.[8] Many approaches have been used to elucidate the relationship of this virus to the diseases in which it is detected. Mechanisms of pathogenesis have been sought through in vitro culturing, transmission, sequence analysis, gene expression, and recombinant DNA techniques. Determination of causality—largely limited to the relationship of KSHV to KS, since the lymphoproliferative disorders are exceedingly rare diseases—has been investigated through epidemiologic studies using polymerase chain reaction (PCR) and serology-based assays.

CLINICAL AND EPIDEMIOLOGICAL FEATURES OF TUMORS LINKED TO KSHV

Since its discovery in KS lesions in 1994, KSHV has been linked to several different tumors involving different cells of origin. A unifying feature of these tumors, however, is their propensity to occur in immunocompromised hosts.

Kaposi's Sarcoma

KS (Figure 8.1) is a tumor of vascular or lymphatic endothelial cells that is seen in a variety of clinical settings. The sporadic or classical form, which frequently presents as multifocal skin lesions on the legs of elderly men, is considered a low-grade malignancy usually displaying an indolent clinical course (mean survival of 13 years). In the 1970s, an increase in the incidence of KS was noticed in organ transplant recipients. Surveys now show that KS accounts for more than 3% of all neoplasms in North American transplant recipients,[9] representing a risk of developing KS five- to nine-fold greater in these patients than in the general population.[10] In addition, individuals on immunosuppressive or cytotoxic therapy for a variety of chronic disorders also have an increased risk of developing KS.[11] Reduction or withdrawal of therapy in cases of iatrogenically induced immunosuppression has resulted in clinical remission of the tumor in some patients.[9,12] This association of KS with immunosuppression first led to the notion that KS may be caused by an infectious agent.

Although KS was seen more frequently as a result of wider use of immunotherapy, it was nevertheless considered rare in North America and Europe until the occurrence of the AIDS epidemic in the 1980s. Presently, KS is the most common AIDS-related malignancy and is disproportionately found in HIV-seropositive gay men, in whom there is a 20% to 30%

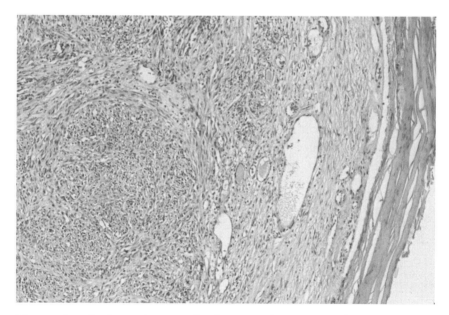

Figure 8.1. A photomicrograph of a Kaposi's sarcoma skin biopsy with tumor composed of irregular fascicles of spindle cells forming random, abnormal vascular channels in the dermis. Overlying epidermis is uninvolved and intact. (Hematoxylin and eosin stain)

lifetime risk of developing the disease.[13] In central and eastern Africa where KS was considered endemic and relatively common even prior to the AIDS epidemic, a parallel epidemic of KS is now seen. The Kampala Cancer Registry in Uganda shows that between 1989 and 1991, KS accounted for up to one half of all malignancies reported.[14]

Body Cavity±Based or Primary Effusion Lymphomas (PELs)

Two lymphoproliferative disorders related to KS have been found to be associated with KSHV. The first is a rare subtype of non-Hodgkin's B-cell lymphoma referred to as primary effusion lymphoma (PEL).[6,7] PELs have unique clinical and pathologic features (Figure 8.2): they usually occur in patients with AIDS, have immunoblastic or anaplastic morphologic features, usually are devoid of surface immunoglobulin and B-cell antigens, and demonstrate no *c-myc* gene rearrangements.[6,7] When they occur in AIDS patients, PELs respond poorly to therapy and are usually rapidly fatal, with a median survival of 2 to 3 months.[7] In contrast, these lymphomas may have a much less aggressive course in HIV-seronegative patients.[15] Although all AIDS-related cases identified thus far have been co-infected with clonal Epstein-Barr virus (EBV), cases of EBV-negative PEL have been reported to occur in HIV-negative patients.[15,16] Similar to KS, PELs have a strong association to an HIV transmission subgroup: All

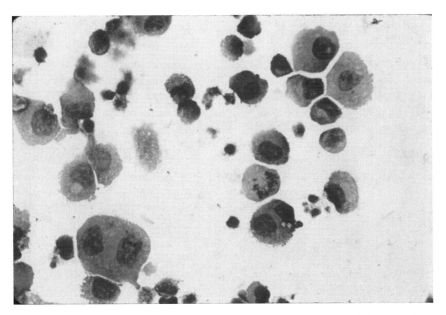

Figure 8.2. Malignant cells of a Kaposi's sarcoma±associated herpesvirus (KSHV)-infected body cavity±based/primary effusion lymphoma showing marked anaplasia, nuclear and cytoplasmic pleomorphism. Mitotic activity is high and large multinucleated cells are identifiable. (Giemsa stain)

AIDS-related cases reported to date have been found in gay men. Several EBV coinfected[17,18] and uninfected[19-21] KSHV cell lines have been established from PEL and have been used in characterizing the virus.[22,23] These cell lines have immunoglobulin gene rearrangements identical to those of their parental lymphomas, indicative of a B-cell origin, and are stably infected with 50 to 150 KSHV genome copies per cell.[17,24]

Castleman's Disease

Another lymphoproliferative disorder associated with KSHV is one form of Castleman's disease: plasma cell variant or multicentric Castleman's disease (MCD).[8] Castleman's disease, also known as angiofollicular lymphoid hyperplasia, is a rare, non-neoplastic, lymphoproliferative disorder related to excess interleukin (IL)-6–like activity (Figure 8.1c). Histologically and clinically, Castleman's disease can be divided into two subtypes: hyaline-vascular and plasma cell variants. The majority of cases of Castleman's disease are of the hyaline-vascular variant, which presents as solitary lymph node hyperplasia, typically in the mediastinum. Other than isolated lymph node enlargement, patients usually have no other symptoms and surgical excision is curative. In contrast, the plasma cell variant has an abundance of polyclonal plasma cells and frequently has a multicentric or generalized presentation that is poorly responsive to treatment.[25] Plasma cell variant MCD is associated with systemic symptoms including fever, anemia, hypergammaglobulinemia, and hypoalbuminemia. This subtype has been reported to be associated clinically with development of KS and of immunoblastic large-cell lymphomas.

Because KSHV encodes a homologue of IL-6 (discussed later) and because IL-6–like activity is believed to play a pathogenic role in Castleman's disease, Parravicini and colleagues examined the expression of KSHV vIL-6 by immunohistochemistry among HIV-seronegative patients with Castleman's disease. A subset of patients with plasma cell variant MCD demonstrated KSHV vIL-6 expression in their lesions, and had a rapidly fatal clinical course frequently associated with autoimmune hemolytic anemia and poly/oligoclonal gammopathy.[26] This finding supports the notion that Castleman's disease is a syndrome of multiple etiologies involving aberrant IL-6 activity. Although Castleman's disease infected with KSHV is only a subset of all Castleman's lesions, this subset is the first recognized disorder that is likely to be, in part, caused by a virus-encoded cytokine.

Multiple myeloma is another lymphoproliferative disorder characterized by plasma cell proliferation thought to be driven in part by dysregulated expression of IL-6. Unlike that in Castleman's disease, the plasma cell dyscrasia found in multiple myeloma is monoclonal and neoplastic in nature, but because of the superficial similarities of plasma cell and IL-6 involvement in these two disorders, Rettig and colleagues searched for the presence of KSHV in multiple myeloma. They reported the detection of

KSHV by PCR and *in situ* hybridization in cultured bone marrow stromal cells from patients with multiple myeloma, but not in similar cell populations from control patients.[27] Serologic studies and direct PCR analysis of bone marrow cell populations performed by other groups do not support a link between KSHV and multiple myeloma (unpublished results, S. Olsen, K. Tarte, B. Klein, Y. Chang; personal communication, T. Scultz, C. Parravicini, D. Ablashi).

EPIDEMIOLOGICAL ASSOCIATIONS

Finding an infectious agent in tumor tissue does little to prove a causal role for the organism in carcinogenesis.[28] To prove this role, a combination of epidemiological, microbiological, and, in the case of KSHV, molecular biological studies must be employed. The first hint that KS might be caused by an infectious agent came from epidemiological studies that showed KS to be 20-fold more common in homosexual or bisexual HIV-infected patients than in HIV-infected hemophiliacs.[13] This suggested that a factor other than HIV alone was critical for the development of KS. Subsequent studies, described here, then confirmed this cofactor to be KSHV.

PCR and Southern Hybridization of KSHV Sequences in Tissues

A steadily accumulating body of evidence suggests that KSHV causes KS in conjunction with other infectious and noninfectious risk factors. Initial studies using both PCR and Southern blot hybridization techniques demonstrated that KSHV DNA is present in most, if not all, KS lesions from people with AIDS but is rarely found in tissues from people without KS or AIDS.[1] Subsequent studies demonstrated near universal KSHV infection in KS lesions from classic KS, KS in HIV-seronegative gay men,[2,4,29] African endemic KS,[3,5] and KS in immunosuppressed patients.[4,30] Overall, nearly 95% of KS lesions examined in a variety of studies by PCR have detectable KSHV DNA[31] and those lesions that are negative for the viral DNA probably result from misdiagnosis or DNA degradation. Although viral DNA generally is not found in nontumor tissues from KS patients by single primer pair PCR,[1] more sensitive nested PCR techniques can detect virus in certain tissues not involved by KS.[32,33]

Because other human herpesviruses, with the exception of herpes simplex type 2, are near-ubiquitous infections of humans,[34] it has been suggested that KSHV is also ubiquitous[35] and therefore is unlikely to be causal for KS and related disorders. Some support for this notion has been derived from a few studies of transplant patients with skin tumors other than KS.[36] Although Rady and colleagues found KSHV DNA by PCR in non-KS skin tumors from four immunosuppressed transplant recipients,[35] these results were not replicated in larger studies of immunosuppressed[37,38] and nonimmunosuppressed[39] skin tumor patients. One of these studies initially detected virus DNA in non-KS skin tumors, but careful reexamination demonstrated that these positive results were due to PCR contamination,[37] a problem common to use of PCR in epidemiological studies. False positive PCR results also appear to have plagued some analyses of semen and prostate tissues.[40-42] Subsequent studies demonstrated only low virus detection rates in semen and prostate tissues from KS patients and no evidence of genitourinary tract infection among tissues or semen samples from control patients using nested and non-nested PCR.[43-47]

Examination of Peripheral Blood Mononuclear Cells (PBMC)

The issue of KSHV ubiquity has been further addressed by examination of peripheral blood mononuclear cells (PBMC) of KS patients by PCR. Using nested PCR, two studies came to similar conclusions regarding viral DNA in PBMC: (1) the sensitivity of detecting virus DNA in PBMC of patients with KS is only approximately 50%; (2) detection of virus DNA is predictive of eventual development of KS in HIV-infected patients; and (3) control patients generally do not have detectable virus DNA in PBMC.[48,49] The low sensitivity of this technique is not unexpected, for examination of PBMC establishes only the current level of viremia and since the percentage of infected cells in the bulk population of PBMC is low.

Serologic Assays for KSHV Infection

Serologic studies avoid the confounding effect of PCR contamination and have the potential benefit of detecting lifetime exposure to the virus rather than current viral burden. AIDS–KS patients develop a specific antibody response directed against KSHV-infected cell lines derived from PEL,[22] and investigators have found two specific immunoblot markers for KSHV infection using one of these cell lines, BC-1. Employing n-butyrate to induce KSHV lytic antigen expression, Miller and colleagues identified a 40-kD antigen present in BC-1 cells but not in other EBV-infected KSHV-negative cell lines.[50] Immunoblotting for p40 reactivity found that 67% of AID–KS patients were p40 positive compared to 13% of AIDS patients without KS. Gao and associates identified a high-molecular-weight antigen doublet (224 and 236 kD) localized to the nucleus of resting BC-1 cells.[51] These antigens appear to be expressed during latent infection, because synthesis of the antigen doublet is not affected by the phorbol ester, 12-O-tetradecanoylphorbol-13-acetate (TPA), which promotes herpesvirus lytic gene expression, nor by phosphonoacetic acid, which inhibits herpesvirus lytic gene expression. They have been designated as latency-associated nuclear antigens (LANA), and the gene encoding these proteins has been identified as KSHV open reading frame (ORF) 73.[52] Immunoblotting for LANA reactivity demonstrated that 32 (80%) of 40 AIDS–KS patients were positive for LANA antibodies immediately prior to KS onset, compared to only 7 (18%) of 40 gay men with AIDS who did not develop KS and to none of 20 HIV-infected hemophiliacs. In addition, none of 122 healthy blood donors or of 22 patients with elevated titers to EBV antigens were seropositive for the LANA doublet.[51]

Researchers have obtained similar results using a more sensitive indirect immunofluorescence assay (IFA) based on EBV-negative, KSHV-infected PEL cell lines.[20,53] Immunofluorescence staining of these cell lines demonstrates a specular nuclear pattern present primarily when sera from patients with KS is used (Figure 8.3). Reexamining the patient sera used for the LANA Western blot studies, Gao and colleagues showed that IFA end-point titers of greater than 1:160 were present in 90% of sera from AIDS–KS patients but were not present in any of the sera from HIV-positive hemophiliacs, HIV seronegative blood donors, or EBV–high titered patients.[20] However, 30% of the gay men with AIDS but without KS had positive test results at dilutions greater than 1:160 compared to only 17% by the LANA assay. In general, the LANA and the IFA assays were concordant, although the IFA appeared to be more sensitive. Among HIV-positive and HIV-negative KS patients from Italy, 79% and 100% were positive by IFA, respectively; in a small study of Italian blood donors, two of 54 (4%) were found to be seropositive by both the IFA and the LANA immunoblot. This slightly higher seropositivity rate than that among North

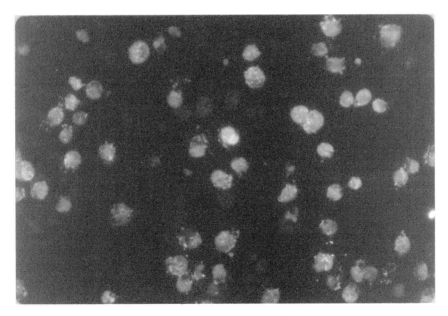

Figure 8.3. Characteristic immunofluorescence staining of the KSHV-infected BCP-1 cell line with serum from a patient with Kaposi's sarcoma. The nuclear speckling corresponds to the major KSHV latency-associated nuclear antigen (LANA) encoded by ORF73.

American blood samples may account in part for the higher rate of classic KS in Italy compared to the United States.[54,55]

Most AIDS–KS patients appear to seroconvert to KSHV seropositivity during adulthood, a finding that is also inconsistent with KSHV infection being ubiquitous. By examining sera longitudinally collected from AIDS patients prior to development of KS, Gao and colleagues[51] found that 53% of the patients had seroconversion to persistent LANA seropositivity, 28% were positive on entry into the study, and 20% were either persistently seronegative or seroreverted to a negative LANA test. LANA seropositivity rates increased linearly with time for the KS patients prior to KS onset, with the median duration prior to KS onset being 33 months. Repeating these studies with the IFA test showed a longer median duration of seropositivity (46 months) with 31% of patients having an seroconversion date earlier than that shown by immunoblotting.[20]

Lennette and colleagues, using a modified IFA protocol based on phorbol ester–induced lytic phase antigens in conjunction with latent antigens in a KSHV-infected cell line, found all patients with African endemic KS and 96% of American patients with AIDS-associated KS to be seropositive for KSHV. They also found 25% of North American blood donors and 2% to 8% of children to have antibodies to lytic and latent phase antigens.[56] The seropositivity rate is higher in all populations examined with this assay in comparison to that found using latent antigens alone. Whether this method is more sensitive or is detecting cross-reactive lytic antigens of other herpesviruses remains to be determined. Other assays using truncated or whole recombinant ORF 65 protein in immunoblot or ELISA formats are reported to have similar seropositivity results.[57,58]

Despite some differences in absolute numbers using different antigen preparation, all these studies consistently demonstrate that KSHV seropositivity is primarily found in people at risk for KS and that specific antibodies can be detected several years prior to KS onset.[20,51] Improvement in these assays may markedly increase their sensitivity and ability to detect primary infection. Although it is possible that widespread KSHV infection occurs without detectable immune response as measured by current assays, the ability to detect seroconversion years prior to KS onset for many patients makes this hypothesis unlikely.

KSHV Localization in Tissues

Localization of the virus to the KS tumor among those patients infected with the virus is another supportive piece of evidence for a causative role for KSHV in KS. Semiquantitative PCR[29] and PCR *in situ* hybridization[59] localize viral genome to KS lesions. Studies by Boshoff and colleagues suggest that endothelial/spindle cells within lesions are the primary site of infection.[59] In an examination of the pattern of KSHV gene expression in KS, Zhong and colleagues have identified two small transcripts, designated T1.1 and T0.7, which correspond roughly to the lytic and latent states of the KSHV life cycle, respectively. T0.7 is expressed in the vast majority of KS endothelial/spindle cells whereas T1.1 transcripts primarily localize to the nucleus in high copy number (approximately 25,000 copies of RNA) and are present in only 0.5% to 1% of cells.[60,61] These data suggest that the majority of the KSHV in tumor cells of KS lesions are in a latent or nonproductive cycle.

PATHOGENETIC MECHANISMS OF CARCINOGENESIS

Controversy still exists regarding whether KS is a true neoplasm or is simply a hyperplastic angioproliferative disorder. Histopathologic examination cannot resolve this question because the microscopic appearance of KS can vary significantly from case to case. In some biopsies—usually of early-stage KS—lesions resemble granulation tissue with a proliferation of vessels, a heterogeneous population of spindle cells, and an infiltrate of inflammatory cells. In advanced nodular lesions, densely packed fascicles of highly malignant appearing cells with marked cellular pleomorphism and high mitotic activity are seen. Likewise, the clinical behavior of KS can be indolent in some individuals yet can be aggressive in others. Support for a malignant nature of KS, however, comes from understanding pathogenic mechanisms of KSHV and related herpesviruses.

Clonality Studies of KS Lesions

One line of evidence that KS lesions in an individual may have a monoclonal origin is the preliminary finding by Rabkin and colleagues of highly unbalanced methylation patterns representing the same allele of the androgen-receptor gene (HUMARA) in multiple lesions from the same individual.[62] Unfortunately, this technique, which is PCR based, is difficult to apply to early KS lesions in which abundant amounts of normal tissue are infiltrated by sparse collections of tumor cells. Therefore, a progression from polyclonal hyperplasia in early lesions to monoclonal neoplastic expansion in advanced, multicentric lesions cannot be ruled out.

Sequencing Studies of KSHV: Phylogeny, Genome Organization, and Similarities to Other Oncogenic Herpesviruses

A major challenge in the KSHV field remains the lack of a system that allows for high-titer transmission of virus. As a result, traditional virological experiments that might provide insights into mechanisms of patho-

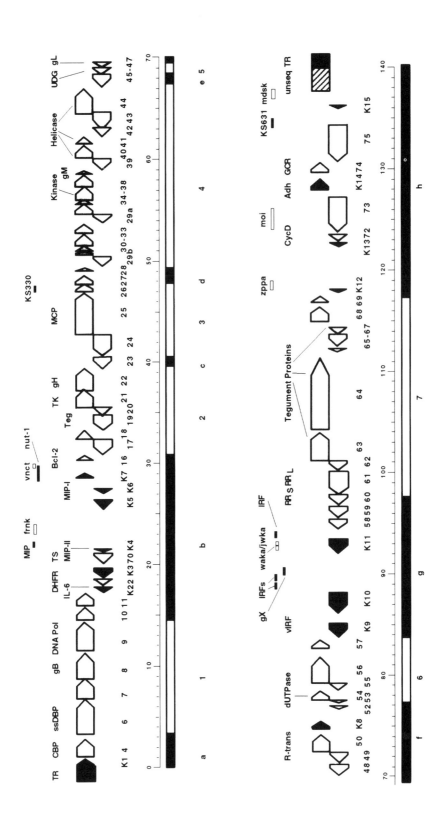

genesis are difficult to perform. An alternate approach to dissecting out the pathogenic process of this virus is to examine its genomic substrates by sequence analysis. In fact, sequencing has helped to elucidate the KSHV genomic structure and has identified specific genes that may contribute to tumorigenesis in KSHV-related disorders. Starting from clones that hybridized to the KS330Bam and KS631Bam fragments originally generated by representational difference analysis, researchers have mapped, sequenced, and annotated the long coding region of KSHV using a contiguous set of 7 lambda phage and 3 cosmids screened from PEL cell line genomic libraries (Figure 8.4).[63]

Analysis of the KSHV genome indicates that the virus is a member of Gammaherpesviridae, a lymphotrophic subfamily of Herpesviridae. Gammaherpesviruses are further divided into two genera: Lymphocryptovirus, which includes EBV, and Rhadinovirus, which includes herpesvirus saimiri (HVS). The genomic organization of genes, as well as phylogenetic studies, suggest that KSHV is a Rhadinovirus.[22] For example, parsimony analysis of the amino acid composition of the hypothetical KSHV major capsid protein compared to major capsid proteins of other human herpesviruses, as well as to those of some animal herpesviruses, shows KSHV to be most closely related to HVS. The KSHV genome has an internal long unique coding sequence of approximately 140 kb flanked by reiterated, high G + C–content terminal repeat sequences of approximately 800 base pairs in size. Within the long unique coding sequence, many ORFs show colinear and sequence homology to other herpesviral genes; however, some ORFs appear unique to KSHV.[63]

Similarities in genes and organizational structure to HVS may provide instructive comparison and guidelines for future KSHV studies. HVS is a T-lymphotrophic virus that naturally infects New World squirrel monkeys. Although HVS is commonly isolated from the squirrel monkey, in which it does not cause apparent clinical disease, it produces lymphomas and leukemias of T-cell derivation in New World primates other than its natural host. Different HVS strains have different degrees of oncogenic potential.[64] Two strains designated A and C have been shown to be capable of transforming a variety of cells in vitro and of causing neoplasms in animal

---

Figure 8.4. The KSHV±140.5 kb long unique region (LUR) encodes at least open 81 open reading frames and is flanked by the terminal repeat region composed of multiple terminal repeat units. Genes with homology to other herpesviruses (white filled) fall into regions that are well-characterized gene blocks (1 to 7 white segments) conserved among herpesviruses. Genes unique to KSHV and related rhadinoviruses are designated with a K prefix (black filled) and lie largely in intervening non-conserved gene blocks. The KSHV genome encodes many homologues to cellular genes that are involved with cell cycle control, apoptosis, immune regulation, and cell proliferation. (Reprinted with permission from reference 63.)

hosts; however, strain B does not appear to have this capability.[65] The genetic basis of this difference in transforming potential resides in the leftmost ORF of HVS's long unique coding sequence, which displays a surprising degree of variation from strain to strain. In the oncogenic strains, ORFs referred to as saimiri transforming proteins (STPs) have been mapped, and functional domains conferring transformation potential have been identified.[66] The STPs are characterized by the presence of repetitive collagen motifs of the Gly-Pro-Pro type, and by a Tip subunit that interacts with cellular Ras.[67]

The KSHV genome has reading frames in its leftmost long unique coding region that may have analogous function to the HVS STPs. The variation is marked even between HVS strains in this region, thus it is not surprising that initial comparison to KSHV has not resulted in the identification of KSHV homologues to STP based on sequence data. The presence of collagen motifs, however, is a promising characteristic of KSHV ORFs in this region, suggesting a function similar to that of the STPs. The KSHV genome appears not to contain sequence homologues to Epstein-Barr nuclear antigen or latent membrane protein genes—genes that have been implicated in the immortalization and transformation potential of EBV.

KSHV and Molecular Mimicry

Although no homologues to EBV or HVS transforming genes have been identified by sequence analysis, the KSHV genome encodes homologues to human intra- and intercellular regulatory genes, including two proto-oncogenes (*cyclin D* and *bcl-2*), two cyto-/chemokines [IL-6 and macrophage inflammatory protein (MIP)-1α], a G-protein coupled receptor (GCR), and an interferon regulatory factor (IRF).[63,68-70] This extensive degree of molecular mimicry by KSHV encoded genes suggest that the virus may modify the host cell environment markedly by directly affecting cell cycle, programmed cell death, cell proliferation, and possibly immunoregulatory functions. Single gene-transfection experiments support the role of these virally encoded genes in KSHV pathogenesis and oncogenesis.

Homologues to cellular protooncogenes include the KSHV *v-cyclin* and the KSHV *v-bcl-2*.[71-73] Both EBV and HVS also carry homologs to human *bcl-2*; however, only HVS has a homolog to human cyclin in its genome. Cyclins constitute a family of proteins, largely defined by sequence homology, that is involved in the regulation of the cell cycle and DNA replication. The cyclins function by binding to and stimulating the activities of specific cyclin-dependent kinases (cdks), and this interaction is facilitated by a highly conserved 100-amino-acid region found in all cyclins, called the cyclin box.

Subtypes of cyclins have been defined according to where they act in the cell cycle (for review, see reference 74). The D-type cyclins, to which the KSHV v-cyclin shows strongest amino acid similarity, function during

G_1 and have very short half-lives. Their synthesis is highly growth-factor dependent, and they may play an important role in the switch between proliferation and differentiation. D-type cyclin–cdk complexes phosphorylate retinoblastoma tumor suppresser protein (pRb), which, in its hypophosphorylated form, blocks cells in the G_1 phase and binds a variety of proteins, including a family of transcription factors collectively known as E2F. Phosphorylation of pRb causes release of E2F, a step necessary for transcription of genes required for DNA synthesis. Several types of human tumors display abnormalities in cyclin. Chromosomal rearrangements that lead to increased and constitutive expression of human cyclin D1 have been found in parathyroid tumors and in mantle cell lymphomas.[75]

The KSHV ORF 72 encodes a protein with 74% amino acid similarity to the HVS cyclin and 61% to 67% amino acid similarity to human D-type cyclins. This KSHV protein is 257 amino acids in length and has a region containing the conserved cyclin box motif.[75] KSHV ORF 72 is expressed in primary biopsies of all clinical subtypes of KS and cell lines derived from PEL, as determined by RT-PCR and Northern hybridization studies, suggesting a functional role of this gene in maintaining the neoplastic phenotype.[71,76,77] In vitro studies using an expression vector with an epitope-tagged KSHV v-cyclin gene show that the v-cyclin protein localizes predominantly to the nuclei of transfected cells where it functions by binding to cdk6. Binding results in activation of kinase activity and phosphorylation of pRb at authentic sites.[70] The KSHV v-cyclin may also have broader specificity than cellular D-type cyclins in that it can mediate phosphorylation of histone H1 as well.[78,79] In a functional assay, KSHV v-cyclin can rescue pRb-mediated senescence when coexpressed with pRb in SAOS-2 osteosarcoma cells.[71]

The second protooncogene identified in the KSHV genome, KSHV ORF 16, possesses significant homology to human bcl-2 and to other members of the bcl-2 family. This family of genes is involved in the regulation of apoptosis, a process of programmed cell death.[80,81] Some members of this family, such as bcl-2, function to prevent apoptosis; other members, such as Bax, function to promote apoptosis. Although the exact mechanism has not been delineated, it is clear that the functional effect derives from the ability of members of this family to bind to each other in stereotypic homodimerization or heterodimerization interactions.[82] These interactions are thought to be mediated by two conserved regions of less than 10 base pairs, each referred to as BH1 and BH2.[83] The bcl-2 gene is normally expressed in mammalian tissues during embryogenesis but shows dysregulated expression in a variety of human cancers and contributes to neoplastic cell expansion by functioning as an anti-apoptotic factor in enhancing cell survival, rather than by accelerating rates of cellular proliferation. In human follicular lymphomas, excessive production of Bcl-2 mRNA and protein is caused by a chromosomal translocation t(14:18), which juxtaposes the bcl-2 gene with the immunoglobulin heavy-chain locus, resulting in a bcl-2 immunoglobulin fusion gene.[84,85]

The KSHV *v-bcl-2* ORF is 525 bp in length and encodes a putative protein with 58.7% and 62.3% amino-acid similarity to human Bcl-2 and Bax,
respectively. It contains the conserved BH1 and BH2 motifs important for
functional binding between members of the family and possesses a hydrophobic C-terminal domain necessary for membrane localization.[72,73] To determine whether KSHV v-Bcl-2 functions as a Bcl-2 homologue rather
than as a Bax homolog (sequence data alone is unable to discriminate
between the two possibilities), we undertook studies using a yeast model.[73]
Different combinations of human *bcl-2*, KSHV *v-bcl-2*, and human *bax* constructs were cotransfected into a host yeast strain that responds to *bax*
transfection by demonstrating a toxic phenotype to growth that can be
rescued by a Bcl-2 functional homolog. With this system, KSHV v-Bcl-2 was
shown to neutralize Bax toxicity similar to human Bcl-2. The ability to
neutralize Bax toxicity was further demonstrated in mammalian cells by
experiments with transient cotransfection of *bax* and KSHV *v-bcl-2* into
human fibroblasts. Using a yeast two-hybrid system, we found that KSHV
v-Bcl-2 formed heterodimers with human Bcl-2, thereby demonstrating
the ability of KSHV v-Bcl-2 to interact directly with other members of the
Bcl-2 family via stereotypic binding reactions that characterize this family
of proteins.[73] Several DNA viruses, including HVS and EBV, carry apoptosis-inhibiting genes.[86] The presence of these genes may represent a viral
strategy to prolong host cell survival by abrogating the natural host mechanism of programmed cell death in the presence of lytic infection; alternatively, expression of an anti-apoptotic gene can be postulated to contribute to a latency-associated transformed state by prolonging survival of
infected tumor cells that are no longer under normal and controlled programmed cell death.

Although KSHV *v-cyclin* and *v-bcl* are homologues to cellular protooncogenes, single-gene transfection experiments with vectors expressing
these genes do not result in transformation. The first KSHV gene shown
to have transformation potential when expressed in NIH3T3 cells is the
KSHV ORF K9, which encodes a 449-amino-acid protein with sequence
similarity to the IRF family of proteins involved in interferon (IFN) signal
transduction.[68] IFNs function by binding to designated cell surface receptors that activate the JAK-tyk pathway. This results in the formation of a
trimeric complex consisting of two "signal tranducer and activator of transcription" (STAT) proteins and a p48 protein; this complex translocates
to the nucleus and binds to specific DNA sequences in the promoter regions of interferon stimulated genes (ISGs). Transcriptional transactivation of ISGs produces a repertoire of antiviral responses, including MHC
upregulation, cell cycle shutdown, and p53-independent apoptosis. This
pathway is regulated to some extent by IRF proteins, which either positively or negatively affect this cascade of events by binding competitively
to ISG promoter elements (for review see reference 87). KSHV v-IRF acts
in a similar fashion to cellular IRF-2, which inhibits IFN activity and which
also has been shown to transform NIH3T3 cells. When these *v-IRF* trans

formed NIH3T3 cells are injected into nude mice, they rapidly produce tumors. However, in contrast to IRF-2, KSHV v-IRF has not been shown to bind to ISG promoter elements and its mechanism of interferon pathway suppression or of transformation remains to be determined.[88]

A KSHV ORF 74 encodes a protein with features of the seven transmembrane superfamily of GCRs.[76] GCRs comprise the largest family of cell surface receptors and mediate cellular responses, including growth and differentiation, to a diverse group of molecules via trimeric GTP-binding proteins (G proteins). Arvanitakis and colleagues have demonstrated that KSHV v-GCR appears to be a constitutively activated signaling receptor that acts through the phosphoinositide–inositoltriphosphate–protein kinase C pathway downstream to the G proteins. Transfection of KSHV *v-GCR* into normal rat kidney fibroblasts, NRK-49F, caused enhanced cellular proliferation.[89]

Taken together, the variety of functional effects demonstrated by pirated genes in the KSHV genome suggests that a combination of cell proliferation, antiapoptosis, and immune modulation is required for the in vivo transformation seen in KSHV-related neoplasms. In the broader context, the degree of molecular piracy in KSHV makes this newly discovered pathogen a useful and transparent model for viral tumorigenesis.

KS and the Cytokine Hypothesis of Pathogenesis

A large number of studies have suggested that KS is a cytokine-mediated disorder and that, at least in the initial stages, development of these lesions is dependent on angiogenic factors. The basis for this hypothesis has derived largely from cultured KS spindle cells taken from pleural effusions or skin lesions.[90] Ensoli and colleagues reported expression of a large range of factors in this cell culture model that have autocrine and paracrine growth effects. These factors include basic fibroblast growth factor (bFGF), acidic fibroblast growth factor (aFGF), platelet-derived growth factor (PDGF), IL-1α, IL-1β, IL-6, granulocyte-macrophage colony-stimulating factor (GM-CSF), and transforming growth factor (TGF)-β.[90] In particular, bFGF and IL-1 mRNAs were found to be highly expressed. bFGF, an angiogenic factor, directly affects growth of mesodermally derived cells, including endothelial cells, and IL-6 can interact with other cytokines to promote angiogenesis. Specific antisera to these cytokines was shown to inhibit the in vitro growth of cultured AIDS–KS cells.[90] Moreover, extensive vascularization occurred when cultured spindle cells were placed on chorioallantoic membranes, and nude mice injected subcutaneously with these cells developed mouse-derived, KS-like lesions.[91]

The more aggressive course of KS in AIDS patients has been attributed to the effects of HIV-1 Tat protein released by infected T cells and its interaction with bFGF.[92,93] Cultured KS cells were found to respond to HIV-1 Tat by proliferation, adhesion, migration, and invasion.[94,95] These effects are attributed, in part, to a Tat Arg-Gly-Asp (RGD) recognition region that interacts with integrin receptors of fibronectin and vitronectin.[95] These integrin receptors, in turn, can be up-regulated by bFGF-induced angiogenesis. This model does not take into consideration the recent finding of KSHV in virtually all types of KS lesions. Most important, virtually all work on cytokines has been performed on KS-derived spindle cell cultures that do not contain KSHV. Lebbe and colleagues found KSHV DNA in three of six primary cultures, but in none of 17 cultures passaged three or four times. Likewise, Dictor and colleagues[38] did not find KSHV DNA by PCR in 17 cultures, including one primary culture (range of passages, 1 to 16). This result may be due to negative selection of virus-infected cells in culture; however, the ability of PEL B-lymphocyte cell lines to propagate virus stably suggests a more complicated virus–host interaction.

Two homologues to members of the human CC chemokine family (v-MIP-I and v-MIP-II) and a homologue to human interleukin-6 (huIL-6) have been identified in the KSHV genome.[63] Transcripts of these cytokines are expressed in latently infected PEL derived cell lines under standard conditions and can be induced with phorbol esters.[77] The two chemokine homologs, v-MIP-I and v-MIP-II, show highest sequence similarity to hu-MIP-1a, a member of the MIP/RANTES family of chemoattractant cytokines (chemokines) that plays an important role in virus infection–mediated inflammation. Recently, chemokine receptors have been identified as coreceptors to CD4 in mediating HIV-1 entry into cells, and members of the MIP/RANTES family have been shown to inhibit HIV-cell fusion through specific competitive binding to CC and CXC chemokine receptors.[96] Using synthetic peptides of the viral homologues, Kledal and colleagues found binding of v-MIP-II to a number of chemokine receptors,[97] and Boshoff and colleagues demonstrated that v-MIP-II produced modest blocking of HIV infection by way of CCR3.[98] These findings not only identify a candidate for anti-HIV therapeutics but also hint at possible interactions between HIV-1 and KSHV in AIDS patients. In addition, viral MIPs elicited prominent angiogenesis in *in ovo* chick chorioallantoic membrane assays,[98] and may drive the vascular pathology, which is a prominent component of KS and MCD.

The cytokine hu-IL-6 has pleiotropic effects on a wide variety of cells. Elevated levels of this cytokine has been linked etiologically to several hematolymphoid diseases, including posttransplantation lymphoproliferative disorders,[99] multiple myeloma,[100] and MCD.[101,102] Tosato and colleagues have shown that IL-6 is an important factor in the establishment and maintenance of EBV-immortalized B cells and in increasing EBV lymphoblastoid cell tumorigenicity in athymic mice.[103,104] Sequence homology suggesting functional homology is supported by hu-IL-6–like activity of the KSHV v-IL-6 in maintaining B9 mouse plasmacytoma cells, which are dependent on exogenous IL-6.[68] Similar to hu-IL-6, the viral homologue also activates Jak-STAT pathway signaling; however, unlike hu-IL-6, v-IL-6 does not require the IL-6Rα receptor subunit and can directly interact with just the gp130 receptor subunit.[105] Immunohistochemical localization studies using rabbit polyclonal antibodies developed against v-IL-6 peptides demonstrate that this protein is expressed in tumor cells of PEL[68] and in a subset of hematopoietic cells in KSHV-infected, plasma-cell-variant MCD.[26] Examination of over 50 KS lesions showed that v-IL-6 is apparently not expressed in the spindle cells of KS lesions, indicating a cell lineage–specific expression of this protein.

CONTROL AND IMPLICATIONS FOR CLINICAL MANAGEMENT

KSHV is strongly associated with KS as well as with related lymphoproliferative disorders, and is probably causal for these diseases. Epidemiological studies suggest that, at least in North America, KSHV infection is not ubiquitous; it predominantly affects a group of high-risk patients: gay men. In this population, KSHV infection appears to occur in adulthood, as reflected by seroconversion studies in KS patients; however, risk factors for transmission have not yet been identified. Prevention policies and practices based on identification of these risk factors are anticipated.

A growing list of antiherpesviral drugs now available or in clinical development may be evaluated in the near future for their effect on KSHV-related disorders. The vast majority of these agents target either directly or indirectly the herpesvirus DNA polymerase, which is functionally active only during lytic virus replication. Morfeldt and Torssander[106] demonstrated clinical improvement in four AIDS–KS patients treated with foscarnet (phosphonoacetic acid), a drug used to treat ganciclovir-resistant cytomegalovirus infections that is also active against oral hairy leukoplakia caused by lytic-phase EBV infection.[107] Although this uncontrolled study was unable to prove a clear effect of the drug on the course of AIDS–KS, the findings have been bolstered subsequently by two large retrospective studies of foscarnet in AIDS patients.[108,109] The surprising conclusions of these studies are that Foscarnet, but not acyclovir or ganciclovir, may have some preventive efficacy on AIDS–KS independent of its effects on HIV infection. Studies on the susceptibility of KSHV to antiviral drugs in culture demonstrate that Foscarnet and Cidofovir [(S)-1-(3-hydroxy-2-phosphonylmethoxyproply) cytosine] are capable of inhibiting late but not latent viral mRNA expression,[110] as would be expected for most herpesviruses.[111] Using DNA polymerase inhibitors to treat KSHV-related neoplasia is counterintuitive, because lytic virus replication presumable kills the host cell[34] and would not be expected to contribute significantly to the tumor. However, there is some evidence that whole virions and lytic cycle replication occur in a small minority of infected KS cells. It is possible that virus production is required continually to recruit newly infected cells into the "neoplastic" lesion, and that DNA polymerase inhibitors interrupt this process. Although promising, specific therapies based on KSHV replication inhibition will require conservative and well-designed trials before their value is known. Standardized therapies—including excision, radiation, and use of intralesional interferon—as well as new therapies, such as encapsulated doxorubicin, are likely to remain the primary therapeutic choices for treatment of KS until virus-specific therapies are evaluated and fully understood.

As reflected by the increasing incidence of KS concomitant with increasing immunosuppression, clinical manifestations of KS must be under exquisite immunologic control. This notion is further supported by the effectiveness of triple anti-HIV therapy, including protease inhibitors, in causing KS resolution in parallel with decreased HIV viral load and reversal of immunosuppression. Thus, first and foremost, treatment of KS in the HIV-seropositive patient is intimately tied to the success of HIV antiviral treatment. With guarded optimism for effective anti-HIV therapy, we can now entertain the notion that the majority of KS in the United States can be controlled. Control of classic KS or KS in people whose immunosuppression cannot be reversed, however, must await development of more specific therapies.

REFERENCES

1. Chang Y, Cesarman E, Pessin MS, Lee F, Culpepper J, Knowles DM, Moore PS. Identification of herpesvirus-like DNA sequences in AIDS-associated Kaposi's sarcoma. Science 1994;265:1865–1869.
2. Moore PS, Chang Y. Detection of herpesvirus-like DNA sequences in Kaposi's sarcoma lesions from persons with and without HIV infection. N Engl J Med 1995;332:1181–1185.
3. Schalling M, Ekman M, Kaaya EE, Linde A, Biberfeld P. A role for a new herpesvirus (KSHV) in different forms of Kaposi's sarcoma. Nature Med 1995;1:707–708.
4. Boshoff C, Whitby D, Hatziionnou T, Fisher C, van der Walt J, Hatzakis A, Weiss R, Schulz T. Kaposi's sarcoma-associated herpesvirus in HIV-negative Kaposi's sarcoma. Lancet 1995;345:1043–1044.
5. Chang Y, Ziegler JL, Wabinga H, Katongole-Mbidde E, Boshoff C, Whitby D, Schulz T, Weiss RA, Jaffe HA, Group UKsSS, Moore PS. Kaposi's sarcoma-associated herpesvirus and Kaposi's sarcoma in Africa. Arch Intern Med 1996;156:202–204.
6. Cesarman E, Chang Y, Moore PS, Said JW, Knowles DM. Kaposi's sarcoma-associated herpesvirus-like DNA sequences are present in AIDS-related body cavity based lymphomas. N Engl J Med 1995;332:1186–1191.
7. Ansari MQ, Dawson DB, Nador R, Rutherford C, Schneider NR, Latimer MJ, Picker L, Knowles DM, McKenna RW. Primary body cavity-based AIDS-related lymphomas. Am J Clin Pathol 1996;105:221–229.
8. Soulier J, Grollet L, Oskenhendler E, Cacoub P, Cazals-Hatem D, Babinet P, d'Agay M-F, Clauvel J-P, Raphael M, Degos L, Sigaux F. Kaposi's sarcoma-associated herpesvirus-like DNA sequences in multicentric Castleman's disease. Blood 1995;86:1276–1280.

9. Penn I. Kaposi's sarcoma in organ transplant recipients: Report of 20 cases. Transplantation 1979;27:8–11.

10. Piette WW. The incidence of second malignancies in subsets of Kaposi's sarcoma. J Am Acad Dermatol 1987;16:855–861.

11. Klepp O, Dahl O, Stenwig JT. Association of Kaposi's sarcoma and prior immunosuppressive therapy. A 5-year material of Kaposi's sarcoma in Norway. Cancer 1978;42:2626–2630.

12. Trattner A, Hodak E, David M, Sandbank M. The appearance of Kaposi sarcoma during corticosteroid therapy. Cancer 1993;72:1779–1783.

13. Beral V, Peterman TA, Berkelman RL, Jaffe HW. Kaposi's sarcoma among persons with AIDS: a sexually transmitted infection? Lancet 1990;335:123–128.

14. Wabinga HR, Parkin DM, Wabwire-Mangen F, Mugerwa J. Cancer in Kampala, Uganda, in 1989–91: changes in incidence in the era of AIDS. Int J Cancer 1993;54:5–22.

15. Strauchen JA, Hauser AD, Burstein DA, Jiminez R, Moore PS, Chang Y. Body cavity-based malignant lymphoma containing Kaposi sarcoma-associated herpesvirus in an HIV-negative man with previous Kaposi sarcoma. Ann Intern Med 1996;125:822–825.

16. Nador RG, Cesarman E, Knowles DM, Said JW. Herpes-like DNA sequences in a body cavity-based lymphoma in an HIV-negative patient. N Engl J Med 1995;333:943.

17. Cesarman E, Moore PS, Rao PH, Inghirami G, Knowles DM, Chang Y. In vitro establishment and characterization of two AIDS-related lymphoma cell lines (BC-1 and BC-2) containing Kaposi's sarcoma-associated herpesvirus-like (KSHV) DNA sequences. Blood 1995;86:2708–2714.

18. Gaidano G, Cechova K, Chang Y, Moore PS, Knowles DM, Dalla-Favera R. Establishment of AIDS-related lymphoma cell lines from lymphomatous effusions. Leukemia 1996;10:1237–1240.

19. Renne R, Zhong W, Herndier B, McGrath M, Abbey N, Kedes D, Ganem D. Lytic growth of Kaposi's sarcoma-associated herpesvirus (human herpesvirus 8) in culture. Nature Med 1996;2:342–346.

20. Gao SJ, Kingsley L, Li M, Zheng W, Parravicini C, Ziegler J, Newton R, Rinaldo CR, Saah A, Phair J, Detels R, Chang Y, Moore PS. KSHV antibodies among Americans, Italians and Ugandans with and without Kaposi's sarcoma [see comments]. Nature Med 1996;2:925–928.

21. Arvanitakis L, Mesri EA, Nador RG, Said JW, Asch AS, Knowles DM, Cesarman E. Establishment and characterization of a primary effusion (body cavity-based) lymphoma cell line (BC-3) harboring Kaposi's sarcoma-associated herpesvirus (KSHV/HHV-8) in the absence of Epstein-Barr virus. Blood 1996;88:2648–2654.

22. Moore PS, Gao S-J, Dominguez G, Cesarman E, Lungu O, Knowles DM, Garber R, McGeoch DJ, Pellett P, Chang Y. Primary characterization of a herpesvirus agent associated with Kaposi's sarcoma. J Virol 1996;70:549–558.

23. Renne R, Lagunoff M, Zhong W, Ganem D. The size and conformation of Kaposi's sarcoma-associated herpesvirus (human herpesvirus 8) DNA in infected cells and virions. J Virol 1996;70:8151–8154.

24. Boshoff C, Gao S-J, Healy L, Matthews S, Thomas AJ, Warnke RA, Strauchen JA, Matutes E, Kamel OW, Weiss RA, Moore PS, Chang Y. Establishing a KSHV positive cell line (BCP-1) from peripheral blood and characterizing its growth in Nod/SCID mice. Blood 1997;91:1671–1679.

25. Frizzera G, Peterson BA, Bayrd ED, Goldman A. A systemic lymphoprolifera-
    tive disorder with morphologic features of Castleman's disease: clinical find-
    ings and clinicopathologic correlations in 15 patients. J Clin Oncol 1985;3:
    1202–1216.
26. Parravicini C, Corbellino M, Paulli M, Magrini U, Lazzarino M, Moore PS,
    Chang Y. Expression of a virus-derived cytokine, KSHV vIL-6, in HIV se-
    ronegative Castleman's disease. Am J Pathol 1997;151:1517–1521.
27. Rettig MB, Ma HJ, Vescio RA, Põld M, Schiller G, Belson D, Savage A,
    Nishikubo C, Wu C, Fraser J, Said JW, Berenson JR. Kaposi's sarcoma-associ-
    ated herpesvirus infection of bone marrow dendritic cells from multiple mye-
    loma patients. Science 1997;276:1851–1854.
28. Moore PS, Chang Y. Kaposi's sarcoma (KS), KS-associated herpesvirus, and
    the criteria for causality in the age of molecular biology. Am J Epidemiol
    1998;147:217–221.
29. Dupin N, Grandadam M, Calvez V, Gorin I, Aubin JT, Harvard S, Lamy F,
    Leibowitch M, Huraux JM, Escande JP, Agut H. Herpesvirus-like DNA in pa-
    tients with Mediterranean Kaposi's sarcoma. Lancet 1995;345:761–762.
30. Gluckman E, Parquet N, Scieux C, Dplanche M, Taineau R, Betheau P, Mor-
    inet F. KS-associated herpesvirus-like DNA sequences after allogeneic bone-
    marrow transplantation. Lancet 1995;346:1558–1559.
31. Strathdee SA, Veugelers PJ, Moore PS. The epidemiology of HIV-associated
    Kaposi's sarcoma: the unraveling mystery. AIDS 1996;10:S51–S57.
32. Corbellino M, Parravincini C, Aubin JT, Berti E. Kaposi's sarcoma and her-
    pesvirus-like DNA sequences in sensory ganglia. N Engl J Med 1996;334:
    1341–1342 (letter).
33. Corbellino M, Poirel L, Bestetti G, Pizzuto M, Aubin JT, Capra M, Bifulco C,
    Berti E, Agut H, Rizzardini G, Galli M, Parravicini C. Restricted tissue distri-
    bution of extralesional Kaposi's sarcoma-associated herpesvirus-like DNA se-
    quences in AIDS patients with Kaposi's sarcoma. AIDS Res Hum Retrovirus
    1996;12:651–657.
34. Roizman B. The family Herpesviridae, in Roizman B, Whitley RJ, Lopez C
    (eds): The Human Herpeviruses. New York, Raven Press;1993:1–9.
35. Levy JA. A new human herpesvirus: KSHV or HHV8? Lancet 1995;346:8978.
36. Rady PL, Yen A, Rollefson JL, Orengo I, Bruce S, Hughes TK, Tyring SK.
    Herpesvirus-like DNA sequences in non-Kaposi's sarcoma skin lesions of
    transplant patients. Lancet 1995;345:1339–1340.
37. Boshoff C, Talbot S, Kennedy M, O'Leary J, Schulz T, Chang Y. HHV8 and
    skin cancers in immunosuppressed patients. Lancet 1996;347:338–339.
38. Dictor M, Rambech E, Way D, Witte M, Bendsöe N. Human herpesvirus 8
    (Kaposi's sarcoma-associated herpesvirus) DNA in Kaposi's sarcoma lesions,
    AIDS Kaposi's sarcoma cell lines, endothelial Kaposi's sarcoma simulators,
    and the skin of immunosuppressed patients. Am J Pathol 1996;148:2009–
    2016.
39. Adams V, Kempf W, Schmid M, Müller B, Briner J, Burg G. Absence of her-
    pesvirus-like DNA sequences in skin cancers of non-immunosuppressed pa-
    tients. Lancet 1995;346:1715.
40. Lin J-C, Lin S-C, Mar E-C, Pellett PE, Stamey FR, Stewart JA, Spira TJ. Is
    Kaposi's sarcoma-associated herpesvirus detectable in semen of HIV-infected
    homosexual men? Lancet 1995;346:1601–1602.

41. Monini P, de Lellis L, Fabris M, Rigolin F, Cassai E. Kaposi's sacoma-associated herpesvirus DNA sequences in prostate tissue and human semen. N Engl J Med 1996;334:1168–1172.

42. Monini P, de Lellis L, Cassai E. Absence of HHV-8 in prostate and semen (letter). N Engl J Med 1996;335:1238–1239.

43. Howard MR, Whitby D, Bahadur G, Suggett F, Boshoff C, Tenant FM, Schulz TF, Kirk S, Matthews S, Weller I, Tedder RS, Weiss RA. Detection of human herpesvirus 8 DNA in semen from HIV-infected individuals but not healthy semen donors. AIDS 1997;11:F15–F19.

44. Lebbé C, Pellet C, Tatoud R, Agbalika F, Dosquet P, Desgrez JP, Morel P, Calvo F. Absence of human herpesvirus 8 sequences in prostate specimens. AIDS 1997;11:270.

45. Gupta P, Singh MK, Rinaldo C, Ding M, Farzadegan H, Saah A, Hoover D, Moore P, Kingsley L. Detection of Kaposi's sarcoma herpesvirus DNA in semen of homosexual men with Kaposi's sarcoma. AIDS 1996;10:1596–1598.

46. Tasaka T, Said JW, Morosetti R, Park D, Verbeek W, Nagai M, Takahara J, Koeffler HP. Is Kaposi's sarcoma–associated herpesvirus ubiquitous in urogenital and prostate tissues? Blood 1997;89:1686–1689.

47. Corbellino M, Bestetti G, Galli M, Parravicini C. Absence of HHV-8 in prostate and semen [letter; comment]. N Engl J Med 1996;335:1238–1239.

48. Whitby D, Howard MR, Tenant-Flowers M, Brink NS, Copas A, Boshoff C, Hatziouannou T, Suggett FEA, Aldam DM, Denton AS, Miller RF, Weller IVD, Weiss RA, Tedder RS, Schulz TF. Detection of Kaposi's sarcoma-associated herpesvirus (KSHV) in peripheral blood of HIV-infected individuals predicts progression to Kaposi's sarcoma. Lancet 1995;364:799–802.

49. Moore PS, Kingsley L, Holmberg SD, Spira T, Conley LJ, Hoover D, Gupta P, Jaffe H, Chang Y. Kaposi's sarcoma-associated herpesvirus infection prior to onset of Kaposi's sarcoma. AIDS 1996;10:175–180.

50. Miller G, Rigsby MO, Heston L, Grogan E, Sun R, Metroka C, Levy JA, Gao SJ, Chang Y, Moore P. Antibodies to butyrate-inducible antigens of Kaposi's sarcoma-associated herpesvirus in patients with HIV-1 infection. N Engl J Med 1996;334:1292–1297.

51. Gao S-J, Kingsley L, Hoover DR, Spira TJ, Rinaldo CR, Saah A, Phair J, Detels R, Parry P, Chang Y, Moore PS. Seroconversion to antibodies against Kaposi's sarcoma-associated herpesvirus-related latent nuclear antigens before the development of Kaposi's sarcoma. N Engl J Med 1996;335:233–241.

52. Rainbow L, Platt GM, Simpson GR, Sarid R, Gao S-J, Stoiber H, Herrington S, Moore PS, Schulz TF. The 226- to 234-kilodalton latent nuclear protein (LNA) of Kaposi's sarcoma-associated herpesvirus (KSHV/HHV8) is encoded by ORF73 and is a component of the latency-associated nuclear antigen. J Virol 1997;71:5915–5921.

53. Kedes DH, Operskalski E, Busch M, Kohn R, Flood J, Ganem D. The seroepidemiology of human herpesvirus 8 (Kaposi's sarcoma-associated herpesvirus): distribution of infection in KS risk groups and evidence for sexual transmission. Nature Med 1996;2:918–924.

54. Geddes M, Franceschi S, Barchielli A, Falcini F, Carli S, Cocconi G, Conti E, Crosignani P, Gafa L, Giarelli L. Kaposi's sarcoma in Italy before and after the AIDS epidemic. Br J Cancer 1994;69:333–336.

55. Geddes M, Franceschi S, Balzi D, Arniani A, Gaf'a L, Zanetti R. Birthplace and classic Kaposi's sarcoma in Italy. J Natl Cancer Inst 1995;87:1015–1017.

56. Lennette ET, Blackbourne DJ, Levy JA. Antibodies to human herpesvirus type 8 in the general population and in Kaposi's sarcoma patients. Lancet 1996; 348:858–861.

57. Lin SF, Sun R, Heston L, Gradoville L, Shedd D, Haglund K, Rigsby M, Miller G. Identification, expression, and immunogenicity of Kaposi's sarcoma-associated herpesvirus-encoded small viral capsid antigen. J Virol 1997;71:3069–3076.

58. Simpson GR, Schulz TF, Whitby D, Cook PM, Boshoff C, Rainbow L, Howard MR, Gao S-J, Bohensky RA, Simmonds P, Lee C, de Ruiter A, Hatziakis A, Tedder RS, Weller IVD, Weiss RA, Moore PS. Prevalence of Kaposi's sarcoma associated herpesvirus infection as measured by antibodies to recombinant capsid protein and latent immunofluorescence antigen. Lancet 1996;348: 1133–1138.

59. Boshoff C, Schulz TF, Kennedy MM, Graham AK, Fisher C, Thomas A, McGee JO, Weiss RA, O'Leary JJ. Kaposi's sarcoma-associated herpesvirus infects endothelial and spindle cells. Nature Med 1995;1:1274–1278.

60. Zhong W, Wang H, Herndier B, Ganem D. Restricted expression of Kaposi sarcoma-associated herpesvirus (human herpesvirus 8) genes in Kaposi sarcoma. Proc Natl Acad Sci USA 1996;93:6641–6646.

61. Staskus KA, Zhong W, Gebhard K, Herndier B, Wang H, Renne R, Beneke J, Pudney J, Anderson DJ, Ganem D, Haase AT. Kaposi's sarcoma-associated herpesvirus gene expression in endothelial (spindle) tumor cells. J Virol 1997;71:715–719.

62. Rabkin CS, Janz S, Lash A, Coleman AE, Musaba E, Liotta L, Biggar RJ, Zhuang ZP. Monoclonal origin of multicentric Kaposi's sarcoma lesions. N Engl J Med 1997;336:988–993.

63. Russo JJ, Bohenzky RA, Chien MC, Chen J, Yan M, Maddalena D, Parry JP, Peruzzi D, Edelman IS, Chang Y, Moore PS. Nucleotide sequence of the Kaposi sarcoma-associated herpesvirus (HHV8). Proc Natl Acad Sci USA 1996; 93:14862–14867.

64. Medveczky MM, Szomolanyi E, Hesselton R, DeGrand D, Geck P, Medveczky RG. Herpesvirus saimiri strains from three DNA subgroups have different oncogenic potentials in New Zealand White rabbits. J Virol 1989;63:3601–3611.

65. Jung JU, Trimble JJ, King NW, Biesinger B, Fleckenstein BW, Desrosiers RC. Identification of transforming genes of subgroup A and C strains of Herpesvirus saimiri. Proc Natl Acad Sci USA 1991;88:7051–7055.

66. Jung JU, Desrosiers RC. Distinct functional domains of STP-C488 of herpesvirus saimiri. Virology 1994;204:751–758.

67. Jung JU, Desrosiers RC. Association of the viral oncoprotein STP-C488 with cellular ras. Mol Cel Biol 1995;15:6506–6512.

68. Moore PS, Boshoff C, Weiss RA, Chang Y. Molecular mimicry of human cytokine and cytokine response pathway genes by KSHV. Science 1996;274:1739–1744.

69. Nicholas J, Ruvolo V, Zong J, Ciufo D, Guo HG, Reitz MS, Hayward GS. A single 13-kilobase divergent locus in the Kaposi sarcoma-associated herpesvirus (human herpesvirus 8) genome contains nine open reading frames that are homologous to or related to cellular proteins. J Virol 1997;71:1963–1974.

70. Nicholas J, Ruvolo VR, Burns WH, Sandford G, Wan X, Ciufo D, Hendrick-

son SB, Guo HG, Hayward GS, Reitz MS. Kaposi's sarcoma-associated human herpesvirus-8 encodes homologues of macrophage inflammatory protein-1 and interleukin-6 Nature Med 1997;3:287–292.

71. Chang Y, Moore PS, Talbot SJ, Boshoff CH, Zarkowska T, Godden-Kent D, Paterson H, Weiss RA, Mittnacht S. Cyclin encoded by KS herpesvirus. Nature 1996;382:410.

72. Cheng EH, Nicholas J, Bellows DS, Hayward GS, Guo HG, Reitz MS, Hardwick JM. A Bcl-2 homolog encoded by Kaposi sarcoma-associated virus, human herpesvirus 8, inhibits apoptosis but does not heterodimerize with Bax or Bak. Proc Natl Acad Sci USA 1997;94:690–694.

73. Sarid R, Sato T, Bohenzky RA, Russo JJ, Chang Y. Kaposi's sarcoma-associated herpesvirus encodes a functional Bcl-2 homologue. Nature Med 1997;3:293–298.

74. Pines J. Cyclins and cyclin-dependent kinases: themes and variations. Adv Cancer Res 1995;66:181–212.

75. Motokura T, Arnold A. PRAD1/Cyclin 1 proto-oncogenes: genomic organization, 5' DNA sequence, and sequence of a tumor-specific rearrangement breakpoint. Chrom Cancer 1993;7:89–95.

76. Cesarman E, Nador RG, Bai F, Bohenzky RA, Russo JJ, Moore PS, Chang Y, Knowles DM. Kaposi's sarcoma-associated herpesvirus contains G protein-coupled receptor and cyclin D homologs which are expressed in Kaposi's sarcoma and malignant lymphoma. J Virol 1996;70:8218–8223.

77. Sarid R, Flore O, Bohenzky RA, Moore PS, Chang Y. Transcription mapping of the Kaposi's sarcoma-associated herpesvirus (KSHV/HHV8) genome in a body cavity-based lymphoma cell line (BC-1). J Virol 1998;72:1005–1012.

78. Li M, Lee H, Yoon DW, Albrecht JC, Fleckenstein B, Neipel F, Jung JU. Kaposi's sarcoma-associated herpesvirus encodes a functional cyclin. J Virol 1997;71:1984–1991.

79. Godden-Kent D, Talbot SJ, Boshoff C, Chang Y, Moore PS, Weiss RA, Mittnacht S. The cyclin encoded by Kaposi's sarcoma associated herpesvirus (KSHV) stimulates cdk6 to phoshorylate the retinoblastoma protein and Histone H. J Virol 1997;71:4193–4198.

80. Vaux DL, Cory S, Adams JM. Bcl-2 gene promotes haemopoietic cell survival and cooperates with c-myc to immortalize pre-B cells. Nature 1988;335:440–442.

81. Garcia I, Martinou I, Tsujimoto Y, Martinou JC. Prevention of programmed cell death of sympathetic neurons by the bcl-2 proto-oncogene. Science 1992;258:302–304.

82. Hanada M, Aime'-Sempe' C, Sato T, Reed JC. Structure-function analysis of Bcl-2 protein T J Biol Chem 1995;270:11962–11969.

83. Yin XM, Oltvai ZN, Korsmeyer SJ. BH1 and BH2 domains of Bcl-2 are required for inhibition of apoptosis and heterodimerization with Bax. Nature 1994;369:321–323.

84. Tsujimoto Y, Croce CM. Analysis of the structure, transcripts, and protein products of bcl-2, the gene involved in human follicular lymphoma. Proc Natl Acad Sci USA 1986;83:5214–5218.

85. Cleary ML, Smith SD, Sklar J. Cloning and structural analysis of cDNAs for bcl-2 and a hybrid bcl-2/immunoglobulin transcript resulting from the t(14;18) translocation. Cell 1986;47:19–28.

86. Henderson S, Huen D, Rowe M, Dawson C, Johnson G, Rickinson A. Epstein-Barr virus-coded BHRF1 protein, a viral homologue of Bcl-2, protects human

B cells from programmed cell death. Proc Natl Acad Sci USA 1993;90:8479–8483.

87. Taniguchi T, Harada H, Lamphier M. Regulation of the interferon system and cell growth by the IRF transcription factors. J Cancer Res Clin Oncol 1995;121:516–520.

88. Gao S-J, Boshoff C, Jayachandra S, Weiss RA, Chang Y, Moore PS. KSHV ORF K9 (v-IRF) is an oncogene that inhibits the interferon signaling pathway. Oncogene 1997;15:1979–1986.

89. Arvanitakis L, Geras RE, Varma A, Gershengorn MC, Cesarman E. Human herpesvirus KSHV encodes a constitutively active G-protein-coupled receptor linked to cell proliferation. Nature 1997;385:347–350.

90. Ensoli B, Nakamura S, Salahuddin SZ, Biberfeld P, larsson L, Beaver B, Wong-Staal F, Gallo RC. AIDS Kaposi's sarcoma derived cells express cytokines with autocrine and paracrine growth effects. Science 1989;243:223–226.

91. Salahuddin SZ, Nakamura S, Biberfeld P, Kaplan MH, Markham P-D, Larsson L, Gallo RC. Angiogenic properties of Kaposi's sarcoma-derived cells after long-term culture in vitro. Science 1988;242:430–433.

92. Ensoli B, Barillari G, Salahuddin SZ, Gallo RC, Wong-Stahl F. Tat protein of HIV-1 stimulates growth of cells derived from Kaposi's sarcoma lesions of AIDS patients. Nature 1990;345:84–86.

93. Ensoli B, Buonaguro L, Barillari G, Fiorelli V, Gendelman R, Morgan RA, Wingfield P, Gallo RC. Release, uptake, and effects of extracellular human immunodeficiency virus type 1 Tat protein on cell growth and viral transactivation. J Virol 1993;67:277–287.

94. Ensoli B, Gendelman R, Markham P, Fiorelli V, Colombini S, Raffeld M, Cafaro A, Chang HK, Brady JN, Gallo RC. Synergy between basic fibroblast growth factor and HIV-1 Tat protein in induction of Kaposi's sarcoma. Nature 1994;371:674–680.

95. Barillari G, Gendelman R, Gallo RC, Ensoli B. The Tat protein of human immunodeficiency virus type 1, a growth factor for AIDS Kaposi sarcoma and cytokine-activated vascular cells, induces adhesion of the same cell types by using integrin receptors recognizing the RGD amino acid sequence. Proc Natl Acad Sci USA 1993;90:7941–7945.

96. Cocchi F, DeVico AL, Garzino DA, Arya SK, Gallo RC, Lusso P. Identification of RANTES, MIP-1 alpha, and MIP-1 beta as the major HIV-suppressive factors produced by CD8+ T cells. Science 1995;270:1811–1815.

97. Kledal TN, Rosenkilde MM, Coulin F, Simmons G, Johnsen AH, Alouani S, Power CA, Luttichau HR, Gerstoft J, Clapham PR, Clark-Lewis I, Wells RNC, Schwartz TW. A broad-spectrum chemokine antagonist encoded by Kaposi's sarcoma-associated herpesvirus. Science 1997;277:1656–1659.

98. Boshoff C, Endo Y, Collins PD, Takeuchi Y, Reeves JD, Schweickart VL, Siani M, Sasaki T, Williams TJ, Gray PW, Moore PS, Chang Y, Weiss RA. Angiogenic and HIV inhbitory functions of KSHV-encoded chemokines. Science 1997;278:290–294.

99. Tosato G, Jones K, Breinig MK, McWilliams HP, McKnight JLC. Interleukin-6 production in posttransplant lymphoproliferative disease. J Clin Invest 1993; 91:2806–2814.

100. Klein B, Zhang XG, Lu ZY, Bataille R. Interleukin-6 in human multiple myeloma. Blood 1995;85:863–872.

101. Yoshizaki K, Matsuda T, Nishimoto N, Kuritani T, Taeho L, Aozasa K, Na-

kahata T, Kawai H, Tagoh H, Komori T, Kishimoto S, Hirano T, Kishimoto T. Pathogenic significance of interleukin-6 (IL-6/BSF-2) in Castleman's disease. Blood 1989;74:1360–1367.

102. Beck JT, Hsu SM, Wijdenes J, Bataille R, Klein B, Vesole D, Hayden K, Jagannath S, Barlogie B. Brief report: alleviation of systemic manifestations of Castleman's disease by monoclonal anti-interleukin-6 antibody. N Engl J Med 1994;330:602–605.

103. Tosato G, Tanner G, Jones KD, Revel M, Pike SE. Identification of interleukin 6 as an autocrine growth factor for Epstein-Barr virus immortalized B cells. J Virol 1990;64:3033–3041.

104. Tanner J, Tosato G. Impairment of natural killer functions by interleukin 6 increases lymphoblastoid cell tumorigenicity in athymic mice. J Clin Invest 1991;88:239–247.

105. Molden J, Chang Y, Yun Y, Moore PS, Goldsmith MA. A Kaposi's sarcoma-associated herpesvirus-encoded cytokine homolog (vIL-6) activates signaling through the shared gp130 receptor subunit. J Biol Chem 1997;272:19625–19631.

106. Morfeldt L, Torsander J. Long-term remission of Kaposi's sarcoma following foscarnet treatment in HIV-infected patients. Scand J Infect Dis 1994;26:749.

107. Albrecht H, Stellbrink HJ, Brewster D, Greten H. Resolution of oral hairy leukoplakia during treatment with foscarnet. AIDS 1994;8:1014–1016.

108. Jones J, Peterman T, Chu S, Jaffe H. AIDS-associated Kaposi's sarcoma. Science 1995;267:1078–1079.

109. Glesby MJ, Hoover DR, Weng S, Graham NMH, Phair JP, Detels R, Ho M, Saah A. Use of antiherpes drugs and the risk of Kaposi's sarcoma: data from the Multicenter AIDS Cohort Study. J Infect Dis 1996;173:1477–1480.

110. Kedes DH, Ganem D. Sensitivity of Kaposi's sarcoma-associated herpesvirus replication to antiviral drugs. J Clin Invest 1997;99:2082–2086.

111. Pagano JS. Epstein-Barr virus: therapy of active and latent infection. In: Jeffries DJ, De Clercq E, eds. Antiviral Chemotherapy. New York: John Wiley and Sons; 1995:155–195.

9
Hepatitis B Virus and Hepatocellular Carcinoma

WILLIAM S. ROBINSON

Although numerous examples of cancer caused by virus infection (natural virus infections, as well as experimental infections) have been recognized in animals since almost 100 years ago,[1] and although intense, investigation of several cancers has led to identification of molecular mechanisms of viral carcinogenesis,[2] there are relatively few examples of human virus infections with irrefutable evidence for a causal association with cancer. In all cases of virus–cancer associations in humans, the strongest evidence for a causal relationship is epidemiological. One of the strongest cases is that chronic or persistent hepatitis B virus (HBV) infection predisposes to the development of primary hepatocellular carcinoma (HCC).[3–5] HCC is one of the most common cancers of humans and evidence suggests that persistent HBV infection is the most important risk factor for its development. HBV infections commonly occur at an early age and become persistent in populations in which this virus is highly endemic, such as those in eastern Asia and sub-Saharan Africa.[4] Such persistent HBV infections may be associated with chronic hepatitis; macronodular cirrhosis develops in a significant fraction of persistently infected individuals, usually over many years.[4,6] Long-standing persistent HBV infection is associated with a greatly increased risk of HCC, compared with the risk in uninfected populations,[5,7,8] and the presence of macronodular cirrhosis in HBV-infected individuals appears to increase further the risk of HCC by at least a factor of 10.[5]

Recently, scientists have discovered in certain rodent and avian species viruses that share ultrastructural, molecular, epidemiological, and pathogenetic features with HBV, including association with HCC. These viruses, like HBV, are members of the hepadnavirus family.[9–11] It was the recognition of chronic hepatitis and HCC in woodchucks in the United States,[12] and in ducks in China,[13] that prompted a search for and discovery of hepadnaviruses in these hosts. The association of HCC with persistent hepadnavirus infection in woodchucks[12,14,15] and in Beechey ground squirrels[16] is even stronger than the association of HBV infection with HCC in humans. These strong associations of HCC with persistent hepadnavirus infections in a variety of mammals suggest an important role for these infections in the development of hepatic malignancy. Moreover, the finding of a clonal pattern of hepadnavirus DNA integration in cellular DNA of many HCC in humans[17-21] and in other hosts naturally infected with hepadnaviruses[16,22-25] indicates that these tumors arise from a single cell with integrated virus. This finding has stimulated interest in whether viral integration plays a role in HCC.

The World Health Organization has estimated that 80% of all HCCs in the world occur in HBV-infected individuals,[26] and careful prospective studies have indicated that 40% or more of middle aged Chinese males with chronic HBV infection die of HCC.[5] Chronic infection can occur in 10% or more of the population in high prevalence areas,[4,6] thus the number of liver cancers in those populations is very great. Among all cancers of humans associated with environmental risk factors, only the number of cigarette smoking–associated lung cancers appears to exceed HBV-associated HCC. In the remaining 20% of HCC cases that are not linked to HBV, other important risk factors have been identified. Risk factors that cause chronic necroinflammatory liver disease and cirrhosis include chronic alcohol-induced liver disease,[27,28] chronic hepatitis C,[29-36] hemochromatosis,[37,38] alpha 1 antitrypsin deficiency,[39] cryptogenic cirrhosis,[40] primary biliary cirrhosis,[41] hereditary tyrosinemia,[28] and other causes of cirrhosis. Chemical carcinogens linked to HCC include dietary aflatoxin (toxins produced by fungal organisms that infest improperly stored grain, peanuts, and other foods)[42-44] androgenic-anabolic steroids[45] and oral-contraceptive steroids,[46-48] undefined substances (possibly pesticides[49]) in polluted groundwater used for drinking in parts of China,[49-51] and possibly other chemical carcinogens (Table 9.1).

Chronic hepadnavirus infection in three different mammalian hosts (humans, woodchucks, and ground squirrels) has been shown to be strongly associated with development of HCC. Described here are relevant features of the hepadnavirus family, epidemiological evidence of the association of these viruses with HCC, and current understanding of molecular mechanisms that may contribute to the development of hepadnavirus-associated HCC in these three hosts.

THE HEPADNAVIRUS FAMILY

Hepadnaviruses comprise a family of closely related viruses that have similar biological, molecular, and epidemiological features, and that are associated with similar disease syndromes, including HCC. The family name (hepadnaviruses) indicates the DNA genome and hepatotropism of these

Table 9.1 Established and possible risk factors for hepatocellular carcinoma in humans

Risk factor	Cause of inflammation and cirrhosis?	Well-established or possible risk factor[a]	References
HBV	Yes	Well-established	4, 5, 7, 12, 14–16, 22, 92, 149–153
HCV	Yes	Well-established	29–36
Alcohol	Yes	Well-established	27, 28, 154–156
Cryptogenic cirrhosis	Yes	Possible	40, 157
Primary biliary cirrhosis	Yes	Possible	41
Autoimmune CAH	Yes	Possible	158, 159
Membranous obstruction of the inferior vena cava	Yes	Possible	160, 161
Alpha-1-antitrypsin deficiency	Yes	Possible	39, 162–167
Hemochromatosis	Yes	Possible	37, 38
Wilson's disease	Yes	Possible	168, 169
Glycogen storage disease	Yes	Possible	170, 171
Hereditary tyrosinemia	Yes	Possible	28, 172–175
Parasitic infections of the liver[b]	Yes	Possible	176–179
Methotrexate therapy	Yes	Possible	180, 181
Aflatoxin B_1	No	Possible	42–44, 182
Polluted drinking water in China	No	Possible	49–51
Contraceptives and anabolic steroids	No	Possible	45–48, 183, 184
Cigarette smoking	No	Possible	185–187

[a]"Well-established" signifies that there is clinical, laboratory and epidemiological evidence for a causal association between the risk factor and cancer. "Possible" signifies that strong epidemiological and/or laboratory evidence for an *independent* role of the factor in HCC is lacking.
[b]There is strong evidence for a role for parasitic infection in cholangiocarcinomas of the liver (see Chapter 13).

viruses.[9–11] The hepadnavirus family includes HBV of humans, the woodchuck hepatitis virus (WHV) of *Marmata monax*,[12] the ground squirrel hepatitis virus (GSHV) of *Spermophilus beecheyi*,[52] the duck HBV (DHBV) found in several varieties of domestic ducks,[13] and similar viruses in tree squirrels,[53] and herons.[54] Less well documented findings in other rodents, in marsupials, and in cats suggest that other hepadnaviruses may exist.

Common features of hepadnaviruses include virion (virus particle) size and ultrastructure with an envelope surrounding an electron-dense spherical nucleocapsid, or characteristic polypeptide and antigenic composition; common virion DNA size, structure, and genetic organization; the presence of DNA polymerase (reverse transcriptase) activity in the virion; and an unusual mechanism of viral DNA replication that includes reverse transcription of a greater-than-genome-length viral RNA transcript of the viral DNA genome.[55] Hepadnaviruses appear to be related to retroviruses and cauliflower mosaic virus in that all share regions of DNA sequence homology; all share features of gene number, function and organization; and all utilize a reverse transcriptase mechanism in viral genome replication,[56,57] suggesting these viruses evolved from a common ancestor.

Two characteristics of persistent as well as of acute hepadnavirus infection are that the liver is the principle site of infection, and that viral envelope (surface) antigen (HBsAg) particles and sometimes virions are continuously present in high concentrations in the blood. The presence of HBsAg in the blood is diagnostic of active HBV infection. Hepadnaviruses are commonly transmitted from infected mothers to their newborn infants or to young children; under this circumstance (infection at a very young age) infections commonly persist, often for many years and commonly for the life of the patient. More than 90% of neonatal HBV infections persist.[58,59] In contrast, primary HBV infection in older children and adults leads to persistent infection in less than 10% of cases.[60-62] Other routes of transmission for these infections include percutaneous (e.g., by needle stick) and mucous membrane exposure to blood or some other body fluids and by sexual contacts with HBV-infected individuals.

VIRAL GENOME STRUCTURE, REPLICATION, AND INTEGRATION

The hepadnavirus DNA genome is among the smallest of all known animal viruses; it consists of an approximately 3200-base-pair circular molecule that contains a single-stranded region of different length in different molecules (see Figure 9.1), reflecting the fact that DNA molecules are packaged into virions before viral DNA replication (i.e., synthesis of the DNA plus strand) is complete.[55,63,64]

The genomes of the three mammalian hepadnaviruses have four long open reading frames (ORFs) in the complete or long (minus) virion DNA strand. These ORFs have similar locations in each virus with respect to the cohesive ends of the DNAs (Figure 9.1) and encode the viral polypeptides of (1) the viral envelope, which contains HBsAg specificity; (2) the viral nucleocapsid or core, which contains both hepatitis B core antigen (HBcAg) specificity and a soluble protein with hepatitis B e antigen (HBeAg) specificity that is a truncated form of the major core protein; (3) the largest polypeptide, which has reverse transcriptase activity, has RNAase activity, and is the protein primer for synthesis of the viral minus DNA strand; and (4) the small X protein, which has the capacity to transactivate transcription regulated by both homologous and heterologous regulatory elements. Hepadnaviruses do not encode an integrase protein, like that of retroviruses, to facilitate viral genome integration.

Other functionally important elements in hepadnavirus genomes in-

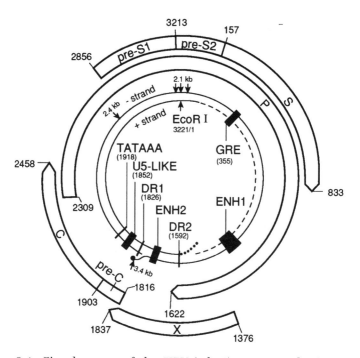

Figure 9.1. Circular map of the HBV (adw2) genome. The inner circles represent the virion DNA strands and the broken (dashed) line in the short (+) DNA strand represents the region within which the 3' end of the + strand may occur in different molecules, and the corresponding region of the long strand is that which may be single-stranded in different molecules. A line of dots represents the oligoribonucleotide primer covalently attached to the 5' end of the + DNA strand and a single dot represents the protein primer covalently attached to the 5' end of the − DNA strand. The large arrows represent the recognized functional open reading frames (ORF) with the direction of transcription from the minus DNA strand indicated. The small arrows indicate the 5'-ends of the three major size classes of transcripts of 3.4, 2.4 and 2.1 Kb, all of which are identically terminated near the poly A addition signal (TATAAA). The nucleotide sequence locations of the initiation and termination codons of each ORF are given with reference to map position 1 at the single EcoRI cleavage site in this DNA. The map position of the first nucleotide of the glucocorticoid-responsive element (GRE), DR2, DR1, the U5-like sequence and the poly A addition sequence (TATAAA) are indicated, as is the general region exhibiting enhancer 1 (ENH 1) and enhancer 2 (ENH 2) activity.

clude 11 bp direct repeat sequences, designated DR1 and DR2 (involved in viral DNA replication), which are approximately 225 bp apart in the mammalian viruses; four promoter elements for transcription; two transcriptional enhancer elements (enhancers 1 and 2); and a polyadenylation signal that is used by all major transcripts and that lies within the beginning of the C-gene.

The hepadnavirus genome is unusually compact and efficiently organized in that much of the genome is utilized for multiple functions; genes overlap so that the same nucleotide sequence encodes more than one protein, and all cis-acting regulatory sequences (e.g., transcriptional enhancer and promoter elements) are contained in genomic sequences that also encode protein (see Figure 9.1).

Hepadnaviral genome replication involves conversion of infecting-virion DNA molecules into covalently closed circular molecules in liver cell nuclei; formation of a greater-than-genome length RNA transcript with a terminally repeated sequence and shorter transcripts that function as messenger RNAs; packaging of the long transcript, newly made viral reverse transcriptase, and protein primer in viral core particles found in hepatocyte cytoplasm; and synthesis of new viral DNA molecules by reverse transcription of the long RNA transcript utilizing a viral-encoded protein primer in forming the first synthesized viral DNA (minus) strand and a capped oligoribonucleotide derived from the 5' end of the long RNA template as primer for synthesis of the second DNA (plus) strand[65-67] (see Figure 9.2). This last step occurs exclusively within cytoplasmic viral core particles. There is a nine-nucleotide terminal redundancy in the minus strand that may cause strand switching by the DNA polymerase during viral DNA replication. A reverse-transcription step in replication of DNA is unusual and is a characteristic feature that defines the hepadnavirus family.

Liver cells are most readily infected and permissive for hepadnavirus replication, at least in part because the viral transcriptional enhancers and certain viral promoters are active in liver cells but are not at all or are only poorly active in other cell types.[68] HBV has been detected irregularly in blood mononuclear cells[69-71] and in pancreatic cells[72] but appears to replicate poorly in such cells.

Ordered integration of viral DNA in cellular DNA is not an intrinsic part of hepadnavirus replication as it is for replication of retroviruses. However, sporadic viral integration by a mechanism such as illegitimate recombination does take place, and integrated viral DNA has been found in cellular DNA of infected livers as well as in HCCs. In hepadnavirus-infected hosts, many HCC contain viral integrations with a clonal pattern. It follows that these tumors must have arisen by clonal expansion of an original cell with that viral integration. The possible role of such integrations in development of HCC has been investigated intensively. Much of the evidence of the fine structure of hepadnavirus integrations comes from investigation of human[73-75] and woodchuck[25] HCCs; there has been much less investigation of viral integrations in nontumorous livers. It is not known whether viral integration occurs in every hepadnavirus infected cell in vivo, or in only a proportion of cells. However, no apparent difference in the structure of viral integrations of HCC and nontumorous liver have been identified.

Researchers have identified general features of hepadnavirus integra

Hepadnavirus Replication

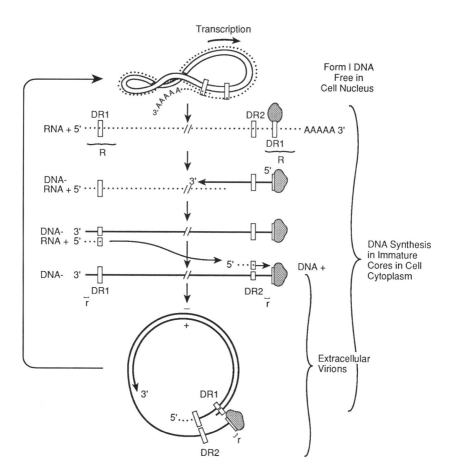

Figure 9.2. Scheme of proposed mechanism of hepadnavirus DNA replication. DR1 and DR2 represent 11 nucleotide pair direct repeat sequences. R represents the approximately 200 nucleotide terminal redundancy in the long RNA transcript and r represents the short terminal
redundancy of the−DNA strand. Solid lines represent DNA strands, dot-
ted lines RNA, and the stippled area the protein primer for DNA strand
synthesis.

tions[63,64,73-75] by comparing the structure of viral and flanking cellular DNA
of many published examples (almost all being HBV integrants in human
HCC). HCCs containing integrated virus sometimes have a single clonal
integrant, but more often there are multiple clonal integrants (most often
three to four but rarely 10 or more), each at a different cellular DNA site.
These integrants appear to arise from separate viral integration events.
The apparent cellular DNA sites of integration have been different in

every human HCC studied. Most HCCs with integrated virus do not contain replicating viral DNA forms, suggesting that cells of such HCCs are nonpermissive for virus replication by an unknown mechanism.

Some integrants consist of simple contiguous linear sequences of HBV DNA without rearrangement; others are complex and may have arisen by integration of multiple viral genomes at one site, or by rearrangement after integration by recombination between viral sequences of different integrants.[74] The complex integrants contain one or more virus–virus junctions. Complete viral genomes have not been found in any integrants. Thus, deletion of some viral sequence has been found in all integrants that have been sequenced, whether they arose from single or multiple genome integrations. The long, terminally redundant HBV transcript that serves as a template for viral genomic DNA synthesis cannot be synthesized from incomplete viral integrations, so natural integrants are defective for virus replication. This contrasts with the integrated DNA provirus of retroviruses, which does allow functional virus replication.

There appear to be preferred sites for integration within the viral genome.[63,64,73–75] More than 50% of viral integrants in HCC and non-HCC liver tissue appear to have one viral DNA end that joins cellular DNA (or viral DNA in the case of virus–virus DNA junctions) near or between the cohesive 5' ends, which are within the direct repeat (DR) sequences of viral DNA (see Figure 9.1). The other end of viral DNA joins cellular DNA (or viral DNA in the case of virus–virus junctions) at variable positions in the viral genome.[63,64,73–75] This variability suggests random recombination with cell DNA, although there may be a slight preference for the pre-S region of the viral genome as a site of integration.

The patterns of viral integration suggest that the cohesive end region of viral DNA is involved in viral DNA integration into cellular DNA. Therefore, the replication intermediates are probably linear molecules with single-stranded DNA at the cohesive end region (Figure 9.2), rather than closed circular viral DNA molecules. That linear molecules are the substrates for integration suggests that recombinations occur at a stage of infection when virus replication is proceeding and appropriate replication intermediates are present.

Although there are preferred sites for integration within the hepadnavirus genome (e.g., the cohesive end region), viral DNA appears to be integrated at many different sites of cellular DNA and in many different chromosomes. Whether there may be somewhat preferred cellular sites of HBV integration—as appears to be case for some retroviruses[76]—is not yet clear. There may be some preference for HBV integration within repeating sequences, such as Alu DNA,[73] satellite III DNA,[73,77] -satellite DNA,[78] and minisatellite or VNTR DNA.[73,75–78]

There are common structural alterations in host chromosomal DNA at sites of viral integrations.[73,74,78] First, all HBV integrations are associated with microdeletions (e.g., 10 bp) in cellular DNA at the site of integration.[74] The consistency of this finding suggests that microdeletions are an integral part of the integration mechanism as for integration of some other DNA viruses by illegitimate recombination. Second, in sporadic HCC, larger deletions of chromosomal DNA have been described at sites of viral DNA integration.[79,80] These large deletions appear to be formed by a mechanism different from the one responsible for microdeletions. Third, translocations involving cellular DNA from two different chromosomes joined to the respective ends of a viral DNA sequence have been described; no two have involved the same chromosomal DNA region.[80,81] Fourth, inverted duplication of integrated virus and flanking cellular DNA is a common rearrangement of host chromosomal DNA found in human HCC. Such structures suggest that an initial simple integration was amplified, and then two copies underwent head-to-tail recombination. Head-to-tail repeats of integrated viral DNA have also been described.[74] In all such integrated-viral-DNA rearrangements, the viral cohesive end region is commonly found at virus–cell and virus–virus junctions. Fifth, amplification of a region of chromosomal DNA at the site of integrated HBV DNA has been described.[82] Sixth, alterations in host chromosomal DNA have also been detected in HCC without virus integration or at host DNA sites a great distance from a viral integration. These alterations include allelic deletions and point mutations. The alterations are not topographically near viral integrations; therefore, it seems unlikely that hepadnavirus integration could play a direct role in their occurrence.

Thus, HBV can act as a sequence-nonspecific, host-DNA insertional mutagen and cause secondary rearrangements of host chromosomal DNA. HCCs, however, frequently appear to contain chromosomal DNA alterations (e.g., point mutations and allelic deletions) with no apparent relationship to hepadnavirus integrations.

THE RISK OF HCC IN CHRONIC HEPADNAVIRUS INFECTION

The strongest evidence that chronic hepadnavirus infection plays an important role in development of HCC is the epidemiological association in all of the well-studied hepadnavirus–host systems.

Geographic Correlation of HBV Infection and HCC

Geographic correlation of the relative frequencies of HBV infection and HCC in human populations has been shown.[4] There is an uneven geographic distribution of HCC in the world[4] because the most important risk factors for HCC are unevenly distributed. Although HCC is rare in most parts of the world, it occurs commonly in populations in sub-Saharan Africa, southeast and eastern Asia, the Arctic, Oceania, Greece, and Italy. Geographic areas with the highest incidence of HCC are also areas where HBV infection is common and where persistent HBV infections occur at the highest known frequencies. Unusual exceptions to this close correspondence in high HCC regions[83] suggest the possibility of important additional factors, such as dietary aflatoxin, in these populations. In certain areas of Asia and Africa, where the prevalence of chronic HBV infection is the highest, HCC is the most common cancer in males. The incidence of HCC is much lower in the United States and western Europe, where HBV infections are much less common. In these regions, more important risk factors for HCC are alcoholic liver disease and, probably, chronic hepatitis C (see Chapter 10).

High Incidence of HCC in Hepadnavirus-Infected Hosts

The incidence of HCC has been shown to be much higher in hepadnavirus-infected than in uninfected humans,[4,5] woodchucks,[12,84,85] and ground squirrels.[16,86]

Studies in Humans

In humans, the association between HBV and HCC is found both in populations with high and in those with low prevalence of HBV infection.[4] A prospective study of more than 22,000 male government workers in Taiwan has demonstrated that the incidence of HCC is more than 100-fold higher in HBsAg-positive than in HBsAg-negative individuals.[5,87] Prospective studies in Japan,[7,88] China,[89] and Alaska (natives)[90] have indicated 30- to 100-fold higher risks of HCC among HBsAg carriers. The few cases of HCC in HBsAg-negative patients in the Taiwanese study[5,87] had serum anti-HBc, indicating past HBV infection. Together, these studies document that HBV infection precedes the development of HCC and that increasing duration of infection magnifies the risk. Most HBV infections in this population occurred early in life and had continued for 30 years or more before development of HCC. Few cases of HCC occur in children. HCC incidence in HBsAg carriers in high-risk populations rises steeply after age 40 years. Furthermore, cirrhosis in HBsAg carriers increases the risk of HCC by more than 10-fold compared with noncirrhotic HBV carriers.[4,5,87] Up to 90% of HCC patients have coexisting cirrhosis.[5,87] The risk of HCC is significantly higher in male than in female carriers,[4,87] and this sex difference is greatest in the presence of cirrhosis.

Animal Models

The association of HCC with hepadnavirus infection is even stronger in animal models than in humans. One-hundred percent of both wild-caught WHV-infected and colony-born experimentally-infected woodchucks died of HCC within 3 years; no HCC developed in animals that had never been infected.[84,85] The animals with HCC had active hepatitis with significant components of inflammation and regeneration, but cirrhosis was not observed.[15] In a colony of captive ground squirrels infected with GSHV in the wild, no HCC was seen before 4.5 years; by 7 years, however, more than two thirds of the infected animals had died of HCC.

Table 9.2. Three mammalian hosts in which chronic hepadnavirus infection is associated with hepatocellular carcinoma

Host (age at infection)	Time after infection to first HCC	HCC incidence in infected host	References
Woodchuck (birth)	< 1 year	100% at 2 years	84, 85
Beechey ground squirrel (birth)	4.5 years	67% at 6.5 years	86
Human (1/3 at birth, 2/3 in childhood)	30 years[a]	40% lifetime risk[b]	5

[a]HBV-associated HCCs infrequently occur before age 30 years.
[b]Data on lifetime risk are from Chinese males; risk may differ in other racial/ethnic groups and in women.

No HCC was observed in animals without serologic evidence of current or past infection.[16,86] Like woodchucks, infected ground squirrels had significant hepatitis but no cirrhosis. The absence of cirrhosis in these animals may be related to an intrinsic difference in the response to chronic liver injury in rodents and primates. In contrast to observations in humans, the prevalence of the carrier state and the incidence of HCC in these models appears to be the same for males and females. In both the woodchuck and ground squirrel colonies, HCC developed in a few serum viral surface antigen negative, anti-core/anti-surface positive animals (evidence of past infection) but in no animals without any serum viral marker.

These studies indicate that chronic hepadnavirus infection alone, without a recognizable cofactor, can result in HCC. This process appears to be most rapid and efficient in WHV-infected woodchucks (Table 9.2). The risk of developing HCC is significantly higher among mammals with evidence of chronic hepadnavirus infection (serum viral surface-antigen positive) than among those with past infection; past infection, in turn, imparts significantly greater risk for HCC than no hepadnavirus infection at all.

The association of DHBV infection and HCC in ducks is less well established. DHBV was first found in small brown domestic ducks with HCC by Summers and colleagues in Qidong county, China (personal communication), where HCC is common both in ducks[91] and in humans.[83] In addition, there appears to be a high content of aflatoxin in many human and animal foods in that region—a factor that complicates the assessment of the role of hepadnaviruses in HCC. No careful study correlating virus infection with HCC has been reported in this location, however, and HCC occurs in ducks without evidence of DHBV infection. Infected brown ducks (and no uninfected animals) from this region of China, followed prospectively in Japan, were noted to develop HCC.[92] On the other hand, in the United States, white Peking ducks infected with DHBV (found in most commercial flocks) have not been observed to develop HCC. Whether this apparent difference is related to a critical difference in virulence of Chinese and U.S. DHBV strains or in susceptibility of different hosts (e.g., Chinese brown versus Peking ducks) or to other nonviral factors is not clear.

The apparent differences in incidence and time of onset of HCC in the different hepadnavirus–mammalian host systems are summarized in Table 9.2. Such differences could be due to differences in viral virulence or in host susceptibility factors that determine the development of HCC. As will be described later, different genetic changes have been found in HCCs of the three different species, raising the possibility that different mechanisms of hepatocarcinogenesis in the different hepadnavirus–host systems could account for the differences in incubation period and incidence of HCC. The ability to infect woodchucks with GSHV has permitted the demonstration that woodchucks chronically infected with GSHV develop HCC an average of 18 months later than do woodchucks chronically infected with WHV.[93] Furthermore, a recent study showed different genetic changes in HCC arising during chronic infection with each of the two viruses in the woodchuck.[94] These findings indicate that there are important differences in the oncogenic effects of the two viruses within the same animal host.

HEPADNAVIRUSES IN CIRRHOTIC LIVER AND HCC

In approximately 85% of HCC, hepadnavirus DNA has been detected, most often integrated into the host genome and only rarely in episomal forms. In the remaining 15% of surface antigen carrier humans, woodchucks, and ground squirrels, hepadnavrius DNA is not found.[63,64] Thus, persistence of viral DNA in tumor cells, as detected by Southern blot analysis, does not appear to be essential for the development of HCC in hepadnavirus-infected livers.

In humans, 60% to 90% of patients with HCC have underlying cirrhosis.[63,64] In such cirrhotic livers, HCCs arise in adenomatous foci that form within regenerative nodules of liver cells. Examination of individual cirrhotic nodules of a few HBV-infected cirrhotic livers revealed that the DNA of most cirrhotic nodules contained integrated virus.[95] Other nodules contained a clonal pattern of one or more viral DNA integrations (i.e., viral integrations in the same cellular DNA sites in many cells of the nodule). Such nodules were undoubtedly formed by proliferation and clonal expansion of an original hepatocyte that contained one or more viral integrations. In these nodules, integration events may have imparted a growth advantage to the original cell containing the integrants, and this advantage resulted in clonal expansion of that cell. Other nodules contained a nonclonal pattern of viral integration (many integrations at different cellular DNA sites).[95] Thus, the state of HBV DNA was not the same in all regenerative nodules of these HBV-infected cirrhotic livers.

Most HCC that contain HBV DNA in a clonal integration pattern have multiple viral integrants and only a few have single integrants.[63,64,73,74] In contrast, in most HBV-infected cirrhotic livers, only a small minority of regenerative nodules contain multiple clonal integrants.[95] This discrepancy suggests that HCCs arise preferentially (but not exclusively) from cells of cirrhotic nodules with multiple HBV integrations and, therefore, that the viral integrations could play a role in development of HCC. However, as described later, the role played by viral integrations in development of HCC remains unclear in most cases. The fact that each HBV integration studied has been found at a different cellular DNA site and on any of several different chromosomes in different human tumors appears to rule out a viral-integration-site–specific mechanism for most human HCCs.

Multiple tumors in the same liver usually have the same clonal integration pattern in each tumor nodule, indicating that they are metastases arising from the same original tumor. Occasionally, however, integration sites can be different in different HCC tumors within the same liver.[95] This pattern demonstrates that HCC can be multicentric in origin in cirrhotic liver.

Immunofluorescent and immunoperoxidase staining of HCC tissue has demonstrated that, in patients with HBsAg in the blood and with HBsAg or HBcAg in nontumorous tissue, tumor cells appear most often to be negative for these antigens. Other studies have reported small numbers of HBsAg-positive cells in tumors[96]; HBcAg has been detected even more rarely. Thus, few tumor cells appear to express either viral gene product in amounts that can be detected by IFA staining, and cells within the same tumor do not uniformly express these antigens. These findings, as well as the failure to detect episomal forms of viral DNA, support the concept that HCC cells are nonpermissive for expression of these viral structural genes and for virus replication.

GENETIC ALTERATIONS IN HEPADNAVIRUS-ASSOCIATED HCCS OF HUMANS, BEECHEY GROUND SQUIRRELS, AND WOODCHUCKS

Four different potentially oncogenic genetic alterations have been detected at significant frequencies (e.g., greater than 25%) in HCCs of at least one of the three mammalian species in which hepadnavirus-associated HCCs occur (humans, woodchucks, or Beechey ground squirrels). Each of the genetic changes has been investigated in HCC of all three species. With each host, a different one of the four genetic alterations has been found. Two of the genetic alterations result from a specific viral effect; and the other two appear to be unrelated to a specific viral mechanism.

A genetic change that is found at a high frequency in HCC and is clonally present in all cells of the tumor (indicating an early event that occurred in a single cell from which the tumor arose) suggests the possibility that the genetic change plays a causal or initiating role in oncogenesis. However, it is often difficult to exclude the possibility that such a change is an incidental event not responsible for the neoplastic process or that it represents a commonly occurring secondary genetic change arising during HCC growth and progression.

Viral Insertional Mutagenesis and *Cis*-Activation of Cellular Genes

Viral transcription regulatory elements integrated near a cellular gene have the potential of altering expression (cis-activation) of that gene. WHV integrations appears to function by such a mechanism in approximately 50% of HCC in infected woodchucks. WHV integration in HCCs has been found within or near protooncogenes c-*myc* or N-*myc*, and appears to activate the expression of these genes. Integration of WHV in three woodchuck HCC near the c-*myc* gene and associated with altered c-*myc* expression[81,97–99] and WHV integrations in two N-*myc* genes of woodchuck HCCs[100] have been described in detail. Viral insertion sites were clustered in a short sequence of the third exon of the N-*myc* gene. This location coincides with a preferred retroviral integration site in the murine N-*myc* gene of T-cell lymphomas induced by murine leukemia viruses. Approximately one third of the WHV integrations were upstream and two thirds downstream of a *myc* gene, and interruption of the gene was unusual. Most were associated with increased levels of *myc* transcription, and *myc*–viral fusion transcripts were detected infrequently. Viral enhancer insertion and disruption of normal *myc* transcriptional or posttranscriptional control appeared to be involved in many of the *myc* activations. One third of the integrations have been found near c-*myc* and two thirds near N-*myc*. A study[94] comparing HCC in woodchucks infected with WHV and with GSHV revealed evidence for WHV integration near the N-*myc* gene in 7 of 17 woodchuck HCCs (confirming the previous findings). In contrast, in GSHV-infected woodchucks, evidence for GSHV integration near N-*myc* was found in only 1 of 16 HCCs, suggesting that viral integration at this site is more common for WHV than for GSHV in HCC of woodchucks infected with the different respective viruses.

Thus, activation of c-*myc* and N-*myc* expression in woodchuck HCC by WHV-insertional mutagenesis appears to occur at a much greater frequency than would be expected by chance if viral integrations were to occur in random cellular DNA sites. Such integrations may, therefore, contribute mechanistically to a significant fraction (~50%) of woodchuck HCC. Viral integrations in the other 50% of HCC of WHV-infected woodchucks are apparently not near or within cellular genes, and thus cannot be implicated in cis-activation or mutation of cellular genes.

Viral insertional mutagenesis involving N-*myc* and c-*myc* genes has not been found in HCCs of hepadnavirus-infected humans or Beechey ground squirrels (none in 14 ground-squirrel HCC [101]). In human HCCs, there are very few documented examples of HBV integrations within or near any known cellular gene despite study of well over 100 integrations by several laboratories. Rare exceptions include a single integration in a human HCC that was identified to be fused in frame with the retinoic acid receptor β gene.[102] The tumor tissue was not available for studies to assess the level of expression of this cellular gene, and it is not known whether the integration and the alteration of this gene played any role in the neoplastic change in this HCC. A second HBV integration was reported in an intron of the cyclin A gene.[103] A functional effect on the cyclin A gene was not shown, however, so the significance of this integration for tumorigenesis is unknown. Systematic searches for viral integrations near or within cellular protooncogenes in HCC of humans have yielded negative results.[104] Moreover, when individual integrations have been cloned and analyzed, the results have been unlightening.[63,64,73,74]

These findings suggest that the kind of viral-insertional mutagenesis and viral-promoter/enhancer cis-activation of cellular genes observed for WHV integrations in woodchuck HCC are unusual mechanisms for HBV in human HCC and for GSHV in ground squirrel HCC. However, other oncogenic mechanisms must be considered for HBV integrations in human HCC. HBV integrations are often found in repetitive human genomic sequences including minisatellite DNA,[63,64] which consists of repeating units of 10 to 100 base pairs.[105] Minisatellites are associated frequently with cellular genes and gene clusters within chromosomes.[106] They have been shown to be capable of activating and repressing transcription[107,108] and to bind transcription regulatory proteins.[108,109] Certain mutations in minisatellite DNA appear to cause disease, and some are associated with specific cancers.[110] It is important to investigate HBV integrants in repetitive cellular DNA to determine whether the mutations caused by such integrants alter normal regulation by the repetitive sequence of nearby cellular genes in a way that exerts an oncogenic effect.

Viral Transactivation of Cellular Genes in HCC–The X Gene

Mammalian hepadnaviruses, like certain retroviruses and larger DNA viruses, contain a regulatory gene that can function as a transcriptional transactivator. This smallest gene of mammalian hepadnaviruses is called the X gene because its precise role in virus infection is not known. The HBV X gene is expressed in the liver of HBV-infected patients and apparently in a significant number of HCCs with integrated HBV DNA.[63,64] The X protein, when expressed in hepatocytes in culture, can transactivate transcription by a number of unrelated *cis*-acting DNA elements that normally regulate transcription of various cellular and viral genes. These include the enhancer I of HBV; the KB sequence, which binds and is activated by the transcription factor NFkB (known to be involved in regulation of the immunoglobulin kB chain gene, the β-interferon gene, HIV-1, SV40, and several other viral and cellular genes); the c-*myc* gene promoter; the Rous sarcoma virus LTR binding sites for AP1 (fos/jun) and AP2 transcription factors; SV40 enhancer; and others.[63,64] Genes activated by the X protein when expressed in cells include: β-interferon, HIV class I major histocompatibility complex gene, c-*myc*, and c-*jun*.[63,64] The variety of different X protein–responsive transcription-regulatory elements, the failure of the X protein to bind any DNA sequence directly, and the cell specificity of the X-transactivation effect[111] suggest that the transactivation mechanism does not involve a direct sequence-specific interaction with DNA. Instead, it may be mediated through an effect on cellular transcription factors.

There has been much recent interest in whether transactivation of cellular genes by the hepadnavirus X gene could play a role in HCC. In HCC, the X gene can be expressed by episomal or replicating forms of HBV-DNA (found infrequently in HCC) and by integrated HBV- DNA, the form of viral DNA more commonly found in HCC. Because HBV integrations occur frequently at the position of the cohesive ends of the viral DNA, the X gene is often interrupted and truncated, most often as integration pattern II with a short truncation at the 3' end of the gene. However, X-gene transcripts appear to be expressed by some such integrants, and some appear to be in the form of truncated X gene–cell gene-fusion transcripts, which contain a large 5' portion of the X gene and retain the X-gene-transactivating function.[112] The specific X-gene sequences required for the transactivation function have not been established, but clearly removal of five carboxyl-terminal amino acids does not abolish this activity.[112] Approximately one third of HBV integrations contain an intact X-gene and are, therefore, candidates for X-gene expression. The specific percentage of HCC that express the X-protein in a form with transcriptional transactivating activity is not known, but it is undoubtedly less than 50% and perhaps much less. Thus, if HBV X-gene expression plays a role in any HCC, it must do so in only a small fraction of tumors.

Several experimental observations are consistent with the possibility that the X gene has oncogenic properties.[63,64] First, X-gene expression in some cell lines has been reported to activate transcription of certain cellular protooncogenes such as c-*myc* [113] and c-*jun*.[114] Second, X-gene expression in partially transformed cells such as—NIH 3T3[113,115] or a mouse hepatocyte line (FMH 202) expressing SV 40 T antigen[116]—resulted in altered cell growth and rendered the cells able to grow into colonies in soft agar and to form tumors in nude mice. X gene does not so transform primary hepatocytes in cell culture. Third, in one study,[117] transgenic mice with liver-and testis-specific expression of the X gene under control of the HBV enhancer and X promoter developed multifocal areas of altered hepatocyte morphology, followed by adenomas and finally HCC between 9 and 21 months of age (earlier in males than in females). In other studies, transgenic mice containing the X gene under control of other transcription regulatory elements were not shown to express X or expressed X during the first 4 weeks of life only. In no case was HCC observed.

These findings suggest the possibility that in some cases, continuous expression of the hepadnavirus X gene in hepatocytes can transactivate cellular genes that play a role in development of hepadnavirus-associated HCC. However, the X gene does not appear to have the properties usually associated with viral oncogenes—such as rapid transformation of primary cells in which the X gene is expressed or rapid tumor formation in vivo. X-gene expression in primary cultured hepatocytes does not lead to rapid neoplastic transformation. Hepadnaviruses appear to infect and replicate (including expression of the X gene) in many hepatocytes for prolonged periods (months or years) without apparent cell transformation or HCC formation. The extended period (9 to 21 months) of X gene expression in liver in transgenic mice before the appearance of HCC[117] suggests that other events that require a long period for their appearance (e.g., mutations affecting cellular genes) were necessary for development of HCC in that model. More investigation is required to determine how many HCCs express the X gene, what cellular genes in HCC may be activated by X, and whether such an action of X plays a role in any HCC.

Another HBV gene product that has also been reported to transactivate transcription is a truncated form of the pre-S2/S gene product.[118] The proportion of HCC that express a truncated pre-S/S protein with transcriptional transactivating activity is not known, but published structures of viral integrants suggests that it is small. Thus, such a mechanism is unlikely to play a role in most HCC.

Cellular Oncogene Amplification

In contrast to the insertional mutagenesis mechanism of c-*myc* and N-*myc* activation by WHV, amplification of c-*myc* (without apparent c-*myc* rearrangement or viral integration in c-*myc*) and increased levels of c-*myc* transcription were found in six of 14 HCCs of ground squirrels with active or past GSHV infection, and in one HCC of a single animal without evidence of active or prior GSHV infection.[101] Amplification of c-*myc* was not found in HCCs of three animals treated with aflatoxin B_1. Only two of the six HCCs with c-*myc* amplification had GSHV integrations detected by Southern blotting; neither of these integrations was near or within the c-*myc* gene. The mechanism of c-*myc* amplification in ground squirrel HCC is not clear. It does not, however, appear to depend on GSHV integration in the tumor, or even on GSHV active or past infection of the host. Amplification of the c-*myc* gene was not found in woodchuck HCC[101] and appears to be rare in human HCC.[119] These results indicate that c-*myc* activation can be demonstrated in a significant fraction of both woodchuck and ground-squirrel HCCs, but it occurs by different mechanisms in the two hosts. Only in the woodchuck is a direct viral mechanism (insertional mutagenesis) apparent. N-*myc* activation, which appears to be common in woodchuck HCC by WHV insertional mutagenesis, may not occur (or may occur less frequently) in ground squirrel HCC.

Increased levels of c-*myc* transcripts and c-*myc* (but not N-*myc*) gene product in some cells have been reported in human HCCs.[63,64] The mechanism and significance of this apparent activation are unknown. Enhanced c-*myc* expression in HCC appears to be independent of the presence of HBV in the tumor, and HBV integration within or near *myc* genes has not been reported. Enhanced c-*myc* expression is not specific for HCC; it has also been observed in cirrhotic liver and regenerating liver. It is unlikely that altered expression of c-*myc* or N-*myc* alone by any mechanism could result in oncogenic transformation of liver cells and HCC formation; additional events, such as altered expression or function of one or more additional cellular genes, might be required for development of HCC.

Tumor Suppressor Genes

The most common genetic alterations found in human cancers are mutations in, or allelic deletion of, the tumor suppressor gene *p53*.[120,121] Recent evidence indicates that such alterations are also common in human HCC. The *p53* gene is on human chromosome 17p13. Loss of one allele of the *p53* gene has been found in 30% to 60% of HCC in different studies.[63,64] Although the HBV status of the patients from whom these HCCs were obtained was not reported, many were undoubtedly infected. Deletions and rearrangements of the *p53* gene have also been reported in some HCC cell lines, and altered expression of *p53* was found in cell lines without deletion of the gene. The mechanism for allelic deletions of *p53* in HCC is not known. HBV integrations can be associated with deletions in cellular DNA near the site of integration.[63,64] Two HCCs have been reported with deletions in 17p13 with loss of *p53* and HBV integrations at that site.[80,122] No other deletions at that chromosomal site have been reported to be accompanied by HBV integrations and p53 deletions do not occur more frequently in HCCs with HBV integrations than in those without.

More recently, nucleotide sequencing of p53 exons 5 to 8, which contain highly conserved sequences and in which most of the *p53* mutations have been found in other human tumors,[63,64] has revealed single point mutations in the *p53* gene of HCC.[123,124] In two studies, mutations were found in *p53* in 13 of 26 human HCC examined.[123,124] Although the HBV status of the patients from whom the HCCs were obtained was not reported, many were undoubtedly infected. Remarkably, in eight of 16 HCCs from Qidong Province in China, mutations were found in the third nucleotide of codon 249 (seven G-to-T transversions, and one G-to-C

transversion, all arginine to serine).[123] Among 10 HCCs from southern
Africa, three had G-to-T transversions in the third base of codon 249, one
had a G-to-T transversion in the third base of codon 157, and one had an
8 base-pair deletion resulting in a frame-shift mutation at codon 286.[124] In
more than 50% of other human carcinomas—such as breast, lung, and
colon—mutations in the p53 gene have been found in many different
codons, although they are clustered in four highly conserved regions of
exons 5 through 10.[63,64,120,121] The finding of mutations in the third nucleotide of codon 249 (all resulting in arginine to serine changes) in 11 of
13 HCCs with *p53* mutations appears to represent a "mutation hot spot"
unique to these HCCs (mutations in this codon have been found infrequently in other tumors). This specificity suggests that such mutations
may confer a selective advantage to cells that form HCC.

   Other studies of HCC of unspecified populations have found point mutations in other sites in the *p53* gene, but not in codon 249, or have found
no point mutations[125] in the p53 genes of 10 HCCs.[63,64]

   That HBV plays a direct role in *p53* mutations in HCC seems unlikely.
There is no known mechanism by which HBV might produce point mutations—such as the G-to-T and G-to-C transversions found in the third base
of codon 249—without viral integration near that site. G-to-T transversions can result from aflatoxin B$_1$,[126-128] which has been found in the diets
of people in Qidong and other parts of China,[89] and in those of native
peoples in southern Africa.[129] Aflatoxin has been thought to be a possible
causal factor in HCC in some populations.[89] In addition, G to T and G to
C transversion can result from oxidants such as H$_2$O$_2$,[130,131] which may arise
in the liver during the inflammatory reaction associated with chronic hepatitis. The explanation for the finding of frequent *p53* codon 249 mutations in HCC of some studies[123,124] and not in others[125] is unclear. It has
been suggested[132] that human populations with HCC p53 codon 249 mutations are exposed to aflatoxin B1 or some other carcinogen that can
cause such specific mutations and that populations without such mutations are not exposed: this possibility deserves further investigation.

   No mutations were found in any exon of the *p53* genes of HCC of 11
WHV carrier woodchucks, eight GSHV carrier ground squirrels, and six
ground squirrels with evidence of past GSHV infection.[133] A G-to-T transversion resulting in a change in a cysteine codon to a phenylalanine codon was found in exon 5 in one of six HCCs in aflatoxin B$_1$–treated
ground squirrels. This finding is consistent with—but does not prove—
that the mutation was caused by aflatoxin B$_1$. More work is required to
establish or disprove a role for aflatoxin in *p53* gene mutations of HCC.

   Evidence for the possible role of other tumor suppressor genes in human HCC is the finding of loss of heterozygosity by deletion at several
chromosomal sights in HCC.[63,64] Whether any or all of these deletions result in functional loss that is important in development of HCC awaits
further analysis. It also has not been established that such loss of hetero-

zygosity precedes tumor formation rather than appearing during tumor growth.

Less Common Genetic Changes in HCC

Investigations of human HCC have identified several genetic changes[63,64] that appear to occur much less frequently than the four changes described in the previous sections; thus, they apparently do not represent common or general mechanisms contributing to the pathogenesis of human HCC. These changes include rare chromosomal translocations,[80,81] and mutations in N-*ras*[134] and other genes. Certain cellular genes are expressed at higher levels in hepadnavirus-associated HCC than in adult liver in woodchucks and humans, including c-*myc*, c-*fos*, c-*fms*, H-*ras*, N-*ras*, and insulin-like growth factor II gene.[63,64] This finding may reflect altered gene expression associated with hepatocellular proliferation, rather than being mechanistically related to HCC, for these genes have been shown to be overexpressed in regenerating and cirrhotic liver without HCC. In human HCC, these changes are not specific for HCC containing HBV-DNA, and no viral integrations in or near these genes have been reported. The altered expression of these genes in human HCC does not appear to result from cis-activation by viral promoter/enhancer insertion. Although the X protein has been shown to transactivate expression of at least the c-*myc* gene[131] and the c-*jun* gene,[114] HCCs without HBV integration appear to show the same pattern of cellular protooncogene gene expression as HCC containing HBV-DNA. Thus, transactivation by an HBV gene product apparently is not required to alter expression of these genes in HCC.

Activation of previously unrecognized protooncogenes in some HCCs has been suggested by cell transformation assays. NIH 3T3 cells appeared to be transformed by DNA of a few, but not most, HCCs, suggesting that cellular genes with transforming activity not present in normal liver may have been detected.[63,64] The cellular (HCC) genes involved appeared not to be related to previously recognized oncogenes, and they have not been related to HBV integrations. What role such cellular genes may play in HCC is unclear. It is also unclear whether hepadnavirus infection plays a role in the mutations in such genes. These and other experimental approaches need to be extended to identify one or more common tumorigenic mutations in HCC, and to determine what, if any, role is played by hepadnaviruses.

Some evidence suggests that hepadnaviral integrations may be unstable and can undergo postintegration rearrangement, including deletions involving both viral and cellular sequences.[135,136] It has been suggested that viral sequences could be completely lost or deleted at some such sites of rearranged or mutated cell DNA.[74,137] If oncogenic mutations arose by such a mechanism, the resulting HCC might have no detectable viral integrant (as is the case for approximately 15% of hepadnavirus-associated

HCC) or might have one or more viral integrations away from the site of the critical mutation. Whether or how often this may occur in HCC is unknown.

A CHRONIC LIVER INJURY±RESPONSE MODEL INVOLVING NO HEPADNAVIRUS-SPECIFIC MECHANISMS

Indirect evidence suggests the possibility that most HCCs in hepadnavirus-infected hosts do not arise through one of the direct viral mechanisms reviewed here but instead may be a response to more general effects of persistent viral infection and resulting chronic liver injury (see Chapters 2 and 3). Both the failure to find a specific viral mechanism for most HCC in hepadnavirus-infected hosts (as reviewed here), and the pathologic process (necroinflammatory response to chronic liver injury) common to numerous different risk factors for HCC, raise this possibility.

Evidence pointing to a nonvirus-specific mechanism includes, first, the finding that approximately 15% of HCCs in hepadnavirus-infected hosts do not contain enough viral DNA to be detected by DNA hybridization. If, in fact, these HCCs do not contain viral DNA, then mechanisms requiring the presence of a viral integrant—such as insertional mutagenesis and transcriptional transactivation of cellular genes by viral gene products—cannot be involved in production of the tumors. Of the remaining approximately 85% of HCCs in hepadnavirus-infected hosts, almost all tumors contain integrated viral DNA in a clonal pattern (the same viral sequence integrated at the same cellular DNA site in many, and probably all, cells of the tumor). However, the cellular site of HBV integration is different in each HCC, and the integrations are usually not within or near cellular genes.

Second, important risk factors for HCC—including chronic HBV, chronic hepatitis C (resulting from infection with an RNA virus that does not integrate in cellular DNA and thus is not an insertional mutagen—see Chapter 10), alcoholic liver disease, hemochromatosis, cryptogenic cirrhosis, biliary cirrhosis, autoimmune hepatitis, and certain other metabolic disorders—all lead to common pathologic effects of chronic liver injury, including hepatocellular necrosis, inflammation and liver regeneration (necroinflammatory liver disease). The process continuing for many years commonly leads to cirrhosis.[138] Sixty to 90% of HCCs associated with different risk factors occur in the setting of cirrhosis, and the risk of HCC appears to be related to the severity of the cirrhosis.[139] HCCs appear to arise in adenomatous foci within the regenerative nodules of cirrhotic liver,[138,140] irrespective of which factor initiated the necroinflammatory liver disease. It is possible that this common pathologic process (chronic necroinflammatory liver disease) is carcinogenic, and that the carcinogenesis does not depend specifically on which of the diverse factors initiates the process of liver injury. If this explanation is true, a specific viral mechanism would not be essential for HCC to arise in hepadnavirus-infected hosts.

Third, transgenic mice carrying HBV sequences encoding pre-S+S polypeptide with liver-specific expression of that polypeptide regulated by the albumin promoter suffer accumulation of the viral polypeptide in hepatocytes because secretion of this polypeptide is blocked (see Chapter 2).[141,142] Different strains of such transgenic mice have different levels of pre-S+S polypeptide accumulation and corresponding degrees of liver injury, hepatocyte necrosis, inflammation and liver regeneration. In one study, all animals of lines with severe liver injury developed HCC between 1 and 2 years of age, 50% of those with moderate injury developed HCC, and none of those with little or no liver injury developed HCC.[141] These data would appear to provide an example of chronic hepatocellular injury leading to reactive inflammation, liver regeneration, and HCC. The only clear role of the virus appears to be in providing a mechanism for chronic liver injury, which initiates other events including the inflammatory response and hepatocellular proliferation associated with liver regeneration. If this chronic liver injury model is applicable to human disease, a carcinogenic mechanism must be one of the processes that accompany continuous liver injury, regardless of which factor causes the necroinflammatory liver disease.

CONTROL OF HCC

Although tumorigenic mechanisms leading to HCC and the precise role of HBV in development of most HCC are not clear, the overwhelming epidemiological evidence described here indicates that persistent HBV infection is the most important risk factor for HCC in humans. Therefore, it can be inferred that prevention of new HBV infections may eventually prevent a majority of HCCs. Although measures such as identification of infected individuals and avoidance of the kind of contacts that result in HBV transmission can reduce infection rates to some extent, effective vaccines for HBV are the most important tool for control of this virus. Vaccines consisting of HBsAg particles purified from the plasma of human HBsAg carriers (the first HBV vaccine developed and no longer manufactured in the United States) and HBsAg produced by recombinant DNA methods in yeast or vertebrate cells in culture have proved to be highly immunogenic and provide excellent protection against HBV infection.[143] Remarkably, these vaccines are highly immunogenic in newborn infants in whom many vaccines are poorly immunogenic. Vaccination of the newborn infants of HBsAg-positive mothers within 7 days of birth, with subsequent vaccine doses given 1 and 6 months later, can reduce perinatal infections by 70 to 80%.[144] When, in addition to vaccination, anti-HBsAg immunoglobulin preparations (HBIG) are administered intramuscularly to infants within a few hours after birth, perinatal infection rates can be reduced by 95% or more.[144,145]

In low-HBV-prevalence countries, at a minimum, newborn infants of all HBsAg positive mothers should be given HBIG and HBV vaccine just after birth to prevent HBV infection. All other susceptible (serum HBsAg, anti-HBs, and anti-HBc negative) children and adults with significant risk of HBV exposure (e.g., health-care workers, intravenous drug users, children in households with an HBV carrier, etc.) also should be given HBV vaccine. In the United States, the Centers for Disease Control and Prevention and the American Academy of Pediatrics Advisory Committee on Vaccines have recommended that all infants be vaccinated against HBV as part of the universal childhood vaccination program.[146] This recommendation was made because the strategy of vaccinating only susceptible individuals at high risk for exposure to HBV had little overall effect on the rate of new HBV infections in the United States over more than a decade.[147,148] Using HBV vaccine universally in infants promises to be the most effective way to control and eventually eliminate HBV and thus prevent HCC.[138]

In geographic regions of high HBV prevalence, the goal of universal HBV vaccination of infants is to interrupt the cycle of infection that leads to viral persistence in 5% to 20% of these populations and thereby prevent the sequelae of HBV, including HCC.[138] Unfortunately, only HBV vaccine alone can be used in many such areas, because of the great expense and limited supply of HBIG; thus, HBIG is not available for optimum protection of infants exposed perinatally by HBV-infected mothers. In high-HBV-prevalence populations, it is expected to take several generations to achieve universal vaccination of all newborns because of difficulties in manufacturing sufficient quantities of vaccine at a feasible cost and in delivering vaccine to all who require it. Moreover, because of the enormous number of existing HBV carriers of all ages in these populations—most of whom will remain infected for life—HBV-associated HCCs can be expected to continue to occur for years after new infections in children have been stopped. A reduction in HCC incidence following reduction in HBV carrier rates from vaccination programs will confirm the importance of HBV infections in development of HCC. Indeed, data from a follow-up study of a universal vaccination program in Taiwan already indicate that vaccination may prevent the rare childhood cases of HCC.[188] Thus, HCC is the only cancer in humans for which the most important approach for control today is vaccination.

SUMMARY AND CONCLUSIONS

Prospective studies have shown that the incidence of HCC is more than 100 times higher in patients with chronic HBV infection than in uninfected individuals. The incidence of HCC is even more pronounced in certain hepadnavirus-infected rodents. This and other epidemiological evidence that implicates chronic hepadnavirus infection with the development of HCC is overwhelming. Most HCCs of hepadnavirus-infected hosts contain viral integrations. Potentially oncogenic viral insertional mutagenic events have been found in a significant number of HCC of WHV-infected woodchucks (e.g., viral integrations activating c-*myc* or N-*myc* genes). In contrast, a direct viral oncogenic mechanism has not been proved for any HCCs of HBV-infected humans. All HBV integrations in human HCC studied thus far have been at different chromosomal DNA sites, and few integrants in human HCC have been found within or near any cellular gene. Thus, the common site-specific viral insertional mutagenic mechanism observed for WHV in woodchuck HCC has not been found for HBV-associated human HCC. There must be either direct viral hepatocarcinogenic mechanisms that have not yet been discovered or demonstrated (e.g., mutations of minisatellite or other repetitive cellular sequences that alter gene regulatory functions, or transactivation of cellular genes by a viral gene product—such as the X protein—encoded by integrated or episomal viral DNA in HCC) or mechanisms not specific to hepadnavirus infection that lead to HCC in hepadnavirus-infected hosts.

Among the three best-studied hepadnavirus-infected mammalian species discussed here, an unexpected finding is that different potentially oncogenic genetic changes were found at a significant frequency in each species. *Cis*-activation of N-*myc* or c-*myc* genes by viral integrants has been found frequently in woodchuck HCCs, but not in human or ground squirrel HCCs; c-*myc* gene amplification has been found frequently in ground squirrel HCCs, but not in human or woodchuck HCCs; and *p53* gene mutations or deletions have been found frequently in human HCCs, but not in ground squirrel or woodchuck HCCs. In addtion, when two different viruses infected the same species, different potentially oncogenic effects were observed. Viral integration near N-*myc* and c-*myc* was common in WHV-infected, but not in GSHV-infected, woodchucks; c-*myc* amplification was common in GSHV-infected, but not in WHV-infected, woodchucks. Thus, hepatocarcinogenic mechanisms are not uniform from species to species or from virus to virus.

A second finding of these studies is that each specific potentially oncogenic change found at a high frequency in HCCs of a particular animal species is not present in all HCCs of that species. This observation indicates that different genetic changes may be involved in hepatocarcinogenesis in different HCCs of the same animal species infected with the same hepadnavirus. In fact, genetic changes have not been found in most HCCs, indicating that causal genetic changes remain to be identified. It is plausible that oncogenic changes common to all HCCs in all mammalian hosts will, in due time, be discovered.

Two of the potentially oncogenic genetic changes found at a significant frequency in HCCs of hepadnavirus-infected hosts represent direct virus effects (viral-enhancer insertion and *cis*-activation of c-*myc* and N-*myc* genes, and *trans*-activation of cellular genes by X protein); the other two appear not to be caused by a direct viral mechanism (e.g., *p53* gene mutations and c-*myc* gene amplification). Thus, genetic events not resulting from direct effects of an hepadnavirus may be important in hepatocarcinogenesis in infected hosts. This finding is consistent with the possibility that a nonvirus-specific oncogenic mechanism is associated with chronic hepadnavirus infection (e.g., that associated with chronic necroinflammatory liver disease of any cause). Such a nonvirus-specific mechanism may play an important role in hepatocarcinogenesis in hepadnavirus-infected hosts more often than do more specific viral mechanisms.

A causal or initiating effect in hepatocarcinogenesis of any genetic change found in HCC is difficult to prove and distinguish from a secondary change arising during HCC growth and progression. The possibility of a causal role in development of HCC appears to be the strongest for WHV-enhancer insertion, which results in *cis*-activation of c-*myc* and N-*myc* genes. A causal role is suggested because these integrants are clonal, indicating that the integrant was introduced into a single infected liver cell from which a tumor arose. The common and repeated selection in HCC of these c-*myc*–*myc* integrants further suggests that such integrants (and not those at other sites) exert a growth advantage to cells that contain them. Other potentially oncogenic genetic changes that have been found infrequently in HCC of some animal species (e.g., viral insertional mutagenesis or chromosomal translocations in human HCC) may contribute to pathogenesis of HCC in these specific cases but do not appear to represent common or general mechanisms in that species. In most tumor systems, however, multiple genetic changes are required for full expression of the malignant phenotype.[189–191] Thus, none of the changes found so far in HCC may be sufficient to cause HCC, but one or more may represent contributing events.

The most important approach for controlling HCC is by prevention through elimination or reduction of risk factors. Universal vaccination against HBV of infants or young children should greatly reduce HBV infections and thus eliminate the most important risk factor for HCC.

REFERENCES

1. Gross L. Oncogenic Viruses. Third ed. New York: Pergamon Press; 1983.
2. Bishop JM. Molecular themes in oncogenesis. Cell 1991;64:235–248.
3. Sherlock, S, Fox, RA, Niazi SP, Scheuer PJ. Chronic liver diseaseand primary liver-cell cancer with hepatitis-associated (Australia) antigen in serum. Lancet 1970;1:1243–1247.
4. Szmuness W. Hepatocellular carcinoma and the hepatitis B virus: evidence for a causal association. Prog Med Virol 1978;24:40–69.
5. Beasley RP, Lin CC, Hwang LY, et al. Hepatocellular carcinoma and hepatitis B virus: a prospective study of 22,707 men in Taiwan. Lancet 1981;2:1129–1133.

6. Liaw YF, Lai DI, Chu CM, Chen TJ. The development of cirrhosis in patients with chronic type B hepatitis: a prospective study. Hepatology 1988;8:493–496.

7. Obata H, Hayashi N, Motoike Y. A prospective study of development of hepatocellular carcinoma from liver cirrhosis with persistent hepatitis B virus infection. Int J Cancer 1980;25:741.

8. Alward WL, McMahon BJ, Hall DB, Heyward WL, Francis DP, Bender TR. The long-term serologic course of asymptomatic hepatitis B virus carriers and the development of primary hepatocellular carcinoma. J Infect Dis 1985;151:604–609.

9. Robinson WS. Genetic variation among hepatitis B and related viruses. Ann NY Acad Sci. 1980;354:371–378.

10. Robinson WS, Marion PL, Feitelson M, Siddiqui A. The hepadnavirus group: hepatitis B and related viruses. In: Szmuness W, Alter JH, JE Maynard, Eds. Viral Hepatitis. Philadelphia: Franklin Institute Press; 1982:57–68.

11. Gust ID, Burrell CJ, Couplis AG, Robinson WS, Zuckerman AJ. Taxonomic classification of human hepatitis B virus. Intervirology 1986;25:14–29.

12. Summers J, Smolec JM, Snyder R. A virus similar to human hepatitis B virus associated with hepatitis and hepatoma in woodchucks. Proc Natl Acad Sci USA 1978;75:4533–4537.

13. Mason WS, Seal G, Summers J. Virus of Pekin ducks with structural and biological relatedness to human hepatitis B virus. J Virol 1980;36:829–836.

14. Popper H, Roth L, Purcell RH, Tennant BC, Gerin JL. Hepatocarcinogenicity of the woodchuck hepatitis virus. Proc Natl Acad Sci USA 1987;84:866–870.

15. Popper H, Shih JW, Gerin JL, Wong DC, Hoyer BH, London WT, Sly DL, Purcell RH. Woodchuck hepatitis and hepatocellular carcinoma: correlation of histologic with virologic observations. Hepatology 1981;1:91–98.

16. Marion PL, Van Davelaar MJ, Knight SS, Salazar FH, Garcia G, Popper H, Robinson WS. Hepatocellular carcinoma in ground squirrels persistently infected with ground squirrel hepatitis virus. Proc Natl Acad Sci USA 1983;83:4543–4546.

17. Brechot C, Pourcel C, Louise A, Rain B, Tiollais P. Presence of integrated hepatitis B virus DNA sequences in cellular DNA of human hepatocellular carcinoma. Nature (London)1980; 286:533–535.

18. Koshy R, Maupas P, Muller R, Hofschneider PH. Detection of hepatitis B virus-specific DNA in the genomes of human hepatocellular carcinoma and liver cirrhosis tissues. J Gen Virol 1981;57:95–102.

19. Shafritz DA, Shouval D, Sherman H, Hadziyannis S, Kew M. Integration of hepatitis B virus DNA into the genome of liver cells in chronic liver disease and hepatocellular carcinoma. N Engl J Med 1981;305:1067–1073.

20. Hino O, Kitagawa T, Koike K, Kobayashi M, Hara M, Mori W, Nakashima T, Hattori N, Sugano H. Detection of hepatitis B virus DNA in hepatocellular carcinoma in Japan. Hepatology 1984;4:90–95.

21. Miller RH, Lee SC, Liaw YF, Robinson WS. Hepatitis B viral DNA in infected human liver and in hepatocellular carcinoma. J Infect Dis 1985;151:1081–1092.

22. Yokosuka O, Omata M, Zhou YZ, Imazeki F, Okuda K. Duck hepatitis B virus DNA in liver and serum of Chinese ducks: integration of viral DNA in a hepatocellular carcinoma. Proc Natl Acad Sci USA 1985;82:5180–5184.

23. Imazeki F, Yaginuma K, Omata M, Okuda K, Kobayashi M, Koike K. Integrated structures of duck hepatitis B virus DNA in hepatocellular carcinoma. J Virol 1988;62:861–865.
24. Summers J, Smolec JM, Werner BG, et al. Hepatitis B virus and woodchuck hepatitis virus are members of a novel class of DNA viruses. Viruses in Naturally Occurring Tumors, Cold Spring Harbor Conference on Cell Proliferation VII. New York: Cold Spring Harbor Press, 1980;459–470.
25. Ogston CW, Jonak GJ, Rogler CE, Astrin SM, Summers J. Cloning and structural analysis of integrated woodchuck hepatitis virus sequences from hepatocellular carcinomas of woodchucks. Cell 1982;29:385–394.
26. World Health Organization. Prevention of liver cancer. WHO Technical Rep Ser 1988;691:8–9.
27. Lee FI. Cirrhosis and hepatoma in alcoholics. Gut 1966;7:77.
28. Omata M, Aschavai M, Liew CT, et al. Hepatocellular carcinoma in the U.S.A. Etiologic considerations. Gastroenterology 1979;76:280.
29. Resnick RH, Stone K, Antonioli D. Primary hepatocellular carcinoma following non-A,non-B posttransfusion hepatitis. Dig Dis Sci 1983;28:908–911.
30. Kiyosawa K, Akahane Y, Nagata A, Furuta S. Hepatocellular carcinoma after non-A, non-B posttransfusion hepatitis. Am J Gastroenterol 1984;79:777–781.
31. Gilliam JH, Geisinger KR, Richter JE. Primary hepatocellular carcinoma after chronic non-A, non-B post-transfusion hepatitis. Ann Intern Med 1984;101:794–795.
32. Dienstag JL, Alter HJ. Non-A, non-B hepatitis: evolving epidemiologic and clinical perspective. Semin Liver Dis 1986;6:67–81.
33. Lefkowitch JH, Apfelbaum TF. Liver cell dysplasia and hepatocellular carcinoma in non-A, non-B hepatitis. Arch Pathol Lab Med 1987;111:170–173.
34. Fevery J, De Groote J, Desmet V, Van Steenbergen W, Verhamme M, Delanote C, Desmyter J. Long-term follow-up of mild chronic active hepatitis. Acta Gastroenterol Belg 1987;50:341–52.
35. Villa E, Baldini GM, Pasquinelli C, Melegari M, Cariani E, Di Chirico G, Manenti F. Risk factors for hepatocellular carcinoma in Italy: male sex, hepatitis B virus, non-A, non-B infection, and alcohol. Cancer 1988;62:611–615.
36. Sakamoto M, Hirohashi S, Tsuda H, Ino Y, Shimosato Y, Yamasaki S, Makuuchi M, Hasegawa H, Terada M, Hosoda Y. Increasing incidence of hepatocellular carcinoma possibly associated with non-A, non-B hepatitis in Japan, disclosed by hepatitis B virus DNA analysis of surgically resected cases. Cancer Res 1988;15;48:7294–7297.
37. Bomford A, Williams R. Long term results of venesection therapy in idiopathic hemochromatosis. Quart J Med 1977;45:617–614.
38. Midler MS, et al. Idiopathic hemochromatosis, an interim report. Medicine 1980;59:34–41.
39. Eriksson S, Hagerstrand I. Cirrhosis and malignant hepatoma in alpha-1–antitrypsin deficiency. Acta Med Scand 1974;195:451–459.
40. Edmondon HA, Craig JR. Neoplasms of the liver. In Diseases of the Liver ed Schiff, L., and Schiff, E.R., J.B. Lippincott Co., Phila. Penn. Sixth Ed., p. 1109–1158.
41. Nakanuma Y, Terada T, Doishita K, Miwa A. Hepatocellular carcinoma in primary biliary cirrhosis: an autopsy study. Hepatology 1990;11:1010–1016.
42. Okuda K, MacKay I. Hepatocellular carcinoma. Tech Rep Ser 1982;74:1.

43. Sun TT, Chu YY. Carcinogenesis and prevention strategy of liver cancer in areas of prevalence. J Cell Physiol Supp. 1984;3:39.

44. Autrup H, Seremet T, Wakhisi J, Wasunna A. Aflatoxin exposure measured by urinary excretion of aflatoxin B_1-guanine adduct and hepatitis B virus infection in areas with different liver cancer incidence in Kenya. Cancer Res 1987;47:3430.

45. Johnson FL, Lerner KG, Siegel M, Feagler JR, Majerus PW, Hartmann JR, Thomas ED. Association of androgenic-anabolic steroid therapy with development of hepatocellular carcinoma. Lancet 1972;2:1273.

46. Fischer G, Hartmann H, Droese M, Schauer A, Bock, KW. Histochemical and immunohistochemical detection of putative preneoplastic foci in women after long-term use of oral contraceptives. Virchows Arch 1986;50:321.

47. Shar SR, Kew MC. Oral contraceptives and hepatocellular carcinoma. Cancer 1982;49:407.

48. Kerlin P, Davis GL, McGill DB, Weiland LH, Adson MA, Sheedy PF. Hepatic adenoma and focal nodular hyperplasia: clinical, pathologic, and radiologic features. Gastroenterology 1983;84:994.

49. Yu SH. Drinking Water and Primary Liver Cancer. Beijing: Springer-Verlag, China Academic Publishers; 1989;30–37.

50. Yu SH. Epidemiology of primary liver cancer. In: Tang ZY, ed.Subclinical Hepatocellular Carcinoma. Beijing: China Academic Publishers; pp. 189–211.

51. Yen FS, Shen KN. Epidemiology and early diagnosis of primary liver cancer in China Adv Cancer Res 1986;47:297–329.

52. Marion PL, Oshiro L, Regnery DC, Scullard GH, Robinson WS. A virus in Beechey ground squirrels that is related to hepatitis B virus of man. Proc Natl Acad Sci USA 1980;77:2941–2945.

53. Feitelson M, Millman I, Blumberg R. The hepadnavirus family: animal hepadnaviruses. Proc Natl Acad Sci USA 1986;83:2994–2997.

54. Sprengel R, Kaleta EF, Will H. Isolation and characterization of a hepatitis B virus endemic in herons. J Virol 1988;62:3832–3839.

55. Robinson WS. Hepadnaviridae and their replication. In: Fundamental Virology, 2nd ed. ed. B. Field, D.M. Knipe, New York: Raven Press, pp. 2137–2169.

56. Toh H, Hayashida H, Miyata T. Sequence homology between retroviral reverse transcriptase and putative polymerases of hepatitis B virus and cauliflower mosaic virus. Nature 1983;305:827–829.

57. Miller RH, Robinson WS. Common evolutionary origin of hepatitis B virus and retroviruses. Proc Natl Acad Sci USA 1986;83:2531–2535.

58. Schweitzer IL, Dunn AEF, Peters RL, et al. Viral hepatitis in neonates and infants. Am J Med 1973;55:762.

59. Tong MJ, Thursby M, Rakela J, et al. Studies of the maternal-infant transmission of the viruses which cause acute hepatitis. Gastroenterology 1981;80:999.

60. Redeker AG. Viral hepatitis: clinical aspects. Am J Med Sci 1975;270:9.

61. Hoofnagle JH, Seeff LB, Bales ZB, et al. Serologic responses in hepatitis B. In: Vyas GN, Cohen SN, SchmidR, eds. Viral Hepatitis: A Contemporary Assessment of Etiology, Epidemiology, Pathogenesis and Prevention. Philadelphia: Franklin Institute Press; 1978:219–242.

62. Norman JE, Beebe GW, Hoofnagle J, et al. Mortality follow-up of the 1942 epidemic of hepatitis B in the U.S. army. Hepatology 1993;18:790–797.

63. Robinson WS. The role of hepatitis B virus in the development of primary hepatocellular caracinoma. Part. I. J Gast Hep 1992;7:622–638.

64. Robinson WS. The role of hepatitis B virus in development of primary hepatocellular carcinoma: Part II. J Gast Hep 1993;8:95–106.

65. Summers J, Mason WS. Replication of the genome of a hepatitis B-like virus by reverse transcription of an RNA intermediate. Cell 1982;29:403–415.

66. Seeger C, Ganem D, Varmus HE. Biochemical and genetic evidence for the hepatitis B virus replication strategy. Science 1986;232:477.

67. Will H, Reiser W, Weimer T, Pfaff E, Buscher M, Spreugal R, Catlaneo R, Schaller H. Replication strategy of human hepatitis B virus. J Virol 1987; 61:904–911.

68. Antonucci TK, Rutter WJ. Hepatitis B virus (HBV) promoters are regulated by the HBV enhancer in a tissue-specific manner. J Virol 1989;63:579–583.

69. Romet-Lemonne JL, McLane MF, Elfassi E, et al. Hepatitis B virus infection in cultured human lymphoblastoid cells. Science 1983;221:667–669.

70. Lie-Injo LE, Balasegaram M, Lopez, CG, et al. Hepatitis B virus DNA in liver and white blood cells of patients with hepatoma. DNA 1983;2:301–308.

71. Bouffard P, Lamelin JP, Zoulim F, et al. Different forms of hepatitis B virus DNA and expression of HBV antigens in peripheral blood mononuclear cells in chronic hepatitis B. J Med Virol 1990;31:312–317.

72. Karasawa T, Tsukagoshi S, Yoshimura M, et al. Light microscopic localization of hepatitis B virus antigens in the human pancreas: possibility of multiplication of hepatitis B virus in the human pancreas. Gastroenterology 1981;81: 998–1005.

73. Nagaya T, Nakamura T, Tokino T, Tsurimoto T, Imai M, Mayumi T, Kamino K, Yamamura K, Matsubara K. The mode of hepatitis B virus DNA integration in chromosomes of human hepatocellular carcinoma. Genes Dev 1987;1: 773–782.

74. Matsubara K, Tokina T. Integration of hepatitis B virus DNA and its implications for hepatocarcinogenesis. Mol Biol Med 1990;7:243–260.

75. Shih C, Burke K, Chou MJ, Zeldis JB, Yang CS, Lee CS, Isselbacher KJ, Wands JR, Goodman HM. Tight clustering of human hepatitis B virus integration sites in hepatomas near a triple-stranded region. J Virol 1987;61:3491–3498.

76. Shih CC, Stoye JP, Coffin JM. Highly preferred targets for retrovirus integration. Cell 1988;53(4):531–537.

77. Shaul Y, Garcia PD, Schonberg S, Rutter WJ. Integration of hepatitis B virus DNA in chromosome-specific satellite sequences. J Virol 1986;59:731–734.

78. Ogata N, Tokino T, Kamimura T, Asakura H. A comparison of the molecular structure of integrated hepatitis B virus genomes in hepatocellular carcinoma cells and hepatocytes derived from the same patient. Hepatology 1990;11: 1017–1023.

79. Rogler CE, Sherman M, Su CY, Shafritz DA, Summers J, Shows TB, Henderson A. Deletion in chromosome lip associated with a hepatitis B integration site in hepatocellular carcinoma. Science 1985;230:319–322.

80. Hino O, Shows IB, Rogler CE. Hepatitis B virus integration site in hepatocellular carcinoma at chromosome translocation. Proc Natl Acad Sci USA 1986;83:8338–8342.

81. Moroy T, Marchio A, Etiemble J, Trepo C, Tiollais P, Buendia MA. Rearrangement and enhanced expression of c-myc in hepatocellular carcinoma of hepatitis virus infected woodchucks. Nature 1986;324:276–279.

82. Hatada I, Tokino T, Ochiya T, Matsubara K. Co-amplification of integrated

hepatitis B virus DNA and transforming gene hst-1 in a hepatocellular carcinoma. Oncogene 1988;3:537–540.

83. Delong S. 1982. The relationship of hepatitis B virus infection to hepatoma: pros and cons. Viral Hepatitis, 1981 (eds) w. Szmuness, H.T. Alter, J.E. Maynard, Franklin Institute Press, Philadelphia, pp. 253–259.

84. Gerin JL. Experimental WHV infection of woodchucks: an animal model of hepadnavirus-induced liver cancer. Gastroenterol Jpn 1990; 25 Suppl. 38–42.

85. Korba BE, Wells FV, Baldwin B, Cote PJ, Tennant BC, Popper H, Gerin JL. Hepatocellular carcinoma in woodchuck hepatitis virus-infected woodchucks: presence of viral DNA in tumor tissue from chronic carriers and animals serologically recovered from acute infections. Hepatology 1989;9:461–470.

86. Marion PL, Robinson WS. Unpublished results.

87. Beasley RP. Hepatitis B virus, the major etiology of hepatocellular carcinoma. Cancer 1988;61:1942–1956.

88. Ijima T, Saitoh N, Nobotumo K, Nambu M, Sakuma K. A prospective cohort study of hepatitis B surface antigen carriers in a working population. Gann. 1984;75:571–573.

89. Yeh F, Yu MC, Mo C-C, Luo S, Tong MJ, Henderson BE. Hepatitis B virus, aflatoxins, and hepatocellular carcinoma in southern Guangxi, China. Cancer Res 1989;49:2506–2509.

90. McMahon BJ, Lanier A, Wainwright RB, Kilkenny JJ. Hepatocellular carcinoma in Alaska Eskimos: epidemiology, clinical features and early detection. Prog Liver Dis 1990;9:643–655.

91. Zhou YZ. A virus possibly associated with hepatitis and hepatoma in ducks. Shanghai Medical Journal 1980;3:641–644.

92. Omata M. Liver diseases associated with hepadnavirus infection: a study in duck model. Cancer Detect Prev 1989;14:231–233.

93. Seeger C, Baldwin B, Hornbuckle WE, Yeager AE, Tennant BC, Cote P, Ferrell L, Ganem D, Varmus HE. Woodchuck hepatitis virus is a more efficient oncogenic agent than ground squirrel hepatitis virus in a common host. J Virol 1991;65:1673–1678.

94. Hansen LJ, Tennant BC, Seeger C, Ganem D. Differential activation of myc gene family members in hepatic carcinogenesis by closely related hepatitis B viruses. Mol Cel Biol 1993;13:659–667.

95. Aoki N, Robinson WS. Hepatitis B virus in cirrhotic and hepatocellular carcinoma nodules. Mol Biol Med 1989;6:395–408.

96. Kew MD. Hepatoma and HBV. In: Viral Hepatitis: A Contemporary Assessment of Etiology, Epidemiology, Pathogenesis and Prevention, Vyas GM, SN Cohen and R Schmid (eds.), Philadelphia: Franklin Institute Press; p. 439.

97. Hsu T, Moroy T, Etiemble J, Louise A, Trepo C, Tiollais P, Buendia, MA. Activation of c-myc by woodchuck hepatitis virus insertion in hepatocellular carcinoma. Cell 1988;55:627–635.

98. Etiemble J, Moroy T, Jacquemin E, Tiollais P, Buendia, MA. Fused transcripts of c-myc and a new cellular locus, hcr in a primary liver tumor. Oncogene 1989;4:51–57.

99. Moroy T, Etiemble J, Bougueleret L, Hadchouel M, Tiollais P, Buendia MA. Structure and expression of hcr, a locus rearranged with c-myc in a woodchuck hepatocellular carcinoma. Oncogene 1989;4:59–65.

100. Fourel G, Trepo C, Bouqueleret L, Hemalein B, Pouzetto A, Tiollaise, Buen-

dia, M. Frequent activation of N-myc gene by hepadnavirus insertion in woodchuck liver tumors. Nature 1990;347:294–298.

101. Transy C, Fourel G, Robinson WS, Tiollais P, Marion PL, Buendia, MA. Frequent amplification of c-myc in ground squirrel liver tumors associated with past or ongoing infection with a hepadnavirus. Proc Natl Acad Sci USA 1992;89:3874–3878.

102. Dejean A, Bougueleret L, Grzeschik KH, Tiollais P. Hepatitis B virus DNA integration in a sequence homologous to v-erb-A and steroid receptor genes in a hepatocellular carcinoma. Nature 1986;322:70–72.

103. Wang J, Chenivesse X, Henglein B, Brechot C. Hepatitis B virus integration in a cyclin A gene in a hepatocellular carcinoma. Nature 1990;343:555–557.

104. Fung G-K, Lai CL, Lok A, Todd D, Varmus HE. Analysis of HBV-associated human hepatocellular carcinoma for oncogene expression and structure rearrangement. In: Molecular Biology of Hepatitis B Viruses: Abstracts of papers presented at the 1985 meeting on molecular biology of hepatitis B viruses, May 2–5, 1985, Varmus, H. (ed.), Cold Spring Harbor, NY: Cold Spring Harbor Laboratory; 1985.

105. Jeffreys AJ, Wilson V, Thein SL. Hypervariable 'minisatellite' regions in human DNA. Nature 1985;314:67–73.

106. Dover GA. DNA fingerprints: victims or perpetrators of DNA turnover? Nature. 1989;342:347–348.

107. Takeda J, Ishii S, Seino Y, Imamoto F, Imura H. Negative regulation of human insulin gene expression by the 5'-flanking region in non-pancreatic cells. FEBS Lett 1989;247:41–45.

108. Idem. IGH minisatellite suppression of USF-binding-site-and Eμ-mediated transcriptional activation of the adenovirus major late promoter. Nucleic Acids Res 1993;21:977–985.

109. Trepicchio WL, Krontiris TG. Members of the rel/NF-kB family of transcriptional regulatory factors bind the HRASI minisatellite DNA sequence. Nucleic Acids Res 1992;20:2427–2434.

110. Gusella JF. Elastic DNA elements—boon or blight? New Engl J Med 1993; 329:571–572.

111. Seto E, Zhou D-X, Peterlin BM, Benedictyen TS. Trans-activation by the hepatitis B virus X protein shows cell-type specificity. Virology 1989;173:764–766.

112. Takada S, Koike K. Trans-activation function of a 3' truncated X gene-cell fusion product from integrated hepatitis B virus DNA in chronic hepatitis tissues. Proc Natl Acad Sci USA 1990;87(15):5628–5632.

113. Koike K, Shrakata Y, Yaginuma K, Arii M, Takada S, Nakamura I, Hayashi Y, Kawada M, and Kobayashi M. Oncogenic potential of hepatitis B virus. Mol Biol Med 1989;6:151–160.

114. Twu JS, Lai M-Y, Chen D-H, Robinson WS. Activation of protooncogene C-jun by the x protein of hepatitis B virus. Virology 1993;192:346–350.

115. Robinson WS, Klote L, Aoki N. Hepadnaviruses in cirrhotic liver and hepatocellular carcinoma. J Med Virol 1990;31:18–32.

116. Hohne M, Schaefer S, Seifer M, Feitelson MA, Paul D, Gerlich WH. Malignant transformation of immortalized transgenic hepatocytes after transfection with hepatitis B virus DNA. EMBO J 1990;9:1137–1145.

117. Kim C-M, Koike K, Saito I, Miyamura T, Jay G. HBx gene of hepatitis B virus induces liver cancer in transgenic mice. Nature 1991;351:317–320.

118. Kekule AS, Lauer U, Meyer M, Caselmann WH, Hofschneider PH, Koshy R.

The preS2/S region of integrated hepatitis B virus DNA encodes a transcriptional transactivator. Nature 1990;343:457–61.

119. Trowbridge R, Fagan EA, Davison F, Eddleston ALWF, Williams R, Linskens MHK, Farzaneh F. Viral Hepatitis and Liver Disease, ed. Zuckerman, A.J. (Liss, New York) pp. 764–768.

120. Levine AJ, Momand J, Finlay CA. The p53 tumor suppressor gene. Nature 1991;351:1991;453–456.

121. Hollstein M, Sidranksky D, Vogelstein B, Harris CC. p53 mutations in human cancers. Science 1991;253:49–53.

122. Slagle BL, Zhou Y-Z, Butel JS. Hepatitis B virus integration event in human chromosome 17p near the p53 gene identifies the region of the chromosome commonly deleted in virus-positive hepatocellular carcinomas. Cancer Res 1991;51:49–54.

123. Hsu IC, Metcalf RA, Sun T, Welsh JA, Wang NJ, Harris CC. Mutational hotspot in the p53 gene in human hepatocellular carcinomas. Nature 1991; 350:427–428.

124. Bressac B, Kew M, Wands J, Ozturk M. Selective G to T mutations of p53 gene in hepatocellular carcinoma from southern Africa. Nature 1991;350: 429–431.

125. Hosono S, Lee CS, Chou MJ, Yang CS, Shih CH. Molecular analysis of the p53 alleles in primary hepatocellular carcinomas and cell lines. Oncogene 1991;6:237–243.

126. Foster PL, Eisenstadt E, Miller JH. Base substitution mutations induced by metabolically activated aflatoxin B1. Proc Natl Acad Sci USA 1983;80:2695–2698.

127. McMahon G, Davis EF, Huber LJ, Kim Y, Wogan GN. Characterization of c-Ki-ras and N-ras oncogenes in aflatoxin B1–induced rat liver tumors. Proc Natl Acad Sci USA 1990;87:1104–1108.

128. Sambamurti K, Callahan J, Luo X, Perkins CP, Jacobsen JS, Humayun MZ. Mechanisms of mutagenesis by a bulky DNA lesion at the guanine N7 position. Genetics 1988;120:863–873.

129. Van Rensburg SJ, Cook-Mozaffari P, Van Schalkwyk DJ, Van der Watt JJ, Vincent TJ. Hepatocellular carcinoma and dietary aflatoxin in Mozambique and Transkei. Brit J Cancer 1985;51:713–726.

130. Moraes EC, Kayes SM, Tyrrell RM. Mutagenesis by hydrogen peroxide treatment of mammalian cells: a molecular analysis. Carcinogenesis 1990;11:283–293.

131. Moraes EC, Keyse SM, Pidoux M, Tyrell RM. The spectrum of mutations generated by passage of a hydrogen peroxide damaged shuttle vector plasmid through a mammalian host. Nucleic Acids Res 1989;17:8301–8312.

132. Ozturk M, et al. p53 mutation in hepatocellular carcinoma after aflatoxin exposure. Lancet 1991;338:1356–1359.

133. Rivkina MB, Cullen JM, Robinson WS, Marion PL. State of the p53 gene in hepatocellular carcinomas of ground squirrels and woodchucks with past and ongoing infection with hepadnaviruses. Cancer Research 1994;54:5430–5437.

134. Gu JR. Molecular aspects of human hepatic carcinogenesis. Carcinogenesis. 1988;9:697.

135. Unoura M, Kobayashi K, Fukuoka K, Matsushita F, Motimoto H, Oshima T, Kameko S, Hattori N, Murakami S, Yoshikawa H. Establishment of a cell line from a woodchuck hepatocellular carcinoma. Hepatology 1985;6:1106–1111.

136. Hino O, Nomura K, Ohtahe K, Kitagawa T, Sugano H, Kimura S, Yokoyamo M, Katsuki M. Rearrangement of integrated HBV DNA in descendants of transgenic mice. Proc Jpn Acad Ser B 1986;62:355–358.

137. Wang HP, Rogler CE. Deletions in human chromosome arms 11p and 13q in primary hepatocellular carcinomas. Cytogenet Cell Genet 1988;48:72–78.

138. Peters RL. Pathology of hepatocellular carcinoma. In: Okuda K, Peters RL, eds. Hepatocellular Carcinoma. New York: John Wiley & Sons, 1976;107–168.

139. Leevy CM, Gellene R, Nina M. Primary liver cancer in cirrhosis of the alcoholic. Ann NY Acad Sci 1964;114:1026–1031.

140. Arakawa M, Kage M, Sugihara S, et al. Emergence of malignant lesions within an adenomatous hyperplastic nodule in a cirrhotic liver: observations in five cases. Gastroenterology 1986;91:198–208.

141. Chisari FV, Filippi P, Buras J, McLachlan A, Popper H, Pinkert CA, Palmiter RD, Brinster RL. Structural and pathological effects of synthesis of hepatitis B virus large envelope polypeptide in transgenic mice. Proc Natl Acad Sci USA 1987;84:6909–6913.

142. Chisari FV. New model systems for hepatitis B virus research. Lab Invest 1988;59:155–157.

143. Advisory Committe for Immunization Practices. Recommendations for protection against viral hepatitis. MMWR. 1990;39(RR-2):1–26.

144. Beasley RP, Hwang LY, Lee GC, et al. Prevention of perinatally transmitted hepatatitis B virus infections with hepatitis B virus infections with hepatitis B immune globulin and hepatitis B vaccine. Lancet. 1983;2:1099–1102.

145. Beasley RP, Hwang LY, Lee GC, et al. Prevention of perinatally transmitted hepatitis B virus infections with hepatitis B immunoglobulin and hepatitis B vaccine. Lancet 1983;2:1099.

146. Advisory Committee for Immunization Practices. Hepatitis B virus: A comprehensive strategy for eliminating transmission in the United States through universal childhood vaccination. MMWR 1991;40:(PR-13).

147. Centers for Disease Control and Prevention. Hepatitis Surveillance Report No. 52. Atlanta: US Department of Health and Human Services, Health Service; 1989.

148. Centers for Disease Control and Prevention. Hepatitis Surveillance Report No. 51. Atlanta: U.S. Department of Health and Human Services, Public Health Service; 1987;9–22.

149. Beasley RP. Hepatitis B virus, the major etiology of hepatocellular carcinoma. Cancer 1988;61:1942–1956.

150. Ijima T, Saitoh N, Nobotumo K, Nambu M, Sakuma K. A prospective cohort study of hepatitis B surface antigen carriers in a working population. Gann. 1984;75:571–573.

151. Yeh F, Yu MC, Mo C-C, Luo S, Tong MJ, Henderson BE. Hepatitis B virus, aflatoxins, and hepatocellular carcinoma in southern Guangxi, China. Cancer Res 1989;49:2506–2509.

152. McMahon BJ, Lanier A, Wainwright RB, Kilkenny JJ. Hepatocellular carcinoma in Alaska Eskimos:epidemiology, clinical features and early detection. Prog Liver Dis 1990;9:643–655.

153. Gerin JL. Experimental WHV infection of woodchucks: an animal model of hepadnavirus-induced liver cancer. Gastroenterol Jpn 1990;25 Suppl. 38–42.

154. Leevy CM, Gellene R, Nina M. Primary liver cancer in cirrhosis of the alcoholic. Ann NY Acad Sci 1964;114:1026–1031.

155. Misslbeck NG, Campbell TC. The role of ethanol in the etiology of primary liver cancer. Adv Nutr Res 1985;7:129–153.

156. Bassendine MF. Alcohol a major risk factor for hepatocellular carcinoma? J Hepatol 1986;2:513–519.

157. Zaman SN, Johnson PJ, Williams R. Silent cirrhosis in patients with hepatocellular carcinoma: implications for screening in high-incidence and low-incidence areas. Cancer 1990;65:1607–610.

158. Wang KK, Czaja AJ. Hepatocellular carcinoma in corticosteroid-treated severe autoimmune chronic active hepatitis. Hepatology 1988;8:1679–1683.

159. Thung SN, Bach N, Fasy TM, Jordon D, Schaffner F. Hepatocellular carcinoma associated with autoimmune chronic active hepatitis. Mt Sinai J Med 1990;57:165–168.

160. Kew MC, McKnight A, Hodkinson J, Bukofzer S, Esser JD. The role of membranous obstruction of the inferior vena cava in the etiology of hepatocellular carcinoma in Southern African blacks. Hepatology 1989;9:121–125.

161. Hautekeete ML, Brenard R, Hadengue A, Degott C, Babany G, Arrive L, Lebrec D, Menu Y, Erlinger S, Benhamou JP. Membranous obstruction of the inferior vena cava and hepatocellular carcinoma in a Caribbean patient. J Clin Gastroenterol 1990;12:214–217.

162. Berg NO, Eriksson S. Liver disease in adults with alpha$_1$- antitrypsin deficiency. N Engl J Med 287:1264–1267.

163. Eriksson S, Hagerstrand I. Cirrhosis and malignant hepatoma in α_1-antitrypsin deficiency. Acta Med Scand 1974;195:451–458.

164. Eriksson S, Carlson J, Valez R. Risk of cirrhosis and primary liver cancer in alpha$_1$-antitrypsin deficiency. New Engl J Med 1986;314:736–739.

165. Carlson J, Eriksson S. Chronic cryptogenic liver disease and malignant hepatoma in intermediate alpha 1–antitrypsin deficiency identified by a Pi Z-specific monoclonal antibody. Scand J Gastroenterol 1985;20:835–842.

166. Marwick TH, Cooney PT, Kerlin P. Cirrhosis and hepatocellular carcinoma in a patient with heterozygous (MZ) alpha-1–antitrypsin deficiency. Pathology 1987;17:649–652.

167. Reid CL, Wiener GJ, Cox DW, Richter JE, Geisinger KR. Diffuse hepatocellular dysplasia and carcinoma associated with the Mmalton variant of alpha 1–antitrypsin. Gastroenterology 1987;93:181–187.

168. Guan R, Oon CJ, Wong PK, Foong WC, Wee A. Primary hepatocellular carcinoma associated with Wilson's disease in a young woman. Postgrad Med J 1985;61:357–359.

169. Polio J, Enriquez RE, Chow A, Wood WM, Atterbury CE. Hepatocellular carcinoma in Wilson's Disease: case report and review of the literature. J Clin Gastroenterol 1989;11:220–224.

170. Limmer J, Fleig WE, Leupold D, Bittner R, Ditschuneit H, Beger HG. Hepatocellular carcinoma in type I glycogen storage disease. Hepatology 1988;8:531–537.

171. Shiomi S, Saeki Y, Kim K, Nishiguchi Seki S, Kuroki T, Kobayashi K, Harihara S, Owada M. A female case of type VIII glycogenosis who developed cirrhosis of the liver and hepatocellular tumor. Gastroenterol Jpn 1989;24:711–714.

172. Dehner LP, Snover DC, Sharp HL, Ascher N, Nakhleh R, Day DL. Hereditary tyrosinemia type I (chronic form): pathologic findings in the liver. Hum Pathol 1989;20:149–158.

173. Esquivel CO, Mieles L, Marino IR, Todo S, Makowka L, Ambrosino G, Na-

kazato P, Starzl TE. Liver transplantation for hereditary tyrosinemia in the presence of hepatocellular carcinoma. Transplant Proc 1989;21:2445–2446.

174. Gilbert-Barness E, Barness LA, Meisner LF. Chromosomal instability in hereditary tyrosinemia type I. Pediatr Pathol 1990;10:243–252.

175. Menowski Z, Silver MM, Roberts EA, Superina RA, Phillips MJ. Liver cell dysplasia and early liver transplantation in hereditary tyrosinemia. Mod Pathol 1990;3:694–701.

176. Nakashima T, Sakamoto K, Okuda K. A minute hepatocellular carcinoma found in a liver with clonorchis sinensis infection; report of two cases. Cancer 1977;39:1306–1311.

177. Kim YI. Liver carcinoma and liver fluke infection. Arzneimittelforschung. 1984;34:1121–1126.

178. Choi BI, Kim HJ, Han MC, Do YS, Han MH, Lee SH. CT findings of clonorchiasis. Am J Roentgenol 1989;152:281–284.

179. Kojiro M, Kakizoe S, Yano H, Tsumagari J, Kenmochi K, Nakashima T. Hepatocellular carcinoma and schistosomiasis japonica: a clinicopathologic study of 59 autopsy cases of hepatocellular carcinoma associated with chronic schistosomiasis japonica. Acta Pathol Jpn 1986;36:525–532.

180. Ruymann FB, Mosijczuk AD, Sayers RJ. Hepatoma in a child with methotrexate induced hepatic fibrosis. JAMA 1977;238:2631–2633.

181. Fried M, Kalra J, Ilardi CF, Sawitsky A. Hepatocellular carcinoma in a long-term survivor of acute lymphocytic leukemia. Cancer 1987;60:2548–2552.

182. Vogel CL, Linsell CA. International symposium on hepatocellular carcinoma—Kampala, Uganda (July 1971). J Natl Cancer Inst 1972;48:567–571.

183. Forman D, Vincent TJ, Doll R. Cancer of the liver and the use of oral contraceptives. Br Med J 1986;292:1357–1361.

184. Neuberger J, Forman D, Doll R, Williams R. Oral contraceptives and hepatocellular carcinoma. Br Med J 292:1355–1357.

185. Trichopoulos D, MacMahon B, Sparros L, Merikas G. Smoking and hepatitis B-negative primary hepatocellular carcinoma. J Natl Cancer Inst. 1980;65:111–114.

186. Lam KC, Yu MC, Leung JW, Henderson BE. Hepatitis B virus and cigarette smoking: risk factors for hepatocellular carcinoma in Hong Kong. Cancer Res 1982;42:5246–5248.

187. Yu MC, Henderson BE. Correspondence re: Harland Austin et al. A case-control study of hepatocellular carcinoma and the hepatitis B virus, cigarette smoking, and alcohol consumption. Cancer Res 1982;47:654–655.

188. Chang MH, Chen CJ, Lai MS, et al. Universal hepatitis B vaccination in Taiwan and the incidence of hepatocellular carcinoma in children. Taiwan Childhood Hepatoma Study Group. N Engl J Med 1997;336:1855–1859.

189. Cerutti PA. Response modification creates promotability in multistage carcinogenesis. Carcinogenesis 1988;9:519–526.

190. Vesselinovitch SD, Mihailovich N. Kinetics of diethylnitrosamine hepatocarcinogenesis in the infant mouse. Cancer Res 1983;43:4253.

191. Scherer E. Neoplastic progression in experimental hepatocarcinogenesis. Biochim Biophys Acta 1984;738:219

10
Hepatitis C Virus
and Hepatocellular Carcinoma

RAYMOND T. CHUNG AND T. JAKE LIANG

Hepatitic C virus (HCV) is an important cause of morbidity and mortality worldwide, responsible for a spectrum of liver disease ranging from the asymptomatic carrier state to end-stage liver disease. Compared to other hepatotropic viruses, HCV carries a higher rate of chronicity after infection, with at least 70% of those infected developing chronic liver disease. In addition to chronic liver dysfunction, HCV has also been linked to the development of hepatocellular carcinoma. Between 30% and 70% of patients with hepatitis B virus (HBV)-negative hepatocellular carcinoma (HCC) are seropositive for HCV; in the United States, as many as 40% of all cases of HCC may be associated with HCV. Efforts to control this infection with antiviral agents have been disappointing. The use of interferon-alfa (IFN-α), currently the only agent licensed for primary therapy of HCV infection in the United States, is limited by a high rate of relapse after discontinuation of therapy, with a sustained response rate of only 5% to 25% 1 year after completion of therapy. At the present time, an effective HCV vaccine is not available.

EPIDEMIOLOGY OF HCV INFECTION

HCV infection is present in more than 1% of the U.S. population, creating as many as 4 million carriers, and the estimated number worldwide is equally, if not more, alarming. Because acute HCV infection is typically mild, it is often not diagnosed and may be recognized only in its chronic stages. The full impact of disease may not be apparent for many years. In contrast to HBV (see Chapter 9), as many as 85% of HCV infections appear to become persistent and to lead to chronic liver disease.[1,2] Based on limited testing, there may be as many as 150,000 new acute infections each year in the United States.

Although HCV accounts for most posttransfusion hepatitis, the increased accuracy of tests for HCV infection has largely eliminated blood transfusions as a source of HCV infection in the United States.[3,4] Nevertheless, elimination of posttransfusion HCV infection is unlikely to have a major influence on reducing the overall frequency of this infection, for only 5% of all cases of HCV infection are transfusion-related. Transmission among intravenous-drug users, through sharing of needles, is responsible for about 30% to 40% of identified cases. Health care employment has been identified in about 2% of cases.[5] Heterosexual activity with multiple sexual partners and household contact that includes exposure to a sexual partner or other household member who has hepatitis C may be responsible for about 10% of recognized infections. Maternal–infant transmission has also been documented as a mode of spread.[5] However, these last two modes of transmission are much less important than they are for HBV. In about 40% of HCV cases, no risk factor can be identified. Like persistent HBV infection, HCV infection also results in chronic hepatitis, cirrhosis, and HCC.

HCV INFECTION AND HEPATOCELLULAR CARCINOMA

Ever since the postulated existence of the non-A, non-B hepatitis virus, the responsible viral agent has been suspected to be an etiologic agent of HCC. Not until its identification in 1989 was the role of HCV in the development of HCC accepted. Because there are no convenient animal models or tissue-culture systems in which HCV infection can be studied in detail, the most convincing evidence for the association of HCV with HCC comes from a large body of epidemiological studies. In this section, we summarize the large body of evidence in support of the linkage of HCV infection and HCC development.

Using serologic and molecular assays developed from the cloning of HCV, several studies from various countries in Europe and Asia documented a strong association between anti-HCV seropositivity and HCC.[6] In Japan, anti-HCV antibodies are present in 0.9% to 1.2% of adults. The rate of anti-HCV seropositivity in patients who had non-A, non-B hepatitis–related HCC is 80% to 94%.[7] In one Japanese study, antibodies to HCV were detected in 94.4% of patients with non-A, non-B hepatitis–related HCC, compared with only 35% seropositivity in patients with hepatitis B–related HCC, providing strong evidence of an independent association between HCV and HCC in that population.[7,8] A case-control study from Italy showed that 71% of patients with HCC were anti-HCV positive as determined by enzyme-linked immunosorbent assay (EIA), compared with only 5% of controls.[9] In this study, anti-HCV positivity was a risk factor for HCC, independent of HBV infection, alcohol intake, age, or gender. A study from Spain reported that 63% of 70 patients with HCC had anti-HCV positivity by the second-generation EIA, and 62% of those tested had HCV RNA detected by reverse transcriptase–polymerase chain reaction (RT-PCR).[10] In addition, 54% of these patients had evidence of past or current infection with HBV, and 14% had evidence of coinfection with HBV and HCV. However, coinfection did not appear to result in a more aggressive clinical course than that seen with infection with either virus alone. In this population, HCV is more prevalent than HBV in patients who have HCC. Using both first- and second-generation anti-HCV EIAs, Zavitsanos and colleagues found that the prevalence of antibodies to HCV among 181 Greek patients with HCC was only 13.3%, and suggested that the association of anti-HCV with HCC had been inflated in previous studies that used less specific anti-HCV detection systems.[11] However, the discrepancy between Zavitsanos's study and others may be related less to methodology than to geographic or racial differences. Studies from other regions of Europe also demonstrated a high prevalence of HCV markers in patients who had HCC.[12]

Epidemiological investigations from other parts of the world have resulted in similar findings. A study from Taiwan confirmed a significantly increased risk of HCC with anti-HCV seropositivity, revealing a multivariate adjusted odds ratio of 23.7 for patients positive for anti-HCV antibodies.[13] In this study, there appeared to be a synergistic effect on HCC development for anti-HCV positivity with hepatitis B surface antigen (HBsAg) carrier status, as well as with cigarette smoking and alcohol intake. A recent study from Korea confirmed these findings, identifying anti-HCV antibodies in almost half of all patients with HBsAg-negative HCC. Overall, HBV remained the most important etiologic agent for HCC in this population; of 336 consecutive patients with HCC, 95.8% had serologic evidence of HBV infection. Anti-HCV seropositivity was present in only 17% of all patients with HCC but was documented in 43% of 103 patients with HBsAg-negative HCC. The importance of HCV as a risk factor for HCC was most obvious in older patients (greater than 61 years of age) in whom the prevalence of HBV and HCV infection were roughly equal.[14] In South Africa, 20% to 29% of patients with HCC have been shown to have antibodies to HCV, but HBV remains the major etiologic agent of HCC in that region.[15,16]

The association between chronic HCV infection and HCC is now well established in regions where the incidence of HCC is high, such as in Asia and parts of Africa. In the United States, however, where the incidence of HCC is low, accounting for only 2% of all cancers, this association has been less evident. Nevertheless, linkage between HCV and HCC has been explored recently in several large case-control studies, confirming a significant role for HCV in the development of HCC in the United States.

Two studies, one using the first-generation anti-HCV assay, and the second using a second-generation assay and molecular techniques, have been conducted to assess the prevalence of HCV infection in HBsAg-negative patients with HCC evaluated at the University of Miami Liver Center.[17,18] Over 150 patients with HCC were included in these studies. Of them, 20% to 30% had a history of blood transfusion. Greater than 95% had biopsy-confirmed cirrhosis. No patients had evidence of other risk factors for HCC, including alcohol abuse or autoimmune or metabolic liver disorders. In both studies, greater than 50% of the patients had evidence of HCV infection. Furthermore, many of the patients were seropositive for HBV (anti-HBs or anti-hepatitis B core antigen [HBc]) and harbored low-level HBV detected by PCR. However, a significant proportion of patients (20% to 30%) had no markers of HBV or HCV infection, despite the sensitive assays used in these studies, indicating that a substantial minority of patients with HCC in the United States have no defined viral risk factors. These studies documented a strong association between HCV and HCC, as well as between HCV and so-called cryptogenic cirrhosis.

In another study, Yu and colleagues examined the prevalence of HBV and HCV markers in 51 patients with histologically confirmed HCC who were residents of Los Angeles County, California[19]; 128 subjects from another, unrelated study were included as controls. Anti-HCV (first-generation EIA) positivity was significantly more prevalent in HCC patients than in controls, with a relative risk of 10.5. The presence of HBV markers was also associated with an increased risk of HCC, with a calculated relative risk of 7.0. Overall, a total of 15 (29%) of 51 patients with HCC demonstrated anti-HCV seropositivity, and 22 (43%) of 51 showed evidence of prior infection with HBV. Of the controls, 3.9% were anti-HCV seropositive. Based on these findings, the authors estimated that 47% of HCC occurring in black and white residents of Los Angeles County, California, could be attributed to HCV or HBV infection; 9% were related to HCV alone, 20% to HBV alone, and 18% to coinfection with HCV and HBV. The presence of either marker alone was significantly associated with increased risk of HCC, but a higher risk was observed when both markers were present.

A study from Johns Hopkins, however, provided evidence that HCV plays a lesser role in the development of HCC in some parts of the United States.[20] In this retrospective, case-control study, 99 consecutive HCC patients evaluated at the Johns Hopkins Oncology Center were compared with 98 consecutive adult patients with other malignant tumors evaluated over a 14-month period. A comparison of clinical and serologic features of these two groups revealed several significant differences. Of patients in the HCC group, 7% had HBsAg and 8% had IgM anti-HBc in their serum, indicating the presence of HBV infection, whereas none of the controls had either marker present in their serum. Anti-HCV, as measured by a first-generation radioimmunoassay, was documented in the serum of 13% of the HCC patients, compared to 2% of the controls. The relative risk of HCC in HBsAg-positive patients was 17.3 and that in HCV-positive patients was 7.3. Unlike the previous studies, this study reported a low rate of coinfection with HCV and HBV in the HCC population. These findings were subsequently confirmed by the same group using the more sensitive second-generation RT-PCR assay and PCR.[21] Little demographic information about the two groups was provided, so this difference may reflect an intrinsic bias between the selected populations. Although this study suggests an association between HCV and HCC development, it provided little information with respect to other possible etiologic factors, such as alcohol consumption, metabolic disorders, or environmental toxins.

For several reasons, it is difficult to compare these studies on the role of HCV in the development of HCC within the United States. Because of the heterogeneity of the study populations, it is not possible to determine whether the differences seen across various centers are based on true geographic variations or on selection bias. Several studies failed to consider patients who had other risk factors for HCC, such as alcohol abuse, metabolic liver disease, or occult HBV infection. It is clear that in the United States, there is geographic variation in the prevalence of HCV infection in HBsAg-negative patients with HCC. Much of this variation probably is due to differences in the prevalence of occult HBV infection. In Chicago, where the prevalence of HBV infection is low, the prevalence of HCV in HBsAg-negative patients with HCC is 60%. In New York City, occult HBV infection probably accounts for many HBsAg-negative HCC cases, as the prevalence of HCV infection is only 35%. Similarly, in San Francisco, less than 20% of HBsAg-negative HCC patients have evidence of HCV; many of the remaining 80% are likely to have occult HBV infection.

Another source of confusion in comparing these studies is the use of different methods to document the presence of HCV infection. Most of the early studies relied on the first-generation anti-HCV assay, which is based on antigens from both the core region of HCV (c22–3) and the nonstructural NS-3/NS-4 region (c200). The second-generation EIA and the confirmatory recombinant immunoblot assays (RIBA-II) were further developed and incorporate the c33–C (from NS-3) and c22–3 recombinant antigens as well as the 5-1-1 and c100–3 antigens. Recent studies have documented the superiority of the second-generation assays over the first, showing greater sensitivity without sacrifice of specificity.[22,23].

Although there has been no direct proof linking HCV to development of HCC, the vast body of epidemiological evidence supporting the role of HCV in HCC is irrefutable. Although these studies do not clarify the mechanism of carcinogenesis, it is clear that most, if not all, HCC in the setting of HCV infection is superimposed on a background of established cirrhosis, probably induced by chronic hepatocellular injury and inflammation.

HEPATITIS C VIRUS: THE VIRAL AGENT

Hepatitis C virus (HCV) was cloned in 1989[24,25] from the infectious sera of individuals with posttransfusion hepatitis, and much information about the virus has accumulated since then. Although suitable animal models or tissue culture systems have not yet been identified, studies using genetic and biochemical approaches have yielded substantial insights into the biology of HCV infection.

Genomic Organization and Viral Polypeptides

The single (+)-stranded 9.4 kb RNA genome of HCV contains a single open reading frame that encodes a polyprotein of 3011 amino acids.[26,27] The polyprotein is subsequently posttranslationally processed to yield several mature structural and nonstructural proteins (Figure 10.1, Table 10.1). The overall organization of the HCV polyprotein bears strong resemblance to sequences from the pestivirus and flavivirus families.[28]

In general, the genome is flanked in its 5'-untranslated region by a highly conserved (greater than 98%) 341 nucleotide sequence that appears to play a key role in translational control.[27] The coding region encodes structural proteins in its N-terminal portion that include a nonglycosylated core protein (p22), which associates with genomic RNA to form the nucleocapsid. The C-terminal 20 amino acids of the core protein are highly hydrophobic and may act as a signal sequence for processing of adjacent polypeptides.[29-31]

Immediately downstream of the core are two proteins, E1 and E2/NS1, which correspond to the putative envelope glycoproteins, designated gp33 and gp70, respectively. These latter proteins are extensively N-glycosylated and appear to function as membrane-associated proteins essential for virion assembly. The presence of a hypervariable region (HVR-1) in the N-terminal portion of the E2/NS1 domain to which an active humoral response is directed in infected individuals suggests that this region is subjected to immune selection.[32-34] This region exhibits significant variation not only among HCV isolates but also within infected individuals over the course of time.[35] In addition, the virus has been shown to exist simultaneously as a set of related but immunologically distinct variants, called quasispecies.[36] The existence of quasispecies may offer the virus an effective mechanism for escape from the host immune response (described later).

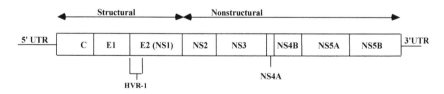

Figure 10.1. Schematic representation of the HCV RNA genome. Structural and nonstructural domains of the long open reading frame are indicated. HVR-1 indicates the hypervariable region.

Table 10.1 Features of HCV-encoded proteins

Protein	Nucleotide position	Name	Function
Core	1–573	p22	Virus nucleocapsid, strong RNA-binding activity. Highly conserved
E1	574–1149	gp33	Integral membrane envelope glycoprotein. Highly variable
E2/NS1	1150–2430	gp70	Membrane-anchored envelope glycoprotein. Highly variable; possesses hypervariable region
NS2	2431–3078	p23	Zinc-dependent autocatalytic metalloproteinase
NS3	3079–4971	p72	N-terminal, serine protease; C-terminal, NTPase/helicase
NS4A	4972–5133	p10	Stabilizes NS3. Cofactor for trans-cleavage of NS4B-NS5A. Modulates hyperphosphorylation of NS5A
NS4B	5134–5916	p27	Unknown
NS5A	5917–7260	p56–p58	Possible regulatory role in replication. Present in phosphorylated and hyperphosphorylated forms. Sequence variations associated with interferon response
NS5B	7261–9033	p66	RNA-dependent RNA polymerase

The nonstructural or C-terminal portion of the HCV polyprotein en-codes proteins with functions generally involved in protein processing and replication of the viral genome. The NS2 region has a high degree of hydrophobicity but its precise function is as yet unknown. Evidence exists that NS2 (p23), in concert with the N-terminal 20 amino acids of NS3, may function as a zinc-dependent metalloproteinase in the *cis*-cleavage of the NS2–NS3 junction.[37]

The NS3 protein, or p72, appears to harbor at least two distinct en-zymatic activities. The N-terminal one third of NS3 contains a trypsinlike serine protease that is essential for the processing of the downstream por-tion of the viral polyprotein. In addition to being needed for *cis* cleavage of the NS3–NS4A junction, NS3 is necessary for *trans* cleavage of the NS4A-NS4B, NS4B-NS5A, and NS5A-NS5B junctions.[38–40] These cleavage sites share common features that are likely to determine the substrate specificity of the NS3 protease. The C-terminal portion of the NS3 protein possesses a domain that bears strong resemblance to, and the enzymatic function of, a nucleoside triphosphate-binding helicase that presump-tively participates in the unwinding of the double-stranded RNA replica-tive intermediate.[41]

The function of NS4, which is cleaved into NS4A and NS4B, is still being elucidated. Both peptides possess strongly immunogenic epitopes and several predicted transmembrane regions. Failla and colleagues dem-onstrated that in addition to NS3, NS4A (p10) must be present to mediate the cleavage at the NS4B/NS5A junction.[42] This finding has been reinforced by the demonstration that the N-terminal portion of NS3 forms a stable complex in vivo with NS4A.[43-45] Further evidence for a functional interaction between NS4A and NS5A has come from recent studies demonstrating that NS4A is required for the hyperphosphorylation of NS5A.[46] These data suggest that in addition to its role as a cofactor for NS3 protease activity, NS4A also acts as a modulator of cellular kinase activity. Little is understood about the function of NS4B (p27).

The NS5 protein is processed into NS5A (p56–58) and NS5B (p66) peptides. The function of NS5A is as yet unknown, but the expressed protein appears to be present in both phosphorylated (p56) and hyperphosphorylated (p58) forms[47,48]; the phosphorylation and hyperphosphorylation occur at serine residues at the C-terminus and midportion of NS5A, respectively. The hyperphosphorylated form of NS5A appears to depend on the presence of NS4A.[46] A retrospective analysis of a cohort of HCV-infected patients from Japan demonstrated an independent association between the presence of multiple substitutions in a 40-amino acid region in NS5A and increased responsiveness to interferon therapy.[49] The finding of lower viral levels among isolates harboring these mutations raises the possibility that NS5A is involved in the control of RNA strand replication. These finding have not been confirmed in studies from Europe, however.[50,51]

The NS5B peptide (p66) appears to play a critical role in RNA strand replication. The viral genome does not replicate through a DNA intermediate form; therefore, it must employ a direct RNA-to-RNA copying mechanism that is encoded virally [an RNA-dependent RNA polymerase (RdRp)], as no such counterpart exists in eukaryotic cells. In fact, sequence analysis of the NS5B protein reveals significant homology with the RdRp domains of pesti- and flaviviruses, including conservation of the presumptive catalytic tripeptide Gly-Asp-Asp motif, which is characteristic of RdRps of all (+)-strand RNA viruses. Preliminary studies have identified an RdRp activity in association with expressed NS5B.[52]

Immediately following the termination codon of the polyprotein is a short 3'-untranslated stretch of nucleotides that is likely to play a critical role in the initiation of new RNA strand synthesis by the HCV replication complex. This stretch has been reported to be variable in size among many groups and to possess a long poly(U) stretch; most recently, it has been demonstrated to possess a highly conserved 98 nucleotide 3'-terminus downstream of the poly(U) tract that forms a hairpin structure.[53,54]

The Viral Life Cycle

The events following entry of the HCV agent into the circulation can be inferred from our understanding of the life cycle of members of the flavivirus and pestivirus families. The virus is likely to enter the hepatocyte via interaction with certain cell-surface molecules (viral receptors). The

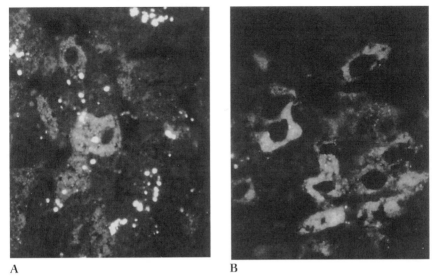

A   B

Figure 10.2. Immunohistochemical staining of HCV-infected liver. Hepatitis C virus antigen staining in the cytoplasm of hepatocytes identified by
FITC-labeled polyclonal IgG anti-HCV Ag (A) Variable intensity of powder-
like and granular fluorescence of HCV Ag in several positive liver cells of
an infected chimpanzee. (B) Liver biopsy specimens from an HCV-
infected patient with prominent deposits of HCV Ag showing a distinct
granular pattern in scattered hepatocytes. (Reprinted with permission
from publisher and Krawczynski et al.[55])

patchy and scanty distribution of infection (Figure 10.2), as determined
by immunohistochemical techniques,[55] suggests that the virus is not particularly efficient in its productive infection of hepatocytes. Following uptake
of the viral particle, the single (+)-stranded genome is released into the
cytoplasm, where it is translated by host cell ribosomes into the viral polyprotein. The polyprotein is subsequently cleaved proteolytically to yield
functional structural and nonstructural proteins. These events are believed to be confined to the host cytoplasm. Together with host proteins
yet to be identified, the nonstructural proteins involved in RNA strand
replication (NS5B and possibly NS5A, NS3) are likely to form a replication complex that initiates new (−) or antigenomic strand synthesis from
the 3'-terminus of the genomic (+) RNA strand. This direct RNA-to-RNA
copying function must be carried out by a virally encoded RdRp. The
antigenomic strand in turn serves as the template for new genomic strand
synthesis. The signals that govern genomic and antigenomic strand synthesis are not yet understood. Once a critical level of structural proteins
has accumulated, a signal yet to be elucidated triggers the association of
the genomic RNA with the core and envelope proteins and the assembly
of the viral particle, which is released by either cell lysis or exocytosis.
    The reliance of HCV on an RdRp to perform RNA-to-RNA copying has

two important implications. First, because of the absence of a DNA intermediate, the integration of HCV genetic sequences into the host chromosomal DNA is not possible, excluding viral integration as a mechanism for HCV-related hepatocarcinogenesis. Second, because the viral RdRp—unlike *DNA*-dependent *RNA* polymerases or *DNA*-dependent *DNA* polymerases—does not possess a proofreading function, a substantial rate of misincorporation can be seen. Researchers have estimated that, on average, between 0.9 and 1.92×10^{-3} base substitutions per genome site per year takes place throughout the genome.[35,56] This mutation rate is likely to be responsible for the rapid emergence of extensive sequence heterogeneity both among isolates and within infected individuals.

HCV Genotypes

The extensive sequence heterogeneity described from viral isolates worldwide has led to the classification of HCV into at least six different genotypes. The most recent classification system is based on sequence alignment of HCV sequences from different regions of the genome, including the 5'-UTR, core, NS3, and NS5 (57–60). The generation of a phylogenetic tree has led to classification of HCV isolates into types and subtypes (Figure 10.3).[59,61,62] Isolates from the same subtype possess greater than 90% nucleotide homology, those from differing subtypes possess about 80%, and isolates from different types share less than 70% sequence identity.[32,60,62] Under the proposed revised nomenclature (Table 10.2), genotype 1b appears to be the most frequent genotype worldwide, being particularly prevalent in Japan and western Europe (Figure 10.4). Genotypes

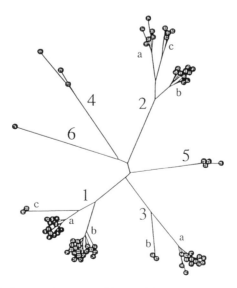

Figure 10.3. Phylogenetic tree of hepatitis C virus genotypes according to the revised classification system.

Table 10.2 Nomenclatures for genotyping of HCV

Simmonds[102]	Chiron[59]	Enomoto[58]	Mori/Okamoto[57]
1a	I	K-PT	I
1b	II	K-1	II
1c	NC	NC	NC
2a	III	K-2a	III
2b	III	K-2b	IV
3a	IV	NC	V
3b	IV	NC	VI
4	NC	NC	NC
5a	V	NC	NC
6a	NC	NC	NC

NC = not classified.

1a and 1b are about equally prevalent in the United States. Genotype 2 is more commonly identified in Japanese and Chinese populations. Genotypes 3 to 6 have been identified more recently and their precise distribution is less clear at present. Undoubtedly, studies of additional viral strains will reveal further sequence diversity.

Different HCV genotypes may lead to the production of type-specific antibody responses in infected individuals. Genotype-specific antibodies have been found to be reactive to the HCV core protein,[63] to the NS4 protein,[64-66] and to the E1 protein. The extent of overlap of serotyping with genotyping is largely unknown, and the specificity of these methods remains to be established.

Less clear than the ability of HCV to mutate and to generate extensive genetic heterogeneity is the clinical significance of this diversity. Several

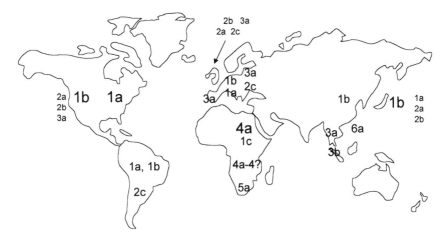

Figure 10.4. Geographic distribution of the hepatitis C virus genotypes.

groups have suggested that certain genotypes are associated with variable responses to interferon therapy.[61,67,68] A group in Europe has identified an association between genotype 1b and more severe forms of liver disease, including cirrhosis and HCC.[69] However, it is possible that because this genotype predominated among the older patients studied, it was over-represented in the group that developed complications. Recently, a case-control study of prevalences of various genotypes in HCV-infected patients with or without HCC in the United States showed that there was no increased risk of HCC development in patients infected with specific genotypes of HCV.[65] It will be necessary to study patients prospectively, however, to determine whether certain genotypes display more virulent long-term clinical behavior. Given the long-term natural history of chronic infection, it may be years before a definitive answer to this question is forthcoming. Thus, while genotyping is a useful marker for the genetic diversity of HCV, its clinical relevance remains to be established.

VIRAL PATHOGENESIS AND ONCOGENESIS

The mechanisms that underlie hepatocellular injury in chronic HCV infection have not been fully delineated. HCV-induced liver disease appears to rely on both viral and host factors as determinants of injury.

Infection with HCV stimulates both the humoral and cellular immune responses; however, this immunity appears to be variable. Humoral responses have been detected against all of the viral antigens. Certain viral polypeptides, such as the core, appear to be highly immunogenic. Neutralizing antibodies directed against the envelope proteins have also been detected.[70] Despite this broadly directed antibody response, protective immunity based on humoral response does not seem to exist. It is also not clear whether any of the antibodies plays an adverse role in the pathogenesis of hepatitis, such as antibody-directed cell cytolysis. Cytotoxic, CD8+ T lymphocytes broadly directed at HCV-specific antigens have been demonstrated in the liver and peripheral blood of chronically infected individuals.[71,72] These effector cells presumably participate in the lysis of virus-infected hepatocytes and in clearance of virus; however, if this response is incomplete, then not only will the virus persist, but cytokines liberated by these lymphocytes will lead to nonspecific inflammatory changes that are characteristic on histopathologic examination of infected livers.

One of the most prominent clinical features underlying the association of HCV with long-term complications such as HCC is the virus's ability to cause persistent infection in the host (see Chapter 1). Because viral integration into the host genome is not observed in HCV infection, the mechanism of persistence appears to reside in the virus's ability to mutate rapidly under immune pressure. The disproportionately high degree of envelope glycoprotein variability supports (but does not prove) the hypothesis that changes in these genes alter the antigenicity of the virus to permit "immune escape" from neutralizing antibodies. In addition, the existence of quasispecies provides a rapid and efficient means for the virus to escape the immune response by replacing one dominant strain, to which the host generates a neutralizing antibody response,[70,73] with another coexisting strain. This phenomenon has been elegantly demonstrated both in vitro and in vivo.[70,74] Within the RNA genome, the 5'-untranslated region, core, NS3, and NS4 are relatively well conserved, whereas E1, E2/NS1, NS2, and NS5 are the most variable regions. In practice, the relatively ineffective humoral antibody response raises the distinct possibility that the cellular immune response, in the form of cytotoxic T lymphocyte (CTL) reactivity, plays a more important role in clearance of virus infection. In this situation, viral mutations within CTL epitopes may also lead to a loss of recognition by the CTL specific for that epitope contributing to immune escape. Single amino-acid substitutions within CTL epitopes have been shown to result in loss of recognition by virus-specific CTL in lymphochoriomenigitis virus,[75] HBV,[76] human immunodeficiency virus,[77] and Epstein-Barr virus[78] infection. Recently, in the chimpanzee model of infection, persistent HCV infection was associated with the emergence of a mutation within a CTL epitope and subsequent loss of HCV-specific CTL responses.[79] Whether virus variation resulting in mutations within key epitopes is a result of true immune selection or is simply a random event remains controversial.[80]

It is also possible that the high mutation rate results in the production of defective interfering particles that are capable of adsorbing potentially neutralizing antibodies and thereby preventing these antibodies' access to actively replicating particles. The observed high particle-to-chimpanzee infectious dose ratio for HCV (M. Houghton, personal communication) supports the notion that a large percentage of particles are defective.

Another means of establishing persistence may lie in the ability of HCV to down-regulate translation of its polyprotein and hence to limit its overall copy number and subsequent recognition by the host immune system. This down-regulation has been well described as a means of establishment of persistence in latent infections with herpes simplex virus. Studies of the highly conserved HCV 5'-untranslated region have demonstrated the presence of a large conserved stem-loop structure known as an internal ribosome entry site (IRES). As is true of picornaviruses, it appears that HCV translation is cap-independent and initiates at an IRES within the 5'-untranslated region. Further, in vitro studies reveal that initiation of translation appears to be inhibited basally.[81] Taken together, the limitations of viral protein expression and copy number could serve to limit recognition and, subsequently, clearance by the cellular immune system.

Another level of regulation could reside at the synthesis and processing of nonstructural proteins. Pulse-chase studies demonstrate that NS5B appears to be the least stable of the bioactive proteins produced by proteolytic cleavage.[39] In vitro studies of RNA-dependent RNA polymerase function also suggest that the polymerase activity is far less robust than that of the comparable protein from poliovirus (Chung RT, personal communication). A replication apparatus with attenuated activity may in turn lead to decreased levels of genomic RNA and infectious virion copy number. A low level of replication may serve HCV in an adaptive manner by allowing the virus to evade detection by the host immune system as well as by limiting direct cytopathic destruction by intracellular virus.

Viral persistence could also be accomplished by nonvirally mediated mechanisms. For instance, researchers have observed that circulating HCV strongly associates with lipoprotein particles.[82,83] This association may contribute to viral persistence by shielding the virion from circulating antibody and from other effector arms of the immune system. Furthermore, this lipid association may provide the means by which HCV infects the liver, given the routine uptake of lipoproteins into hepatocytes.

Like several other chronic liver diseases associated with an increased risk of development of HCC, nearly all cases associated with chronic HCV infection appear in the setting of preexisting cirrhosis.[84] Indeed, an indolent, linear progression from chronic active hepatitis to cirrhosis to HCC has been well documented in a Japanese posttransfusion cohort followed over several decades.[7] In the absence of genomic integration, it is therefore likely that the emergence of malignant transformation reflects a multifactorial process of inflammation, necrosis, and cellular regeneration. Although hepatic iron concentrations are typically elevated in chronic HCV infection,[9] the extent of tissue deposition rarely approaches that seen in homozygous genetic hemochromatosis, so increased iron is a less likely causal agent of malignant transformation.

Whether HCV itself directly contributes to hepatocarcinogenesis is the subject of ongoing investigation. Case reports of HCC in noncirrhotic or near-normal livers have raised the provocative possibility that HCV may be able to cause HCC without evoking chronic injury and regeneration.[85] Analysis of HCV sequences fails to reveal proteins that are similar to known classical oncogenes or to tumor suppressor genes. Unfortunately, the absence of a suitable animal model for chronic infection and HCC formation makes an in vivo approach difficult. Although no data exist for the expression of core protein in the nuclei of infected hepatocytes, in vitro studies have shown that core interacts with cellular oncogenes at the cellular level,[86] cooperates with ras to transform primary rat embryo fibroblasts,[87] and suppresses apoptotic cell death.[88]

It will also be intriguing to determine whether one of the unassigned functions of the nonstructural portion of the genome will include transformation of the host cell. A provocative report recently demonstrated that the N-terminal (or serine-protease–containing) portion of the NS3 protein is capable of transforming fibroblasts in tissue culture.[89] Moreover, NIH3T3 cells that express a carboxy-terminally truncated NS3 are resistant to actinomycin D–induced apoptosis than are controls; this may be mediated by decreased expression of p53.[90] Indeed, Muramatsu and col-

leagues subsequently showed that the N-terminus of NS3 possesses a nuclear localization signal and that wild-type, but not mutant, p53 enhances
nuclear accumulation of NS3, suggesting a direct interaction between
NS3 and p53.[91] It is tempting to speculate that NS3 binding sequesters
p53 from its role in mediating apoptosis induced by genotoxic insult.
Whether such a dynamic interplay between HCV NS3 and cellular p53
underlies the development of the transformed phenotype in hepatocytes
awaits further study.

Although it is possible that the NS3 protease acts to cleave and activate
a cellular oncogene, it is not at all clear whether this action can be as-
cribed to the protease function itself. Another study has demonstrated an
interaction between the HCV core protein and several tumor-necrosis–
factor receptor family members,[92] raising the possibility that HCV may
interrupt the usual signal transduction pathways of these receptors, including CTL-induced lysis of infected hepatocytes. Similar studies directed at other viral gene products may shed further light on potential
viral transforming activities.

PREVENTION AND TREATMENT

The greatest advance in prevention of HCV infection has been the development of screening tests for use by blood transfusion services. Screening
has dramatically reduced the incidence of posttranfusion hepatitis to less
than 0.025% per unit of blood.[93] Blood transfusion, however, is not the
major source of HCV infection and other prevention methods are imperative to prevent this epidemic problem. Encouraging safe sex practices and
distributing clean needles to intravenous drug users could ostensibly prevent a small number of cases. One study has recommended giving postexposure prophylaxis with immunoglobulin after known exposure.[94] The efficacy of postexposure prophylaxis has not been confirmed in animal
models,[95] however, and is not currently advised by the Centers for Disease
Control and Prevention as a routine practice.[96] Moreover, 40% of HCV
infection occurs without a recognized exposure; thus, it is unlikely that
traditional prevention practices will have a momentous impact on viral
transmission. Given the occult source of most infection, interest in vaccine development has been intense.

Development of vaccines against HCV will be problematic for several
reasons. The first is the inability to produce large amounts of immunogen
in vitro, either for use in an inactivated vaccine or as the basis of a live
attenuated strain. Second, the correlates of protective immunity in HCV
infection remain undefined, in part because of the low rate of spontaneous elimination of HCV in infected humans and the lack of a small-
animal model. In the chimpanzee model, recent data show that re-
challenge with either homologous or heterologous virus in once-infected
animals can result in recurrent infection, suggesting that protective im-

munity induced by natural infection is low.[97,98] Studies attempting to induce immunity in chimpanzees by inoculation of proteins from the envelope and core region of HCV (analogous to the region used to induce immunity to HBV) have failed to produce high titer antibodies in the animals and are equally unsuccessful in conferring protection against subsequent exposure to virus. In addition, there is considerable genetic heterogeneity of this virus so, even if protective immunity is produced, the virus may be able to circumvent readily the host response and protection may be only transient. For similar reasons, transfer of passive immunity with standard immunoglobulin after needle-stick exposure is unlikely to be effective.

Treatment of chronic HCV infection with 3 million units of interferon alfa, given subcutaneously three times a week, is an FDA-approved treatment but normalizes serum ALT in less than 40% of patients. Only about one half of these patients continue to have normal ALT after stopping therapy. Long-term virological remission is rare. Presence of cirrhosis and high levels of pretreatment HCV RNA are associated with a reduced responsiveness to interferon. New therapeutic approaches to the treatment of chronic HCV infection (for example, use of interferon in combination with ribavirin, recently approved by the FDA for relapses following initial IFN-α response) may improve this response rate.

Patients with clinically decompensated HCV-related liver cirrhosis should be considered candidates for liver transplantation. Recurrent HCV infection is common in tranplanted livers (more than 90% of patients with pretransplant infection). However, recurrence is typically associated with relatively mild disease; histologic hepatitis is seen on biopsy in approximately 50% of patients at 1 year, with cirrhosis in only 10% at 3 years. Graft failure from reinfection is rare.[99,100]

In summary, with the exception of the blood screening programs in transfusion centers, there are currently no practical strategies for prevention of HCV infection. Moreover, therapeutic options in patients with chronic viral diseases are limited. Improvement in liver disease is typically transient and attainable in the minority of patients. Furthermore, most treatment trials have used the intermediate yardsticks of inhibition of viral replication and decrease in liver damage to assess efficacy, so that long-term impact of treatment on progressive liver failure and death are largely unknown. Thus, although much has been learned in the 8 years since the discovery of HCV, much more work is needed before this important cause of HCC is contained and cured.

REFERENCES

1. Dienstag JL. Non-A, non-B hepatitis: recognition, epidemiology, and clinical features. Gastroenterology 1983;85:439–462.

2. Alter MJ, Margolis HS, Krawczynski K, Judson F, Mares A, Alexander W, Hu P-Y, Miller JK, Gerber MA, Sampliner RE. The natural history of community-acquired hepatitis C in the United States. N Engl J Med 1992;327:1899–1905.

3. Alter HJ, Purcell R, Shih J, Melpolder J, Houghton M, Choo Q-L, Kuo G. Detection of antibody to hepatitis C virus in prospectively followed transfusion recipients with acute and chronic non-A, non-B hepatitis. N Engl J Med 1989;321:1494–1500.

4. Gonzalez A, Esteban JI, Madoz P, Viladomiu L, Genesca J, Muniz E, Enriquez J, Torras X, Hernandez JM, Quer J, Vidal X, Alter HJ, Shih JW, Esteban R, Guardia J. Efficacy of screening donors for antibodies to the hepatitis C virus to prevent transfusion-associated hepatitis: final report of a prospective trial. Hepatology 1995;22:439–445.

5. Alter MJ. Transmission of hepatitis C virus—route, dose, and titer [editorial; comment]. N Engl J Med 1994;330(11):784–786.

6. Blum HE. Does hepatitis C virus cause hepatocellular carcinoma? Hepatology 1994;19:251–255.

7. Kiyosawa K, Sodeyama T, Tanaka E, et al. Interrelationship of blood transfusion, non-A, non-B hepatitis and hepatocellular carcinoma: analysis by detection of antibody to hepatitis C virus. Hepatology 1990;12:671–675.

8. Okuda K. Hepatocellular carcinoma: recent progress. Hepatology 1992;15: 948–963.

9. Simonetti RG, Camma C, Fiorello F, et al. Hepatitis C virus as a risk factor for hepatocellular carcinoma in patients with cirrhosis. Ann Intern Med 1992; 116:97–102.

10. Ruiz J, Sangro B, Cuende JI, Beloqui O, Riezu-Boj JI, Herrero JI, Prieto J. Hepatitis B and C viral infections in patients with hepatocellular carcinoma. Hepatology 1992;16:637–641.

11. Zavitsanos X, Hatzakis A, Kaklamani E, Tzonou A, Toupadaki N, Broeksma C, Chrispeels J, Troonen H, Hadziyannis S, Shieh C-C, Alter H, Trichopoulos D. Association between hepatitis C virus and hepatocellular carcinoma using assays based on structural and nonstructural hepatitis C virus peptides. Cancer Res 1992;52:5364–5367.

12. Paterlini P. Persistence of hepatitis B and hepatitis C viral genomes in primary liver cancers from HBsAg-negative patients: a study of a low-endemic area. Hepatology 1993;17:20–29.

13. Yu M-W, You SL, Chang A-S, Lu S-N, Liaw Y-F, Chen C-J. Association between hepatitis C virus antibodies and hepatocellular carcinoma in Taiwan. Cancer Res. 1991;51:5621–5625.

14. Lee H-S, Han C-J, Kim CY. Predominant etiologic association of hepatitis C virus with hepatocellular carcinoma compared with hepatitis B virus in elderly patients in a hepatitis B-endemic area. Cancer 1993;72:2563–2567.

15. Kew MC, Houghton M, Choo Q-L, Kuo G. Hepatitis C antibodies in southern African blacks with hepatocellular carcinoma. Lancet 1990;335:873–874.

16. Bukh J, Miller RH, Kew MC, Purcell RH. Hepatitis C virus RNA in southern African blacks with hepatocellular carcinoma. Proc Natl Acad Sci USA 1993; 90:1848–1851.

17. Hasan F, Jeffers LJ, De Medina M, Reddy KR, Parker T, Schiff ER, Houghton M, Choo Q-L, Kuo G. Hepatitis C-associated hepatocellular carcinoma. Hepatology 1990;12:589–591.

18. Liang TJ, Jeffers L, Reddy KR, Medina M, Parker T, Cheinquer H, Idrovo V,

Rabassa V, Schiff E. Viral pathogenesis of hepatocellular carcinoma in the United States. Hepatology 1993;18:1326–1333.

19. Yu MC, Tong MJ, Coursaget P, Ross RK, Govindarajan S, Henderson BE. Prevalence of hepatitis B and C viral markers in black and white patients with hepatocellular carcinoma in the United States. J Natl Cancer Inst 1990;82: 1038–1041.

20. DiBisceglie AM, Order SE, Klein JL, Waggoner JG, Sjogren M, Kuo G, Houghton M, Choo Q-L, Hoofnagle JH. The role of chronic viral hepatitis in hepatocellular carcinoma in the United States. Am J Gastroenterol 1991;86: 335–338.

21. Mangia A, Vallari DS, DiBisceglie AM. Use of confirmatory assays for diagnosis of hepatitis C viral infection in patients with hepatocellular carcinoma. J Med Virol 1994;43:125–128.

22. Nakatsuji Y, Matsumoto A, Tanaka E, Ogata H, Kiyosama K. Detection of chronic hepatitis C virus infection by four diagnostic systems: first-generation and second-generation enzyme-linked immunosorbent assay, second-generation recombinant immunoblot assay and nested polymerase chain reaction analysis. Hepatology 1992;16:300–305.

23. Sugitani M, Inchauspe G, Chindo M, Prince AM. Sensitivity of serological assays to identify blood donors with hepatitis C viremia. Lancet 1992;339: 1018–1019.

24. Choo Q-L, Kuo G, Weiner AJ, et al. Isolation of a cDNA clone derived from a blood-borne non-A, non-B viral hepatitis genome. Science 1989;244:359–362.

25. Kuo G, Choo Q-L, Alter HJ, et al. An assay for circulating antibodies to a major etiologic virus of human non-A, non-B hepatitis. Science 1989;244: 362–364.

26. Choo Q-L, Kuo G, Weiner AJ, Overby LR, Bradley DW, Houghton M. Genetic organization and diversity of the hepatitis C virus. Proc Natl Acad Sci USA 1991;88:2451–2455.

27. Kato N, Hijikata M, Ootsuyama Y, et al. Molecular cloning of the human hepatitis C virus genome from Japanese patients with non-A, non-B hepatitis. Proc Natl Acad Sci USA 1990;87:9524–9528.

28. Miller RH, Purcell RH. Hepatitis C virus shares amino acid sequence similarity with pestiviruses and flaviviruses as well as members of two plant virus supergroups. Proc Natl Acad Sci USA 1990;87:2057–2061.

29. von Heijne G. A new method for predicting signal sequence cleavage sites. Nucleic Acids Res 1986;14:4683–4690.

30. Takeuchi K, Kubo Y, Boonmar S, et al. The putative nucleocapsid and envelope protein genes of hepatitis C virus determined by comparison of the nucleotide sequences of two isolates derived from an experimentally infected chimpanzee and healthy human carriers. J Gen Virol 1990;71:2027–2033.

31. Takeuchi K, Kubo Y, Boonmar S, et al. Nucleotide sequence of core and envelope genes of the hepatitis C virus genome derived directly from healthy human carriers. Nucleic Acids Res 1990;18:4626.

32. Weiner AJ, Brauer M, Rosenblatt J, et al. Variable and hypervariable domains are found in regions of HCV corresponding to the flavivirus envelope and NS1 proteins and the pestivirus envelope glycoproteins. Virology 1991;180: 842–848.

33. Weiner AJ, Geysen HM, Cristopherson C, et al. Evidence for immune selec-

tion of hepatitis C virus putative envelope glycoprotein variants: potential role in chronic HCV infection. Proc Natl Acad Sci USA 1992;89:3468–3472.

34. Lesniewski RR, Boardway KM, Casey JM, et al. Hypervariable 5'-terminus of hepatitis C virus E2/NS1 encodes antigenically distinct variants. J Med Virol 1993;40:150–156.

35. Okamoto H, Kojima M, Okada S, et al. Genetic drift of hepatitis C virus during an 8.2-year infection in a chimpanzee: variability and stability. Virology 1992;190:894–899.

36. Martell M, Esteban JI, Quer J, et al. Hepatitis C virus circulates as a population of different but closely related genomes: quasispecies nature of HCV genome distribution. J Virol 1992;66:3225–3229.

37. Hijikata M, Mizushima M, Akagi T, et al. Two distinct proteinase activities required for the processing of a putative nonstructural precursor of hepatitis C virus. J Virol 1993;67:4665–4675.

38. Grakoui A, McCourt DW, Wychowski C, et al. Characterization of the hepatitis C virus-encoded serine proteinase: determination of proteinase-dependent polyprotein cleavage sites. J Virol 1993;67:2832–2843.

39. Grakoui A, Wychowski C, Lin C, et al. Expression and identification of hepatitis C virus polyprotein cleavage products. J Virol 1993;67:1385–1395.

40. Tomei L, Failla C, Santolini E, DeFrancesco R, LaMonica N. NS3 is a serine protease required for processing of hepatitis C virus polyprotein. J Virol 1993;67:4017–4026.

41. Suzich JA, Tamura JK, Palmer-Hill P, et al. Hepatitis C virus NS3 protein polynucleotide-stimulated nucleoside triphosphatase and comparison to the related pestivirus and flavivirus enzymes. J Virol 1993;67:6152–6158.

42. Failla C, Tomei L, DeFrancesco R. Both NS3 and NS4A are required for proteolytic processing of hepatitis C virus nonstructural proteins. J Virol 1994;68:3753–3760.

43. Satoh S, Tanji Y, Hijikata M, Kimura K, Shimotohno K. The N-terminal region of hepatitis C virus nonstructural protein 3 is essential for stable complex formation with NS4A. J Virol 1995;69:4255–4260.

44. Failla C, Tomei L, DeFrancesco R. An amino-terminal domain of the hepatitis C virus NS3 protease is essential for interaction with NS4A. J Virol 1995; 69:1769–1777.

45. Bartenschlager R, Lohmann V, Wilkinson T, Koch JO. Complex formation between the NS3 serine-type proteinase of the hepatitis C virus and NS4A and its importance for polyprotein formation. J Virol 1995;69:7519–7528.

46. Asabe S-I, Tanji Y, Satoh S, Kaneko T, Kumura K, Shimotohno K. The N-terminal region of hepatitic C virus-encoded NS5A is important for NS4A-dependent phosphorylation. J Virol 1997;71:790–796.

47. Kaneko T, Tanji Y, Satoh S, et al. Production of two phosphoproteins from the NS5A region of the hepatitis C viral genome. Biochem Biophys Res Commun 1994;205:320–326.

48. Tanji Y, Kaneko T, Satoh S, Shimotohno S. Phosphorylation of hepatitis C virus-encoded nonstructural protein NS5A. J Virol 1995;69:3980–3986.

49. Enomoto N, Sakuma I, Asahina Y, et al. Mutations in the nonstructural protein 5A gene and response to interferon in patients with chronic hepatitis C virus 1b infection. N Engl J Med 1996;334:77–81.

50. Zeuzem S, Lee J-H, Roth WK. Mutations in the nonstructural 5A gene of

European hepatitis C virus isolates and response to interferon alpha. Hepatology 1997;25:740–744.

51. Squadrito G, Leone F, Satori M, Nalpas B, Berthelot P, Raimondo G, Pol S, Brechot C. Mutations in the nonstructural 5A region of hepatitis C virus and response of chronic hepatitis C to interferon alpha. Gastroenterology 1997; 113:567–572.

52. DeFrancesco R, Behrens S-E, Tomei L. Identification and properties of the RNA-dependent RNA polymerase of hepatitis C virus. Hepatitis C Keystone Symposium. Burlington, VT, 1996.

53. Tanaka T, Kato N, Cho M-J, Shimotohno K. A novel sequence found at the 3' terminus of hepatitis C virus genome. Biochem Biophys Res Commun 1995; 215:744–749.

54. Kolykhalov AA, Feinstone SM, Rice CM. Identification of a highly conserved sequence element at the 3' terminus of hepatitis C virus genome RNA. J Virol 1996;70:3363–3371.

55. Krawczynski K, Beach MJ, Bradley DW, et al. Hepatitis C virus antigen in hepatocytes: immunomorphologic detection and identification. Gastroenterology 1992;103:622–629.

56. Ogata N, Alter HJ, Miller RH, Purcell RH. Nucleotide sequence and mutation rate of the H strain of hepatitis C virus. Proc Natl Acad Sci USA 1991;88:3392–3396.

57. Okamoto H, Sugiyama Y, Okada S, et al. Typing hepatitis C virus by polymerase chain reaction with type-specific primers: application to clinical surveys and tracing infectious sources. J Gen Virol 1992;73:673–679.

58. Enomoto N, Takada A, Nakao T, Date T. There are two major types of hepatitis C virus in Japan. Biochem Biophys Res Commun 1990;170:1021–1025.

59. Cha TA, Beall E, Irvine B, et al. At least five related, but distinct, hepatitis C viral genotypes exist. Proc Natl Acad Sci USA 1992;89:7144–7148.

60. Stuyver L, Rossau R, Wyseur A, et al. Typing of HCV isolates and characterization of new (sub)types using a line probe assay. J Gen Virol 1993;1993:1093–1102.

61. Simmonds P. Variability of hepatitis C virus. Hepatology 1995;21:570–583.

62. Bukh J, Miller RH, Purcell RH. Genetic heterogeneity of hepatitis C virus: Quasispecies and genotypes. Sem Liv Disease 1995;15:41–63.

63. Machida A, Ohnuma H, Tsuda F, et al. Two distinct subtypes of hepatitis C virus defined by antibodies directed to the putative core protein. Hepatology 1992;16:886–891.

64. Simmonds P, Rose KA, Graham S, et al. Mapping of serotype-specific, immunodominant epitopes in the NS-4 region of hepatitis C virus: use of type-specific peptides to serologically differentiate infections with HCV types 1,2, and 3. J Clin Microbiol 1993;31:1493–1503.

65. Stuyver L, van Arnhem W, Wyseur A, DeLeys R, Maartens G. Analysis of the putative E1 envelope and NS4a epitope regions of the HCV type 3. Biochem Biophys Res Commun 1993;192:635–641.

66. Tsukiyama-Kohara K, Yamaguchi K, Maki N, et al. Antigenicities of group I and II hepatitis C virus polypeptides—molecular basis of diagnosis. Virology 1993;192:430–437.

67. Takada N, Takase S, Enomoto N, Takada A, Date T. Clinical backgrounds of the patients having different types of hepatitis C virus genomes. J Hepatol 1992;14:35–40.

68. Yoshioka K, Kakumu S, Wakiti T, et al. Detection of hepatitis C virus by polymerase chain reaction and responses to interferon-alfa therapy: relationship to genotypes of hepatitis C virus. Hepatology 1992;16:293–299.
69. Nousbaum J-B, Pol S, Nalpas B, et al. Hepatitis C virus type 1b infection in France and Italy. Ann Intern Med 1995;122:161–168.
70. Shimizu YK, Hijikata M, Iwamoto A, et al. Neutralizing antibodies against hepatitis C virus and the emergence of neutralization escape mutant viruses. J Virol 1994;68:1494–1500.
71. Koziel MJ, Dudley D, Afdhal N, et al. Hepatitis C virus-specific cytotoxic T lymphocytes recognize epitopes in the core and envelope proteins of HCV. J Virol 1993;67:7522–7532.
72. Botarelli P, Brunetto MR, Minutello MA, et al. T-lymphocyte response to hepatitis C virus in different clinical courses of infection. Gastroenterology 1993;104:580–587.
73. Kato N, Sekiya H, Ootsuyama Y, Nakazawa T, Hijikata M, Ohkoshi S, Shimotohno K. Humoral immune response to hypervariable region 1 of the putative envelope glycoprotein (gp70) of hepatitis C virus. J Virol 1993;67(7):3923–3930.
74. Farci P, Alter HJ, Wong DC, et al. Prevention of HCV infection in chimpanzees following antibody-mediated in vitro neutralization. Proc Natl Acad Sci USA 1994;91:7792–7796.
75. Aebischer T, Moskophidis D, Rohrer U, Zinkernagel R, Hengartner H. In vitro selection of lymphocytic choriomeningitis escape mutants by cytotoxic T lymphocytes. Proc Natl Acad Sci USA 1991;88:11047–11051.
76. Bertoletti A, Sette A, Chisari F, Penna A, Levrero M, De Carli M, Fiaccadori F, Ferrari C. Natural variants of cytotoxic epitopes are T-cell receptor antagonists for antiviral cytotoxic T cells. Nature 1994;369:407–410.
77. Takahashi H, Merli S, Putney SD, Houghten R, Moss B, Germain RN, Berzofsky JA. A single amino acid interchange yields reciprocal CTL specificities for HIV-1 gp160. Science 1989;246(4926):118–121.
78. de Campos-Lima P-O, Gavioli R, Zhang Q-J, Wallace L, Dolcetti R, Rowe M, Rickinson AB, Masucci MG. HLA-A11 epitope loss isolates of Epstein-Barr virus from a highly A11+ population. Science 1993;260:98–100.
79. Weiner A, Erickson AL, Kansopon J, Crawford K, Muchmore E, Hughes AL, Houghton M, Walker CM. Persistent hepatitis C virus infection in a chimpanzee is associated with emergence of a cytotoxic T lymphocyte escape variant. Proc Natl Acad Sci USA 1995;92(7):2755–2759.
80. Chen ZW, Shen L, Miller M, Ghim S, Hughes A, Letvin N. Cytotoxic T lymphocytes do not appear to select for mutations in an immunodominant epitope of simian immunodeficiency virus gag. J Immunol 1992;149:4060–4066.
81. Han JH, Shyamala V, Richman KH, et al. Characterization of the terminal regions of hepatitis C virus RNA: identification of conserved sequences in the 5'-untranslated region and poly(A) tails at the 3' end. Proc Natl Acad Sci USA 1991;88:1711–1715.
82. Miyamoto H, Okamoto H, Sato K, Tanaka T, Mishiro S. Extraordinarily low density of hepatitis C virus estimated by sucrose density gradient centrifugation and the polymerase chain reaction. J Gen Virol 1992;73:715–718.
83. Thomssen R, Bonk S, Thiele A. Density heterogeneities of hepatitis C virus in human sera due to the binding of beta-lipoproteins and immunoglobulins. Med Microbiol Immunol 1993;182:329–334.

84. Sallie R, DiBisceglie AM. Viral hepatitis and hepatocellular carcinoma. Gastroenterol Clin North Am 1994;23:567–579.
85. De Mitri M, Poussin K, Baccarini P, Pontisso P, D'Errico A, Simon N, Grigioni W. HCV-associated liver cancer without cirrhosis. Lancet 1995;345:413–415.
86. Ray RB, Lagging LM, Meyer K, Steele R, Ray R. Transcriptional regulation of cellular and viral promoters by the hepatitis C virus core protein. Virus Res 1995;37:209–220.
87. Ray RB, Lagging LM, Meyer K, Ray R. Hepatitis C virus core protein cooperates with *ras* and transforms primary rat embryo fibroblasts to tumorigenic phenotype. J Virol 1996;70:4438–4443.
88. Ray RB, Meyer K, Ray R. Suppression of apoptotic cell death by hepatitis C virus core protein. Virology 1996;226:176–182.
89. Sakamuro D, Furukawa T, Takegami T. Hepatitis C virus nonstructural protein NS3 transforms NIH 3T3 cells. J Virol 1995;69:3893–3896.
90. Ishido S, Muramatsu S, Fujita T, et al. Wild-type but not mutant-type p53 enhances nuclear accumulation of the NS3 protein of hepatitis C virus. Biochem Biophys Res Commun 1997;230:431–436.
91. Muramatsu S, Ishido S, Fujita T, Itoh M, Hotta H. Nuclear localization of the NS3 protein of hepatitis C virus and factors affecting the localization. J Virol 1997;71:1301–1309.
92. Matsumoto M, Hsieh T-Y, Zhu N, VanArsdale T, Hwang SB, Jeng K-S, Gorbalenya AE, Lo S-Y, Ou J-H, Lai MMC. Hepatitis C virus core protein interacts with the cytoplasmic tail of lymphotoxin-B receptor. J Virol 1997;71:1301–1309.
93. Nishioka K. Hepatitis C virus screening and intravenous immunoglobulin safety in Japan. Clin Ther 1996;18 Suppl B:83–92.
94. Piazza M, Sagliocca L, Tosone G, et al. Sexual transmission of the hepatitis C virus and efficacy of prophylaxis with intramuscular immune serum globulin: a randomized controlled trial. Arch Intern Med 1997;157:1537–1544.
95. Krawczynski K, Alter MJ, Tankersley DL, et al. Effect of immune globulin on the prevention of experimental hepatitis C virus infection. J Infect Dis 1996;173:822–828.
96. The Centers for Disease Control and Prevention. Recommendations for follow-up of health-care workers after occupational exposure to hepatitis C virus. JAMA 1997;278:1056–1057.
97. Prince A, Brotman B, Hiuma T, Pascual D, Jaffery M, Inchauspe G. Immunity in hepatitis C infection. J Infect Dis 1992;165:438–443.
98. Farci P, Alter H, Govindarajan S, Wong D, Engle R, Lesniewski R, Mushahwar I, Desai S, Miller R, Ogata N, Purcell RH. Lack of protective immunity against reinfection with hepatitis C virus. Science 1992;258:135–140.
99. Wright T, Donegan E, Hsu H, Ferrell L, Lake J, Kim M, Combs C, Fennessy S, Roberts J, Ascher N, Greenberg H. Recurrent and acquired hepatitis C viral infection in liver transplant recipients. Gastroenterology 1992;193:317–322.
100. Feray C, Gigou M, Samuel D, Paradis V, Wilber J, David MF, Urdea M, Reynes M, Brechot C, Bismuth H. The course of hepatitis C virus infection after liver transplantation. Hepatology 1994;20:1137–1143.
101. Simmonds PE, Alberti A, Alter HJ, Bonino F, Bradley DW, Brechot C, Brouwer JT, et al. A proposed system for the nomenclature of hepatitis C viral genotypes. Hepatology 1994;19:1321–1324.

11

Human C-type Oncoviruses
and T-cell Leukemia/Lymphoma

MITSUAKI YOSHIDA

Human T-cell leukemia viruses (HTLVs), also called human C-type oncoviruses or human T-cell lymphotropic viruses, include two human pathogens: HTLV type 1 (HTLV-1) and HTLV type 2 (HTLV-2).[1-4] HTLV-1, the
better characterized of the two viruses, is the etiologic agent of adult
T-cell leukemia (ATL)—the subject of this chapter.[2,3,5] HTLV-1 also causes
a slowly progressive myelopathy [HTLV-1–associated myelopathy, or tropical spastic paraparesis (HAM/TSP)][6,7] and uveitis.[8] HTLV-1 infection has
also been reported to induce a mild immunodeficiency, thereby increasing the incidence of both cancers[9] and opportunistic parasitic infections,
such as stronglyloidiasis.[10] An association of HTLV-1 infection with rheumatoid arthritis has been proposed but, as yet, has found little epidemiological support.[11] Closely related retroviruses include bovine leukemia
virus (BLV)[12] and simian T-cell leukemia viruses (STLVs).[13-15] These latter
viruses have been isolated from various species of Old World monkeys,
including the Japanese macaque, African green monkey, pig-tailed macaque, gorilla, and chimpanzee. The STLVs show 90% to 95% homology
with the genomic sequence of HTLV-1 and are also similar to each other.[16]
Their pathogenic effects are not clearly described.

THE VIRUS

Like retroviruses in general, HTLVs carry their genetic information in
single-stranded RNA. The genomic RNA is reverse-transcribed into DNA
by viral reverse transcriptase. Then, complementary viral DNA is transcribed, forming double-stranded viral DNA that is integrated into the
host chromosome. The site of integration is not specific to any locus in

the cellular DNA. Moreover, all cells infected with HTLV harbor the proviruses in their genome irrespective of whether or not the proviruses are expressed. The proviruses become a template for transcription to generate the original viral RNA genome and also to express the mRNA.

The proviral HTLV genome is 9032 bp long and, unique among the retroviruses, does not require any helper virus for its replication. Like other retroviruses, however, HTLVs have *gag*, *pol*, and *env* genes in their genome, encoding viral core proteins, reverse transcriptase, and surface glycoprotein for receptor binding, respectively. In addition to these three genes, the viral genome has an extra sequence, the pX region, that is situated between the *env* gene and the 3' long terminal repeat (LTR).[17] In HTLV-1, this 1.6 kilobase (kb) pX region contains three overlapping genes[18,19]: *tax*, *rex*, and a third gene, encoding p40[tax], p27[rex], and p21[x], respectively (Figure 11.1). As we shall discuss in detail, Tax is a transcriptional activator that enhances HTLV-1 gene expression,[20,21] and is thus essential for viral replication. Rex protein is a trans-regulator of RNA processing and modulates the expression of subgenomic mRNA; it is, thus, also essential for viral replication.[22,23] The p21 protein has unknown function. The pX region has little sequence similarity to the human genome, indicating that it does not contain a known oncogene homologue.

Expression of HTLV-1 genes is mediated by three major mRNA species (Figure 11.2). Transcription starts from the 5' LTR and terminates at the 3' LTR, and the transcripts, like the original genomic RNA, are 9 kb in length. The genomic RNA serves as mRNA for Gag and Gag-pol polyproteins. To express Env and Tax/Rex/p21 in the pX region, the primary transcript is spliced into two other species.[24] The first splicing removes the *gag* and *pol* sequences generating 4.2 kb subgenomic mRNA that encodes the Env protein. The second splicing removes the *env* sequence generating 2.1 kb mRNA that encodes Tax, Rex, and p21.[25] Numerous other RNA

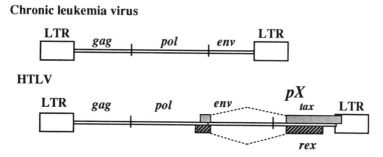

Figure 11.1. Genomic structures of HTLV and general chronic retroviruses. HTLV types 1 and 2 have similar genomic arrangements containing genes for nonstructural regulatory proteins, *tax*, *rex*, and some others. These regulatory genes are unique to a group of HTLV.

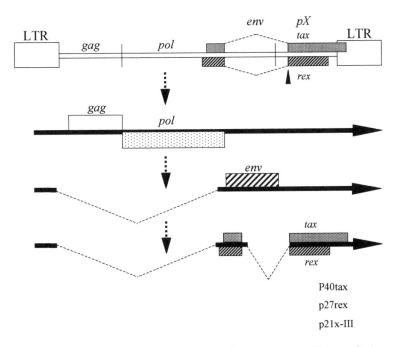

Figure 11.2. Mechanism of expression of HTLV genes. Two splicings are required for the expression of basal genes of HTLV. Alternative splicings for other minor proteins such as p12 and p30 are not indicated. Transcription of the genome is *trans*-activated by Tax protein and splicings into *gag-pol* mRNA and into pX mRNA are down-regulated by Rex protein. These positive and negative regulations by two viral proteins make the viral expression transient.

species produced by splicing pX sequences have been identified. The physiological significance of these species, however, remains unknown.

HTLV-1±ASSOCIATED DISEASES

Adult T-cell leukemia (ATL) is a malignancy of CD4-positive T cells.[26] This malignancy occurs most frequently in people in their forties and fifties but can occur in people as young as 20 and as old as 70 years of age.[27,28] The incidence of ATL is somewhat higher in men than in women (male-to-female ratio 1.4 to 1). Symptoms of ATL are varied; infiltration of leukemic cells into various organs can result in skin lesions or in enlargement of lymph nodes, liver, or spleen. On laboratory testing, patients usually show an increased level of serum LDH and suffer from hypercalcemia. Most have antibodies to HTLV-1 proteins.

In addition to the typical, acute form of ATL, smoldering, chronic, and lymphoma types have been recognized.[29] In smoldering ATL, patients have a few morphologically abnormal T cells in their peripheral blood, but do not show particular signs of severe illness for a long period. The subsequent acute phase of ATL, like primary acute ATL, is aggressive and resistant to any treatment. Most patients die within 6 months of its onset.

In all forms of ATL, leukemic cells are T cells with the CD4[+] phenotype; they usually have a highly lobulated nucleus.[30] These cells always contain integrated HTLV-1 proviruses,[2] with the site of integration being clonal in any given ATL patient.[5] In most cases of ATL, one complete copy of the provirus is integrated into each leukemic cell. In some instances, however, these proviruses are defective.[5] The leukemic cells express a high level of the alpha chain of the interleukin-2 receptor (IL-2Rα) on their surface.[31] Production of parathyroid hormone–related protein (PTHrP),[32] interleukin (IL)-1β,[33] or granulocyte-macrophage colony-stimulating factor (GM-CSF)[34] by tumor cells has been reported. In almost all cases, leukemic cells carry aberrant chromosomes, often with multiple abnormalities, but no common abnormality has been described.[35] Infiltration of these leukemic cells into the skin and other organs and tissues completes the complicated phenotype of ATL.

Interestingly, HTLV-1 also causes a completely distinct disease: a slowly progressive myelopathy known in tropical zones as tropical spastic paraparesis (TSP)[7] and in endemic areas of Japan as HTLV-1-associated myelopathy (HAM).[6] Symptoms of HAM/TSP reflect chronic, symmetrical, bilateral involvement of the pyramidal tracts, mainly at the thoracic level of the spinal cord, resulting in progressive spastic paresis with spastic bladder and minimal sensory deficit. HTLV-1–infected T cells infiltrate into the cerebrospinal fluid and spinal cord. No specific neurotropic HTLV-1 subtypes have been identified; the virus that causes HAM/TSP appears to be identical to the one that causes ATL.[36] Most patients with HAM/TSP have titers of HTLV-1 antibodies much higher than those of asymptomatic carriers and ATL patients, however.[37] Yet, despite this strong antibody response to HTLV-1 infection, most HAM/TSP patients have populations of infected cells much larger than those of HTLV-1 carriers.[38] These patients have been reported to have particular types of human leukocyte antigens (HLA).[39]

EPIDEMIOLOGY OF HTLV-1

HTLV-1 antibodies are recognized in 5% to 15% of adults in southwestern Japan,[3] the Caribbean islands, South America, Central Africa,[28] Papua New Guinea, and the Solomon islands.[40] The ATL patients and healthy carriers found sporadically elsewhere in the world are mostly individuals who moved from endemic areas. Within endemic areas, however, the prevalence of infection in healthy adults varies significantly from district to district, and even from village to village. The reason for such a scattered distribution is unknown; perhaps the unique mode of viral transmission and the host-related factors that affect responses to infection explain it.

The HTLV-1 genome within the separate endemic areas is highly conserved,[41] and differences are limited to only 1% to 3%. Even these small differences, however, allow the HTLV-1 viruses to be classified into subtypes. Two different schema based on restriction length polymorphisms differentiate the viruses into subtypes A and B or subtypes I, II, and III.[42,43] HTLV-2 has also been classified into two subtypes: A and B.[44] These subtypes are useful for our understanding of epidemiology and evolution of HTLVs, but they do not correlate with infectivity, replication capacity, or pathogenicity.

HTLV-1 prevalence is somewhat higher (1.6-fold) in females than in males. Its prevalence is also age dependent; the frequency of viral carriers increases after age 20 years, reaching a maximum in people between 40 and 60 years of age. Although HTLV-1 may infect adults through sexual contact and blood transfusion, the vast majority of infection is acquired in infancy. Thus, the highly significant increase in prevalence of seropositivity after 20 years of age requires specific explanation. One hypothesis is that HTLV-1 infection through breast milk results in latent infection, with viral replication delayed for the next 20 to 30 years; no plausible mechanism for this delayed presentation has been proposed. It is more likely that the age-dependent increase of seroprevalence reflects changing rates of viral transmission over the past 20 to 50 years (a birth-cohort effect). In other words, the transmission of HTLV-1 50 years ago was high, but the rate has subsequently decreased with a precipitous drop 20 years ago. More studies will be needed to resolve this epidemiological question definitively.

Familial aggregation is another epidemiological feature of HTLV-1 infection.[45] Viral transmission from mother to child was originally suggested by epidemiological studies; most mothers of seropositive children were seropositive, and about 30% of the children of seropositive mothers were themselves seropositive. In the laboratory, breast milk has been confirmed to be a source of transmissible virus.[46,47] Milk taken from seropositive mothers can induce antibodies in adult marmosets.[48] More direct evidence of breast-milk transmission was obtained from a clinical trial demonstrating that cessation of breast feeding by seropositive mothers drastically reduced the seropositive rate of their children (S. Hino et al., personal communication).

Other modes of HTLV-1 transmission are blood transfusion and sexual contact. Retrospective studies of blood transfusions showed that 60% to 70% of recipients of fresh seropositive blood became infected with HTLV-1,[49] but no recipients of seropositive plasma were infected. Thus, the transfer of infected cells from donor to recipient is required for viral transmission. In support of sexual transmission, the wives with seropositive husbands are usually seropositive. Conversely, the husbands of seropositive wives show the same frequency of seropositivity as do men in the local population.[50] Thus, the virus appears to be transmitted frequently from husband to wife, but infrequently from wife to husband. Infected T cells have been detected in semen and are thought to mediate the viral transmission from male to female. Taken together, the data suggest that high-efficiency HTLV-1 transmission from husband to wife results in an infected woman who then transmits HTLV-1 to her child through breast milk. This transmission pathway can explain both familial aggregation and the strong association of infection with specific populations.

EPIDEMIOLOGICAL ASSOCIATION BETWEEN HTLV-1 AND ATL

The etiologic role of HTLV-1 in the development of ATL has been demonstrated convincingly by seroepidemiological, molecular biological, and experimental studies. These studies support a causal association at four levels. First, at an ecologic level, ATL and HTLV-1 have identical geographic distributions.[51] Second, at the level of the individual, almost all ATL patients are infected with HTLV-1 and only a few cases of ATL are reported in uninfected populations.[3] Third, at a cellular level, leukemic cells from ATL patients are all infected with HTLV-1 and show monoclonal integration of proviral DNA, indicating that leukemic cells originate from a single HTLV-1-infected cell.[2,5] Fourth, at an experimental level, infection by HTLV-1 can immortalize CD4-positive T cells, but not other cell types in vitro.[52] Immortalized T cells show phenotypes similar to some of those of leukemic cells,[30,31] indicating the transforming capacity of HTLV-1. These observations on the association of HTLV-1 infection and ATL or transformation at different levels demonstrate convincingly that HTLV-1 is a critical etiologic agent in the leukemogenic process of ATL development.

Several cases of ATL "unrelated to HTLV-1 infection" have been described.[53] These leukemias are phenotypically indistinguishable both clinically and hematologically from typical ATL, but sufferers have no HTLV-1 antibodies and their leukemic cells carry no HTLV-1 proviral DNA. There has been debate about whether the proviruses in tumor cells were excised during or after malignant transformation. If these seronegative ATL cases were caused by HTLV-1 infection, however, nonmalignant cells in these patients should be infected and antibodies to HTLV-1 should be present. Because neither finding is observed in HTLV-1–negative ATLs, the hypothesis that provirus is excised is untenable. It should be emphasized, however, that the vast majority of ATL cases are associated with HTLV-1 infection.

HTLV-1 has been isolated from patients diagnosed as having Sézary syndrome[54] or mycosis fungoides.[1] The association of HTLV-1 infection with these specific T-cell malignancies has not been established because, in some of these cases, the diagnosis was not clearly distinguished from ATL.

The incidence of ATL in HTLV-1 carriers during their lifetimes is estimated as 2% to 5%.[55] Although most infection begins in childhood, the associated disease ATL starts to develop at 20 to 70 years of age, most frequently from 40 to 60.[56] Thus, the latency for ATL is as long as 60 years. There are approximately 1 million carriers of HTLV-1 in Japan alone; given the 2% to 5% ATL rate, 20,000 to 50,000 infected Japanese would be expected to develop ATL at some point in their lives. Why only a small percentage develops disease remains unknown. In any infectious disease, however, only a portion of the infected population develops clinical illness. No significant difference in incidence of ATL has been reported in two endemic areas of Japan—Kyushu (south) and Hokkaido (north)—where the environments and lifestyles are different, suggesting that no other exogenous factors are involved in the development of ATL. Investigators have reported, however, that some HLAs are linked to the immunologic response to HTLV-1 infection[39]; thus, the incidence of ATL in HTLV-1 infected persons might differ across races for genetic reasons.

Interestingly, HTLV-1 infection through transfusion does not induce ATL but does induce HAM/TSP. Similarly, HTLV-1 transmitted sexually in adulthood does not result in ATL. This may explain why the incidence of ATL is almost the same in females and males despite the 1.6-fold higher rate of HTLV-1 seropositivity in females. Because females are more likely than males to acquire HTLV-1 through sexual contact, they have a disproportionately low proportion of infection leading to malignancy.

HTLV-2 is not associated with ATL. Although type 2 virus was originally isolated from a patient with hairy T-cell leukemia,[4] only a few subsequent leukemia patients with HTLV-2 infection have been described. Thus, no association with any specific leukemia or other cancers has been established. Identification of HTLV-2–associated diseases has been hampered by an insufficient understanding of HTLV-2 epidemiology. Although sporadic carriers of HTLV-2 have been detected among drug users and among people coinfected with HIV, the distribution of HTLV-2 is far less well understood than is that of HTLV-1. A recent survey for serum antibodies to HTLV-2 infection identified clusters of HTLV-2 carriers in small villages in Central Africa[57] and in high-altitude areas in South America.[58] Further studies on cancers in these areas should identify diseases associated with HTLV-2 infection.

PATHOGENIC AND ONCOGENIC MECHANISMS

The target cells in vivo for HTLV-1 infection and malignant transformation are almost exclusively T cells with the CD4$^+$ phenotype.[30] The receptor for HTLV-1 infection has not yet been identified, so the viral tropism for CD4-positive T cells is not well understood. In vitro, cell-free viral particles of HTLV-1 show extremely low infectivity and usually cannot establish infection. HTLV-1 can be transmitted to CD4-positive T cells, however, by cocultivation with virus-producing cells. In this system, HTLV-1 can also be transmitted to a variety of human cells including T and B cells, macrophages, fibroblasts, and epithelial cells; within these cells, HTLV-1 proteins will be expressed. Thus, the cocultivation system does not appear to mimic the natural in vivo process. HTLV-1 can also be transmitted to various animals, but, unfortunately, not to mice.

Despite the many cells that are potentially infectable, only CD4-positive T cells are immortalized on infection. The immortalized cells mimic some characteristics of in vivo ATL cells, expressing high levels of IL-2Rα and proliferating in an IL-2R–dependent fashion.[30,59] These observations indicate that HTLV-1 transforms with cell-type specificity for CD4-positive T cells. Such specificity might not be strict, however, because transgenic mice carrying HTLV-1 genes suffer from mesenchymal tumors.[60]

Without exception, provirus integration in malignant ATL cells is clonal.[16] This clonality clearly indicates a single infected-cell origin of ATL, strongly supporting a causative role for HTLV-1 in ATL induction. No common site of integration has been observed among ATL patients, however.[61] Therefore, the role of HTLV-1 in leukemogenesis is independent of HTLV-1's site of integration. In this respect, HTLV-1 differs from the chronic retroviruses of other animals in which the virus usually integrates adjacent to a protooncogene (cis-acting effect). To explain the consistent oncogenic effects of HTLV-1 despite random integration, we must posit a trans-acting function of HTLV-1 in the leukemogenic process. Consistent with this proposal, HTLV-1 infection is able to immortalize CD4-positive T cells in vitro, however, other chronic retroviruses which do not carry the putative function are unable to immortalize cells in vitro culture.

Trans-acting factors of HTLV-1 have thus became a central issue of HTLV-1 study. What is this factor? What is its function? The Tax protein (p40^{tax}), encoded by pX region, was identified as a trans-acting factor. In activating transcription of HTLV-1 genome,[20,21,62,63] Tax is essential for viral gene expression and replication. The Rex protein (p27^{rex}) is also a trans-acting modulator of RNA processing; it is required for the expression of unspliced gag and env mRNAs, and thus is also essential for HTLV-1-gene expression and replication.[22,23] Of these two trans-acting viral products, Tax protein is thought to be the critical factor in ATL induction (Figure 11.3).

PUTATIVE ONCOGENIC PROPERTIES OF TAX

Observations supporting the role of Tax in ATL causation are Tax's abilities to immortalize human CD4-positive T cells in an IL-2–dependent fashion,[64] to transform rodent fibroblastic cell lines in vitro,[65] and to induce mesenchymal tumors in Tax transgenic mice.[60] How it effects these malignant changes is unclear. Multiple potential transforming functions of Tax have been identified, including (1) activation of cellular transcription factors, (2) suppression of transcriptional inhibitory protein, and (3) suppression of cell cycle inhibitors. These activations and suppressions, described below, all result from Tax binding to cellular target proteins that are involved in transcription or in cell cycle control.

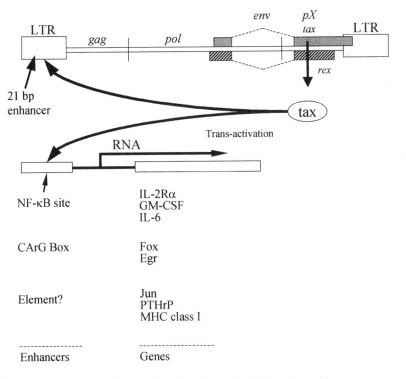

Figure 11.3. Transcriptional activation of cellular genes by Tax protein. Tax protein *trans*-activates the viral transcription responding to the 21-bp enhancer containing cyclic AMP-response element (CRE). The protein also *trans*-activates various cellular genes responding to NF-κB binding site and to CArG box in serum response element (SRE).

Activation of Cellular Transcription Factors

Tax binds to cellular transcription factors to activate transcription of specific genes. The genes that are activated include lymphokines (IL-2,[66] IL-3,[67] IL-5,[68] GM-CSF,[33] tumor necrosis factor−β,[69] transforming growth factorβ,[70] PTHrP[31], lymphokine receptors (IL-2Rα[66,71−73] and IL-2Rγ (K. Sugamura, personal communication)), cell-surface proteins (MHC class I[74] and gp36 (OX40 ligand)[75]), and a group of nuclear oncogenes (c-*fos*,[76] c-*egr*,[77] and c-*jun*).[77] All these gene expressions are activated through augmentation of the enhancer to which a specific transcription factor binds. Tax does not bind to these enhancer DNAs directly but does bind to the enhancer binding proteins. The enhancer binding proteins identified to date are (1) cyclic AMP-response element binding protein (CREB)[78−80] and, for activation of the 21-enhancer in the LTR of HTLV-1, CRE modulator protein (CREM)[79]; (2) for activation of the NF-κB binding site in IL-2 receptor α gene, NF-κB family proteins including NF-κB p50,[81] p52,[82] p65,[83,84] and c-Rel[83]; and (3) for activation of serum response element in c-*fos* gene, p67SRF.[85] Tax protein, thus, forms a complex with specific enhancer DNA through its binding proteins. Generally, these transcription factors are regulated strictly by cellular machinery—for example, by signal-dependent phosphorylation. Tax protein in HTLV-1–infected cells, however, can bind to these transcription factors and activate the specific transcription without any stimulatory signals. Thus, HTLV-1–infected cells exhibit specific phenotypes or undergo continuous proliferation as though they were being stimulated. Tax is also known to bind to TATA binding protein (TBP), a factor in the basic transcription machinery.[86] This finding strongly suggests that Tax serves as a bridging factor between the enhancer and the TATA box for formation of the initiation complex.

Suppression of Transcriptional Inhibitory Protein

Tax binds to IχB proteins, inhibitory proteins of NF-χB, and suppresses their inhibitory activity on NF-χB (Figure 11.4).[87,88] The IχB family consists of IχBα, β, and γ, and NF-χB precursors, p100 and p105. Among these, IkBα is the major component in human T cells. In resting cells, NF-χB proteins are bound to IχB proteins in the cytoplasm and are kept as an

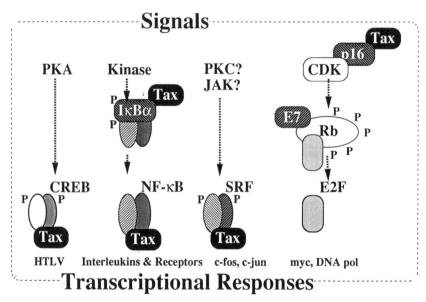

Figure 11.4. Summary of mechanisms by which Tax affects cellular function. Tax protein binds to transcription factors, CREB, NF-χB family proteins, SRF, which are all enhancer binding proteins. Tax also binds to IχBα which inhibits NF-χB proteins in cytoplasm and suppresses its inhibitory function. Tax further binds to p16, a tumor suppressor protein and an inhibitor of CDK-4 and -6. Through this binding, Tax activates CDK-4 and -6 and results in phosphorylation of Rb protein.

inactive form. On stimulation of cells, IκBα is phosphorylated and desta-bilized. The released NF-κB proteins are consequently translocated into the nucleus to activate transcription. In HTLV-1-infected T cells, Tax binds to IκBα and continuously destabilizes IκBα/ NF-κB complex, thus resulting in constitutive activation of NF-κB. Tax has also been shown to bind to IκBγ,[87] p100,[89] and p105.[90]

In the regulation of the NF-κB system, an interesting mechanism has been characterized. Activated NF-κB activates expression of IkBα gene, thus producing more inhibitory protein IκBα.[91] This feedback mechanism activation makes activation of NF-κB transient. In HTLV-1–infected T cells, however, Tax binds to and destabilizes IκBα protein. Thus, func-tional IκBα protein is maintained at a low level,[88] although IkBα mRNA is expressed at a high level. These low levels of IκBα in the face of high gene expression have also been demonstrated in primary leukemic cells from some cases of ATL.[92] These results demonstrate that destabilization of IκBα protein is constitutively taking place in leukemic cells in vivo, activating many genes that are regulated by NF-κB.

Suppression of Cell-Cycle Inhibitors

Tax binds to p16INK4A, a cell cycle inhibitor, and suppresses the latter's inhibitory activity (Figure 11.4).[93] The tumor suppressor protein, p16INK4A, binds to cell-cycle–dependent kinase 4 (Cdk4) and inactivates the kinase activity that phosphorylates Rb protein. Unphosphorylated Rb binds to and keeps inactive E2F, whose function is required for the ex-pression of a series of genes necessary for G_1 progression into S phase. Therefore, p16INK4A arrests the cell cycle at G_1 through the Rb-signaling pathway. Binding of Tax to p16INK4A has been found to suppress the latter's inhibitory effect on Cdk4 activity, and thus to result in activation of the kinase.[93] In p16INK4A-deficient cells, overexpression of p16INK4A in-duced G_1 arrest of cells, but coexpression of Tax rescued the cells from G1 arrest. Thus, Tax can compete successfully with the growth inhibitory activity of p16INK4A.[93]

In human cancer cells, p16INK4A is frequently deleted. This deletion is observed most commonly in cells that have no defect in the Rb gene, indicating that this signaling pathway is critical for normal cells. It is well known that transforming proteins of DNA tumor viruses bind to Rb and inactivate the Rb signaling pathway (see Chapters 4 and 6). If the same complementary inactivation of p16INK4A and Rb is used by different vi-ruses, that suggests a critical role for this pathway in viral oncogenesis, and specifically for the ATL leukemogenic process.

Tax and Cell Transformation

Which of the functions described here is responsible for transformation? Tax has been demonstrated to activate specific transcription through two independent mechanisms; activation of transcription factors and suppression of transcriptional inhibitory factors. Furthermore, Tax suppresses a cell-cycle inhibitor and directly affects the cell cycle. It is unknown whether one specific function of Tax, however, can be deemed sufficient for T-cell immortalization or transformation. Some mutants of Tax are active in the CREB pathway but not in the NF-κB pathway, and vice versa (the effects of these mutants on the SRF pathway are unknown). These mutants have been used for transformation assay of rodent fibroblasts and also in the study of immortalization of T cells. Two groups[94,95] reported that the Tax mutant that is active in the CREB pathway, but not in the NF-κB pathway, transformed rodent fibroblasts and immortalized human T cells, suggesting that the CREB pathway is responsible for immortalization or transformation. Unfortunately, another group[96] reported exactly the opposite observation. More investigations are required along this line. Before the picture can be clarified, however, the independent contributions of cell-cycle modulation and the SRF pathway in transformation must also be evaluated. In the end, Tax expression may not be sufficient for induction of final ATL. Multistep processes involving many genes are typically required before cancers can occur. It may be most appropriate to expect that the pleiotropic effects of Tax contribute at various steps, promoting cells into more malignant phenotypes or accelerating the process.

The level of Tax expression in leukemic cell in vivo also belies the critical role observed in vitro. In quantitative assays, 90% of leukemic cells in vivo are completely negative for expression of HTLV-1 messages, as determined by reverse transcriptase-mediated polymerase chain reaction.[97] Such low expression is also seen in HTLV-1–infected nonleukemic cells in vivo. This discrepancy with the in vitro results is not due to defects of the proviruses in vivo: once cells are taken out of plasma and placed in culture in the presence of calf or bovine serum, the HTLV-1 proviruses efficiently begin expression within several hours. Instead, the lower expression in vivo suggests the presence of a suppressive factor in the blood of infected individuals. This factor appears not to be antibodies against viral proteins, but it has not been characterized further. Even a low level of Tax expression, however, is sufficient to maintain the transformed phenotypes in vivo. Moreover, since ATL cells do not replicate in peripheral blood, low levels of Tax expression in blood do not negate a role for Tax in cell transformation and growth. Viral expression must be analyzed carefully in lymph nodes or spleen or skin, where ATL cells replicate efficiently.

It is also possible that Tax is critical at a specific stage of leukemogenesis—perhaps at an early stage—but plays no role later on. It is not easy to prove this so-called "hit-and-run model," but several facts support it. For example, although only a portion of leukemic cells in vivo express HTLV-1 message, the great majority of these cells express IL-2Rα at their cell surface at a high level. Thus, Tax alone may not be able to explain the high expression of IL-2Rα. Furthermore, a fibroblast cell line established from a transgenic mouse carrying *tax* gene showed growth properties dependent on NF-ϰB, but not on Tax. Although this observation was made in an artificial cell line, it suggests the dispensable situation of Tax in proliferation of this cell line. The possibility that Tax is not obligatory for transformation contrasts with the transforming proteins of DNA tumor viruses. For example, E6/7 genes are uniformly required for cell transformation by human papillomaviruses (see Chapter 6). In addition, antisense RNA of E6/7 inhibited growth of HeLa cells that had been maintained in culture for many years. The inhibition was specific to E6/7-expressing cells, strongly suggesting the requirement of E6/7 in the maintenance of transformed phenotypes of cancer cells. No such strong evidence for an essential role in transformation has been reported for Tax.

CONTROL OF INFECTION AND CLINICAL MANAGEMENT

With virally induced cancers, we can generally focus on three ways to control the specific cancers: primary prevention through prevention of the viral infection; secondary prevention through inhibition of the viral replication in infected individuals; and tertiary prevention by treatment of cancer patients. In ATL induced by HTLV-1 infection, only the first of these—primary prevention—has been well studied.

As mentioned, transmission of HTLV-1 occurs by three routes: (1) nursing of infants by infected mothers, (2) blood transfusion, and (3) sexual relations. Because transmission patterns are known, prevention of HTLV-1 infection is feasible. The major, natural route of viral transmission is from mother to child via infected T cells in breast milk. Therefore, stopping breast-feeding should prevent infection of children. This possibility is being tested in Nagasaki City, Japan (S. Hino, personal communication). After providing informed consent, pregnant women are surveyed for HTLV-1 antibodies; those who are seropositive are asked to avoid breast-feeding. The trial is still in progress, but the results thus far available indicate a drastic reduction in the prevalence of childhood infection, from about 30% to just a few percent. The early success of this trial provides direct evidence for viral transmission through milk and suggests the possibility of eliminating ATL in the next few generations. Unfortunately, not all children of seropositive mothers who did not breast-feed remained seronegative.

Transfusion of seropositive blood transmits HTLV-1 to two thirds of the recipients. With the introduction of HTLV-1 screening systems in blood banks, seropositive blood is now discarded in Japan, and viral transmission through transfusion has been greatly reduced. Application of these systems to populations in all endemic areas is an urgent measure to prevent HTLV-1 infection.

Unfortunately, we have thus far learned little about secondary or tertiary prevention. Other than the routine chemotherapeutic treatment regimens for leukemias and lymphomas, no specific therapy is currently available for treatment of HTLV-1 or ATL. Specific strategies—such as using monoclonal antibodies against cell surface markers of activated T cells or injecting toxin-conjugated antibodies—have been tested; none of them showed great efficacy. Other strategies, such as targeting the viral antigens, are not promising, because the vast majority of leukemic cells do not express HTLV-1 antigens at a significant level. These problems seem to be difficult to overcome.

FUTURE DIRECTIONS

It is generally accepted that tumorigenesis progresses through a multistep process, and such a process apears to occur in ATL as well. At the initial stage, a regulatory gene, *tax*, is responsible for abnormal growth of HTLV-1–infected cells, but apparently is not sufficient for the malignant transformation of infected T cells. The additional molecular events that allow for a clonal, malignant expansion of infected cells remain unknown.

Advanced studies on HTLV-1 and modern technologies have made it possible to prevent much viral transmission; such techniques, however, may not be feasible everywhere that HTLV-1 is endemic. For example, cessation of breast-feeding might result in serious nutritional deficiencies in children in developing countries. Development of an efficient vaccine is imperative for the complete eradication of HTLV-1 and its associated diseases.

REFERENCES

1. Poiesz BJ, Ruscetti FW, Gazdar AF, Bunn PA, Minna JD, Gallo RC. Detection and isolation of type C retrovirus particles from fresh and cultured lymphocytes of a patient with cutaneous T-cell lymphoma. Proc Natl Acad Sci USA 1980;77:7415–7419.
2. Yoshida M, Miyoshi I, Hinuma Y. Isolation and characterization of retrovirus from cell lines of human adult T cell leukemia and its implication in the diseases. Proc Natl Acad Sci USA 1982;79:2031–2035.
3. Hinuma Y, Nagata K, Misaka M, Nakai M, Matsumoto T, Kinoshita K, Shirakawa S, Miyoshi I. Adult T cell leukemia: antigen in an ATL cell line and detection of antibodies to the antigen in human sera. Proc Natl Acad Sci USA 1981;78:6476–6480.
4. Kalyanaraman VS, Sarngadharan MG, Robert-Guroff M, Miyoshi I, Blayney D, Golde D, Gallo RC. A new subtype of human T cell leukemia virus (HTLV-II) associated with a T cell variant of hairy T cell leukemia. Science 1982;218:571–573.
5. Yoshida M, Seiki M, Yamaguchi K, Takatsuki K. Monoclonal integration of HTLV in all primary tumors of adult T-cell leukemia suggests causative role of HTLV in the disease. Proc Natl Acad Sci USA 1984;81:2534–2537.
6. Osame M, Matsumoto M, Usuku K, Izumo S, Ijichi N, Amitani H, Tara M, Igata A. Chronic progressive myelopathy associated with elevated antibodies to

human T-lymphotropic virus type 1 and adult T-cell leukemia-like cells. Ann Neurol 1987;21:117–22.

7. Gessain A, Barin F, Vernant JC, Gout O, Maurs L, Calender A, De The G. Antibodies to human T lymphotropic virus type 1 in patients with tropical spastic paraparesis. Lancet 1985;2:407–410.

8. Mochizuki M, Watanabe T, Yamaguchi K, Takatsuki K, Yoshimura K, Shirao M, Nakashima S, Mori S, Araki S, Miyata N. HTLV-I uveitis: a distinct clinical entity caused by HTLV-I. Gan (Jpn J Cancer Res) 1992;83:236–239.

9. Miyazaki K, Yamaguchi K, Tohya T, Ohba T, Takatsuki K, Okamura H. Human T-cell leukemia virus type I infection as oncogenic and prognostic risk factor in cervical and vaginal carcinoma. Obstet Gynecol 1991;77:107–110.

10. Nakada K, Yamaguchi K, Furugen S, Nakasone T, Nakasone K, Oshiro Y, Kohakura M, Hinuma Y, Seiki M, Yoshida M, Matutes E, Catovsky D, Ishii T, Takatsuki K. Monoclonal integration of proviral DNA in patients with strongyloidiases. Int J Cancer 1987;40:145–148.

11. Iwakura Y, Tosu M, Yoshida E, Takiguchi M, Sato K, Kitajima I, Nisioka K, Yamamoto K, Takeda T, Hatanaka M, Yamamoto H, Sekiguchi T. Induction of inflammatory arthropathy resembling rheumatoid arthritis in mice transgenic for HTLV-I. Science 1991; 253:1026–1028.

12. Sagata N, Yasunaga T, Tsuzuku-Kawamura J, Ohishi K, Ogawa Y, Ikawa Y. Complete nucleotide sequence of the genome of bovine leukemia virus. Its evolutionary relationship. Proc Natl Acad Sci USA 1985;82:677–681.

13. Miyoshi I, Fujishita M, Taguchi H, Matsubayashi K, Miwa N, Tanioka Y. Natural infection in non-human primates with adult T-cell leukemia virus or a closely related agent. Int J Cancer 1983;32:333–336.

14. Komuro A, Watanabe T, Miyoshi I, Hayami M, Tsujimoto H, Seiki M, Yoshida M. Detection and characterization of simian retroviruses homologous to human T-cell leukemia virus type I. Virology 1984;138:373–378.

15. Guo HG, Wong-Stall F, Gallo RC. Novel viral sequences related to human T-cell leukemia virus in T cells of a seropositive baboon. Science 1984;223:1195–1197.

16. Watanabe T, Seiki M, Tsujimoto H, Miyoshi I, Hayami M, Yoshida M. Sequence homology of the simian retrovirus (STLV) genome with human T-cell leukemia virus type I (HTLV-I). Virology 1985;144:59–65.

17. Seiki M, Hattori S, Hirayama Y, Yoshida M. Human adult T cell leukemia virus: complete nucleotide sequence of the provirus genome integrated in leukemia cell DNA . Proc Natl Acad Sci USA 1983;80:3618–3622.

18. Yoshida M, Seiki M. Recent advances in the molecular biology of HTLV-1: transactivation of viral and cellular genes. Annu Rev Immunol 1987;5:541–559.

19. Yoshida M. HTLV-1 Tax: regulation of gene expression and disease. Trends Microbiol 1993;1:131–135.

20. Sodroski JG, Rosen CA, Haseltine WA. Trans-acting transcriptional activation of the long terminal repeat of human T lymphotropic viruses in infected cells. Science 1984;226:177–179.

21. Fujisawa J, Seiki M, Kiyokawa T, Yoshida M. Functional activation of long terminal repeat of human T-cell leukemia virus type I by trans-activator. Proc Natl Acad Sci USA 1985;82:2277–2281.

22. Hidaka M, Inoue M, Yoshida M, Seiki M. Post-transcriptional regulator (rex) of HTLV-1 initiates expression of viral structural proteins but suppresses expression of regulatory proteins. EMBO J 1988;7:519–523.

23. Inoue J, Itoh M, Akizawa T, Toyoshima H, Yoshida M. HTLV-1 Rex protein accumulates unspliced RNA in the nucleus as well as in cytoplasm. Oncogene 1991;6:1753–1757.

24. Seiki M, Hikikoshi A, Taniguchi T, Yoshida M. Expression of the pX gene of HTLV-1: general splicing mechanism in the HTLV family. Science 1985;-228:1532–1534.

25. Nagashima K, Yoshida M, Seiki M. A single species of pX mRNA of HTLV-1 encodes trans-activator p40x and two other phosphoproteins. J Virol 1986;-60:394–399.

26. Uchiyama T, Yodoi J, Sagawa K, Takatsuki K, Uchino H. Adult T cell leukemia. Clinical and hematologic features of 16 cases. Blood 1977;50:481–491.

27. Tajima K, Tominaga S, Suchi T, Kawagoe T, Komoda H, Hinuma Y, Oda T, Fujita K. Epidemiological analysis of the distribution of antibody to adult T cell leukemia virus associated antigen: possible horizontal transmission of adult T cell leukemia virus. Gan (Jpn J Cancer Res) 1982;73:893–901.

28. Blattner W, Kalyanaraman VS, Robert-Guroff M, Lister TA, Galton DA, Sarin PS, Crawford MH, Catovsky D, Greaves M, Gallo RC. The human type C retrovirus, HTLV in Blacks from the Caribbean region, and relationship to adult T-cell leukemia/lymphoma. Int J Cancer 1982;30:257–264.

29. Kawano F, Yamaguchi K, Nishimura H, Tsuda H, Takatsuki K. Variation in the clinical courses of adult T-cell leukemia. Cancer 1985;55:851–856.

30. Hattori T, Uchiyama T, Tobinai K, Takatsuki K, Uchino H. Surface phenotype of Japanese adult T-cell leukemia cells characterized by monoclonal antibodies. Blood 1981;58:645–647.

31. Uchiyama T, Hori T, Tsudo M, Wano Y, Umadome H, Tamori S, Yodoi J, Maeda M, Sawami H, Uchino H. Interleukin-2 receptor (Tac antigen) expressed on adult T-cell leukemia cells. J Clin Invest 1985;76:446–453.

32. Watanabe T, Yamaguchi K, Takatsuki K, Osame M, Yoshida M. Constitutive expression of parathyroid hormone-related protein (PTHrP) gene in HTLV-1 carriers and adult T cell leukemia patients which can be trans-activated by HTLV-1 tax gene. J Exp Med 1990;172:759–765.

33. Wano Y, Hattori T, Matsuoka M, Takatsuki K, Chua AO, Gubler U, Greene WC. Interleukin 1 gene expression in adult T-cell leukemia. J Clin Invest 1987;80:911–916.

34. Miyatake S, Seiki M, Malefijt RD-W, Heike T, Fujisawa, J-I, Takebe Y, Nishida J, Shilomai J, Yokota T, Yoshida M, Arai K-I, Arai N. Activation of T cell-derived lymphokine genes in T cells and fibroblasts; effects of human T cell leukemia virus type I p40^x protein and bovine papilloma virus encoded E2 protein. Nucleic Acids Res 1988;16:6547–6566.

35. Kamada N, Sakurai M, Miyamoto K, Sanada I, Sadamori N, Fukuhara S, Abe S, Shiraishi Y, Abe T, Kaneko Y, Shimoyama M. Chromosome abnormalities in adult T-cell leukemia/lymphoma: a karyotype review committee report. Cancer Res 1992;52:1481–1493.

36. Yoshida M, Osame M, Usuku K, Matsumoto M, Igata A. Viruses detected in HTLV-1-associated myelopathy and adult T-cell leukemia are identical in DNA blotting. Lancet 1987;1:1085–1086.

37. Nakamura M, Kuroki M, Kira J, Itoyama Y, Shiraki H, Kuroda N, Washitani Y, Nakano S, Nagafuchi S, Anzai K, et al. Elevated antibodies to synthetic peptides of HTLV-1 envelope transmembrane glycoproteins in patients with HAM/TSP. J Neuroimmunol 1991;35:167–177.

38. Yoshida M, Osame M, Kawai H, Toita M, Kuwasaki N, Nishida Y, Hiraki Y, Takahashi K, Nomura K, Sonoda S, Eiraku N, Ijichi S, Usuku K. Increased replication of HTLV-1 in HTLV-1-associated myelopathy. Ann Neurol 1989; 26:331–335.

39. Usuku K, Sonoda S, Osame M, Yashiki S, Takahashi K, Matsumoto M, Sawada T, Tsuji K, Tara M, Igata A. HLA haplotype-linked high immune responsiveness against HTLV-1 in HTLV-1-associated myelopathy: comparison with adult T-cell leukemia/lymphoma. Ann Neurol 1988;23:143–150.

40. Yanagihara R, Nerurkar VR, Ajdukiewicz AB. Comparison between strains of human T lymphotropic virus type I isolated from inhabitants of the Solomon islands and Papua New Guinea. J Infect Dis 1991;164:443–449.

41. Watanabe T. HTLV type I (U.S. isolate) and ATLV (Japanese isolate) are the same species of human retrovirus. Virology 1984;133:238–241.

42. Komurian F, Pelloquin F, De Thé G. In vivo genomic variability of human T-cell leukemia virus type I depends more upon geography than upon pathologies. J Virol 1991;65:3770–3778.

43. Miura T, Fukunaga T, Igarashi T, Yamashita M, Ido E, Funahashi S, Ishida T, Washio K, Ueda S, Hashimoto K, Yoshida M, Osame M, Singhal BS, Zaninovic V, Cartier L, Sonoda S, Tajima K, Ina Y, Gojobori T, Hayami M. Phylogenetic subtypes of human T-lymphotropic virus type I and their relations to the anthropological background. Proc Natl Acad Sci USA 1994;91:1124–1127.

44. Hall WW, Takahashi H, Liu C, Kaplan MH, Scheewind O, Ijichi S, Nagashima K, Gallo RC. Multiple isolates and characteristics of human T-cell leukemia virus type II. J Virol 1992;66:2456–2463.

45. Miyoshi I, Taguchi H, Fujishita M, Niiya K, Kitagawa T, Ohtsuki Y, Akagi T. Asymptomatic type C virus carriers in the family of an adult T cell leukemia patient. Gan (Jpn J Cancer Res) 1982;73:339–340.

46. Hino S, Yamaguchi K, Katamine S, Sugiyama H, Amagasaki T, Kinoshita K, Yoshida Y, Doi H, Tsuji Y, Miyamoto T. Mother to child transmission of human T cell leukemia virus type I. Gan (Jpn J Cancer Res) 1985;76:474–480.

47. Kusuhara K, Sonoda S, Takahashi K, Tokunaga K, Fukushige J, Ueda K. Mother to child transmission of human T cell leukemia virus type I (HTLV-I): a fifteen year follow up in Okinawa. Int J Cancer 1987;40:755–757.

48. Kinoshita K, Amagasaki T, Hino S, Dio H, Yamanouchi K, Ban N, Momita S, Ikeda S, Kamihira S, Ichimaru M, Katamine S, Miyamoto T, Tsuji Y, Ishimaru T, Yamabe T, Ito M, Kamura S, Tsuda T. Milk-borne transmission of HTLV-1 from carrier mothers to their children. Gan (Jpn J Cancer Res) 1987;78:674–680.

49. Okochi K, Sato H, Hinuma Y. A retrospective study on transmission of adult T cell leukemia virus by blood transfusion: seroconversion in recipients. Vox Sang 1983;46:245–253.

50. Tajima K, Tominaga S, Suchi T, Kawagoe T, Komoda H, Hinuma Y, Oda T, Fujita K. Epidemiological analysis of the distribution of antibody to adult T cell leukemia virus associated antigen: possible horizontal transmission of adult T cell leukemia virus. Gan (Jpn J Cancer Res) 1982;73:893–901.

51. Tajima K, Ito S-I, Tsushima ATL Study Group. Prospective studies of HTLV-I and associated diseases in Japan. In: Blattner WA, ed. Human Retrovirology: HTLV. New York: Raven Press, 1990;267–279.

52. Miyoshi I, Kubonishi I, Yoshimoto S, Akagi T, Ohtsuki Y, Shiraishi Y, Nagata K, Hinuma Y. Type C virus particles in a cord T cell line derived by cocultivating

normal human cord leukocytes and human leukemic T cells. Nature 1981; 294:770–771.

53. Shimoyama M, Kagami Y, Shimotohno K, Miwa M, Minato K, Tobinai K, Suemasu K, Sugimura T. Adult T-cell leukemia/lymphoma not associated with human T-cell leukemia virus type I. Proc Natl Acad Sci USA 1986;83:4524–4528.

54. Poiesz BJ, Ruscetti FW, Reitz MS, Kalyanaraman VS, Gallo RC. Isolation of a new type-C retrovirus (HTLV) in primary uncultured cells of a patient with Sezary T-cell leukemia. Nature 1981;294:268–271.

55. Tajima K. The 4th nation-wide study of adult T-cell leukemia/lymphoma (ATL) in Japan: estimates of risk of ATL and its geographical and clinical features. The T- and B-cell Malignancy Study Group. Int J Cancer 1990;45: 237–243.

56. Tajima K, Kamura S, Ito S, Ito M, Nagatomo M, Kinoshita K, Ikeda S. Epidemiological features of HTLV-I carriers and incidence of ATL in an ATL-endemic island: a report of the community-based co-operative study in Tsushima, Japan. Int J Cancer 1987;40:741–746.

57. Garin B, Gosselin S, de The G, Gessain A. HTLV-I/II infection in a high viral endemic area of Zaire, Central Africa: comparative evaluation of serology, PCR, and significance of indeterminate western blot pattern. J Med Virol 1994;44:104–109.

58. Cartier L, Araya F, Castillo JL, Zaninovic V, Hayami M, Miura T, Imai J, Sonoda S, Shiraki H, Miyamoto K, Tajima K. Southernmost carriers of HTLV-I/II in the world. Gan (Jpn J Cancer Res) 1993;84:1–3.

59. Arima N, Daitoku Y, Ohgaki S, Fukumori J, Tanaka H, Yamamoto Y, Fujimoto K, Onoue K. Autocrine growth of interleukin 2 producing leukemic cells in a patient with adult T cell leukemia. Blood 1986;68:779–782.

60. Nerenberg M, Hinrichs SH, Reynolds RK, Khoury G, Jay G. The tat gene of human T lymphotropic virus type I induces mesenchymal tumors in transgenic mice. Science 1987;237:1324–1329.

61. Seiki M, Eddy R, Shows TB, Yoshida M. Nonspecific integration of the HTLV provirus genome into adult T-cell leukemia cells. Nature 1984;309:640–642.

62. Felber BK, Paskalis H, Kleinman-Ewing C, Wong-Staal F, Pavlakis GN. The pX protein of HTLV-1 is a transcriptional activator of its long terminal repeats. Science 1985;229:675–679.

63. Chen ISY, Slamon DJ, Rosenblatt JD, Shah NP, Quan SG, Wachsman W. The x gene is essential for HTLV replication. Science 1985;229:54–58.

64. Grassman R, Dengler C, Muller-Fleckenstein I, Fleckenstein B, McGuire K, Dokhelar M, Sodroski J, Haseltine W. Transformation to continuous growth of primary human T lymphocytes by human T cell leukemia virus type I X-region genes transduced by a Herpesvirus saimiri vector. Proc Natl Acad Sci USA 1989;86:3351–3355.

65. Tanaka A, Takahashi C, Yamaoka S, Nosaka T, Maki M, Hatanaka M. Oncogenic transformation by the tax gene of human T cell leukemia virus type I in vitro. Proc Natl Acad Sci USA 1990;87:1071–1075.

66. Inoue J, Seiki M, Taniguchi T, Tsuru S, Yoshida M. Induction of interleukin 2 receptor gene expression by p40x encoded by human T-cell leukemia virus type I. EMBO J 1986;5:2883–2888.

67. Wolin M, Kornuc M, Hong C, Shin SK, Lee F, Lau R, Nimer S. Differential effect of HTLV infection and HTLV Tax on interleukin 3 expression. Oncogene 1993;8:1905–1911.

68. Yamashita I, Katamine S, Moriuchi R, Nakamura Y, Miyamoto T, Eguchi K, Nagataki S. Transactivation of the human interleukin-6 gene by human T-lymphotropic virus type 1 Tax protein. Blood 1994;84:1573–1578.

69. Kobayashi N, Hamamoto Y, Yamamoto N. Production of tumor necrosis factor by human T cell lines infected with HTLV-1 may cause their high susceptibility to human immunodeficiency virus infection. Med Microbiol Immunol (Berl) 1990;179:115–122.

70. Nakajima T, Kitamura K, Yamashita N, Sakane T, Mizushima Y, Delespesse G, Lal RB. Constitutive expression and production of tumor necrosis factor-beta in T-cell lines infected with HTLV-I and HTLV-II. Biochem Biophys Res Commun 1993;191:371–377.

71. Maruyama M, Shibuya H, Harada H, Hatakeyama M, Seiki M, Fujita T, Inoue J, Yoshida M, Taniguchi T. Evidence for aberrant activation of the interleukin-2 autocrine loop by HTLV-1 encoded by p40^x and T3/Ti complex triggering. Cell 1987;48:493–500.

72. Cross SL, Feinberg MB, Wolf JB, Holbrook NJ, Wong-Staal F, Leonard WJ. Regulation of the human interleukin-2 receptor a chain promoter: activation of a nonfunctional promoter by the trans-activator gene of HTLV-1. Cell 1987;49:47–56.

73. Bours V, Villalobos J, Burd PR, Kelly K, Siebenlist U. Cloning of a mitogen-inducible gene encoding a kB DNA-binding protein with homology to the *rel* oncogene and to cell-cycle motifs. Nature 1990;348:76–80.

74. Sawada M, Suzumura A, Yoshida M, Marunouchi T. Human T-cell leukemia virus type I *trans* activator induces class I major histocompatibility complex antigen expression in glial cells. J Virol 1990;64:4002–4006.

75. Baum PR, Gayle RB III, Ramsdell F, Srinivasan S, Sorensen RA, Watson ML, Seldin MF, Baker E, Sutherland GR, Clifford KN, Alderson MR, Goodwin RG, Fanslow WC. Molecular characterization of murine and human OX40/OX40 ligand systems: identification of a human OX40 ligand as the HTLV-1–regulated protein gp34. EMBO J 1994;13:3992–4001.

76. Fujii M, Sassone-Corsi P, Verma IM. C-fos promoter trans-activation by the tax$_1$ protein of human T-cell leukemia virus type I. Proc Natl Acad Sci USA 1988;85:8526–8530.

77. Fujii M, Niki T, Mori T, Matsuda T, Matsui M, Nomura N, Seiki M. HTLV-1 Tax induces expression of various immediate early serum responsive genes. Oncogene 1991;6:1023–1029.

78. Zhao L-J, Giam C-Z. Interaction of the human T-cell lymphotrophic virus type I (HTLV-I) transcriptional activator Tax with cellular factors that bind specifically to the 21-base-pair repeats in the HTLV-I enhancer. Proc Natl Acad Sci USA 1991;88:11445–11449.

79. Suzuki T, Fujisawa J-I, Toita M, Yoshida M. A trans-activator Tax of human T-cell leukemia virus type 1 (HTLV-1) interacts with AP-responsive element (CRE) binding and CRE modulator proteins that bind to the 21-base-pair enhancer of HTLV-1. Proc Natl Acad Sci USA 1993;90:610–614.

80. Zhao L-J, Giam C-Z. Human T-cell lymphotropic virus type I (HTLV-I) transcriptional activator, Tax, enhances CREB binding to HTLV-I 21-base-pair repeats by protein-protein interaction. Proc Natl Acad Sci USA 1992;89:7070–7074.

81. Suzuki T, Hirai H, Fujisawa J, Fujita T, Yoshida M. A trans-activator Tax of human T-cell leukemia virus type 1 binds to NF-κB p50 and serum response

factor (SRF) and associates with enhancer DNAs of the NF-κB site and CArG box. Oncogene 1993;8:2391–2397.

82. Murakami T, Hirai H, Suzuki T, Fujisawa J, Yoshida M. HTLV-1 Tax enhances NF-κB2 expression and binds to the products p52 and p100, but does not suppress the inhibitory function of p100. Virology 1995;206:1066–1074.

83. Suzuki T, Hirai H, Yoshida M. Tax protein of HTLV-1 interacts with the Rel homology domain of NF-κB p65 and c-Rel proteins bound to the NF-κB binding site and activates transcription. Oncogene 1994;9:3099–3105.

84. Pepin N, Roulston A, Lacoste J, Lin R, Hiscott J. Subcellular redistribution of HTLV-1 Tax protein by NF-kappa B/Rel transcription factors. Virology 1994; 204:706–716.

85. Fujii M, Tsuchiya H, Chuhjo T, Akizawa T, Seiki M. Interaction of HTLV-1 Tax1 with p67^{SRF} causes the aberrant induction of cellular immediate early genes through CArG boxes. Genes Dev 1992;6:2066–2076.

86. Caron C, Rousset R, Beraud C, Moncollin V, Egly JM, Jalinot P. Functional and biochemical interaction of the HTLV-I Tax1 transactivator with TBP. EMBO J 1993;12:4269–4278.

87. Hirai H, Suzuki T, Fujisawa J, Inoue J, Yoshida M. Tax protein of human T-cell leukemia virus type I binds to the ankyrin motifs of inhibitory factor kB and induces nuclear translocation of transcription factor NF-κB proteins for transcriptional activation. Proc Natl Acad Sci USA 1994;91:3584–3588.

88. Suzuki T, Hirai H, Murakami T, Yoshida M. Tax protein of HTLV-1 destabilizes the complexes of NF-κβ and Iκβ-α and induces nuclear translocation of NF-κβ for transcriptional activation. Oncogene 1995;10:1199–1207.

89. Beraud C, Sun S, Ganchi P, Ballard DW, Greene WC. Human T-cell leukemia virus type 1 Tax associates with and is negatively regulated by the NF-κB2 p100 gene product: implication for viral latency. Mol Cell Biol 1994;14:1374–1382.

90. Hirai H, Fujisawa J, Suzuki T, Ueda K, Muramatsu M, Tsuboi A, Arai N, Yoshida M. Trans-activator Tax of HTLV-1 binds to the NF-κB precursor p105. Oncogene 1992;7:1737–1742.

91. Sun SC, Ganchi PA, Ballard DW, Greene WC. NF-κ B controls expression of inhibitor I κ B alpha: evidence for an inducible autoregulatory pathway. Science 1993;259:1912–1915.

92. Inoue M, Matsuoka M, Yamaguchi K, Takatsuki K, Yoshida M. Characterization of mRNA expression of IκB α and NF-κB subfamilies in primary adult T-cell leukemia cells. Jpn J Cancer Res 1998;89:53–59.

93. Suzuki T, Kitao S, Matsushime H, Yoshida M. HTLV-1 Tax protein interacts with cyclin-dependent kinase inhibitor p16INK4A and counteracts its inhibitory activity to CDK4. EMBO J 1996;15:1607–1614.

94. Smith MR, Greene WC. Type I human T cell leukemia virus tax protein transforms rat fibroblasts through the cyclic adenosine monophosphate response element binding protein/activating transcription factor pathway. J Clin Invest 1991;88:1038–1042.

95. Rosin O, Koch C, Radant I, Semmes O, Jeang K-T, Grassmann R. The capacity of HTLV-1 Tax to induce NFkB activity is not required for T-cell immortalization. J AIDS Hum Retrovirol 1995;10:215.

96. Yamaoka S, Inoue H, Sakurai M, Sugiyama T, Hazama M, Yamada T, Hatanaka M. Constitutive activation of NF-κB is essential for transformation of rat fibroblasts by the human T-cell leukemia virus type I Tax protein. EMBO J 1996;15:873–887.

97. Kinoshita T, Shimoyama M, Tobinai K, Ito M, Ito S, Ikeda S, Tajima K, Shim-otohno K, Sugimura T. Detection of mRNA for the tax_1/rex_1 gene of human T cell leukemia virus type I in fresh peripheral blood mononuclear cells of adult T-cell leukemia patients and viral carriers by using the polymerase chain reaction. Proc Natl Acad Sci USA 1989;86:5620–5624.

III
INFECTIONS
AND CANCER:
PARASITES
AND BACTERIA

12

Schistosomiasis, Bladder and Colon Cancer

MIRIAM P. ROSIN AND LORNE J. HOFSETH

Schistosomiasis is a parasitic disease of worldwide importance, second only to malaria in its effect on human populations.[1] It is endemic in 74 tropical and subtropical countries, with 600 million people at risk and over 200 million currently infected. The infection is associated with significant morbidity and mortality.[2,3] Among the severe complications of the disease is the development of cancer.

Of the five species of *Schistosoma* that infect humans, three are responsible for the majority of schistosomal disease: *S. haematobium*, *S. mansoni*, and *S. japonicum*. Each of these infections has been associated with an increased rate of cancer. *S. mansoni* infections have been associated with the development of follicular lymphomas of the spleen, colorectal and hepatocellular cancers, and cholangiocarcinomas;[4–8]; however, epidemiological studies of these relationships tend either to have negative findings or to be inconclusive.[9,10] In contrast, there is strong, consistent evidence of causal relationships between *S. haematobium* infection and urinary bladder cancer[11] and between *S. japonicum* infection and colorectal cancer.[11] *S. japonicum* infections have also been associated with an increase in mortality from hepatocellular cancers, but the latter relationship is inconsistent, being seen in only a portion of epidemiological studies.[12,13] This chapter will focus on the relationship of *S. haematobium* and *S. japonicum* infections to urinary bladder and colorectal cancers, respectively, and will summarize the epidemiological evidence for these associations. The review includes a description of pathobiological changes occurring in tissues of infected individuals, and provides a mechanistic framework for the involvement of this disease in the genesis of these cancers. Before beginning these reviews, we briefly present the schistosome life cycle.

THE SCHISTOSOME LIFE CYCLE

Although humans are the definitive host for the schistosome species, the parasite spends a portion of its life cycle in an intermediate host: a snail. Human infection with this parasite occurs through contact of an individual with water containing cercariae that have been released from the snail. The cercariae penetrate the human's skin and transform into schistosomulum larvae, which migrate through the bloodstream to the hepatic portal system. There, the male and female worms undergo sexual maturation, pair up, and migrate into the venules draining the bladder and ureters (*S. haematobium*) or into the small intestine (*S. japonicum*) and large gut (*S. mansoni*). In these sites, adult worms live up to 30 years (average 3 to 8 years), with the female schistosomes laying ova (from about 300 per day per worm pair in the case of *S. haematobium* and *S. mansoni* to about 500 to 3500 per day per worm pair for *S. japonicum*), one half of which pass into the lumen of the bladder or intestine.[14] The eggs remaining in the submucosa elicit a chronic inflammatory reaction with associated pathology (granuloma formation, fibrosis). The eggs that do pass through the blood-vessel walls and epithelium into the lumen are assisted by lytic enzymes that are released by the miracidium, a larva that has matured inside the eggs.[15] These miracidia are released when the eggs are shed with the urine or feces into fresh water; they either infect an appropriate snail host within hours or die. The miracidium transforms into a sporocyst and matures to produce cercariae (several million for each miracidium) in the tissues of the snail. The cercariae are shed from the snail to infect a new human host.

Much of the significant pathology that occurs in schistosomiasis patients results from the retention of parasite eggs by the host tissue. These eggs release soluble antigens that incite a granulomatous response around them. The granuloma is composed of a complex mixture of cells that can include lymphocytes, eosinophils, macrophages, fibroblasts, neutrophils, plasma cells, sporadic mast cells, and multinucleated giant cells. The lymphocytes and macrophages secrete cytokines and other factors that promote fibrogenesis. Granulomatous lesions caused by *S. haematobium* eggs retained in the urinary bladder can lead to filling defects, stenosis, and eventual obstruction of the ureters—restricting urine flow and creating a condition that is associated with hydroureter, hydronephrosis, and failure of the ureteric sphincter. These changes are conducive to the development of ascending bacterial infection of the ureters and kidneys. The retention of *S. mansoni* and *S. japonicum* eggs in the submucosa of the intestine elicits a granulomatous reaction in this tissue, leading to hemorrhagic polyps, colitis, and colonic dysfunction. Finally, many of the eggs fail to lodge in the submucosa and are swept upstream into the hepatic portal vein, where they elicit a granulomatous reaction that can lead to periportal fibrosis, the presence of obstructive vascular lesions, portal hypertension, ascites, and fatal bleeding from esophago-gastric varices.

GEOGRAPHICAL DISTRIBUTION OF SCHISTOSOMIASIS

The geographic distribution of the three schistosomal species largely depends on the availability of specific intermediate host snails in different regions.[2] S. japonicum is transmitted by amphibious prosobranch snails of the genus Oncomelania, and S. mansoni and S. haematobium are transmitted by pulmonate aquatic snails of the genus Biomphalaria and Bulinus, respectively.[15]

The species S. haematobium is widely distributed in Africa, both north and south of the Sahara, extending across the Mediterranean region from Morocco to Turkey and into Arabia and Asia Minor. There is a small focus of infection in India, but none in the Americas. S. mansoni has a similar distribution in Africa and the eastern Mediterranean area, but in addition is present in South America and the Caribbean. S. mansoni is the most widespread species, affecting 52 countries. Current estimates are that approximately 95% of human schistosomal infections are caused by S. mansoni and S. haematobium. Note that because mixed infections of these two species are common, they could interact in producing pathological changes in the host; studies examining such interactions and their effect on cancer development have not been done. Infection with S. japonicum is restricted to the Far East, where it is endemic in three countries: China, the Philippines, and Indonesia.

EPIDEMIOLOGICAL EVIDENCE FOR A LINK BETWEEN SCHISTOSOMIASIS AND CANCER

Table 12.1 presents a summary of the extent to which the data available on S. haematobium and S. japonicum infections support a causal relation-

Table 12.1 Evidence of causality for relationship of schistosomiasis infections and cancer[a]

| Criteria for causality | S. haematobium | S. Japonicum | |
	Bladder cancer	Liver cancer	Colorectal cancer
Consistency of relationship	Yes	No	Yes
Dose-response	No data available	No data available	Yes, but limited
Specificity	Yes	No	Yes
Temporal sequence	Yes, but limited	No data available	Yes, but limited
Strength of association	Strong	Varied	Strong
Biological plausibility	Yes	Yes	Yes
Experimental support	Yes	Yes	Yes

[a]For references see Tables 2 and 3.

ship for development of urinary bladder and colorectal cancer, respectively. For comparison, Table 12.3 includes data available on liver cancer in association with *S. japonicum* infection, a relationship considered to be inconclusive. The references supporting this summary are provided in Table 12.2 for *S. haematobium* and in Table 12.3 for *S. japonicum* and are described briefly in this chapter. (For an extensive review of the schistosomiasis literature with respect to cancer risk, see IARC Monograph 6, which contains the summary statement of the IARC Working Group on the evaluation of schistosome infection.[11]

Table 12.2 Evidence in support of an association of *S. haematobium* infection[a] **with urinary bladder cancer**

Type of study	Observation	Reference
Descriptive studies	Urinary bladder cancer higher in geographic regions with a high prevalence of infection	17–22
	Number of urinary bladder cancer cases increased in populations with greater exposure to contaminated water due to occupation (for example, farmers in Egypt) or to gender (for example, males do most of agriculture work)	23–26
	Alteration in bladder cancer morphology to greater frequency of squamous-cell carcinomas rather than transitional-cell carcinomas in countries with high prevalence of infection. Also increased proportion of squamous-cell cancers in bladder cancer specimens containing eggs	22,27,28
	Low proportion of squamous-cell tumors and low prevalence of infection at high elevations near Mount Kilimanjaro, Tanzania, associated with decrease in distribution of snail vectors	29
Case reports	Preponderance of squamous-cell bladder tumors among cases with infection	29–31
	Rare occurrence of tumours in bladder trigone compared to Western tumors	26
	Younger age for cases of bladder cancer that are infected	32–35
Case-control studies	Six of 7 hospital-based studies that examined the relationship between infection and bladder cancer reported significant association. Odds ratios from 2 to 14	31,36–41
Molecular studies	Different mutation patterns in *p53* gene of urinary bladder cancers of infected individuals in Egypt compared to Western bladder cancers	42–44
	Altered frequencies of loss of heterozygosity (LOH) for putative suppressor genes in Egyptian compared to Western urinary bladder cancers	45

[a]Infection ascertained indirectly by questionnaire or medical history or measured directly by examining urine, biopsies of urinary bladder tissue, or digests of bladder tissue for the presence of eggs.

Table 12.3 Evidence in support of an association of *S. japonicum* infection with colorectal cancer

Type of study	Observation	Reference
Descriptive studies	Correlation between schistosomiasis mortality rate and geographic variation in colorectal cancer rate (China)	13,46,47
	Correlation between colorectal cancer mortality rate and prevalence of infection (China)	13,48,49
	Correlation of colorectal cancer mortality rate and incidence rate of infection (China)	50
Case reports	Case reports of colorectal cancer associated with infection (Japan and Philippines)	51–53
	Younger age for cases of colorectal cancer that are infected	50,54
	Infection associated with chronic schistosomal colitis and dysplastic changes in colonic membrane	55,56
Case-control studies	Comparison of infection rates (based on eggs in pathological specimens) for colon cancer and non-cancer patients. Odds ratio 1.2 (Japan)	53
	Comparison of exposure (based on medical history) of colorectal cancer cases (1973–79) and non-gastrointestinal cancer patients or healthy neighbors. Odds ratio: for colon, 1.2 with cancer controls and 0.64 with neighbors; for rectum, 8.3 with cancer controls and 4.5 with neighbors (China)	48
	Comparison of exposure (based on medical history) of colon cancer deaths (1981–83) and lung cancer patients or healthy persons. Odds ratio, 2.1 and 4.2 for early- and late-stage disease with lung cancer controls, and 2.4 and 5.7 with healthy controls (China)	57
Cohort studies	Duration of residence in endemic region correlated with liver cancer in men (>9 but <50 years) and colorectal cancer in women (>50 years) (Japan)	58

S. Haematobium Infection and Urinary Bladder Cancer

In 1965, an epidemiologist, Sir A. Bradford Hill, established seven criteria for deciding whether a disease is caused by a specific exposure.[16] These criteria include finding (1) a strong statistical association between the exposure and the disease, (2) a consistent association in different types of studies from different populations, (3) a specific association between the factor and disease, (4) the correct temporal sequence (exposure preceding disease), (5) a dose–response relationship, (6) plausible mechanisms by which the exposure could cause disease (including coherence with other knowledge about the disease), and (7) experimental proof of causation either in humans, animals or in vitro models. Applying these widely used criteria to *S. haematobium* and urinary bladder cancer provides convincing evidence that there is a causal association between the infection and later development of malignancy.

Strength and Consistency of Relationship

There are obvious limitations to performing epidemiological studies in developing countries such as those in which *S. haematobium* is endemic. For example, population-based cancer incidence rates are often unavailable and mortality rates are unreliable. Most studies report the frequency of urinary bladder cancer relative to other malignant tumors using hospital-based reports—a source with inherent biases. Indices of exposure to the parasite are also variable, ranging from a direct assessment of egg presence (in urine or bladder biopsies or through use of pelvic x-ray examinations) to self-reports suggestive of infection (for example, presence of hematuria, frequency and urgency of micturition) or medical histories from clinics or hospitals. Despite these limitations, the data supporting the association between *S. haematobium* infection and bladder cancer are viewed as strong and consistent. They come from a combination of descriptive studies, clinical and pathological case reports, and case-control studies (Table 12.2).

Perhaps the most striking support of a relationship between *S. haematobium* infection and urinary bladder cancer comes from studies that report a similarity in geographic distribution of bladder cancer and endemic schistosomiasis, especially in those areas where the intensity and prevalence of infection is high, such as in Africa.[2] For example, urinary bladder cancer is 10 times more common among men in Egypt (where there is a high prevalence of infection) than among men in Algeria (a country with a low prevalence of infection).[11] Also, when comparisons are made between regions within a country, bladder cancer frequencies have been shown to be elevated in areas where the parasite is endemic.[17–22,27,28] Finally, the gender ratio of patients with urinary bladder cancer is reported to vary widely in different African countries and to correspond roughly to the relative involvement of men and women in agricultural work and, hence, to their risk of exposure to infection.[23–25]

Seven hospital-based case-control studies have been reported in which an examination was made of the association between *S. haematobium* infection and urinary bladder cancer (Table 12.2). Six of these studies showed a significant positive association between the occurrence of urinary bladder cancer and infection with *S. haematobium*, with an estimated relative risk ranging from 2 to 14. These studies were performed in six different countries, and used several different approaches to identifying infection, yet all produced similar findings. Although there were major sources of bias and confounding in these studies (for example, the failure to consider confounding by age and gender in four studies, or by smoking in all but one study, and the use of different methods of measuring past infection between cases and controls in three studies), these deficiencies are not likely to alter significantly the overall finding of a strong association.[11]

Specificity of the Relationship

Bladder cancer related to schistosomal infection shows distinct histogenic and pathological differences from nonschistosomal bladder cancers observed in Europe and North America.[59] Schistosomal bladder cancers are largely squamous-cell carcinomas. In regions in which *S. haematobium* is endemic, the percentage of tumors that are squamous cell in origin at autopsy or cystectomy is reported to range from 53% to 80% (reviewed in reference 11). Schistosomal tumors occur at an early age. For example, in Egypt, the peak incidence of bladder cancer occurs at around 50 years of age, with 73% of the cases occurring in individuals aged younger than 50 years.[32–35] Finally, the tumors rarely affect the trigone.[26] In contrast, nonschistosomal bladder cancers in the Western world are mainly transitional-cell carcinomas; fewer than 10% are squamous cell carcinomas.[60] The nonschistosomal cancers usually occur in the seventh decade of life, with only 12% of patients under the age of 50 years, and they more often involve the trigone.[60,61] Of interest is the observation that the majority of schistosomal carcinomas present at an advanced stage in endemic countries, in contrast to the situation seen in Western countries, where 60% to 70% of the tumors are in the intraepithelial or lamina propria stage, making the early age at presentation even more striking.[59]

Temporal Sequence

There have been two reports of intensive quantitative postmortem studies in Egypt in which the presence of pathological changes associated with this infection (ureteral fibrosis, hydroureter and hydonephrosis, and urinary bladder carcinoma) were documented.[6,62] These reports indicated that by the age of 9 years, infected individuals already manifest structural abnormalities in the bladder. In another study, Lehman and colleagues reported significant functional and radiological urinary-tract abnormalities in persons over 14 years of age.[63] These data suggest that infection and the pathological changes associated with infection begin early in life and are progressive. Of interest is that some of these early lesions appear to regress, and urinary tract functions to improve, in the absence of reinfection.[64] There are no data on the age distribution of schistosomal premalignant lesions, but cancers, as mentioned, are most common in the fifth decade, suggesting a temporal sequence of events with progressive pathology.

Dose Response

Although it is probable that the intensity or duration of infection with *S. haematobium* alters the risk of development of bladder cancer (because it affects the production of eggs in an individual and the ensuing level of inflammatory and pathological change in the bladder), studies confirming this hypothesis have not been done, mainly because it is difficult to quantify the level or duration of infection in an individual. The quantity of eggs in a urine sample is not a reliable indicator of the intensity of exposure, because the production of such eggs depends on the age of the host. There is a characteristic rapid increase in the number of egg-containing urine samples during the first two decades of life followed by a progressive slow decline.[65] At the chronic stage of the disease, many patients do not pass eggs in their urine.[66] The most widely accepted explanation for this phenomenon is that immune modulation in older individuals regulates the parasite burden, reducing the number of eggs released.

There also is no clear indication of a reduction in bladder cancer rates in those endemic locales that have reported decreases in prevalence of the infection. Researchers have suggested that the parasite may have been eradicated too recently for us to be able to see such a response, because the latency period between infestation and subsequent development of bladder cancer is probably at least 20 years.[26] There are several alternate explanations, however—the chief of which is the difficulty in maintaining environmental control of the parasite because of mobility of individuals and because of increased agricultural expansion occurring in developing countries; both of these facilitate renewed spread of infection.[67] Yet, despite this problem, there is some indication that the clinicopathological patterns of bladder cancer are altering in several previously endemic regions. A recent hospital-based retrospective study in Egypt showed that, during the past 20 years, there has been a shift to fewer squamous-cell cancers (down from 77% to 51%) and to more transitional cell carcinomas (up from 21% to 44%), accompanied by an increase in the peak age incidence (up from 30 to 50 years, now 50 to 70 years).[68] Whether this change in the histogenic type of bladder cancers and the age of the patients reflects a change in the prevalence of the infection or some other parameter in the region is unknown. Other possibilities are that (1) the criteria used to classify bladder tumors have changed, (2) the number and types of cases being identified are altering because of better screening approaches, and (3) the carcinogen exposure in the population being treated in the hospitals is changing—for example, cigarette smoking is becoming more common. All these changing patterns deserve in-depth study.

Biological Plausibility and Experimental Evidence

There has recently been a renewed interest in exploring the association between schistosomiasis and urinary bladder cancer from an experimental viewpoint. Taken together, the data suggest several biological mechanisms by which this infection could lead to the development of bladder cancers. Some investigators posit mechanisms based on alterations to the level of genetic damage in this tissue, produced either by schistosome-related dysregulation of xenobiotic metabolism or by inflammation-related production of endogenous mutagens. Other studies focus on changes that would lead to increased cell turnover and, hence, tumor promotion. The data supporting these postulated mechanisms are described in detail later in this chapter.

With the advent of molecular techniques and their recent application to clinical samples, it is becoming increasingly possible to explore the underlying genetic alterations occurring in schistosomal tumors, and to contrast them to those observed in Western tumors. For example, an examination of the types of mutations in the tumor suppressor gene *p53* in these two types of tumors might provide evidence for the types of causative agents acting in these two populations. Recent data suggest a different mutational spectrum in this gene in schistosomal bladder cancers from Egypt and in nonschistosomal bladder cancers in Western countries. Schistosomal bladder cancers have a higher proportion of base-pair substitutions at CpG dinucleotides ($p = .003$) and an apparent shift in the region of the gene that is mutated, away from mutation in exons 7 and 8 toward mutations in exons 5 and 6,[43,44] suggesting the involvement of different mutagenic agents in schistosomiasis patients than in other patients with bladder cancer. Another recent approach has been to identify regions of loss of heterozygosity (LOH) on specific chromosomes in tumors by using polymerase chain reaction-based technology. This loss represents the deletion of a putative tumor suppressor gene. Of interest is a paper by Gonzalez-Zulueta and coworkers[45] that reports an alteration in the pattern of loss of specific chromosomal arms in tumors from Egypt compared to those from Sweden. This alteration consists of an increase in loss at 9p and a decrease at 9q in the Egyptian tumors. If these data are supported by additional studies, it would suggest that the pathway by which these tumors are induced, and the critical genes that are involved, are different in tumors from regions in which *S. haematobium* is endemic.

S. Japonicum Infection and Colorectal Cancer

Bradford Hill's criteria for causality can also be applied to *S. japonicum* and colorectal cancer. Taken together, however, the accumulated data are not yet as persuasive as those for *S. haematobium* and urinary bladder cancer.

Consistency and Strength of Relationship

A majority of studies that examine the relationship between *S. japonicum* infestation and colorectal cancer has come from China, a country in which there is considerable geographic variation in colon-cancer mortality rates. Six correlation studies have examined this relationship in different provinces, counties, or communes of varying *S. japonicum* endemicity.[13,46–50] Mortality from and, in one study, incidence of colorectal cancer have been strongly and significantly correlated with *S. japonicum* infection in each of these investigations. In one study, there was a high correlation between schistosomiasis prevalence and colon cancer mortality after adjustment for dietary factors. This finding was important because diet could be a significant confounding factor in such correlational research.[47]

In addition to these descriptive studies, two case-control investigations have been conducted in the schistosomiasis-endemic areas of Jiangsu province, China, where the colorectal cancer mortality rate is high. One of these studies compared prevalence of *S. japonicum* in colorectal cancer patients with that in two control groups: patients with other cancers, and healthy neighbors.[48] Controls were matched to cases on age, gender, and occupation, but not on diet; medical histories were used to assess exposure. The estimated relative risks of colon and rectal cancer were 1.2 and 8.3, respectively, when comparisons were made with cancer patient controls, and 0.6 and 4.5 when case patients were compared with healthy neighbors. A second study[57] compared patients who died of colorectal cancer with those who died of lung cancer and with healthy people. In this study, the medical history differentiated between early- and late-stage infection. After adjustment for smoking and for family history of colon cancer (but not for diet), odds ratios in comparison with lung-cancer controls were 2.1 and 4.2 for early- and for late-stage disease, respectively, and 2.4 and 5.7 in comparison with healthy controls.[69]

Specificity of the Relationship

The association between *S. japonicum* infections and colorectal cancers is strongly supported by epidemiological studies; yet, there have also been reports of an association between *S. japonicum* and hepatocellular carcinoma. The association of infection with several forms of cancer casts some doubt on the specificity of the exposure–disease relationship. The reports linking *S. japonicum* infection with hepatocellular cancer, however, are inconsistent. Mortality from liver cancer and prevalence of infection with *S. japonicum* have been found to be positively correlated in Japan, but not consistently in China.[12,13] Moreover, within China, the correlation has been present in certain provinces but not in others, and sometimes is seen in only one gender.[46] In larger correlation studies, involving numerous counties and provinces in China, no correlation between *S. japonicum* and hepatocellular cancer was found. There have been three case-control studies of hepatocellular cancer in Japan and China[57,58,70] that gave estimated relative risks of 2 to 10. These studies did not control for hepatitis viral infection, however, or for dietary nutrients and carcinogenic contaminants such as aflatoxin. Viral hepatitis is thought to play a significant role in hepatocellular cancers in these regions (see Chapter 9) and many reports suggest that it is this virus, rather than schistosomal infections, that is causing the primary hepatocellular carcinomas in endemic regions.[71]

Temporal Sequence

Researchers generally assume that infection with *S. japonicum* precedes the development of cancer in most individuals in endemic regions because individuals usually become infected at an early age. Although there is some suggestion that schistosomal colorectal cancers also occur in people at a younger age than do nonschistosomal cancers,[51,54] little information exists for schistosomal patients on the relative occurrence of premalignant lesions or the age at which they occur. Infection with the parasite often leads to chronic schistosomal colitis, associated with dysplastic changes in the colonic mucosa that resemble those found in long-standing chronic ulcerative colitis, a disease with a significant risk for colon cancer in the West.[72] In a retrospective review of colectomy specimens from schistosomiasis patients, Chen and coworkers[55,56] found mild to severe epithelial dysplasia in 36 of 60 specimens. These lesions occurred in the flat mucosa, in pseudopolyps, or in regenerative epithelium at the edges of ulcers. Unfortunately the incidence of dysplasia in individuals who had no infection was not reported.

Dose Response

Two studies have examined the role of the duration of exposure to *S. japonicum* on the risk for colorectal cancer: a cohort study with a limited sample size in Japan, and a case-control study in China. The cohort study was based on death certificates for natives of a town in Yamanashi Prefecture, Japan.[58] A total of 2067 people were categorized into four groups based on the length of time that they had resided in this locale before 1957, the date at which the parasite was eradicated in this region. The sample size was small: only 16 deaths occurred from colorectal cancer. However, women living in the community for 50 or more years were identified as having a significantly high risk of colorectal cancer. Men had an elevated risk of hepatocellular carcinoma if they had lived in this locale for more than 9 but less than 50 years. Unfortunately, the study was not controlled for hepatitis viral infection.

The Chinese case-control study compared cumulative exposure to schistosomal infection in 197 patients who died of colon cancer, 205 who died of lung cancer, and 200 healthy controls.[69] Data were adjusted for age, gender, smoking habits and family history of colon cancer, but were not adjusted for diet. A stepwise increase in relative risk from 1.2 to 4.3 was observed as the duration of exposure increased from less than 10 to greater than 30 years.

Although *S. japonicum* has been eradicated in several regions in China, no studies have evaluated the influence of this eradication on colorectal-cancer frequencies.

Biological Plausibility and Experimental Evidence

Although there have been fewer mechanistic studies of *S. japonicum* and its role in carcinogenesis than of *S. haematobium*, changes occurring in the colon of infected individuals could certainly play a role in the development of cancers at this site. Experimental evidence from animal models suggests that carcinogen metabolism might be altered significantly in infected individuals as the result of pathological changes in the liver. Other studies have emphasized the role of the inflammatory response, which may act as a stimulant for growth of mucosal cells.[73] These studies will be described in more detail later in this chapter.

PATHOGENETIC MECHANISMS OF CARCINOGENESIS

Several theories have been proposed to explain why schistosome infections predispose to cancer, although none has yet been confirmed. It is likely that the infection acts via several pathways, each of which contributes to the carcinogenic process. Some of the cellular changes observed in animal models or in infected humans appear to be associated with initiation events, such as the endogenous formation of DNA-damaging agents (nitrosamines or reactive oxygen species) or altered metabolism of carcinogens. Others have characteristics normally associated with promotion events (for example, induction of regenerative hyperplasia).

S. Haematobium Infections and Urinary Bladder Cancer

Although clinical studies have long documented an association between inflammation and cancer, the nature of this relationship is as yet unresolved (for reviews, see references 74 and 75). There appears to be little doubt, however, that the eggs released by the S. haematobium play a central role in the pathological changes occurring in the bladder and liver of schistosomiasis patients (Figure 12.1). The infiltration of eggs through the bladder stroma produces tissue damage and stimulates compensatory cell turnover and inflammation, both associated with tumorigenesis. Inflammation, in turn, may play a role in carcinogen bioactivation, reactive-oxygen-species (ROS) release, and nitrosamine formation (see Chapter 2), all of which may increase DNA damage to the urothelium. Egg deposition in the bladder wall and urethral walls can also lead to obstruction, urinary retention, and secondary bacterial infection. Mucosal damage from these processes could increase the absorption of free carcinogens in the bladder.[64] Urinary retention prolongs the exposure of the urothelium to carcinogens in the urine[76] and allows the concentration of endogenous carcinogens in the urine, produced either by bacteria or by inflammatory cells. Finally, investigators have suggested, based mainly on results from experimental animal studies, that schistosomiasis can lead to alterations in carcinogen metabolism and to the presence of relatively high levels of active intermediates that can damage DNA.[77,78]

Formation of Nitrosamines and Other N-Nitroso Compounds

Researchers have devoted much attention to the possible role of N-nitroso compounds in the etiology of schistosomal bladder cancers.[79-82] The involvement of these agents is supported by three pieces of evidence:

First, several studies have reported an elevation in the levels of nitrite and volatile N-nitroso compounds in the urinary bladder of schistosomiasis patients.[83,84] The source of these N-nitroso compounds is as yet unknown. They may be formed endogenously through the action of bacteria involved in secondary infections: some bacterial species can mediate nitrosation reactions between secondary amines and nitrate under the phys-

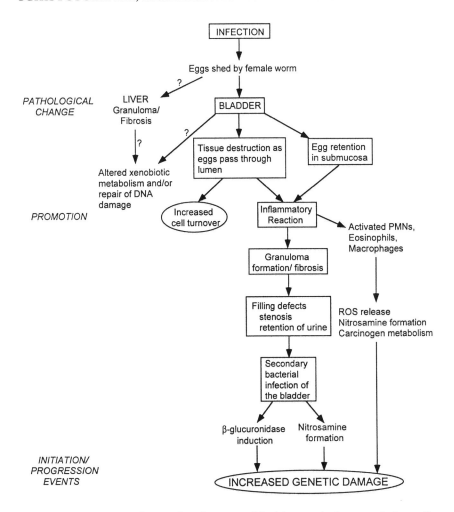

Figure 12.1. Interrelationship between bladder pathology and the cellular changes associated with carcinogenesis in schistosomal bladders.

iological conditions normally encountered in the urinary bladder.[85] Alternatively, inflammatory cells can convert nitrate to nitrite and are capable of inducing nitrosamine formation.[86–89] Macrophages also have the capacity to produce nitric oxide, an oxidant that can set into action a chain of chemical events that induces mutation.[44,90] Finally, N-nitroso compounds could come from exogenous sources such as diet and cigarette smoke.

Second, Badawi and coworkers[80] reported the presence of O^6-methyl-deoxyguanosine (O^6-MedG) in bladder-tissue DNA of Egyptian subjects who had bladder carcinoma and concomitant schistosomiasis. Although nitrosamine levels were not assayed in these patients, it is generally accepted that O^6-MedG is a promutagenic DNA adduct that would be expected in tissue exposed to nitrosamines. O^6-MedG was detected more frequently and at higher levels in the bladder DNA of schistosome-infected patients than in normal bladder tissue from European patients.

Third, Badawi and his colleagues[91] measured the activity of O^6-alkylguanine-DNA-alkyltransferase (ATase), the enzyme that mediates the repair of O^6-MedG adducts, in extracts of 55 bladder-tissue samples from Egyptian patients who had schistosome-associated bladder carcinomas. ATase levels in tissue samples from schistosomiasis patients (both tumor tissue and adjacent uninvolved tissue) were lower than those observed in normal human bladder mucosal tissue from individuals of European origin. These data suggest a lower capacity for repair of alkylation damage in infected individuals and thus a greater risk of DNA damage by *N*-nitroso compounds. The researchers suggest that further investigation is necessary to determine whether the lowered ATase levels are due to the depletion of ATase activity by continuous exposure to high levels of alkylating agents, or to other factors, such as an ethnic variation in enzyme activity.

Inflammation

An association between chronic inflammation and increased risk of cancer is supported by many clinical observations.[74] Probably one of the most convincing associations involves the *S. haematobium*–infected individual. Inflammation may act to increase genetic damage in the urothelium through several pathways. Indirectly, the inflammatory infiltrates and ulceration in areas surrounding the eggs might increase the capacity of the urothelium to absorb carcinogens from the urine.[6] A more direct mechanism involves the production and release of DNA damaging agents from inflammatory cells. Support for this mechanism comes from in vitro studies in which TPA-activated inflammatory cells have been coincubated with a variety of target cells. DNA strand breakage, chromosomal change, micronuclei, and malignant transformation are reported in the target cells.[92–98]

What agents are responsible for these effects is still a subject of debate (see Chapter 2). One possible candidate is the hydroxyl radical, formed by a Haber-Weiss reaction between hydrogen peroxide (released by the inflammatory cell) and chromatin-bound metal ions, or alternatively formed by decomposition of a peroxynitrite radical (produced by interaction of two other products of inflammatory cells: superoxide anions and nitric oxide).[74,92] Another possibility is that the damage could arise from nonenzymatic oxidation of cell-membrane unsaturated fatty acids. This oxidation leads to the release of lipid hydroperoxides and their breakdown products, some of which can damage DNA.[93] Clastogenic factors also appear to be produced via the arachidonic acid cascade in damaged cells.[98] Intermediates from this cascade are involved in free-radical production,[99] bioactivation of carcinogens,[100–104] and direct genetic damage.[105] Finally, the inflammatory cells may also act to increase DNA damage in a tissue by producing nitric oxide and fostering formation of nitrosamines.

Several recent studies, including those originating in our laboratory,

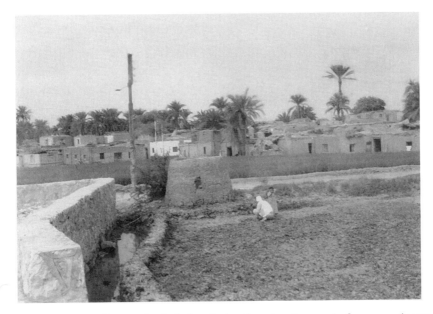

Figure 12.2. Village of Shakshouk in Egypt where study on urinary micronuclei and schistosomiasis was conducted. Persons were infected by exposure to contaminated water in the irrigation canals.

have looked at common biomarkers of the carcinogenic process in schistosomiasis patients and have provided indirect support for inflammation as an etiologic factor in carcinogenesis. For example, our studies examined the level of in vivo chromosomal breakage that occurs in the bladders of schistosomiasis patients.[75,106] The approach used was to evaluate micronucleus frequencies in exfoliated urothelial cells collected by centrifuging urine samples from infected individuals and controls (Figure 12.2). Micronuclei (MN) are formed by damage to chromosomes or to the spindle apparatus in dividing cells. When a cell with such damage divides, the chromosomes or parts of chromosomes are excluded from the main nucleus and form their own membrane. After staining by the Feulgen reaction, they are easily seen as extranuclear bodies under a high power (1000× magnification) microscope (Figure 12.3). MN frequencies were elevated 9.1-fold in urothelial cells of infected individuals and were accompanied by a significant elevation in urinary white-blood-cell levels. Treatment with praziquantel, which killed the parasite, resulted in a reduction of MN frequencies to the level of uninfected controls with a concomitant reduction in urinary white-cell levels. In contrast, the bacterial superinfections routinely found in schistosomiasis patients (but not in controls) remained approximately unchanged before and after praziquantel treatment. This finding suggests that bacterial infections are not responsible for the elevated MN frequencies present in schistosomiasis-infected patients.

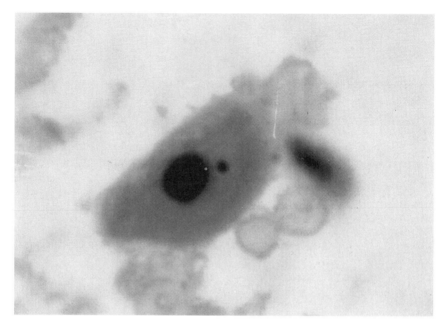

Figure 12.3. A micronucleated urothelial cell obtained from the urine of an Egyptian infected with *S. haematobium*.

This latter observation brings up the question of the relative significance of the schistosomal and bacterial infections in genetic damage and carcinogenesis. Although Western populations are not exposed to schistosomal infection, chronic bacterial infections do occur and have been associated with elevated rates of bladder cancer.[107] We studied a group of patients in Vancouver who had continual long-term urinary catheterization.[108] Such patients have recurrent bacterial infections and chronic bladder inflammation, along with an associated increase in bladder cancer risk.[109] In contrast to the results observed with the Egyptian population, MN frequencies were not elevated above control levels in these patients (Figure 12.4).

In interpreting these results, it is important to keep in mind several critical differences between populations with schistosomiasis and those with chronic urinary catheters. First, there is much less trauma in the catheterized bladder, for there are no eggs penetrating the uroepithelium. Furthermore, the types of inflammatory cells and the depth to which they penetrate the epithelium are different (reviewed in reference 108). The differences between the two populations are further confounded by the higher amounts of vitamins and nonsteroidal anti-inflammatory agents that are consumed by Canadian catheterized patients compared to North African subjects; both vitamins and nonsteroidal anti-inflammatory agents protect cells from DNA damage by reactive oxygen species.

Another approach being used to study schistosomal bladder cancers involves the molecular analysis of mutational spectra in the tumor-

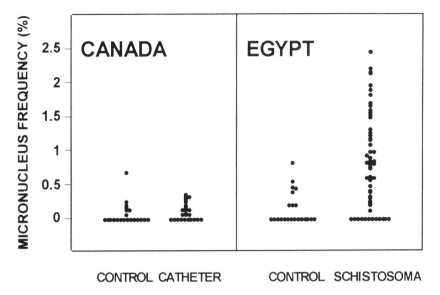

Figure 12.4. Frequency of micronucleated urothelial cells in patients with chronic bladder infections: (1) patients with schistosomiasis in Egypt; (2) Vancouver patients with long-term urinary catheterization.

suppressor gene *p53*. The aim of this approach is to identify unique alterations in critical genes that can be associated with DNA damage by specific agents. Warren and coworkers[44] reported an excess of transitions at CpG dinucleotides in schistosomal bladder cancers as compared with nonschistosomal cancers. Although there is no direct evidence that this change was caused by nitrosamine exposure, laboratory studies with animals have shown that such alterations are characteristic of the molecular events resulting from such an exposure.[110] Warren and associates suggested that the excess in CpG transitions could be due to the action of nitric oxide produced by the inflammatory response. Nitric oxide could either cause direct DNA damage and mutation or interact with other molecules to form N-nitroso compounds that in turn damage the DNA.

Urothelial Cell Proliferation and S. Haematobium

One of the characteristic changes that occur in schistosome-infected bladders is an increased rate of cell turnover due to the release of growth factors, eicosanoids, and "wounding hormones" from activated inflammatory cells and the damaged tissue itself.[111-114] This altered proliferation can be extensive, especially in the early acute phase of infection. We analyzed the expression of proliferating cell nuclear antigen (PCNA) in biopsy samples from patients who had schistosomal cystitis (patients with inflammatory cells and ova, as well as epithelial changes of cystitis cystica, cystitis glandularis, or Brunn's nest).[75] PCNA expression is commonly used as an indicator of the fraction of proliferating cells in a tissue because this antigen is mainly expressed in cycling cells. We found proliferating cells throughout the urothelium, especially in areas of extensive infiltration with inflammatory cells and ova. In contrast, proliferating cells were restricted to a few cycling cells in the basal uroepithelium in biopsies from normal bladders.

Increased epithelial proliferation could have a significant impact on the induction of tumors in an individual (see Chapter 3). It could increase the genetic damage sustained in a tissue by facilitating the interaction of a carcinogen with the DNA, because replicating DNA has an altered structural configuration, or it could decrease the probability of DNA damage being repaired before the damaged cell divides.[114,115] Elevated epithelial proliferation can also increase carcinogenesis by allowing genetic changes such as chromosome loss, duplication, or translocation (which require cell division to be expressed) to occur. Proliferation also allows the selective clonal expansion of "initiated" cells to occur more rapidly.[75]

Animal Carcinogenicity Data and Metabolism Studies

Most experimental animal models using rodents and nonhuman primates support a role of the schistosome infection as either a cocarcinogen (by increasing carcinogen damage) or as a promoter.[116-119] In most cases, however, the data are not sufficient to differentiate between these two possibilities. Many of the experimental models to date have been limited by the difficulty of sustaining an active infection in the animal for a significant portion of its life span. Infection with *S. haematobium* alone has resulted in urinary bladder hyperplasia in a few studies using mice, hamsters, opossums, and nonhuman primates (reviewed in ref. 11), but reports of bladder tumors generally have been restricted to a few nonhuman primates, and these tumors were either papillomas or papillary transitional cell carcinomas. In contrast, animals exposed simultaneously to low, subcarcinogenic doses of a chemical carcinogen developed bladder neoplasms in most studies.[116-119]

A few animal studies have examined whether enzyme activities in infected animals could play a role in the carcinogenic process. Most of these studies have used mice infected with *S. mansoni*, rather than *S. haematobium*, and have focused on alterations occurring in the liver—the main site of carcinogen metabolism. These studies suggest a decreased capability of these animals to process xenobiotics (for review, see reference 78). Among the enzymes affected by the parasite are the phase I enzymes (such as dealkylases, hydroxylases, cytochrome P450s, and electron transport enzymes) that act to insert or reveal an electrophilic substitute group on xenobiotics, and the phase II metabolizers (such as transferases and hydrolases) that act to conjugate this substitute group.[78,120] Phase I enzymes show increased activities in the early stages of infection, changing to reduced levels in the intermediate and late stages of the disease. In contrast, the activities of phase II enzymes are altered in favor of the deconjugation pathways in the late stages.[78]

The extent to which changes in the liver play a role in bladder cancers in schistosomiasis patients is unknown. There are likely to be alterations in carcinogen metabolism in individuals infected with *S. haematobium*, because their livers are affected by the presence of this species of the parasite, albeit to a lesser degree than in *S. mansoni* infections.[121] Furthermore, coinfections are common for these two species. If similar enzyme alterations occur in infected humans as occur in animals, they could lead to an heightened exposure of the bladder to carcinogenic intermediates. An unresolved question is why such changes in liver metabolism would result in specific increases only in *S. haematobium*–related bladder cancers but not in other tumors.

Other Aspects of Host Metabolism That Could Affect Risk

Data suggest that genetic differences in host metabolic capacity might have a significant influence on whether individuals develop schistosomal bladder cancer. This premise comes from the analysis of DNA for specific polymorphisms in genes that encode carcinogen-metabolizing enzymes (reviewed in references 122 and 123). Anwar and coworkers compared 22 Egyptian patients with bladder cancer and 21 control subjects for the presence of genetic polymorphisms to the cytochrome P450 genes CYP2E1 and CYP2D6 and to the glutathione S-transferase gene, GSTM1.[124] The majority of the bladder-cancer patients (86%) had either a clinical or self-reported history of schistosomiasis. Controls had no history of schistosoma infection or malignancy and were matched to cases with respect to age and smoking history. The GSTM1 gene codes for a multifunctional enzyme that catalyzes the conjugation reaction between glutathione (GSH) and a variety of electrophilic and hydrophobic compounds. Egyptian bladder cancer patients showed a significantly higher frequency of the GSTM1 null genotype (deletion of both copies of the gene) compared with controls. Individuals with this genotype would be devoid of GSTM1 activity and thus would be deficient in a critical detoxification process. In contrast, there was no significant difference in the distribution of the CYP2E1 polymorphism, although only one such polymorphism was examined (the *PstI* genotype). There, was, however an increase in the number of patients with extensive metabolizer (EM) genotypes of CYP2D6 relative to the controls (68% versus 48%), although this increase was not significant ($P = 0.15$). Extensive metabolizers would be expected to convert more of a carcinogenic substrate to reactive intermediates than poor metabolizers. The CYP2D6 polymorphism is associated with the polymorphic oxidation of a wide range of agents. Of interest is the observation that there is a magnified risk of bladder cancer in people who harbor both the CYP2E1 extensive metabolizer and the GSTM1 null genotypes; these persons have the misfortune of carrying defects in both phase I and phase II metabolism.

Another enzyme that has received much attention over the past two decades is the deconjugation enzyme, β-glucuronidase. This enzyme acts to split glucuronide conjugates of xenobiotics, thus releasing reactive forms that can induce DNA damage. Several studies have reported elevated levels of this enzyme in the urine of schistosomiasis patients, although the source of this elevation is unresolved.[125-127] The enzyme is present in blood leukocytes, plasma, and epithelial cells of the ureter and bladder and is produced by bacteria that infect schistosomiasis patients, notably *E. coli*. Any one of these cell types could be a source. Alternatively, the elevated urinary levels of this enzyme could be due to release of damaged urothelial cells into the bladder lumen, for the diurnal variation in urinary egg output appears to parallel alterations in urinary β-glucuronidase levels. This excretion pattern has been reported to disappear in praziquantel-treated patients.[127]

Other data suggest an impairment of tryptophan metabolism in schistosomiasis patients that is associated with the presence of elevated levels of tryptophan metabolites in their urine, some of which are known bladder carcinogens (for example, kynurenic acid, acetylkynurenine, kynurenine, 3-hydroxykynurenine, and anthranilic acid and its derivatives).[128,129] Infected patients challenged with 2 g of L-tryptophan showed a significant increase in the secretion of these metabolites.[128] The cause of this altered tryptophan metabolism is unknown, although the elevation has been associated with the induction of hepatocellular dysfunction by the infection, the consumption of tryptophan by the parasite or its eggs, and possibly the involvement of the bladder tumor itself in directly producing the metabolites (reviewed in reference 125).

A final path by which altered metabolism could affect cancer risk in schistosomiasis patients is through an indirect effect on nutritional status. For example, liver damage is associated with an impairment in vitamin A status. Deficiency of this vitamin may play a major role in the predominance of squamous metaplasias and squamous-cell carcinomas that occur in infected patients.[26] It may also increase the overall risk of tumor development, because human and animal studies suggest that this vitamin can inhibit the development of pre- and neoplastic lesions.[130] Schistosomiasis patients also often suffer from other nutritional deficiencies due both to low socioeconomic conditions and to the disease itself. The effect of these deficiencies on cancer development is unknown.

S. Japonicum Infection and Colorectal Cancer

There is little direct information on the role of *S. japonicum* infection in cancer development, because few mechanistic studies have been performed using this species. The available studies involve animal models, primarily mice. These models are only partially successful: although the infection results in metabolic liver dysfunction, the tumors that are induced are not colorectal but rather are restricted to the liver. Our understanding of the mechanism by which this infection could be acting to increase colorectal cancer is largely extrapolated from studies involving *S.*

haematobium infection and bladder cancer, although some information comes from comparisons to ulcerative colitis in Western countries. The latter condition also involves a chronic inflammation in the colon and an increased risk of colon cancer.[131]

S. *japonicum* infection in humans is associated with pathological alterations to the colorectum that are collectively known as *colorectal schistosomiasis*. The S. *japonicum* eggs are released into the venules draining the intestine, where they produce many of the pathological changes observed in the urinary bladders of individuals infected with S. *haematobium*. Eggs retained in the tissue incite the formation of granulomas and polyps and lead to colonic dysfunction. Eggs passing through the epithelium to the lumen induce chronic inflammation, altered cell proliferation, and a disruption of the cellular architecture. Thus, S. *japonicum* infections could act via pathways similar to those of S. *haematobium* to produce genetic and proliferative changes, albeit this time in the colon.

In many ways, the changes to the bowel epithelium associated with this condition parallel those in Western lesions associated with ulcerative colitis or inflammatory bowel disease.[55,56,132] Ming-Chai and colleagues[132] analyzed 454 colectomy specimens with carcinoma, of which 64% were associated with S. *japonicum* infection. The schistosomal specimens displayed increased mucosal thickness, glandular hyperplasia with elongated irregular tubuli, immature cells in the upper two thirds of the crypt, nuclear atypia, pseudopolyps with or without atypia, diminutive polyps with stratification of the epithelium and hyperplastic features, and inverted polyps with isolated islands of hyperplastic epithelium and denudation of epithelial layers. These tissue alterations closely resemble those occurring in individuals with inflammatory bowel disease.

One hypothesis for the elevated risk of colon cancers in patients with ulcerative colitis is that activated inflammatory cells produce nitric oxide and nitrite that in the lowered luminal pH of ulcerative colitis can lead to the formation of *N*-nitroso compounds.[133] Elevated luminal nitrite levels were found in 77% of ulcerative colitis patients. To our knowledge, *N*-nitroso levels have not been assessed in the colons of patients with either ulcerative colitis or schistosomiasis, so this pathway remains hypothetical.

Remaining information that is available on S. *japonicum*–related oncogenesis supports a role for altered carcinogen metabolism in the liver of infected individuals. As with S. *haematobium*, all these data are derived from animal, rather than from human, studies. Gven the extensive liver damage created by the S. *japonicum* parasite, however, it is not unlikely that carcinogen metabolism may be critical in the induction of cancer in these patients.

Liver tumors are induced in mice infected with S. *japonicum* without carcinogen exposure.[134] Liver cancers appear earlier and in larger numbers, however, in infected animals treated with a carcinogen.[135] One hypothesis for this effect is that mutagen-processing potential is reduced in infected animals. Arimoto and his colleagues[136] incubated 3-amino-1-

methyl-5*H*-pyridol[4,3-*b*]indole (Trp-P-2) with liver metabolic enzyme (S9) preparations from infected and uninfected mice and analyzed the conversion into 3-hydroxy-amino-1-methyl-5*H*-pyrido[4,3-*b*]indole (Trp-P-2(NHOH)). They found that S9 preparations from infected mice had a lower ability to convert Trp-P-2 into Trp-P-2(NHOH), the activated form. Using mice infected with *S. japonicum* and injecting the carcinogenic mutagen, Trp-P-2, the same researchers[137] showed that infection results in a decreased metabolism and an increased retention of Trp-P-2 in the liver. They suggested the possibility that pigments in the liver, formed by the schistosome infection, may function as a reservoir for the mutagen. Similarly, Matsuoka and coworkers[138] found reduced levels of mutagen-processing potential by hepatic P450s in the *S. japonicum*-infected mouse liver. Finally, Hasler and associates[139] examined the effect of schistosomiasis on the activation of aflatoxin B$_1$ (AFB1). Microsomes from infected mice mediated the binding of AFB1 to calf thymus DNA less than those from uninfected animals. Taken together, these findings suggest that in infected animals, some carcinogens might be retained for longer periods than in uninfected animals, thereby increasing and prolonging the total exposure level of the animal to the carcinogens.

CONTROL OF SCHISTOSOMIASIS AND REDUCTION IN SCHISTOSOME-RELATED CANCERS

A variety of approaches can be used to combat schistosomiasis, depending on which part of the parasite life cycle is attacked. Transmission is determined by four factors: the degree of contamination of water with schistosome eggs, the number and characteristics of intermediate host snails, the amount of contact people have with infested water, and the longevity of the mature schistosome worms in infected individuals. Thus, the disease can be attacked by the provision of safe water supplies, by eliminating snail hosts with molluscides or altered habitats, by changing human behavior through health education, and by removing adult worms from infected individuals with drugs.

Current evidence suggests control increases exponentially with the use of a combination of these measures. The Japanese use of such an integrated approach has led to the virtual elimination of the parasite from their country.[140] In China, a control campaign combining local involvement and major government projects was launched in 1956.[141] Since then, the disease has been eradicated in four of 12 provinces (Fujian, Guan, Guangzi, and Shanghai) and in 171 of 380 counties, with the prevalence reduced in an additional 101 counties. By 1994, there had been an 87% reduction in the number of people infected, from 12 million to 1.6 million.[141]

Despite these successes and concerted efforts in many endemic regions of the world, there has been no overall reduction in the global number of infections during the past decade.[2] This static level is largely the result of the difficulties in controlling population migration due to numerous factors (war, drought, famine, job availability) but also is associated with demographic increases in younger age groups (the groups with the highest level of infection) and with ecological changes, including water-resource development, that have spread the disease to new areas.

Additional problems have modulated the success of various control measures. Population-based chemotherapy campaigns, with drugs such as praziquantel, are effective at killing the mature worm. The drug is expensive for developing countries, however, and, in the absence of other control measures, it will not significantly reduce transmission, because reinfection is rapid and commonplace. In the past, snail eradication with molluscides has been commonly used concurrently with chemotherapy to achieve control in some areas. However, area-wide mollusciciding is becoming less common because of both high cost and fears of environmental contamination.[142]

Of interest is the developing role of behavioral studies in the design of intervention regimes.[143] These studies provide detailed information on all water-contact activities and yield exposure indices based on the frequency, duration, and intensity of water contact. Identification of heterogeneities in water-contact patterns assist control programs in aiming interventions at heavily used sites, at sites with greater densities of cercariae in the water (focal mollusciciding), or at the minority of individuals making most water contacts (targeted chemotherapy).[144] These studies also create a better understanding of the community's perception of the disease and of how this perception affects control measures. Schistosomiasis is considered to be inevitable in many affected communities, with the development of hematuria (*S. haematobium* infection) viewed as a normal growth stage during childhood. *S. japonicum* and *S. mansoni* are seldom recognized as distinct diseases.[143]

An attractive goal in the past decade has been to develop vaccines capable of conferring long-term protection against infection with this parasite.[145–148] The possibility that such a vaccine could be created is strengthened by two observations. First, infected individuals appear to develop effective acquired immunity to this parasite under conditions of repeated natural exposure, as shown by the characteristic decline in age-specific prevalence and intensity of infection in endemic areas. Second, several protective antigens defined at the molecular level are currently being evaluated in animal models as preludes to clinical trials.[142] These experiments have shown some vaccines to be beneficial. For example, the *S. mansoni* glutathione-S-transferase (Sm28 GST) induces IgE and IgA antibodies in experimental models. Treatment with this vaccine leads to a reduction in worm burden and a decrease in parasite fecundity, accompanied by a significant decrease in the number, size, and volume of liver granulomas.[147] Thus, immunization could act both to reduce transmission (by reducing egg output by worms) and to decrease the pathological consequences of infection (associated with production and retention of eggs in infected individuals).

Although it is likely that the reduction in schistosome-related cancers in populations in which schistosomiasis is endemic will be achieved most effectively through control of the parasite transmission, there are two other possibilities. Screening to detect precancerous lesions in rural communities has already been used in Egypt with some success.[59] In this case, selective screening of urine cytology was done in rural communities heavily infested with *S. haematobium*. An alternate approach would be to screen selected groups of symptomatic patients (for example, those with cystitis or hematuria) who attend outpatient urologic clinics. Unfortunately, such approaches would be expensive and by their very selectivity might have limited influence on the overall population of infected individuals in countries in which schistosomiasis is endemic. Furthermore, we have yet to establish effective strategies for managing patients who have premalignant bladder lesions, even in Western countries.

A final possibility is that we may be able to use our developing knowledge of the mechanism by which these cancers are produced in infected individuals to intervene and prevent their occurrence. One example has been to examine the effect of treatment with praziquantel and an antifibrotic agent, such as β-aminoproprionitrile (BAPN). Using an *S. mansoni* mouse model, Giboda et al.[149] have shown that such a combination of drugs leads to a marked reduction in the tissue egg load compared with treatment with praziquantel alone. In addition, mice receiving this combined treatment retained a high level of resistance to reinfection. These observations suggest that it may be possible to modulate egg granuloma formation in infected individuals, and thereby slow down the pathological sequelae associated with granuloma formation. Whether the same combination would work in humans, and what its effect on cancer development would be, are unknown. Another possible intervention regime could focus on reducing the amount of genetic damage occurring in the urothelium in *S. haematobium*–infected individuals by supplementation with agents that either scavenge nitrite (for example, ascorbate) or trap free radicals or the active electrophiles of carcinogenic agents (for review, see references 74 and 75). These suggestions emphasize again the importance of obtaining a more comprehensive understanding of the pathobiological processes underlying schistosome-related cancers so that we can develop alternate, novel approaches to combating this disease.

REFERENCES

1. Webb G. The six diseases of WHO. Schistosomiasis: some advances. Br Med J 1981;283:1104–1106.
2. WHO. The Control of Schistosomiasis. Geneva: WHO, 1993; Second Report of the WHO Expert Committee (WHO Tech Rep Ser 830).

3. Stephenson L. The impact of schistosomiasis on human nutrition. Parasitology 1993;107:S107–S123.
4. Hashem M. The aetiology and pathogenesis of primary liver cancer and its relation to schistosomiasis. Ain Shams Med J 1971;22:555–567.
5. Nouh MS, Bashi SA, Laajam MA, Mogleh IAA, Al-Aska A. Hepatitis B virus vs schistosomiasis and hepatocellular carcinoma in Saudi Arabia. E Afr Med J 1990;67:139–145.
6. Cheever AW, Kamel IA, Elwi AM, Mosimann JE, Danner R, Sippel JE. *Schistosoma mansoni* and *S. haematobium* infection in Egypt. III. Extrahepatic pathology. Am J Trop Med Hyg 1978;27:55–75.
7. Uthman S, Farhat B, Farah S, Uwayda M. Association of *Schistosoma mansoni* with colonic carcinoma [Letter to the Editor]. Am J Gastroenterol 1991;86: 257–262.
8. Andrade ZA, Abreu WN. Follicular lymphoma of the spleen in patients with hepatosplenic schistosomiasis mansoni. Am J Trop Med Hyg 1971;20:237–243.
9. Edington GM. Schistosomiasis and primary liver cell carcinoma [Letter to the Editor]. Trans R Soc Trop Med Hyg 1979;73:351.
10. Parkin DM, ed. Cancer Occurrence in Developing Countries. Lyon: Iarc, 1986; IARC Scientific Publications No. 75.
11. IARC. Infection with schistosomes (*Schistosoma haematobium, Schistosoma mansoni* and *Schistosoma japonicum*). Lyon: IARC, 1994, 61, 45–119; IARC monographs on the evaluation of carcinogenic risks to humans: Schistosomes, liver flukes and Helicobacter pylori.
12. Inaba Y, Takahashi EY, Maruchi N. A statistical analysis on the mortality of liver cancer and liver cirrhosis in Yamanashi Prefecture, with special emphasis on the relation to the prevalence of schistosomiasis. Jpn J Public Health 1977;24:811–815.
13. Guo ZR, Ni YC, Wu JL. Epidemiological study on relationship between schistosomiasis and colorectal cancer. Jiangsu Med J 1984;4:35.
14. Strickland GT. Gastrointestinal manifestations of schistosomiasis. Gut 1994; 35:1334–1337.
15. Sturrock RF. The parasites and their lifecycles. In: Jordan P, Webb G, Sturrock R, eds. Human Schistosomiasis. Oxon, UK: Cab International; 1993: 1–22.
16. Hill AB. The environment and disease: association or causation? Proc R Soc Med 1965;58:295–300.
17. Talib H. The problem of carcinoma of bilharzial bladder in Iraq [critical review]. Br J Urol 1970;42:571–579.
18. Anjarwalla KA. Carcinoma of the bladder in the coast province of Kenya. E Afr Med J 1971;48:502–509.
19. Bowry TR. Carcinoma of bladder in Kenya. E Afr Med J 1975;52:356–564
20. Malik MOA, Veress B, Daoud EH, El Hassan AM. Pattern of bladder cancer in Sudan and its relation to schistosomiasis: a study of 255 vesical carcinomas. J Trop Med Hyg 1975;78:219–226.
21. Hanash KA. Carcinoma of the bilharzial bladder. Progr Clin Biol Res 1984; 2:249–274.
22. Thomas JE, Bassett MT, Sigola LB, Taylor P. Relationship between bladder cancer incidence, *Schistosoma haematobium* infection, and geographical region in Zimbabwe. Trans R Soc Trop Med Hyg 1990;84:551–553.

23. Makhyoun NA, El-Kashlan KM, Al-Ghorab MM, Mokhles AS. Aetiological factors in bilharzial bladder cancer. J Trop Med Hyg 1971;74:73–78.

24. Prates MD. The rates of cancer of the bladder in the Portuguese East Africans of Lourenco Marques. In: Stewart H, Clemmensen J, eds. Geographical Pathology of Neoplasms of Urinary Bladder. New York: S. Karger; 1963:125–29.

25. Keen P, Fripp PJ. Bladder cancer in an endemic schistosomiasis area: geographical and sex distribution. S Afr J Sci 1980;76:228–230.

26. Tawfik HN. Carcinoma of the urinary bladder associated with schistosomiasis in Egypt: the possible causal relationship. In: Miller RW, Watanabe S, Fraumeni JF, Sugimua R, Rakayama S, Sugano H, eds. Unusual Occurrences as Clues to Cancer Etiology. Tokyo: Japan Scientific Societies Press; 1988: 197–209.

27. Lucas SB. Squamous cell carcinoma of the bladder and schistosomiasis. E Afr Med J 1982;59:345–351.

28. Al-Fouadi A, Parkin DM. Cancer in Iraq: seven years' data from the Baghdad tumor registry. Int J Cancer 1984;34:207–213.

29. Kitinya JN, Lauren PA, Eshleman LJ, Paljarvi L, Tanaka K. The incidence of squamous and transitional cell carcinomas of the urinary bladder in northern Tanzania in areas of high and low levels of endemic Schistosoma haematobium infection. Trans R Soc Trop Med Hyg 1986;80:935–939.

30. Sharfi ARA, El Sir S, Beleil O. Squamous cell carcinoma of the urinary bladder. Br J Urol 1992;69:369–371.

31. Hinder RA, Schmaman A. Bilharziasis and squamous carcinoma of the bladder. S Afr Med J 1969;43:617–618.

32. Aboul Nasr AL, Gazayerli ME, Fawzi RM, El-Sebai I. Epidemiology and pathology of cancer of the bladder in Egypt. Acta Univ Int Cancer 1962;18:528.

33. El-Bolkainy MN, Ghoneim MA, Mansour MA. Carcinoma of the bilharzial bladder in Egypt: clinical and pathological features. Br J Urol 1972;44:561.

34. El-Bolkainy MN, Mokhtar NM, Ghoneim MA, Hussein MH. The impact of schistosomiasis on the pathology of bladder carcinoma. Cancer 1981;48: 2643–2648.

35. Chen MG, Mott KE. Progress in assessment of morbidity due to Schistosoma haematobium infection: a review of recent literature. Trop Dis Bull 1989; 86:R1–R36.

36. Mustachi P, Shimkin MS. Cancer of the bladder and infestation with Schistosoma haematobium. J Natl Cancer Inst 1958;20:825–842.

37. Prates MD, Gillman J. Carcinoma of the urinary bladder in the Portuguese East African with special reference to bilharzial cystitis and preneoplastic reactions. S Afr J Med Sci 1959;24:13–40.

38. Gelfand M, Weinberg RW, Castle WM. Relation between carcinoma of the bladder and infestation with Schistosoma haematobium. Lancet 1967;1:1249–1251.

39. El-Bolkainy MN, Chu EW, Ghoneim MA, Ibrahim AS. Cytologic detection of bladder cancer in a rural Egyptian population infested with schistosomiasis. Acta Cytol 1982;26:303–310.

40. Elem B, Purohit R. Carcinoma of the urinary bladder in Zambia: a quantitative estimation of Schistosoma haematobium infection. Br J Urol 1983;55:275–278.

41. Skinner MEG, Parkin DM, Vizcaino AP, Ndhlovu A. Cancer in the African

Population of Bulawayo, Zimbabwe, 1963–1977, Incidence, Time, Trends and Risk Factors. Lyon: IARC; 1993; IARC Technical Report No.15.

42. Ramchurren N, Cooper K, Summerhayes IC. Molecular events underlying schistosomiasis-related bladder cancer. Int J Cancer 1995;62:237–244.

43. Habuchi T, Takahashi R, Yamada H, Ogawa O, Kakehi Y, Ogura K, Hamazaki S, Toguchida J, Ishizaki K, Fujita J, Sugiyama T, Yoshida O. Influence of cigarette smoking and schistosomiasis on p53 gene mutation in urothelial cancer. Cancer Res 1993;53:3795–3799.

44. Warren W, Biggs PJ, El-Baz M, Ghoneim MA, Stratton MR, Venitt S. Mutation in the p53 gene in schistosomal bladder cancer: a study of 92 tumors from Egyptian patients and a comparison between mutational spectra from schistosomal and nonschistosomal urothelial tumors. Carcinogenesis 1995;16(5): 1181–1189.

45. Gonzalez-Aulueta M, Shibata A, Ohneseit PF, Spruck III CH, Busch C, Shamaa M, Elbaz M, Nichols PW, Gonzalgo ML, Malmstrom P-U, Jones PA. High frequency of chromosome 9p allelic loss and CDKN2 tumor suppressor gene alterations in squamous cell carcinoma of the bladder. J Natl Cancer Inst 1995;87(18):1383–1392.

46. Liu BC, Rong XP, Sun XT, Wu YP, Gao RQ. Study of geographic correlation between colorectal cancers and schistosomiasis in China. Acta Acad Med Sin 1983;5:173–177.

47. Guo W, Xheng, W, Li J-Y, Chen J-S, Blot WJ. Correlations of colon cancer mortality with dietary factors, serum markers and schistosomiasis in China. Nutr Cancer 1993;20:13–20.

48. Xu Z, Su DL. *Schistosoma japonicum* and colorectal cancer: an epidemiological study in the People's Republic of China. Int J Cancer 1984;34:315–318.

49. Guo ZR, Lu QX, Wu JW, Xu J, Yang ML, Wang DW. Schistosomiasis factor in the formation of colorectal cancer. Jiangu Med J 1985;12:41–42.

50. Li Y. Geographical correlation analysis between schistosomiasis and large intestine cancer. Chung Hua Liu Hsing Ping Hsueh Tsa Chih 1988;9:265–268.

51. Abanilla LM. A report on the association of colonic cancer with *Schistosoma japonicum* infection. J Philipp Med Assoc 1986;62:30–32.

52. Sekiguchi A, Shindo G, Okabe H, Aoyanagi N, Furuge A, Oka T. A case of metastatic lung tumor of the colon cancer with ova of *Schistosoma japonicum* in the resected lung specimen. Jpn J Thorac Surg 1989;42:1025–1028.

53. Amano T. Clinicopathological studies on the gastro-intestinal schistosomiasis in the endemic area of Yamanashi Prefecture, with special reference to the carcinogenicity of schistosome infection. Jpn J Parasitol 1980;29:305–312.

54. Chen SC. Carcinoma of the large bowel. Relationship between eggs of schistosome in large bowel and carcinoma of the large bowel. Chin J Pathol 1986;15:69–70.

55. Chen M-C, Chuang C-Y, Chang P-Y, Hu J-C. Evolution of colorectal cancer in schistosomiasis: transitional mucosal changes adjacent to large intestinal carcinoma in colectomy specimens. Cancer 1980;46:1661–1675.

56. Chen M-C, Chang P-Y, Chuang C-Y, Chen Y-J, Wang F-P, Tang Y-C, Chou S-C. Colorectal cancer and schistosomiasis. Lancet 1981;1:971–973.

57. Guo ZR, Lu QX. Parasitic diseases: a case-control study on the relationship between schistosomiasis and liver cancer. Chin J Parasitol Parasit Dis 1987; 5:220–223.

58. Inaba Y. A cohort study on the causes of death in an endemic area of schistosomiasis japonica in Japan. Ann Acad Med 1984;13:142–148.
59. El-Sebai I. Carcinoma of the urinary bladder in Egypt: current clinical experience. In: El Bolkainy MN, Chu EW, eds. Detection of Bladder Cancer Associated with Schistosomiasis. Cairo: Al-Ahram Press, 1981:9–18.
60. Higginson J, Muir CS, Munoz N. Human Cancer: Epidemiology and Environmental Causes. Cambridge, UK: Cambridge University Press; 1992.
61. Payne P. Tumors of the bladder. In: Wallace DM, ed. Edinburgh and London: E.and S. Livingstone; 1959.
62. Smith JH, Kamel IA, Elwi A, von Lichtenberg F. A quantitative postmortem analysis of urinary schistosomiasis in Egypt. I. Pathology and pathogenesis. Am J Trop Med Hyg 1974;23:1054.
63. Lehman JS, Farid Z, Smith JH, Bassily S, El-Masry NA. Urinary schistosomiasis in Egypt: clinical, radiological, bacteriological and parasitological correlations. Trans Roy Soc Trop Med Hyg 1973;67(3):384–399.
64. Young SW, Farid Z, Bassily S, El-Masry NA. Urinary schistosomiasis: a 5-year clinical, radiological, and functional evaluation. Trans R Soc Trop Med Hyg 1973;67(3):379–383.
65. Higashi GI, Aboul-Enein MI. Diagnosis and epidemiology of *Schistosoma haematobium* infections in Egypt. In: El-Bolkainy MN, Chu EW, eds. Detection of Bladder Cancer Associated with Schistosomiasis. Cairo: Al-Ahram Press; 1981:47–69.
66. El-Bolkainy MN, Hammouda F, Raafat M. Urine cytology of bilharzial cystitis. In: El-Bolkainy MN, Chu EW, eds. Detection of Bladder Cancer Associated with Schistosomiasis. Cairo: Al-Ahram Press; 1981:77–83.
67. El-Sebai I. Cancer of the bladder in Egypt. Kasr El-Aini J Surg 1961;2:183.
68. Koraitim M, Metwalli NE, Atta M, Karam M, El-Sadr A. Schistosomal bladder carcinoma: is it changing? J Cancer Inst, Cairo University, in press.
69. Guo ZR, Lu QX, Zhao, LP, Zhang ZH. Schistosomiasis japonicum and colon cancer: an enquiry about the pathogenesis of colon cancer by using a logistic regression model. Chin J Epidemiol 1987;8:21–24.
70. Iuchi M, Nakayama Y, Ishiwa M, Yamada H, Chiba K. Primary cancer of the liver associated with chronic schistosomiasis japonica. Naika 1971;27:761–766.
71. Nakashima T, Okuda K, Kojiro M, Sakamoto K, Kubo Y, Shimokawa Y. Primary liver cancer coincident with schistosomiasis japonica: a study of 24 necropsies. Cancer 1975;36:1483–1489.
72. Taylor BA, Pemberton JH, Carpenter HA, Levin KE, Schroeder KW, Welling DR, Spencer MP, Zinsmeister AR. Dysplasia in chronic ulcerative colitis: implications for colonoscopic surveillance. Dis Col Rectum 1992;35(10):950–956.
73. Li ZM. Colon cancer. In: Internal Medicine, 4th ed. First Shanghai Medical College and Zhongshan Medical College, eds. Beijing: People's Health Publ House; 1981:377–381.
74. Rosin MP, Anwar WA, Ward AJ. Inflammation, chromosomal instability, and cancer: the schistosomiasis model. Cancer Res (suppl) 1994;54:1929s–1933s.
75. Rosin MP, El Din Zaki SS, Ward AJ, Anwar WA. Involvement of inflammatory reactions and elevated cell proliferation in the development of bladder cancer in schistosomiasis patients. Mutation Res 1994;305:283–292.

76. Badr M, Zaher M, Faway R. Further experience with bilharzial bladder neck obstruction. J Egypt Med Assoc 1958;41:624–629.

77. Gentile JM, Brown S, Aardema M, Clark D, Blankespoor H. Modified mutagen metabolism in Schistosoma hematobium-infested organisms. Arch Environ Health 1985;40(1):5–12.

78. Badawi AF, Mostafa MH. Possible mechanisms of alteration in the capacities of carcinogen metabolizing enzymes during schistosomiasis and their role in bladder cancer induction. J Int Med Res 1993;21:281–305.

79. Hicks RM. Nitrosamines as possible etiological agents in bilharzial bladder cancer. In: Magee PN, ed. Banbury report number 12: Nitrosomines and Human Cancer. Cold Spring Harbor, NY: Cold Spring Harbor Laboratory Press; 1981:455–471.

80. Badawi AF, Mostafa MH, Aboul-Azm T, Haboubi NY, O'Connor PJ, Cooper DP. Promutagenic methylation damage in bladder DNA from patients with bladder cancer associated with schistosomiasis and from normal individuals. Carcinogenesis 1992;13(5):877–881.

81. Bartsch H, Ohshima H, Pignatelli B, Calmels S. Human exposure to endogenous N-nitroso compounds: quantitative estimates in subjects at high risk for cancer of the oral cavity, esophagus, stomach and urinary bladder. In: Foorman D, Shuker D, eds. Cancer Surveys: Nitrate, Nitrite and Nitroso Compounds in Human Cancer, Vol. 8; 1989:335–362.

82. Ohshima H, Calmels S, Pignatelli B, Vincent P, Bartsch H. N-Nitrosamine formation in urinary-tract infections. In: Bartsch H, O'Neill IK, Schulte-Hermann RC, eds. The Relevance of N-Nitroso Compounds in Human Cancer: Exposures and Mechanism (IARC Sci. Publ. No. 84). Lyon: IARC, 1987:384–390.

83. Tricker AR, Mostafa MH, Spiegelhalder B, Preussmann R. Urinary excretion of nitrate, nitrite and N-nitroso compounds in schistosomiasis and bilharzia bladder cancer patients. Carcinogenesis 1989;10(3):547–552.

84. Mostafa MH, Helmi S, Badawi AF, Tricker AR, Spiegelhalder B, Preussmann R. Nitrate, nitrite and volatile N-nitroso compounds in the urine of Schistosoma haematobium and Schistosoma mansoni infected patients. Carcinogenesis 1994;15(4):619–625.

85. Calmels S, Ohshima H, Bartsch H. Nitrosamine formation by denitrifying and non-denitrifying bacteria: implication of nitrite reductase and nitrate reductase in nitrosamine catalysis. J Gen Microbiol 1988; 134:221–226.

86. Miwa M, Stueher DJ, Marletta MA, Wishnok JS, Tannenbaum SR. N-Nitrosamine formation by macrophages. In: Bartsch H, O'Neill IK, Schulte-Hermann RC, eds. Relevance of N-Nitroso Compounds to Human Cancer: Exposure and Mechanisms. Lyon: IARC Sci. Publ no. 84, 1987:340–344.

87. Stuehr DJ, Marletta MA. Further studies on murine macrophage synthesis of nitrate and nitrite. In: Bartsch H, O'Neill IK, Schulte-Hermann RC, eds. Relevance of N-Nitroso Compounds to Human Cancer: Exposure and Mechanisms. Lyon: IARC Sci. Publ. no. 83, 1987:335–339.

88. Marletta MA. Mammalian synthesis of nitrite, nitrate, nitric oxide and N-nitrosating agents. Chem Res Toxicol 1988;1:249–257.

89. Roediger WEW, Lawson MJ, Radcliffe BC. Nitrite from inflammatory cells—a cancer risk factor in ulcerative colitis? Dis Colon Rectum 1990;33:1034–1036.

90. Vallance P, Collier J. Biology and clinical relevance of nitric oxide. Br Med J 1994;309:453–457.

91. Badawi AF, Cooper DP, Mostafa MH, Aboul-Azm T, Barnard R, Margison GP, O'Connor PJ. O^6-alkylguanine-DNA alkyltransferase activity in schistosomiasis-associated human bladder cancer. Eur J Cancer 1994;30A(9):1314–1319.

92. Frenkel K. Carcinogen-mediated oxidant formation and oxidative DNA damage. Pharmacol Ther 1992;53:127–166.

93. Gordon LI, Weitzman SA. The respiratory burst and carcinogenesis. In: Sbarra AJ, Strauss RR, eds. The Respiratory Burst and Its Physiological Significance. New York: Plenum; 1988:277–298.

94. Cerutti P. Prooxidant states and tumor promotion. Science 1985;227:375–381.

95. Schacter E, Beecham EJ, Covey JM, Kohn KW, Potter M. Activated neutrophils induce prolonged DNA damage in neighboring cells. Carcinogenesis 1988;9:2297–2304.

96. Schraufstater I, Hyslop PA, Jackson JH, Cochrane CG. Oxidant-induced DNA damage of target cells. J Clin Invest 1988;82:1040–1050.

97. Ward AJ, Olive PL, Burr AH, Rosin MP. A sensitivity to oxidative stress is linked to chromosome 11 but is not due to a difference in single strand DNA breakage or repair. Mutat Res 1993;294:299–308.

98. Lewis JG, Hamilton T, Adams DO. The effect of macrophage development on the release of reactive oxygen intermediates and lipid oxidation products and their ability to induce oxidative DNA damage in mammalian cells. Carcinogenesis 1986;7:813–818.

99. Foegh ML, Thomas G, Ramwell PW. Free Radicals, Arachidonic Acid Metabolites, and Nutrition. JPEN J Parenter Enteral Nutr 1990;14(5):218S–222S.

100. Trush MA, Kensler TW. An overview of the relationship between oxidative stress and chemical carcinogenesis. Free Rad Biol Med 1991;10:201–209.

101. Battista JR, Marnett LJ. Prostaglandin H synthase-dependent epoxidation of aflatoxin B_1. Carcinogenesis 1985;6(8):1227–1229.

102. Dix TA, Marnett LJ. Metabolism of polycyclic aromatic hydrocarbon derivatives to ultimate carcinogens during lipid peroxidation. Science 1983;221:77–79.

103. Marnett LJ. Polycyclic aromatic hydrocarbon oxidation during prostaglandin biosynthesis. Life Sci 1981;29:531–546.

104. Yamazoe Y, Zenser TV, Miller DW, Kadlubar FF. Mechanism of formation and structural characterization of DNA adducts derived from peroxidative activation of benzidine. Carcinogenesis 1988;9(9):1635–1641.

105. Ueda K, Kobayashi S, Morita J, Komano T. Site-specific DNA damage caused by lipid peroxidation products. Biochim Biophys Acta 1985;824:341–348.

106. Rosin MP, Anwar W. Chromosomal damage in urothelial cells from Egyptians with chronic Schistosoma haematobium infections. Int J Cancer 1992;50:539–543.

107. La Vecchia C, Negri E, D'Avanzo B, Savoldelli R, Franceschi S. Genital and urinary tract diseases and bladder cancer. Cancer Res 1991; 51: 629–631.

108. Hofseth LJ, Dunn BP, Rosin MP. Micronucleus frequencies in urothelial cells of catheterized patients with chronic bladder inflammation. Mutat Res (Fundam Mol Mech Mut) 1996; 352/1–2: 65–72.

109. El-Masri WS, Fellows G. Bladder cancer after spinal cord injury. Paraplegia 1981; 19: 265–270.

110. Ohgaki H, Hard GC, Hirota N, Maekawa A, Takahashi M, Kleihues P. Selective mutation of codon 204 and 213 of the *p53* gene in rat tumors induced by alkylating *N*-nitroso compounds. Cancer Res 1992; 52: 2995–2998.

111. El-Bolkainy MN, Eissa S, Mokhtar N. Histopathology of proliferative and metaplastic lesions. In: El-Bolkainy MN, Chu EW, eds. Detection of Bladder Cancer Associated with Schistosomiasis. Cairo: Al-Ahram Press; 1981:84–96.

112. Wahl SM, Wong H, McCartney-Francis N. Role of growth factors in inflammation and repair. J Cell Biochem 1989;40:193–199.

113. Lynch SE, Calvin RB, Antoniades HN. Growth factors in wound healing. J Clin Invest 1989;84:640–646.

114. Ames BN, Gold LS. Too many rodent carcinogens: mitogenesis increases mutagenesis. Science 1990;249:970–971.

115. Preston-Martin S, Pike MC, Ross RK, Jones PA, Henderson BE. Increased cell division as a cause of human cancer. Cancer Res 1990;50:7415–7421.

116. Hashem M, Boutros K. The influence of bilharzial infection on the carcinogenesis of the mouse bladder. J Egypt Med Assoc 1961;44:598–606.

117. James C, Hicks M, Webbe G, Nelson GS. *Schistosoma haematobium* and bladder cancer [abstract]. Parasitology 1974;69:viii–ix.

118. Hicks RM, Walters CL, Elsebai I, El Aasser A-B, El Merzabani M, Gough TA. Demonstration of nitrosamines in human urine: preliminary observations on a possible etiology for bladder cancer in association with chronic urinary tract infections. Proc R Soc Med 1977;70:413–417.

119. Hicks RM, James CL, Webb, G. Effect of *Schistosoma haematobium* and *N*-butyl-N(4-hydroxylbutyl) nitrosamine on the development of urothelial neoplasia in the baboon. Br J Cancer 1980; 42:730–755.

120. Ishii A, Matsuoka H, Aji T, Ohta N, Arimoto S, Wataya Y, Hayatsu H. Parasite infection and cancer: with special emphasis on *Schistosoma japonicum* infections (Trematoda). A review. Mutat Res 1994;305(2):273–281.

121. Farid Z. Schistosomes with terminal-spined eggs: pathological and clinical aspects. In: Jordan P, Webbe G, Sturrock RF, eds. Human Schistosomiasis. Oxon, UK: Cab International; 1993;159–183.

122. Raunio H, Husgafvel-Pursiainen K, Anttila S, Hietanen E, Hirvonen A, Pelkonen O. Diagnosis of polymorphisms in carcinogen-activating and inactivating enzymes and cancer susceptibility—a review. Gene 1995;159:113–121.

123. Wolf CR, Smith CAD, Forman D. Metabolic polymorphisms in carcinogen metabolising enzymes and cancer susceptibility. Br Med Bull 1994;50(3):718–731.

124. Anwar WA, Abdel-Rahman SZ, El-Zein RA, Mostafa HM, Au WW. Genetic polymorphism of GSTM1, CYP2E1 and CYP2D6 in Egyptian bladder cancer patients. Carcinogenesis 1996;17(9):1923–1029.

125. Badawi AF, Mostafa MH, Probert A, O'Connor PJ. Role of schistosomiasis in human bladder cancer: Evidence of association, aetiological factors, and basic mechanism of carcinogenesis. European Journal of Cancer Prevention 1995;4:45–59.

126. Gentile JM, Clark D, Aardema MJ, Hohnson M, Blankespoor HD. Modification of mutagens metabolism in parasite-infected organism. Arch Environ Health 1985;40:5–12.

127. Lemmer LB, Fripp PJ. Schistosomiasis and malignancy. S Afr Med J 1994;84: 211–215.

128. Abdel-Tawab GA, Ibrahim EK, El-Masri A, Al-Ghorab M, Makhyoun N.

Studies on tryptophan metabolism in bilharzial bladder cancer patients. Invest Urol 1968;5:591–601.

129. Bryan GT. Role of tryptophan metabolites in urinary-bladder cancer. Am Ind Hyg Assoc J 1969;30:27–34.

130. Rosin MP. Genetic and proliferation markers in clinical studies of the premalignant process. Cancer Bull 1991;43(6):507–514.

131. Gyde SN, Prior P, Allan RN. Colorectal cancer in ulcerative colitis: a cohort study of primary referrals from three centres. Gut 1988;29:206–217.

132. Ming-Chai C, Chi-Yuan C, Pei-Yu C, Jen-Chun H. Evolution of colorectal cancer in schistosomiasis: transitional mucosal changes adjacent to large intestinal carcinoma in colectomy specimens. Cancer 1980;46:1661–1675.

133. Roediger WE, Lawson MJ, Nance SH, Radcliffe BC. Detectable colonic nitrite levels in inflammatory bowel disease—mucosal or bacterial malfunction? Digestion 1986;35:199–204.

134. Amano T, Oshima T. Hepatoma formation in ddY mice with chronic schistosomiasis japonica. Jpn J Cancer Res 1988;79:173–180.

135. Miyasato M. Experimental study of the influence of *Schistosoma japonicum* infection on carcinogenesis of mouse liver treated with N-2-fluorenylacetamide (2-FAA). Jpn J Parasitol 1984;33:41–48.

136. Arimoto S, Matsuoka H, Aji T, Ishii A, Wataya Y, Hayatsu H. Modified metabolism of a carcinogen, 3-amino-1-methyl-5H-pyrido[4,3-b]indole (Trp-P-2), by liver S9 from *Schistosoma japonicum*-infected mice. Mutat Res 1992;282:177–182.

137. Aji T, Matsuoka H, Ishii A, Arimoto S, Hayatsu H. Retention of a mutagen 3-amino-1-methyl-5H-pyrido[4,3-b]indole (Trp-P-2), in the liver of mice infected with *Schistosoma japonicum*. Mutat Res 1994;305(2):265–272.

138. Matsuoka H, Aji T, Ishii A, Arimoto S, Wataya Y, Hayatsu H. Reduced levels of mutagen processing potential in the *Schistosoma japonicum*-infected mouse liver. Muta Res 1989;227:153–157.

139. Hasler JA, Siwelak AH, Nyathi CB, Chetsanga CJ. The effect of schistosomiasis on the activation of aflatoxin B1. Res Commun Chem Pathol Pharm 1986;51:421–424.

140. Kitani K, Iguchi M. *Schistosomiasis japonica*: a vanishing endemic in Japan. J Gasteroenterol Hepatol 1990;5:160–172.

141. Daren Z, Yuesheng L, Xianming Y. Schistosomiasis control in China. World Health Forum 1994;14:387–389.

142. Taylor MG. Schistosomiasis vaccines: farewell to the god of plague? J Trop Med Hyg 1994;97:257–268.

143. Kloos H. Human behavior, health education and schistosomiasis control: a review. Soc Sci Med 1995;40(11):1497–1511.

144. Chandiwana SK, Woolhouse MEJ. Heterogeneities in water contact patterns and the epidemiology of *Schistosoma haematobium*. Parasitology 1991;103:363–370.

145. Dunne DW, Hagan P, Abath FGC. Prospects for immunological control of schistosomiasis. Lancet 1995;345:1488–1492.

146. Capron A, Riveau G, Grzych J, Boulanger D, Capron M, Pierce R. Development of a vaccine strategy against human and bovine schistosomiasis. Trop Geograph Med 1994;46(4):242–246.

147. Capron M, Capron A. Immunoglobulin E and effector cells in schistosomiasis. Science 1994;264:1876–1877.

148. Ming-gang C, Yao L. Conference procedings: International symposium on schistosomiasis. Chin Med J 1993;106(8):628–234.

149. Giboda M, Smith JM, Prichard RK. Reduction in tissue egg load and maintenance of resistance to challenge in mice infected with *Schistosoma mansoni*, following combined treatment with praziquantel and an antifibrotic agent. Ann Trop Med Parasitol 1994;88(4):385–395.

13

Liver Flukes and Biliary Cancer

WITAYA THAMAVIT, TOMOYUKI SHIRAI, AND NOBUYUKI ITO

Infections with three human liver flukes, *Opisthorchis viverrini*, *Clonorchis sinensis*, and *Opisthorchis felineus*, have long been known to be associated with malignancy. In this chapter, we will emphasize the first two parasites and the evidence linking them to cancer. The malignancies related to these parasites are two forms of liver cancer: cholangiocarcinoma (a cancer derived from bile ducts) and hepatocellular carcinoma (a cancer derived from parenchymal liver cells).

THE THAI LIVER FLUKE: *O. VIVERRINI*

O. viverrini, the Thai liver fluke, is endemic mainly in northeast Thailand and some parts of Laos and is also found sporadically in certain areas of the central and northern Thai provinces.[1-9] Researchers have estimated that 7 millon Thai people harbor infection.[4] The parasite inhabits the bile ducts—and occasionally the pancreatic ducts and gallbladder—of humans, dogs, cats, and other mammals.

O. viverrini is a hermaphrodite measuring 7 to 12 mm long by 1.5 to 3 mm wide. The worm is transparent and elongate, tapering anteriorly and somewhat rounded posteriorly.[5,10] It has two suckers, one oral and one ventral, that are nearly equal in size.[1,5,10,11] The oral sucker connects to a small, bulbous pharynx that leads to a short esophagus. The esophagus then bifurcates to form two ceca extending to the posterior end of the body. Reproductive organs occupy most of the body and, as the name Opisthorchis implies, a pair of lobated testes are located in the posterior quarter of the body (opis = behind, orchis = testis). The uterus is a markedly coiled tubule, and the vitellaria consist of transverse compressed follicles, lying laterally in the middle third of the body.

The life cycle of *O. viverrini* is fully described in many standard textbooks and journals.[2,3,5,10,11] Briefly, two intermediate hosts are required: snails and fish. The adult worm releases ovoid, yellowish-brown 26.7-μm by 15-μm eggs, each with an operculum at the anterior end and a knob posteriorly.[1,12] These eggs, which contain fully developed ciliated miracidia, enter into the biliary system and are then excreted in the feces. The eggs do not hatch, however, unless swallowed by the first intermediate host, one of several species of snails (*Bithynia siamensis goniomphalus, B. funiculata*, or *B. siamensis siamensis*). In the snails, the miracidia are released to develop further to sporocysts, redia, and cercariae within 6 to 8 weeks. Many cercariae leave the snail in search of the second intermediate cyprinoid fish (freshwater, soft-finned fishes including carps and minnows), such as *Cyclocheilichthys siaja, C. tapiensis, Hampala dispar*, and *Puntius orphoides*. After entering the fish, the cercariae lose their tails and develop into infective cysts (metacercariae) in the muscles and connective tissue. Humans and other mammals can be infected by ingestion of raw fish. In Thailand, the native dishes koi-pla and pla-som are the main sources of *O. viverrini* infection. After being eaten by humans, the infective metacercariae excyst in the duodenum. The newly excysted worms, armed with scales and spines around the oral and ventral suckers,[13] move into the bile duct through the ampulla of Vater and develop into adults within 1 month. The life span of mature *O. viverrini*, as deduced from observations of people who have left endemic areas and experienced no reinfection, is 25 to 30 years.[14]

THE CHINESE LIVER FLUKE: *C. SINENSIS*

C. sinensis infection is endemic in China, as well as in Taiwan, South Korea, North Vietnam, and the far-eastern part of Russia; epidemiologists estimate that 7 million people worldwide are infected (see reviews in references 11,15–17). *C. sinensis* resides mainly in the hepatic ducts; in heavy infection, it may also reside in the common bile duct, gallbladder, and pancreatic ducts.[11,15–19] The morphology and life cycle of *C. sinensis* are similar to those of *O. viverrini*. The mature worm is larger, however: 8-mm to 15-mm long, 1.5-mm to 5-mm wide, and about 1-mm thick. The worm is flat and leaf-shaped, and the oral sucker at the anterior end opens into a pharynx that bifurcates into two blind-ended ceca. The ventral sucker is a little smaller and lies about one quarter from the anterior end. The parasite is hermaphroditic, with reproductive organs occupying most of the body. Differentiation can be done simply by examination of the testes,[1,5,10,15] which are strikingly clawlike and branched (hence the derivation of the name Clonorchis: klonos = branch, orchis = testis), in contrast to the lobed structures of *O. viverrini* and *O. felineus*.

The first intermediate snail hosts of *C. sinensis* are *Parafossarulus manchouricus, P. anomalospiralis*, and *Alocinma longicornis; Semisulcospira libertina* and *Thiara granifera* may also be infected. Approximately 95 fish species in the family Cyprinidae serve as the second intermediate hosts for the developmental cycle of the fluke.[17] *Pseudorasbora parva* is the most important in the transmission of the disease because of its large population, wide distribution, and often heavy infection with metacercariae of *C. sinensis.* Exposure occurs by ingestion of a variety of dishes composed of raw or only partly cooked fish containing metacercariae of the fluke. The life span of *C. sinensis* is reported to be 25 to 30 years.[20,21]

THE RUSSIAN LIVER FLUKE: *O. FELINEUS*

Approximately 1.5 millon cases of *O. felineus* infection have been reported in the former USSR, of which about 1.2 million are in the Russia Federation, mainly in western Siberia.[11,22] Infections also occur in the Ukraine and Kazazhstan. The worm resides mainly in the bile ducts, gallbladder, and pancreatic ducts and is about the size of *O. viverrini,*[5] from which it can be differentiated by the characteristics of its sucker, esophagus, ovary and testes, and vitellaria. The relatively localized geographic distribution of the parasite also helps with its identification.[10,15] The life cycle of *O. felineus* is similar to that of *O. viverrini* and *C. sinensis,* with the first intermediate hosts being *Bithynia leachi* and *B. tentaculata,* and the second intermediate hosts being cyprinoid fishes such as *Idus melantous* and *Tinca tinca.*[10] As with the other liver flukes, mammalian infection with *O. felineus* occurs by consumption of raw fish.

CHOLANGIOCELLULAR CARCINOMA

Cholangiocarcinoma is a primary liver cancer that derives from epithelial cells of the intrahepatic bile ducts. It is divided by anatomical location into two types: the hilar type that occurs in the hepatic hilum region and the peripheral type that develops in interlobular ducts of the liver.[23–25] According to the classification of the Japanese Society of Biliary Surgery, cholangiocarcinoma are histologically categorized into several types: papillary, tubular (well, moderately, or poorly differentiated), mucinous, signet ring cell, adenosquamous, squamous, anaplastic, undifferentiated, miscellaneous, and unclassified types.[26,27] Cholangiocarcinoma is pathologically and etiologically different from the more common form of primary liver cancer, hepatocellular carcinoma, which is discussed more fully in Chapters 9 and 10 of this book.

EPIDEMIOLOGICAL ASSOCIATION BETWEEN LIVER FLUKES AND CANCER

In 1994, evidence for the association between liver flukes and cancer was reviewed in detail by the International Agency for Research on Cancer, a branch of the World Health Organization.[11] The agency concluded that *O. viverrini* was a definite cause of cancer in humans (a Group 1 agent), that *C. sinensis* was a probable cause of cancer in humans (a Group 2A agent), and that *O. felineus* had not yet been sufficiently studied to assess its carcinogenicity (a Group 3 agent). Here, we present some of the data on which these conclusions were based. However, some of our new data are in contrast to the previous conclusions.

Opisthorchis Viverrini

Studies that evaluate the association between *O. viverrini* and cancer include hospital-based case series, population-based ecologic studies that correlate the incidence of cancer with prevalence of infection in various geographic areas, and one very convincing case-control study (reviewed in references 10,11,14, 28–32).

Bhamarapravati and Viranuvatti at Siriraj Hospital, Mahidol University, Bangkok, conducted the first large case series that evaluated the relationship between *O. viverrini* and cancer. They analyzed 9694 autopsies conducted between 1954 and 1965, and 1301 liver biopsies obtained between 1960 and 1962. An unusually high incidence of cholangiocarcinoma in *O. viverrini*–infected cases was observed in both the autopsy and biopsy materials.[33] The ratio of hepatocellular carcinoma to cholangiocarcinoma in autopsies without opisthorchiasis was 8 to 1, in contrast to the 1 to 8 ratio in the infected patients. Similarly, the ratio of these two tumors in biopsies was 5 to 1 in uninfected cases and 1 to 2 in the presence of liver fluke infection.

At the same institution in 1978, Koompirochana and associates expanded the autopsy case series to include 15,641 subjects from 1954 to 1974. This larger group included 154 subjects with *O. viverrini* infection.[34] Among these subjects, 85 (55%)—68 males and 17 females (mean age of 46.2 years)—had primary hepatic carcinomas. The majority of these tumors [N = 67 (79%)] were cholangiocarcinomas; the remaining tumors included nine hepatocellular carcinomas, four mixed hepatocholangiocarcinomas, and five tumors that could not be classified. Similarly, Sinawat and Hemsrichart at Khon Kaen Hospital identified 61 cases of peripheral cholangiocarcinoma from 1983 to 1986: 5 from autopsies, 13 surgically resected, and 43 from open biopsies.[35] Fifty-eight of 61 cases were associated with the liver fluke infection.

A huge, nationwide survey of liver pathology in Thailand was conducted by Bunyaratvej and colleagues, who examined 3305 biopsy specimens collected between 1974 and 1978.[36] Their work also disclosed a high incidence of cholangiocarcinoma in association with liver fluke infection in the northeast of Thailand. This association was particularly pronounced in Khon Kaen, where the incidence of this bile duct cancer was twofold that of hepatocellular carcinomas. The average age at diagnosis of cholangiocarcinoma was 48.8 years in males and 48.1 years in females;

more than two thirds of the patients were male. Srivatanakul and associates had reported similar data, noting that the incidence of cholangiocarcinomas was almost twofold that of hepatocellular carcinoma in the *O. viverrini* endemic northeast area. In that study also, cholangiocarcinoma was 2.4 times more common in males[37]

Several clinical series support these pathology findings. Kurathong and colleagues performed a prospective evaluation of 551 patients from Northeast Thailand.[38] Each patient was examined for development of hepatobiliary diseases in association in the setting of *O. viverrini* infection. Liver fluke infection was diagnosed by identification of parasite ova either in stool or in fluid aspirated from the intrahepatic biliary trees. Of 72 patients with clinical evidence of hepatobiliary disease, 28 underwent liver biopsy, revealing cholangiocarcinoma in 11 patients and combined hepatocellular carcinoma and cholangiocarcinoma in one patient. All 12 of these cases were associated with *O. viverrini* infection. Hitanant and colleagues used peritoneoscopy in 5356 patients from 1972 to 1983 to diagnosis opisthorchiasis. They, too, found a strong link between infection and disease. Of 203 proven cases of *O. viverrini* infection, 59 (29%) had cholangiocarcinoma.[39]

From such hospital-based data, Green and associates estimated the incidence of cholangiocarcinoma in the high-risk area of Khon Kaen and the surrounding provinces. Using pathology, ultrasound, and inpatient and outpatient records, they diagnosed a total of 203 cholangiocarcinomas within a one month period of 1988; 75 of the cases were from Khon Kaen province itself; the remainder from other northeastern provinces.[40] From these numbers, the authors estimated the age-standardized incidence rates of cholangiocarcinoma in this region to be 135.4 and 40 per 100,000 in males and females, respectively. The truncated standardized incidence rates (ages 35 to 64 years only) were a remarkable 334.2 per 100,000 in males and 104.3 per 100,000 in females.

In population-based research from the Khon Kaen province cancer registry, Vatanasapt and colleagues found cholangiocarcinoma to be the leading cancer in both men and women in this province.[41] The age-standardized incidence rates for the year 1988 were 89.2 per 100,000 in males and 35.5 per 100,000 in females. Although these population-based numbers are lower than the hospital-based estimates reported by Green, they still represent the highest rates of cholangiocarcinoma in the world. Moreover, clusters of liver cancer appeared to be associated with the prevalence and intensity of *Opisthorchis viverrini* infection in the region. Srivatanakul and colleagues similarly correlated *O. viverrini* prevalence with hepatic-cancer incidence data among five locations in Thailand (Ubol and Korat [northeast], Chiang Mai [north], Bangkok [central] and Songkhla [south]).[42] There was no significant difference across centers in hepatocellular carcinoma incidence. The incidence of cholangiocarcinoma, however, was significantly elevated in Ubol and Korat, where liver flukes were highly endemic. Age-standardized incidences per 100,000 population in the center of the endemic area were 78.8 in males and 30.8 in females, compared to a mere 7.3 in males and 5.3 in females in the low-risk *O. viverrini* region of Chiang Mai..

In 1991, using more traditional observational epidemiological methods, Parkin and colleagues performed a case-control study of cholangiocarcinoma in 103 individuals from northeastern Thailand. Patients with cholangiocarcinoma who had been admitted to one of three hospitals between 1987 and 1988 were compared to control patients matched by age and gender.[43] Diagnoses of cancer were made either by histopathology, or with typical findings on ultrasound examination, or by percutaneous cholangiography with or without an elevated titer of CA 19-9. *O. viverrini* was diagnosed with serology. The results indicated that *O. viverrini* infection increased the risk of cholangiocarcinoma fivefold, with infected males appearing to be at higher risk for cancer than infected females. Parkin estimated that a full two thirds of cholangiocarcinoma cases in Thailand were caused by infection with *O. viverrini*.

Clonorchis Sinensis

Like that for *O. viverrini*, most of the evidence for an association between *C. sinensis* and cancer comes from case series. One of the first of these studies was conducted by Hou, a Hong Kong pathologist, in 1956.[44] He reported that all 30 randomly selected cases of the peripheral-type intrahepatic bile-duct tumors were associated with the Chinese liver fluke. One decade later, Belamaric reviewed autopsy slides from 213 primary hepatic carcinomas diagnosed in Hong Kong, and found 18 of 19 cholangiocarcinomas to be linked with *C. sinensis* infection.[45] Chou and Chan then described 50 cases of hilar and peripheral cholangiocarcinoma, from among 5814 autopsies from 1964 to 1973; 46 of them also harbored *C. sinensis*.[46] Choi and colleagues subsequently chose 16 patients with peripheral cholangiocarcinoma for computed tomography in conjunction with histopathology, stool examination for parasite eggs, and intradermal test for *C. sinensis*. Ten were thus demonstrated to have heavy *C. sinensis* infections.[47]

Cases of cholangiocarcinoma associated with *C. sinensis* infection in Asian immigrants to the United States have been reported frequently.[48–50] Three Laotian cholangiocarcinoma patients, who had lived in Laos and Thailand only, were also reported to have *C. sinensis* infection,[49,50] but these reports are questionable because these countries are thought to be areas for *O. viverrini* only and *C. sinensis* is absent.

Few analytical epidemiological studies on *C. sinensis* and cholangiocarcinoma have been conducted. In a case-control study by Chung and Lee conducted in Pusan, Korea, an area of extremly high *C. sinensis* prevalence, *C. sinensis* eggs were sought in the stools of 36 patients with cholangiocarcinoma, 170 patients with hepatocellular carcionoma, and 559 subjects without known liver disease.[11] *C. sinensis* infection increased the risk of cholangiocarcinoma sixfold, but did not increase the risk of hepato-cellular carcinoma. The analysis exhibited the close assocation of *C. sinensis* infection and cholangiocarcinoma development, while no association between the liver fluke and hepatocellular carcinoma was shown.

Opisthorchis Felineus

Few systematic studies have been conducted specifically concerning the association between *O. felineus* and cancer.[11] Numerous case series, predominantly from the former USSR, do link infection with malignancy.[34,35,38,51-57]. This large number of reported cases cannot be explained easily by chance alone.

PATHOLOGY AND MECHANISMS OF CARCINOGENESIS

Although the incidence of cholangiocarcinoma in populations infected with the three liver flukes is higher than that observed elsewhere, the rates are still low considering the millions of people who harbor the parasites.[17,40-42] The liver flukes, therefore, are probably not sufficient for carcinogenesis in human beings. There are plausible mechanisms, however, by which liver flukes may contribute, as either initiators or promotors and coinitiators, to the oncogenic process.

Pathology in Humans

Consistent pathological findings for chronic fluke infection in humans, with and without cholangiocarcinoma, are desquamation, hyperplasia, and formation of adenomatous structures with goblet-cell metaplasia in the large- and medium-sized, second-order bile ducts where the parasites reside. Dilated thick-walled ducts or periductal fibrosis almost always occur in association with adenomatous hyperplasia.[10,14,15,18,44,45,56,57] Proliferation of the smaller second-order duct epithelium also is present[35,39] with infiltration of neutrophils, eosinophils, lymphocytes, macrophages and plasma cells invariably being seen.[10]

Another hepatic lesion frequently seen with liver fluke infections is obstruction of bile ducts due to large numbers of parasites in the ductal lumen. This obstruction may lead to suppurative cholangitis with abscess formation. These abscesses can involve the surrounding hepatic cells, particularly when ruptures of abscesses occur, leading to cholangiohepatitis.[18] Compression of hepatic parenchyma due to dilated ducts, abscesses, and cyst formation are observed, and egg granulomas are occasionally seen.[14,15]

Pathology in Domestic Animals

Three cases of cholangiocarcinoma have been reported from among 93 cats with *C. sinensis* infection.[58,59] Two of these cats were infected naturally;

at the time of cancer diagnosis at 4 years of age, one cat harbored 150 and the other 200 adult *C. sinesis* flukes The third cat with cholangiocarcinoma was one of the 26 cats infected experimentally by feeding fish flesh containing *C. sinensis* metacercariae. The animal died of bronchopneumonia at age 4 years; at necropsy, cholangiocarcinoma was found and 105 *C. sinensis* were recovered from the bile ducts. In addition, an 8-year-old female chow dog suffering from abdominal enlargement was reported to have a cholangiocarcinoma in association with *C. sinensis* infection.[60] All the intrahepatic bile duct tumors that developed in these domestic animals exhibited histopathological features similar to those found in humans.[10,14,15,18,44,45,56,57]

From the available data for infection of cats and dogs, the liver fluke is also probably not the sole carcinogenic agent in these species.

Pathology in Experimental Animals

Most of what is known about the pathogenesis of liver fluke–related carcinogenesis has been learned from studies in experimental animals. Cholangiocellular lesions in Syrian hamsters have been observed at three levels of the biliary tree[61]: the first-order duct or bile ductules, the second-order ducts, and the second-order main ducts where the parasites reside. Lesions of first-order ducts include bile ductule proliferation, acute and chronic proliferative cholangitis (cholangiolitis), cholangiofibrosis (cholangiolofibrosis), cholangiofibromas (cholangiolofibroma, borderline lesions between cholangiofibrosis and cholangiocarcinomas),[62] cholangiocarcinomas (cholangiolocarcinomas) (Figure 13.1), and all their dilated or cystic counterparts. Lesions derived from the second order ducts are hyperplasia with or without dysplasia, acute and chronic proliferative cholangitis, cholangiofibrosis, mucinous cystadenomas, cholangiofibromas, and cholangiocarcinomas (Figure 13.2). In the main ducts where the parasites reside, infolding and papillary formation, mucinous cystadenomas, and cholangiocarcinomas occur. From our observations, cholangiocellular lesions with the potential to develop into cholangiocarcinoma include cholangiolofibrosis, cholangiolofibromas, bile duct hyperplasia with dysplasia, cholangiofibrosis, mucinous cystadenomas, and cholangiofibromas.

In hamsters infected with *O. viverrini*, early pathologic changes (at 3 to 15 days of infection) include multifocal necrosis of liver parenchyma and inflammatory reactions involving the second-order bile ducts and portal connective tissue.[63] As the flukes mature into the adult forms, they cause hyperplasia and infrequently adenomatous changes in the large bile duct. Multilobular or secondary biliary cirrhosis results from replacement of atrophic and necrotic cells by proliferated bile ductules and fibrous tissues. In the late phase of infection, egg and parasitic granulomas often are present.

In the hamster bile duct, hepatic and bile duct cell death and regeneration occur early after *O. viverrini* infection,[63] partially attributable to bacte-

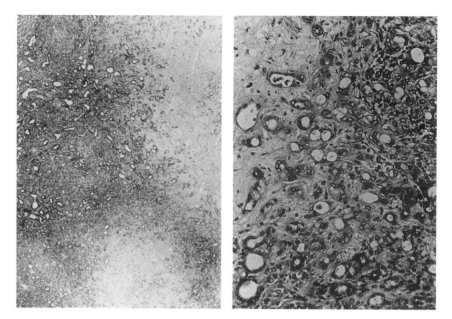

Figure 13.1. Cholangiocarcinoma of a first-order duct or bile ductule (cholangiolocarcinoma) showing varying sizes of bile ductules of small lumen lined with flattened epithelial cells with scant cytoplasm, embedded in loose fibrovascular tissue with a central area of necrosis (left). (2 × 10.) Some of the ductular epithelial cells have escaped through the basement membrane (right). (10 × 10).

ria from the gut being carried into the intrahepatic duct system by parasites during migration.[64] The liver fluke wedged in the main duct also causes enlargement and hyperplasia of intrahepatic second-order ducts and intense proliferation of bile ductules.[61,62,64-70] Obvious hyperplasia of the main-duct epithelium is partly due to compensatory regeneration resulting from multifocal desquamation of ductal epithelium by the action of parasite suckers during their movement (Figure 13.3). Bile-duct cell regeneration is readily demonstrable by immunohistochemical staining of bromodeoxyuridine (BrdU) in hamsters infected with *O. viverrini* for 18 days (Figure 13.4). Regeneration or hyperplasia of the main duct is more obvious in the late stages of infection, as shown by infolding and adenomatous hyperplasia.[59,63] Albino rats infected with *C. sinensis* for 1,2,5, and 15 weeks also exhibit similar changes.[71] It has not been established, however, whether chemicals released by the liver flukes are directly responsible for eliciting hyperplasia of the second order duct epithelium. In support of a direct relationship, proline produced and released by another liver fluke, *Fasciola hepatica*, has been reported to induce bile duct hyperplasia in rats[72,73]; administration of this compound to hamsters, however, did not result in similar promotion effects.[74]

Whereas enlargement of the second-order main ducts may be an ac-

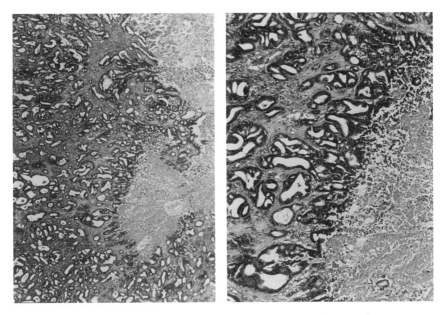

Figure 13.2. Cholangiocarcinoma of a second-order duct with structures composed of varying sizes of bile ducts of larger lumen with cuboidal or columnar lining epithelial cells with more abundant cytoplasm (compared to cholangiolocarcinoma), embedded in desmoplastic tissues with a large area of necrosis in the tumor (left). (2 × 10.) Higher-magnification appearance of the tumor cells is shown on the right. (5 × 10.)

commodation to the parasite growth, the proliferation that first appears about 15 to 30 days after infection[63] probably results from stasis due to mechanical obstruction by the flukes.[61,63] Egg or parasitic granulomas resulting from immune reactions may also play a role in this obstructive process.[61,63] Bile-ductule proliferations in the hamsters infected with liver fluke may be extensive, spanning from one portal area to another. These proliferative cells may eventually die or become quiescent, being replaced by fibrous connective tissues such that a multilobular or secondary biliary cirrhosis results.[63]

Both acute and chronic inflammatory cells—particularly activated macrophages—participate in formation of egg and parasitic granulomas. Macrophages and eosinophils may also be found inside or around the first- and second-order main ducts, evincing immunological reactions against the surface tegument, or against excretory or secretory antigens released by the liver fluke.[75] Toxic products—such as oxygen radicals, nitric oxide, nitrite, and nitrate—might cause cell death with subsequent regeneration of bile ducts and, to a lesser extent, of hepatocytes (Figure 13.4).[76,77]

In addition to the hepatic cell death and regeneration that occurs with early *O. viverrini* infection,[63] changes in the parenchyma also take place indirectly due to compression by enlarged second order main ducts and

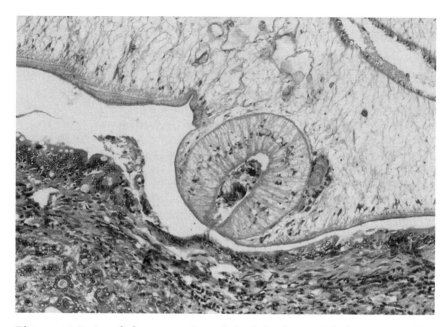

Figure 13.3. Local desquamation of the bile duct epithelium caused by the ventral sucker of *O. viverrini* during its movement. (20 × 10.)

ongoing multilobular (secondary biliary) cirrhosis that renders the adjacent hepatic cells atrophic and finally necrotic. Although the process is slow, compensatory regeneration is a gradual consequence. Infiltration of the both acute and chronic inflammatory cells also contributes to cell death and to regeneration of hepatocytes (Figure 13.4). Since *O. viverrini* infection causes chronically increased cell turnover in both parenchymal and ductular compartments of the liver, it would be expected to act not only as a promoter, but also as a coinitiator in the oncogenic process.[78]

Carcinogenesis in Experimental Animals

The multiple changes associated with infection are not in themselves sufficient to induce tumors. In one study, no cholangiocarcinoma development was seen 70 weeks after 37 Syrian hamsters were infected with 50 *O. viverrini* metacercariae.[79] In a second experiment, hamsters infected with 60 to 80 metacercariae of *O. viverrini* without additional carcinogen exposure also had no bile duct cancers after observation periods ranging from 22 to 45 weeks.[61,62,64–68,80]

In conflict with these studies, two of 18 female Syrian golden hamsters aged 6 to 8 weeks that had received 60 *O. viverrini* metacercariae by intragastric intubation in our laboratory developed cholangiocarcinomas by the end of 38 weeks.[69] Because this finding conflicted with other research, we designed a larger experiment to evaluate metacercarial load and to

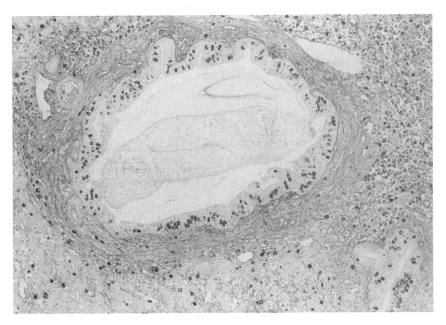

Figure 13.4. Immunoperoxidase staining of 5±bromodeoxyuridine (BrdU) of liver infected with *O.viverrini* for 18 days reveals BrdU-positive bile duct epithelial cells, surrounding inflammatory cells, and hepatic cells, indicating the proliferative state of the liver compartments. (10 × 10.)

mimic the heavy infestation with *O. viverrini* seen in humans. A total of 300 male and female Syrian hamsters, 6 to 8 weeks old, were divided into four groups, and all were infected monthly for 10 months with 0 metacercariae (40 hamsters), 13 metacercariae (80 hamsters), 25 metacercariae (80 hamsters), or 50 metacercariae (100 hamsters) by intragastric intubation. Animals were maintained for 52 weeks. Although the magnitude of proliferative and inflammatory lesions involving the first- and second-order ducts depended on the number of metacercariae inoculated, bile duct tumors were not detected despite the presence of cholangiofibrosis in some animals.[70] Thus, little evidence exists for complete carcinogenicity of the Thai liver fluke, *O. viverrini*.[61,62,64–69,80]

Similarly, bile duct tumors do not arise following experimental infection in rats. In one experiment, 25 male Wistar rats aged 8 to 10 weeks were infected with 50 metacercariae of *C. sinensis*, and then were sacrificed at either 4, 8, 12, 16, 20, 24, or 28 weeks.[81] Necrotic foci and mild inflammatory cell changes were the only lesions seen in the liver. In another experiment, a group of 10 male Fischer rats administered 60 *C. sinensis* metacercariae and killed after 40 weeks[82] demonstrated cholangiocellular lesions, including bile duct proliferation with mucinous metaplasia, extensive ductular proliferation, and periductal inflammation as well as fibrosis. Nevertheless, like in the hamsters, no bile-duct cancers were apparent.

Experimental carcinogenesis has been observed more consistently with two-stage experiments. In one model, Syrian hamsters received a single or double oral or intraperitoneal dose of a hepatocarcinogen (one of di-methylnitrosamine (DMN), diethylnitrosamine (DEN), or dihydroxy-di-n-propylnitrosamine (DHPN)) prior or subsequent to inoculation with *O. viverrini* metacercariae. The animals were then maintained on a basal diet for various periods.[64,67,68,79] In this setting of chemical initiation, *O. viverrini* infection acted as a strong promoter of bile duct cancer and as a weaker promoter of tumor development in the hepatic parenchyma. Most chol-angiocarcinomas found in these experiments were of the peripheral type, probably because the two types of duct epithelium from which they derive (bile ductules and second-order ducts) are most intimately associated with the hepatocytes that metabolize administered carcinogens. These cholan-giolocarcinomas and cholangiocarcinomas are composed of a varying sizes of tubular glands with sporadic mucin-producing cells embedded in stroma ranging from loose fibrous connective tissue to dense desmoplasia (Figures 13.1 and 13.2). Almost all the tumors contain necrotic areas in their centers with an infiltrative pattern and other characteristics of malig-nant change, including transplantability.[61] Cholangiocarcinomas in the main duct are hilar in type and were not seen frequently in our experi-ments.

Promotion of tumors by *O. viverrini* has been demonstrated by the high incidences of preneoplastic and neoplastic cholangiocellular and hepato-cellular lesions attained when a single initiating intraperitoneal dose of 20 mg/kg body weight of DMN was given prior to *O. viverrini* infection in the hamster model.[64] DMN targets both bile duct cells and hepatocytes,[83,84] requiring activation for generation of a methylating species (methyl car-bonium ion).[85] These methylating species then methylate the DNA of the liver cells in which they are generated. They also pass out of the liver cells to initiate adjacent cells, particularly those in the bile ducts.[86] In the same way, cholangiocarcinoma occurred when *O. viverrini*–infected hamsters re-ceived an initiating stimulus with high doses of DHPN, a chemical similar to DMN that give rises to methylating species.[87] In this experiment, be-cause hepatocellular lesions also arose, the parasite may have acted both as a coinitiator and as a promotor.[67,78] In contrast, a hamster experiment performed by Flavell and Lucas resulted in substantially lower rates of cholangiocarcinoma following DMN administration to *O. viverrini* infected hamsters.[79] Although the dose of DMN (1.6 mg orally 41 days before or 4 days after *O. viverrini* metacercariae administration) approximated that used in the hamster experiment described above,[64] incomplete absorption of DMN in the intestine or other unknown factors might have been re-sponsible for the low yield of bile-duct cancer in this experiment.

In an attempt to see whether tumor development due to fluke infection results from the flukes' obstructive effects or from other infection-related processes, the extrahepatic bile duct of the left lateral lobe of uninfected hamsters was ligated following initiation with 20 mg/kg body weight DMN. The bile stasis resulted in mechanical damage and was also associated with increased cellular repair and regeneration. Although cholangiocarcinoma developed, there were no appreciable effects on the hepatocellular compartment. This finding showed that mechanical damage, rather than chemical or immunological damage, was responsible for tumor promotion by the liver flukes.[88]

That the promoting action of *O. viverrini* is limited to carcinogen-initiated cells was shown by an experiment with DEN,[65,68] which specifically targeted hepatocytes for ethylation.[89] In two experiments, one with metacercariae given before and one after DEN initiation, preneoplastic nodules were observed in hepatocellular tissue without significant development of bile duct lesions. The results might explain some cases of hepatocellular carcinoma in liver fluke-infected patients.[10,54,55]

Interestingly, a combination of liver fluke infection and a continuous administration of a hepatocarcinogen in the drinking water or in the basal diet for a certain period in hamsters resulted in an extremely high number of cholangiocarcinomas and other cholangiocellular lesions yet in few or no hepatocellular lesions.[61,62,90,91] The carcinogens used were DMN in the drinking water for 10 weeks plus *O. viverrini*[61,62]; DMN in drinking water for 8 weeks plus *C. sinensis*[90]; or 0.03% N-2-fluorenylacetamide in the basal diet for 40 weeks plus *C. sinensis*.[91] With 100 *O. viverrini* metacercariae plus 25 ppm DMN,[61] more than 50% of the hepatic parenchyma was occupied by cholangiocellular lesions. Similar increases in cholangiocellular lesions, as well as in preneoplastic hepatocellular lesions, were also realized in hamsters receiving continuous administration of combined nitrite and aminopyrine in their drinking water and *O. viverrini* infection.[66] Nitrite and aminopyrine are reported to form DMN in the stomach.[92]

Aflatoxin B_1 exposure is known to augment risk of hepatocellular carcinoma in humans, particularly when the exposure occurs in the presence of hepatitis B infection (see chapter 9). Increased incidence of hepatocellular carcinomas or preneoplastic lesions (glutathione-S-transferase–positive hepatic foci) has been observed in *C. sinensis*–infected rats administered 1 ppm of aflatoxin B_1 in the diet for 12 weeks.[81] In contrast to DMN, which uniquely initiated tumors in bile ducts, aflatoxins induced only hepatocellular and not cholangiocellular lesions, supporting the experimental data indicating that liver fluke infection promotes tumors only in initiated cells.[93,94]

At this point, we conclude that the liver flukes act as promoters and co-initiators of hepatic cancers, rather than as complete carcinogens.[61–69,79,81,82] Unfortunately, many staple foods and foodstuffs of the people in northeast Thailand contain low levels of N-nitroso compounds, N-nitroso compound precursors, and aflatoxins.[95,96] Given the low incidence of bile-duct cancer despite high prevalence of fluke infections, exposure to these initiating carcinogens must be at only a relatively low level. If the liver flukes alone could induce cholangiocarcinomas, or if cocarcinogen exposure were more pronounced, the incidence of this terrible cancer might be substantially higher.

MOLECULAR EVENTS IN CHOLANGIOCARCINOGENESIS

In vitro generation of oxygen radicals, nitric oxide, nitrite, and nitrate from activated macrophages, neutrophils, and other cells, and nitrosamine formation in the presence of nitrosatable amines, are believed to occur in inflammatory sites in humans and experimental animals (see Chapter 2). These reactive and mutagenic species cause DNA damage and adduct formation as well as cell death with subsequent compensatory or increased cell proliferation (see Chapter 3). Taken together, these events may facilitate mutation, activation of oncogenes, or alteration of tumor suppressor genes.[97-105] These processes chronically occur in liver fluke–infected humans and animals and might contribute to an increased risk of cholangiocarcinoma development.[106,107] However, the inflammatory effects of infection may not be sufficient in themselves to cause cancer, at least over the short term. Syrian hamsters that, monthly for ten months, received large doses of *O. viverrini* metacercariae (500 metacercariae in total–an inoculum rarely, if ever, encountered in humans) did not develop tumors by the end of one year, despite the presence of a small number of preneoplastic foci.[70]

With regard to oncogene activation or tumor-suppressor gene inactivation, little is known in either humans or animal models. Mutations of the *p53* tumor suppressor gene without alteration of c-*Ki-ras* oncogene have been described in Thai patients who have cholangiocarcinoma associated with *O. viverrini* infection.[108,109] Investigation is warranted of whether alteration of these two kinds of genes might facilitate differentiation of irreversible cholangiocellular or hepatocellular precancerous lesions from reversible precancerous lesions.[70,80]

FLUKE CONTROL AND IMPLICATIONS FOR CLINICAL MANAGEMENT

Unfortunately, the incidence of cholangiocarcinoma in northeast Thailand has not decreased appreciably since the introduction of an effective anthelmintic drug for the liver fluke (praziquantel) more than 10 years ago (references 40–43 and Banchob Sripa, Khon Kaen University, Thailand, personal communication). The effects of infection in the setting of initiated cells appear to be quickly irreversible, and infection proceeds to cancer regardless of whether further carcinogen exposure occurs or a promoter is present. Indeed, this irreversibility was indicated by our experimental data. When hamsters received DMN initiation prior to *O. viverrini* infection, followed by praziquantel treatment to eliminate the parasites at different time points, only 8 weeks of active liver fluke infection (equivalent to about 5 years in humans) was sufficient to drive initiated cells to give rise to cancers.[69]

Because treatment may not prevent cancer, prevention of infection is the optimal approach to eliminating the adverse consequences of liver flukes. Considering the fluke's life cycle, there are various steps that, in combination with effective treatment of infected people, would achieve marked reduction or local extermination of the parasites. One step is prevention of fecal parasite ova from reaching the waterways or water reservoirs where the first intermediate host snails reside. Other interventions are reduction of the snail hosts and adequate cooking of fish to kill metacercariae.

Control of the Transfer of Fluke Ova from Humans to the Environment

In northeast Thailand where *O.viverrini* is endemic, deforestation proceeded for many decades until a large percentage of the jungle was replaced by rice fields. Concomitant disappearance of natural water resources turned the region into a semi-arid zone. Several large reservoirs were built to supply water for consumption, for irrigation, and for growing various kinds of fish as a food source for the local people. Many dams were also constructed for the same purposes and for generation of electricity. Within these bodies of water, the first intermediate Bithynia snail hosts and the secondary cyprinoid fish hosts are abundantly present. The majority of people in northeast Thailand are poor and have minimal education. For them, fish from the reservoirs has been the main source of protein. Formerly, the houses in the villages in northeast Thailand seldom had latrines, and people defecated directly into the environment, often close to canals, rivers, and reservoirs, or even directly into water from fishing boats. Feces containing *O. viverrini* ova therefore found their way into natural or constructed water bodies, leading to transmission to the Bithynia snails, in turn entering cyprinoid fish where infective metacercariae develop.

At present, however, the proportion of fish containing metacercaria in almost all water resources has been reduced tremendously due to continuous education and treatment projects by the Ministry of Public Health and by university research groups. The majority of people now have latrines at their homes and refrain from defecating outside whenever possible. During the rainy season, however, the rain water stored in prepared rice fields contains an abundance of Bithynia snails and small cyprinoid fishes, and because of the lack of local toilet facilities, the parasite life cycle may not be broken. It is also convenient for farmers to eat raw cyprinoid fish while they work, perpetuating the infection cycle. Moreover, in addition to humans, dogs and cats in the villages may be infected by the liver flukes, and because they deposit their feces indiscrimately, they can be an important source of parasite ova.[1] Most of the northeast Thai people are Buddhist and refrain from killing animals. Thus, while considerable progress has been made to prevent contamination of water resources with feces, more work is still necessary.

Control of the Intermediate Hosts

Extermination of the snail hosts is another way of breaking the life cycle of the parasite. Great reduction or even complete eradication of snail host of *C. sinensis* has been reported in streams contaminated with insecticides or industrial effluents.[15] It is unlikely that the levels of insecticides or molluscicides used in northeast Thailand, however, would have any major effect on the snail population. Moreover, the large reservoirs would require huge amounts of chemicals to kill the snails—amounts that might kill all other living creatures in the water, devastating the environment. Thus, control of the snail population in northeast Thailand is not likely to be feasible in the near future.

Control of Transfer from Fish to Humans

It is not feasible to eliminate the cyprinoid fish because they are the main protein source for the indigenous population. Perfect prevention of infection would be achieved, however, if raw or improperly cooked fish were not consumed. Theoretically, this strategy would appear simple to implement, but it is a most difficult task in practice. The majority of northeast Thai people who live around and outside cities are poor farmers, and their lives mainly depend on fish in the natural and constructed water bodies. They have a tradition of eating raw-fish dishes that dates back for generations. In addition, because liver flukes do not cause any immediate clinical effects, local people have not realized the true hazard presented by the parasites and have tended to ignore the advice of educated personnel from outside their community. These problems have been largely overcome, however, by a continuous nationwide campaign by the Thai government to educate the people about the insidious and hidden danger of liver fluke infections. As part of this campaign, television and radio have been used to discourage people from eating raw fish and from defecating outside latrines. Popular television and movie stars, as well as local notable personalities, have also been employed to attract attention and to inject an entertainment element into the educational programs. The village public-address system, monthly village broadcasting bulletins, and folksongs are all tools used to acquaint people with the harmfulness of the parasite and to promote anti–liver fluke practices.[110] One focus of education is schoolteachers, who pass information on to their students, who then become amenable to altering the traditional lifestyle in their households. All these practices have resulted in the liver fluke being controlled in certain villages.[110] Absolute eradication may not be possible, however, unless economic problems are solved, giving farmers the purchasing power for new kinds of attractive and palatable foods. Japan is a good example in this respect. It is now completely free of *C. sinensis* infection, despite being an endemic area before the war. This success mainly came from economic growth, education, and faith of the people in their leaders.

Although irradiation of fresh fish has been tried by Laoharanu and Sornmani,[111] it does not seem feasible on a large scale. Similar problems in prevention of *O. viverrini* infection have also been encountered with *C. sinensis* infection; the practical difficulties have been reviewed elsewhere.[15,17]

Treatment of Infected Hosts

An effective drug for treatment of liver flukes in infected hosts, praziquantel, has been available for more than 10 years. Prior to the advent of praziquantel, antimony preparations, gentian violet, emetine hydrochloride, dehydroemetine, Entobex (4–7 phenanthroline-5,6 quinone), Faudin, chloroquin, amopyroquin, carbarsone, Atabrine, bithionol, niclofolan, hexachloroparaxylol, hexachloroethane bentonite, and Hetol were all tried but either lacked efficacy or caused unacceptable toxicity.[14,15,112] Praziquantel (Biltricide, EMBAY 8440), a pyrazinoisoquinoline, was firstly introduced for treatment of schistosomes in 1975. In the subsequent period, the drug has been used widely in treatment of both veterinary and human trematodes and cestodes. Its actions on parasites have been reviewed by Day and colleagues.[113]

Treatment of *O. viverrini* or *C. sinensis* infection by praziquantel at 25 mg/kg body weight three times per day for 2 days results in cure in 100% of cases; a 96% to 100% cure rate can be obtained after a 1-day treatment at this dose.[114–116] A single oral administration of 40 mg/kg body weight of the drug yields a 90% to 96% cure rate.[117,118] Combination of praziquantel treatment and integrated health education, along with sanitation improvement, should prevent reinfection.[119] Without such integrated measures, however, a high percentage of hosts are reinfected within one year of treatment.[120] Annual treatments with praziquantel in reinfected people, however, have resulted in a gradual reduction of reinfection rate in subsequent years.[121] due to the decreased shedding of eggs and reduced contamination of the local bodies of water. Although the effects of a reduction in fluke burden on cholangiocarcinoma development may not be large in the short term, in the long term it should bring major benefit, especially if linked to reduced consumption of foods contaminated with carcinogens.

Treatment of cholangiocarcinoma typically involves complete resection of tumors and restoration of bile flow.[122] Five surgical methods are local resection, local resection with hepatic resection, liver transplantation, transtumoral drainage, and paratumoral bypass individually or in conjunction with intraoperative or postoperative radiation, with or without chemotherapy. With all methods, however, the prognosis is poor.

CONCLUSIONS

Cholangiocarcinoma has long been recognized as a serious complication of liver fluke infection. Experimental evidence in animals indicates that the parasites act as both co-initators and as promotors of bile duct transformation. Although the International Agency for Research on Cancer recently considered infections with *O. viverrini* to be carcinogenic and infections with *C. sinensis* to be "probably carcinogenic" to humans,[11] subsequent animal experiments suggest that the liver flukes cannot induce bile duct cancers in the absence of other factors.[70] The flukes stimulate cell division in the bile ducts either by causing mechanical damage to the epithelium and mechanical obstruction when present in large numbers, or by causing immunological occlusion due to the egg or parasite granulomas in the bile ducts. The existence of other parasite-induced chemical or immunologic effects remains a subject for future studies. Similarly, the effect of infection on oncogenes or tumor suppressor genes requires further investigation. Such studies will assist us in elucidating the mechanisms of cholangiocarcinoma development as induced by the combined effects of the liver flukes and of exogenous hepatocarcinogens. The findings of animal experiments will also need to be extended if we are to understand fully liver fluke–associated bile duct cancers in humans.

Although praziquantel, the most effective drug for the treatment of liver flukes, is widely used, the incidence of cholangiocarcinoma has not decreased. A variety of education campaigns will be required to encourage people in endemic areas to avoid eating raw and undercooked fish. Measures must also be taken to eliminate carcinogens from foods and foodstuffs in the affected communities. Such complementary activities are most likely to be successful in eliminating the problem of liver fluke–associated malignancy.

REFERENCES

1. Sadun EH. Studies on Opisthorchis viverrini in Thailand. Am J Hyg 1955;62: 81–115.
2. Wykoff DE, Harinasuta C, Juttijudata P, Winn MM. Opisthorchis viverrini in Thailand—the lifecycle and comparison with O. felineus. J Parasitol 1965; 51:207–214.
3. Harinasuta C. Opisthorchiasis in Thailand: a review. In: Harinasuta C, ed. Proceedings of the 4th Southeast Asian seminar on parasitology and tropical medicine. Schistosomiasis and other snail-transmitted helminthiasis, Manila 24–27 February, Bangkok, Bangkok Vejsarn, 1969:253–264.

4. Preuksaraj S. Public health aspects of opisthorchiasis in Thailand. Arzneim-Forsch/Drug Res 1984; 34 (II):1119–1120.

5. Harinasuta C, Harinasuta T. Opisthorchis viverrini: lifecycle, intermediate hosts, transmission to man and geographical distribution in Thailand. Arzeim-Forsch/Drug Res 1984; 34(II):1164–1167.

6. Haswell-Elkins MR, Satarug S, Elkin DB. Opisthorchis viverrini infection in Northeast Thailand and its relationship to cholangiocarcinoma. J Gastroenterol Hepatol 1992; 7:538–548.

7. Pholsena K, Sayaseng B, Hongvanthong B, Vanisaveth V. The prevalence of helminth infection in Ban Nanin, Laos. Southeast Asian J Trop Med Public Health 1991; 22:137–138.

8. Giboda M, Ditrich O, Scholz T, Viengsay T, Bouaphanh S. Current status of food-borne parasitic zoonoses in Laos. Southeast Asian J Trop Med Public Health (Supp) 1991; 22: 56–61.

9. Giboda M, Ditrich O, Scholz T, Viengsay T, Bouaphanh S. Human Opisthorchis and Haplorchis infections in Laos. Trans Roy Soc Trop Med Hyg 1991; 85:538–540.

10. Tansurat P. Opisthorchiasis. In: Marcial-Rojas PA, ed. Pathology of Protozoal and Helminthic Diseases with Clinical Correlation. Baltimore: Williams & Wilkins; 1971: 536–545.

11. International Agency for Research on Cancr. Infection with liver flukes (Opisthorchis viverrini, Opisthorchis felineus and Clonorchis sinensis). IARC monographs on the evaluation of carcinogenic risks to humans. Vol. 61, Lyon, 1994:121–175.

12. Kaewkes S, Elkin DB, Sithithaworn P, Haswell-Elkins MR. Comparative studies on the morphology of the eggs of Opisthorchis viverrini and lecitho-dendriid trematodes. Southeast Asian J Trop Med Public Health 1991;22:623–630.

13. Sriurairatna S, Thamavit W. Scaning electron microscopy of newly excysted Opisthorchis viverrini. Proc. IVth Asia-Pacific conference and workshop on electron microscopy, Bangkok, 1988: 587–588.

14. Viranuvatti V, Stitnimankarn T. Liver fluke infection and infestation in Southeast Asia. In: Popper H, Schaffner F,eds. Progress in Liver Disease. New York: Grune & Stratton, 1972:537–547.

15. Gibson JB, Sun T. Clonorchiasis. In: Marcial-Rojas PA, ed. Pathology of Protozoal and Helminthic Diseases with Clinical Correlation. Baltimore: Williams & Wilkins; 1971: 546–566.

16. Choi DW. Clonorchis sinensis: lifecycle, intermediate hosts, transmission to man and geographical distribution in Korea. Arzneim-Forsch/Drug Res 1984;34(II):1145–1151.

17. Chen MG, Lu Y, Hua XJ, Mott KE. Progress in assessment of morbidity due to Clonorchis sinensis infection: a review of recent literature. Trop Dis Bull 1994; 91: R7–R65.

18. Hou PC. The pathology of Clonorchis sinensis infestation of the liver. J Pathol Bact 1955;70:53–64.

19. Chan PH, Teoh TB. The pathology of Clonorchis sinensis infestation of the pancreas. J Pathol Bact 1967;93:185–189.

20. Hou PC, Pang LSC. Clonorchis sinensis infestation in man in Hong Kong. J Pathol Bact 1964;87:245–250.

21. Attwood HD, Chou ST. The longevity of Clonorchis sinensis. Pathology 1978;10:153–156.

22. Iarotski LS, Be'er SA. Epidemiology and control of opisthorchiasis in the former USSR. 1993; Geneva, WHO.

23. Edmondson HA, Peters RL. Tumors of the liver: pathologic features. Semin Roentgenol 1983;18:75–83.

24. Mori W, Nagasako K. Cholangiocarcinoma and related lesions. In: Okuda K, Peters RL, eds. Hepatocellular Carcinoma. New York:Wiley; 1976: 227–246.

25. Craig JR. Liver. In: Kissane JM, ed. Anderson's Pathology, 9th ed. St Louis: Mosby; 1990:1293–1300.

26. Nakajima T, Kondo Y, Miyazaki M, Okui K. A histopathologic study of 102 cases of intrahepatic cholangiocarcinoma: histologic classification and modes of spreading. Hum Pathol 1988;19:1228–1234.

27. Shirai T, Pairojkul C, Ogawa K, et al. Histomorphological characteristics of cholangiocellular carcinomas in Northeast Thailand, where a region infection with the liver fluke, Opisthorchis viverrini is endemic. Acta Pathologica Japonica 1992;42:734–739.

28. Schwartz DA. Helminths in the induction of cancer: Opisthorchis viverrini, Clonorchis sinensis and cholangiocarcinoma. Trop Geogr Med 1980;32:95–100.

29. Juttijudata P, Prichanond S, Churnratanakul S, Chiemchaisri C, Palavatana C. Hilar intrahepatic cholangiocarcinoma and its etiology. J Clin Gastroenterol 1984;6:503–504.

30. Haswell-Elkins MR, Sithithaworn P, Elkins DB. Opisthorchis viverrini and cholangiocarcinoma in Northeast Thailand. Parasitology Today 1992;8:86–89.

31. Haswell-Elkins MR, Satarug S, Elkins DB. Opisthorchis viverrini infection in Northeast Thailand and its relationship to cholangiocarcinoma. J Gastroenterol Hepatol 1992;7:538–548.

32. Sithithaworn P, Heswell-Elkins MR, Mairiaing P, et al. Parasite-associated morbidity: liver fluke infection and bile duct cancer in Northeast Thailand. Int J Parasitol 1994;6:833–843.

33. Bhamarapravati N, Viranuvatti V. Liver diseases in Thailand. An analysis of liver biopsies. Am J Gastroenterol 1966;45:267–275.

34. Koompirochana C, Sonakul D, Chinda K, Stitnimankarn T. Opisthorchiasis: a clinocopathologic study of 154 autopsy cases. Southeast Asian J Trop Med Public Health 1978;9:60–64.

35. Sinawat P, Hemsrichart V. A histological study of 61 cases of peripheral intrahepatic cholangiocarcinoma. J Med Assoc Thai 1991;74:448–453.

36. Bunyaratvej S, Meenakanit V, Tantachamrun T, Srinawat P, Susilaworn P, Chongchitnum N. Nationwide survey of major liver diseases in Thailand analysis of 3305 biopsies as to year-end 1978. J Med Assoc Thailand 1981;64:432–438.

37. Srivatanakul P, Sontipong S, Chotiwan P, Parkin DM. Liver cancer in Thailand: temporal and geographic variations. J Gastroenterol Hepatol 1988;3:413–420.

38. Kurathong S, Lerdverasirikul P, Wongpaitoon V, et al. Opisthorchis viverrini infection and cholangiocarcinoma: a prospective, case-control study. Gastroenterology 1985;89:151–156.

39. Hitanant S, Tan-Ngarm Trong D, Damrongsak C, et al. Peritoneoscopic findings in 203 patients with Opisthorchis viverrini infection. Gastrointest Endosc 1987;33:18–20.

40. Green A, Uttaravichien T, Bhudhisawasdi V, et al. Cholangiocarcinoma in North East Thailand: a hospital-based study. Trop Geogr Med 1992;43:193–198.

41. Vatanasapt V, Tangvoraphonkchai V, Titapant V, Pipitgool V, Viriyapap D, Sriamporn S. A high incidence of liver cancer in Khon Kaen province, Thailand. Southeast Asian J Trop Med Public Health. 1990;21:382–387.

42. Srivatanakul P, Parkin DM, Jiang YZ, et al. The role of infection by Opisthorchis viverrini, hepatitis B virus, and aflatoxin exposure in the etiology of liver cancer in Thailand. Cancer 1991;68:2411–2417.

43. Parkin DM, Srivatanakul P, Khlat M, et al. Liver cancer in Thailand. I. A case-control study of cholangiocarcinoma. Int J Cancer 1991;48:323–328.

44. Hou PC. The relationship between primary carcinoma of the liver and infestation with Clonorchis sinensis. J Pathol Bact 1956;72:239–246.

45. Belamaric J. Intrahepatic bile duct cancinoma and C. sinensis infection in Hong Kong. Cancer 1973;31:468–473.

46. Chou ST, Chan CW. Mucin-producing cholangiocarcinoma: an autopsy study in Hong Kong. Pathology 1976;8:321–328.

47. Choi BI, Park JH, Kim YI, et al. Peripheral cholangiocarcinoma and clonorchiasis: CT findings. Radiology 1988;169:149–153.

48. Schwartz DA. Cholangiocarcinoma associated with liver fluke infection: a preventable source of morbidity in Asian immigrants. Am J Gastroenterol 1986;81:76–79.

49. Sher L, Iwatsuki S, Lebeau G, Zajko A. Hilar cholangiocarcinoma associated with clonorchiasis. Dig Dis Sci 1989;34:1121–1123.

50. Ona FV, Dytoc JNT. Clonorchiasis-associated cholangiocarcinoma: a report of two cases with unusual manifestations. Gastroenterology 1991;101:831– 839.

51. Shain AA. Opisthorchiasis and hepatic cancer among the population of the Hanty-Mansy National District. Vopr Onkol 1971;17:34–39.

52. Glumov VY, Kotrikov VV, Tret'yakova NA. Pathogenesis and morphology of primary hepatic cancer developed on a background of opisthorchiasis. Vopr Onkol 1974;20:46–50.

53. Iablokov DD, Ordina OM, Taranov SV, Trotsenko BA, Baiusova ZA. Combination of primary liver cancer with opisthorchiasis. Arkh Patol 1980;42:95–96.

54. Viranuvatti V, Kasemsant D, Bhamarapravati N. Retention cyst of liver caused by opisthorchiasis associated with carcinoma. Am J Gastroenterol 1955;23:442–446.

55. Nakashima T, Sakamoto K, Okuda K. A minute hepatocellular carcinoma found in a liver with Clonorchis sinensis infection. Cancer 1977;39:1306–1311.

56. Sonakul D, Koompirochana C, Chinda K, Stitnimakarn T. Hepatic carcinoma with opisthorchiasis. Southeast Asian J Trop Med Public Health 1978;9:215–219.

57. Riganti M, Pungpak S, Punpoowong B, Bunnag D, Harinasuta T. Human pathology of Opisthorchis viverrini infection: a comparison of adults and children. Southeast Asian J Trop Med Public Health 1989;20:95–100.

58. Hou PC. Primary carcinoma of bile duct of the liver of the cat (Felis catus) infested with Clonorchis sinensis. J Pathol Bact 1964;87:239–244.

59. Hou PC. Pathological changes in the intrahepatic bile ducts of cats (Felis catus) infected with Clonorchis sinensis. J Pathol Bact 1965;89:357–364.

60. Hou PC. Hepatic clonorchiasis and carcinoma of the bile duct in a dog. J Pathol Bact 1965;89:365–367.

61. Thamavit W, Bhamarapravati N, Sahaphong S, Vajrasthira S, Angsubhakorn S. Effects of dimethylnitrosamine on induction of cholangiocarcinoma in Opisthorchis viverrini-infected Syrian golden hamsters. Cancer Res 1978;38: 4634–4639.

62. Thamavit W, Kongkanuntn R, Tiwawech D, Moore MA. Level of Opisthorchis infestation and carcinogen dose-dependence of cholangiocarcinoma induction in Syrian golden hamsters. Virchows Arch B 1987;54:52–58.

63. Bhamarapravati N, Thamavit W, Vajrastira S. Liver changes in hamsters infected with a liver fluke of man, Opisthorchis viverrini. Am J Trop Med Hyg 1978;27:787–794.

64. Thamavit W, Pairojkul C, Tiwawech D, Shirai T, Ito N. Strong promoting effect of Opisthorchis viverrini infection on dimethylnitrosamine-initiated hamster liver. Cancer Lett 1994;78:121–125.

65. Thamavit W, Ngamying M, Boonpucknavig V, Boonpucknavig S, Moore MA. Enhancement of DEN-induced hepatocellular nodule development by Opisthorchis viverrini infection in Syrian golden hamsters. Carcinogenesis 1987;8:1351–1353.

66. Thamavit W, Moore MA, Hiasa Y, Ito N. Generation of high yields of Syrian hamster cholangiocellular carcinomas and hepatocellular nodules by combined nitrite and aminopyrine administration and Opisthorchis viverrini infection. Jpn J Cancer Res 1988;79:909–916.

67. Thamavit W, Moore MA, Hiasa Y, Ito N. Enhancement of DHPN induced hepatocellular, cholangiocellular and pancreatic carcinogenesis by Opisthorchis viverrini infestation in Syrian golden hamsters. Carcinogenesis 1988;9: 1095–1098.

68. Thamavit W, Boonpucknavig V, Boonpucknavig S, Moore MA, Ito N. Secondary enhancing effect of Opisthorchis viverrini infection on development of hepatocellular nodules in Syrian golden hamsters initiated with diethylnitrosamine. Thai J Toxicol 1992;8:35–40.

69. Thamavit W, Moore MA, Sirisinha S, Shirai T, Ito N. Time-dependent modulation of liver lesion development in Opisthorchis-infected Syrian hamster by an anthelminthic drug, praziquantel. Jpn J Cancer Res 1993;84:135–138.

70. Thamavit W, Tiwawech D, Moore, MA, Ito N, Shirai T. Equivocal evidence of complete carcinogenicity after repeated infection of Syrian hamsters with Opisthorchis viverrini. Toxicol Pathol 1996;24:493–497.

71. Hong ST, Kho WG, Kim WH, Chai JY, Lee SH. Turnover of biliary epithelial cells in Clonorchis sinensis infected rats. Korean J Parasitol 1993;31:83–89.

72. Isseroff H, Sawma JT, Reino D. Fascioliasis: role of proline in bile duct hyperplasia. Science 1977;198:1157–1159.

73. Sawma JT, Isseroff H, Reino D. Proline in fascioliasis IV. Induction of bile duct hyperplasia. Comp Biochem Physiol 1978;61A:239–243.

74. Thamavit W, Pairojkul C, Tiwawech D, Shirai T, Ito N. Lack of promoting effect of proline on bile duct cancer development in dimethylnitrosamine-initiated hamster livers. Teratog Carcinog Mutagen 1994;14:169–174.

75. Wongratanacheewin S, Bunnag D, Vaeusorn N, Sirisinha S. Characterization of humoral immune response in the serum and bile of patients with opisthorchiasis and its application in immunodiagnosis. Am J Trop Med Hyg 1988;38:356–362.

76. Flavell DJ, Flavell SU. Opisthorchis viverrini: pathogenesis of infection in im-
    munodeprived hamsters. Parasit Immunol 1986;8:455–466.
77. Cotran RS, Kumar V, Robbins SL. Robbins Pathologic Basis of Disease. 5th
    ed. Philadelphia: WB Saunders; 1994: 51–92.
78. Moore MA, Thamavit W, Tiwawech D, Ito N. Cell death and proliferation in
    Opisthorchis viverrini-DHPN induced carcinogenesis in the Syrian hamster
    hepato-pancreatic axis. In: Columbano et al, eds. Chemical Carcinogenesis 2.
    New York: Plenum Press; 1991:503–510.
79. Flavell DJ, Lucas SB. Promotion of N-nitrosodimethylamine-initiated bile
    duct carcinogenesis in hamster by the human liver fluke, Opisthorchis viver-
    rini. Carcinogenesis 1983;4:927–930.
80. Thamavit W, Moore MA, Ruchirawat S, Ito N. Repeated exposure to Opis-
    thorchis viverrini and treatment with anthelminthic praziquantel lacks carci-
    nogenic potential. Carcinogenesis 1992;13:309–311.
81. Park HK. Effect of Clonorchis sinensis infection on the histopathology of the
    liver in rats administered aflatoxin B_1. Jpn J Parasitol 1989;38:198–206.
82. Jang JJ, Cho KJ, Myong NH, Chai JY. Enhancement of dimethylnitrosamine-
    induced glutathione S-transferase P-positive heptic foci by Clonorchis sin-
    ensis infestation in F344 rats. Cancer Lett 1990;52:133–138.
83. Tomatis L, Cefis F. The effects of multiple and single administration of di-
    methylnitrosamine to hamsters. Tumori 1967;53:447–452.
84. Tomatis L, Magee PN, Shubik P. Induction of liver tumors in Syrian golden ham-
    ster by feeding dimethylnitrosamine. J Natl Cancer Inst 1964;33:341–345.
85. Preussmann R, Stewart BW. N-nitroso carcinogens. In: Searle CE, ed. Chemi-
    cal Carcinogens. 2nd ed, vol 2 (ACS Monograph 182). Washington. DC:
    American Chemical Society; 1984:643–828.
86. Umbenhauer DR, Pegg AE. Alkylation of intracellular and extracellular DNA
    by dimethylnitrosamine following activation by isolated rat hepatocytes. Can-
    cer Res 1981; 41:3471–3474.
87. Gottenplan JB, Kokkinakis D. High mutagenic activity of N-nitrosobis (2-ox-
    opropyl) amine and N-nitrosobis (2-hydroxypropyl) amine in the host-medi-
    ated assay in hamsters: evidence for premutagenic methyl and hydroxypropyl
    adducts. Carcinogenesis 1993; 14:1621–1625.
88. Thamavit W, Pairojkul C, Tiwawech D, Itoh M, Shirai T, Ito N. Promotion of
    cholangiocarcinogenesis in hamster liver by duct ligation after dimethylni-
    trosamine initiation. Carcinogenesis 1993;14:2415–2417.
89. Becker RA, Shank RC. Kinetics of formation and persistence of ethylguanine
    in DNA of rats and hamsters treated with diethylnitrosamine. Cancer Res
    1985;45:2076–2084.
90. Lee JH, Rim HJ, Bak UB. Effect of Clonorchis sinensis infection and dimet-
    hylnitrosamine administration on the induction of cholangiocarcinoma in
    Syrian golden hamsters. Korean J Parasitol 1993;1:21–30.
91. Iida H. Experimental study of the effect of Clonorchis sinensis infection on
    induction of cholangiocarcinoma in Syrian golden hamsters administered
    0.03 percent N-2-fluorenylacetamide (FAA). Jpn J Parasitol 1985;1:7–16.
92. Lijinsky W, Greenblatt M. Carcinogen dimethylnitrosamine produced in vivo
    from nitrite and aminopyrine. Nature New Biol 1972;236:177–178.
93. Craddock VM. Liver carcinomas induced in rats by single administration of
    dimethylnitrosamine after partial hepatectomy. J Natl Cancer Inst 1971;47:
    899–907.

94. Barnes JM, Butler WH. Carcinogenic activity of aflatoxin in rats. Nature 1964;202:1016.

95. Migasena P. Cholangio-carcinogenesis: relationship of liver flukes, bile acids and food contaminants. In: Ruchirawat M, Shank RC, eds. Environmental Toxicity and Carcinogenesis. Bangkok, Thailand; Texts and Journal Corp; 1986: 179–186.

96. Shank RC, Wogan GN, Gibson JB, Nondasuta A. Dietary aflatoxins and human liver cancer. II. Aflatoxins in market foods and foodstuffs of Thailand and Hong Kong. Fd Cosmet Toxicol 1972;10:61–69.

97. Weitzman SA, Weitberg AB. Phagocytes as carcinogens: malignant transformation produced by human neutrophils. Science 1985; 227: 1231–1233.

98. Lewis JG, Hamilton T, Adams DO. The effect of macrophage development on the release of reactive oxygen intermediates and lipid oxidation products, and their ability to induce oxidative DNA damage in mammalian cells. Carcinogenesis 1986; 7: 813–818.

99. Moncada S, Palmer RMJ, Higgs EA. Nitric oxide: physiology, pathophyiology, and pharmacology. Pharmacol Rev 1991;43:109–142.

100. Hibbs JB Jr, Tainter RR, Vavrin Z. Macrophage cytotoxicity: role for L-arginine deiminase and imino nitrogen oxidation to nitrite. Science 1987;235: 473–476.

101. Iyengar R, Stuehr DJ, Marletta MA. Macrophage synthesis of nitrite, nitrate, and N-nitrosamines: precursors and role of the respiratory burst. Proc Natl Acad Sci USA 1987;84:6369–6373.

102. Miwa M, Stuehr DJ, Marletta MA, Wishnok JS, Tannenbaum SR. Nitrosation of amines by stimulated macrophages. Carcinogenesis 1987;8:955–958.

103. Wink DA, Kasprzak KS, Maragos CM, et al. DNA deaminating ability and genotoxicity of nitric oxide and its progenitors. Science 1991;254:1001–1003.

104. Ohshima H, Tsuda M, Adachi H, Ogura T, Sugimura T, Esumi H. L-Arginine-dependent formation of N-nitrosamines by the cytosol of macrophages activated with lipopolysaccharide and interferon-γ. Carcinogenesis 1991;12: 1217–1220.

105. Nguyen T, Brunson D, Crespi CL, Penman BW, Wishnok JS, Tannenbaum SR. DNA damage and mutation in human cells exposed to nitric oxide in vitro. Proc Natl Acad Sci USA 1992;89:3030–3034.

106. Ohshima H, Bandaletova TY, Brouet I, et al. Increased nitrosamine and nitrate biosynthesis mediated by nitric oxide synthase induced in hamsters infected with liver fluke (Opisthorchis viverrini). Carcinogenesis 1994;15:271–275.

107. Haswell-Elkins MR, Satarug S, Tsuda M, et al. Liver fluke infection and cholangiocarcinoma: model of endogenous nitric oxide and extragastric nitrosation in human carcinogenesis. Mutat Res 1994;305:241–252.

108. Kiba T, Tsuda H, Pairojkul C, Inoue S, Sugimura T, Hirohashi S. Mutations of the p53 tumor suppressor gene and the ras gene family in intrahepatic cholangiocellular carcinoma in Japan and Thailand. Mol Carcinog. 1993;8: 312–318.

109. Tsuda H, Satarug S, Bhudhisawasdi V, Kihana T, Sugimura T, Hiroshashi S. Cholangiocarcinomas in Japanese and Thai patients: difference in etiology and incidence of point mutation of the c-Ki-ras proto-oncogene. Mol Carcinog 1992;6:266–269.

110. Sornmani S. Control of opisthorchiasis through community participation. Parasitology Today 1987;3:31–33.

111. Laoharanu P, Sornmani S. Preliminary estimates of economic impact of liver fluke in Thailand and the feasibility of irradiation as a control measure. Southeast Asian J Trop Med Public Health 1991; 22 (suppl): 384–390.
112. Rim HJ. Therapy of fluke infections in the past. Arzneim-Forsch/Drug Res.1984; 34 (II): 1127–1129.
113. Day TA, Bennet JL, Pax RA. Praziquantel: the enigmatic antiparasitic. Parasitology Today 1992;8:342–344.
114. Bunnag D. Harinasuta T. Studies on the chemotherapy of human opisthorchiasis in Thailand: I. Clinical trial of praziquantel. Southeast Asian J Trop Med Public Health 1980;11:528–531.
115. Supanvanich S, Supanvanich K, Pawabut P. Field trial of praziquantel in human opisthorchiasis in Thailand. Southeast Asian J Trop Med Public Health 1981;12:598–602.
116. Chen CY, Hsieh WC. Clonorchis sinensis: epidemiology in Taiwan and clinical experience with praziquantel. Arzneim-Forsch/Drug Res 1984; 34 (II): 1160–1162.
117. Bunnag D, Harinasuta T. Studies on the chemotherapy of human opisthorchiasis: III. Minimum effective dose of praziquantel. Southeast Asian J Trop Med Public Health 1981;12:413–417.
118. Vivatanasesth P, Sornmani S, Schelp FP, et al. Mass treatment of opisthorchiasis in northeast Thailand. Southeast Asian J Trop Med Public Health 1982;13:609–613.
119. Saowakontha S, Pipitgool V, Pariyanonda S, Tesana S, Rojsathaporn K, Intarakhao C. Field trials in the control of Opisthorchis vivierrini with an integrated programme in endemic areas of northeast Thailand. Parasitology 1993;106:283–288.
120. Upatham ES, Viyanant V, Brockelman WY, Kurathong S, Lee P, Kraengraeng R. Rate of re-infection by Opisthorchis viverrini in an endemic northeast Thai community after chemotherapy. Int J Parasit 1988;18:643–649.
121. Pungpak S, Sornmani S, Suntharasamai P, Vivatanasesth P. Ultrasonographic study of the biliary system in opisthorchiasis patients after treatment with praziquantel. Southeast Asian J Trop Med Public Health 1989;20:157–162.
122. Vauthey JN, Blumgart LH. Recent advances in the management of cholangio-carcinomas. Semin Liver Dis 1994;14:109–114.

14

Helicobacter pylori and Gastric Adenocarcinoma

JULIE PARSONNET

Gastric cancer is the fourteenth leading cause of death in the world and the second leading cause of cancer death.[1] In 1990, 752,000 people worldwide died of stomach cancer,[1] approximately 14,000 of them in the United States.[2] Consequently, this disease is seen as an important public health concern, particularly in developing countries. We should feel fortunate, then, that worldwide, age-adjusted gastric cancer mortality is decreasing spontaneously at a remarkable rate of 10% to 20% per 5-year period (Figure 14.1).[3] In the United States, gastric cancer has gone from being the preeminent cause of cancer death in 1900 (causing more deaths than all other cancers combined), to the second leading cause of cancer death in 1945 (behind lung cancer) to a relatively uncommon cancer today.[4] All other countries with thorough cancer registries report similar trends.[3] Yet, despite the continuing global decline in gastric cancer incidence, the actual number of cases is expected to grow over the next several decades. Due to the advances in life expectancy anticipated in developing countries, gastric cancer, a disease of older age groups, is predicted to become the eighth leading cause of death by the year 2020.[5] Even today, gastric cancer is the most common cause of cancer in parts of Asia and Latin America.[6] Moreover, within countries with low rates of gastric cancer, minority groups may still have substantial risk for the disease. In the United States, for example, blacks, Hispanics and Asian Americans all have at least twice the mortality from gastric cancer as do whites.[2]

Gastric adenocarcinoma is really several different diseases that are distinguished by their site of origin within the stomach and by their histopathologic appearance. Noncardia cancers (defined as cancers of the antrum, corpus, and fundus) comprise the most common site for the disease; it is these cancers that are decreasing in frequency worldwide.[7-9]

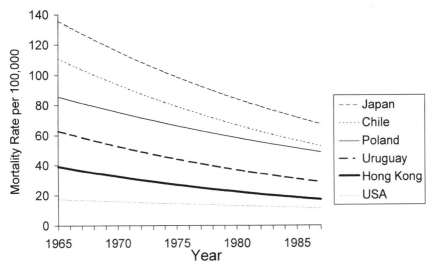

Figure 14.1. Gastric mortality has been declining worldwide at a rate of 10% to 20% percent per decade. Unlike what has been seen for other malignancies, little of this change appears to be due to improvements in treatment; the case-fatality rate for gastric cancer remains high. Instead, the decline in mortality indicates a global decline in gastric cancer incidence. (Data obtained from Coleman MP, et al. Trends in Cancer Incidence and Mortality. Lyon: International Agency for Research on Cancer; 1993:193±224.)

Cancers of the cardia and gastroesophageal junction are less common but appear to be on the increase, particularly in Europe and in the United States. In the mid-twentieth century, cardia carcinomas constituted only 10% of all gastric cancers. Today, as the overall number of cancers has strikingly declined, the proportion of cancers in the cardia has risen to as high as 50% in some areas.[9] Because the epidemiological trends in noncardia and cardia tumors are so divergent, it is assumed that the risk factors for these diseases are either distinct or affect the two tumor sites in paradoxically opposite ways. Unfortunately, in most studies of gastric cancer—particularly those published before 1990—the two sites of tumor are not distinguished but are grouped together. As a consequence, studies of disease risk factors are often biased and difficult to interpret. Throughout this chapter, however, I will focus on noncardia cancers—the more common of the two tumors worldwide and the type of cancer directly associated with *H. pylori* infection.

There are several different schemes for categorizing gastric tumors by histologic appearance. From an epidemiological perspective, the most useful system is that of Laurén, which classifies gastric adenocarcinomas into two histologic types : the intestinal type and the diffuse type.[10] Intestinal-type gastric cancers have the histologic appearance of gastrointestinal tissue, forming glands and often secreting mucus. Most of these tumors occur following a decades-long succession of precancerous lesions, starting with chronic atrophic gastritis and progressing to intestinal metaplasia, dysplasia, and finally cancer.[11] Diffuse-type gastric cancers lack cell cohesion and the cells no longer recapitulate functional gastrointestinal cells. Precursor conditions for diffuse cancer are not well defined. Histologic classification of tumor type is not always clear-cut, and in some instances, tumors may contain a mixture of intestinal and diffuse tissue. Moreover, the tumor types may occasionally be difficult to distinguish. In these instances, immunohistochemical staining for protein e-cadherin—a protein that causes cell cohesion that is absent in diffuse tumors—can be helpful in differentiating the two.[12]

Intestinal-type tumors have been decreasing in frequency as the overall gastric cancer incidence declines.[11,13] Diffuse-type cancer rates have declined but at a much slower rate. Thus, the proportion of diffuse tumors among all cancers has been increasing over time and now makes up approximately 50% of gastric malignancies in the United States and parts of Europe. Intestinal-type cancers still predominate in developing countries.

Regardless of its site or histologic type, gastric adenocarcinoma has a dismal prognosis. The 5-year survival is less than 20% in most series.[2] Almost all long-term survivors are serendipitously diagnosed very early in the course of their disease and are cured by surgical resection of the tumor. In Japan, where gastric cancer is extremely common, routine screening for gastric cancer with barium x-ray maximizes identification of early cases and, consequently, may reduce mortality.[14] In most countries, however, screening is not done and the unfortunate majority of tumors have progressed too far for curative resection to be feasible. In these patients, life expectancy is typically less than 9 months.

Given its bleak prognosis, the rapid decline in gastric cancer is a very happy circumstance, one that investigators have worked hard to understand. The overall consensus before the 1980s was that the decline was largely attributable to improvements in diet, particularly increases in fruits and vegetables and decreases in food preservatives such as nitrates and salts.[4] This healthier type of diet typically parallels an overall improvement in socioeconomic status because fresh foods are accessible year round only in populations that can afford to import food and to provide refrigeration. The exact component of fruits and vegetables that prevents cancer is unknown but is presumed to be some combination of antioxidants. In support of this, a recent study from China showed that supplementation of the diet with beta carotene, vitamin E, and selenium reduced gastric cancer mortality by approximately 21% over 5 years.[15] However, diet can explain only a small proportion of cancer incidence. A significant proportion of disease must relate to other factors. The discovery of *Helicobacter pylori* in 1983 provided new insights into the epidemiology, etiology, and pathogenesis of this disease.

HELICOBACTER PYLORI–THE ORGANISM

H. pylori is a gram-negative, spiral-shaped rod that lives beneath the mucus overlaying the gastric epithelium. First recognized more than 100 years ago, the organism was rediscovered and brought to prominence in 1983 by Barry Marshall and Robin Warren.[16] They initially named the organism *Campylobacter pyloridis* because of its microscopically similar morphology to *Campylobacter* species, and reported its association with both gastric inflammation (chronic gastritis) and with duodenal ulcers. In the fifteen years since these initial reports, the organisms has become one of the most extensively studied human pathogens. Close to 1500 scientific papers were written about it in 1997 alone. This research culminated with the sequencing of the entire *H. pylori* genome, making it the second bacterium to be completely sequenced.[17]

H. pylori is now recognized as one species of approximately two dozen in the genus *Helicobacter*—a group of organisms that infects that gastrointestinal tract of animals and humans.[18] *H. pylori* are between 2.5 and 5.0 microns long and have four to six unipolar flagellae. These flagellae enable the organism to swim in a corkscrew-like fashion through the gastric mucus and take residence adjacent to the surface and pit epithelial cells. Beneath the mucus, most *H. pylori* remain free-living, although approximately one fifth of organisms will attach to the cells.[19] The specific adhesins for this attachment are being actively investigated. In tissue culture, the Lewis blood group b antigen acts an important host receptor,[20] a finding that has not yet been confirmed in vivo.[21] Phosphotidylethanolamine is also a plausible host cell receptor; putative bacterial adhesins are a hemagglutinin and lipopolysaccharide.[22] Whatever the mechanism, when it does adhere, *H. pylori* causes epithelial cell protein phosphorylation resulting in actin polymerization and ultrastructural changes (pedestal formation) in the host cell (see Figure 14.2).[23]

Another salient feature of *H. pylori* is its vast, constitutive production of urease, an enzyme that splits urea into ammonia and carbon dioxide. Urease constitutes up to 5% of the bacterial cell protein.[24] Exactly why the organism produces so much of this enzyme remains unknown. Many believe, however, that the ammonia released by urease enables the organism to survive its initial exposure to the extremely low gastric pH until it can reach a more hospitable environment beneath the gastric mucus.[24] In support of this, *H. pylori* is not able to colonize animal models if the urease gene is made nonfunctional.[25] Urease may also serve nutritional functions for *H. pylori* or directly damage the gastric mucosa, allowing nutrients to be released into its environment.[26] Other salient proteins produced by all *H. pylori* included catalase, oxidase, superoxide dismutase, and two heat shock proteins, HspA and HspB.

In all infected persons, *H. pylori* causes chronic and acute inflammation of the gastric mucosa, but the amount of this inflammation may vary con-

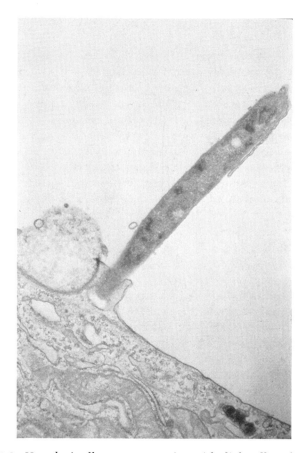

Figure 14.2. *H. pylori* adheres to gastric epithelial cells, often with the formation of epithelial cell pedestals that encircle a portion of the organism. In this electron micrograph (×10,000), note that both morphologic forms of *H. pylori*–the round coccoid form on the left and the slim, flagellated, bacillary form on the right–induce structural changes in the underlying epithelial cell. (Courtesy Ellyn D. Segal and Elsevier Press, Biomed Pharmacother 1997;51:7; with permission).

siderably. Acute inflammation is, in part, mediated by epithelial cell release of interleukin-8 (IL-8) and growth regulated oncogene alpha (Gro-α); these chemokines cause chemotaxis and activation of neutrophils.[27,28] *H. pylori*–associated proteins also causes activation of macrophages and lymphocytes, inducing a TH-1 type immune response. With rare exception, this is accompanied by production of mucosal IgA and serum IgG to *H. pylori* antigens. Some of these antibodies may cross-react with gastric epithelial antigens, leading to the hypothesis that *H. pylori*–related inflammation is partly an autoimmune phenomenon.[29]

The degree of inflammation associated with *H. pylori* appears to vary based on characteristics of the infecting organism. *H. pylori* can be divided into several phenotypes. The most virulent phenotype expresses a 90-kd vacuolating cytotoxin called VacA and contains an extra cassette of genes (the "pathogenicity island").[30] In animal models, instillation of recombinant VacA into the stomach causes gastric inflammation and even ulceration. In humans, those with VacA-expressing infections have higher degrees of inflammation than those without VacA expression. The amount of inflammation and damage caused by the VacA protein may, in turn, be determined by variations in its encoding gene sequence. The pathogenicity island contains 29 open reading frames, most of which code for unknown proteins.[17] Inactivation of several of the pathogenicity island genes, however, reduces IL-8 expression in tissue cultures and might therefore account for the lower amounts of inflammation seen with pathogenicity island–negative infections.[31] Although the gene for VacA is not itself within the pathogenicity island, it depends on signals from this island to be functionally expressed. One gene in the pathogenicity island, the *cagA* gene, encodes a highly antigenic protein that appears to be a relatively good marker for VacA expression.[32] Because of their ease of detection in the serum, CagA antibodies are frequently used to indicate infection with the more inflammatory phenotype of *H. pylori* that produces both VacA and carries the pathogenicity island of genes.[33] In this chapter, the term "CagA positive" will signify these more virulent strains.

H. PYLORI NATURAL HISTORY AND EPIDEMIOLOGY

H. pylori is an extremely common pathogen, chronically infecting 50% of the world's population.[34] In the absence of specific antimicrobial therapy to cure the infection, the organism typically persists throughout life. In many developing countries, *H. pylori* is almost universal in adulthood and 50% of children younger than 10 carry the infection. In contrast, in industrialized countries, infection is present only in 40% to 50% of adults and infection in children is unusual. Yet, belying this higher infection prevalence observed in adults, infection appears to be more readily transmitted and acquired in childhood. The high prevalence and low incidence of infection in adults (approximately 0.4% acquire infection annually[35]) in the face of the current disproportionately low prevalence in children, in part, indicates a "birth cohort effect"—i.e., that acquisition of *H. pylori* infection was common in children years ago but is less common today.[36,37] This pattern resembles that of infections related to community sanitation and hygiene, such as hepatitis A.

 H. pylori prevalence inversely correlates with socioeconomic status, probably due to increased household crowding and lower levels of household sanitation and hygiene that low income engenders. Indeed, socioeconomic status in childhood is one of the strongest predictors of *H. pylori* infection in adults.[38] Yet, even when socioeconomic status is taken into account, certain population subgroups (in the United States, blacks and Hispanics), still manifest higher prevalences of *H. pylori*.[34,39,40] This may be due to genetic predispositions to infection that are as yet poorly understood.[41] Similarly, for unknown reasons, males in some populations have 20% to 30% higher rates of infection than do females.[39]

The mode of acquisition of *H. pylori* is unknown. The most widely held hypothesis is that it is transmitted either in human feces or in regurgitated gastric material in saliva or vomitus.[42] The organism is rarely cultured from stools, however, possibly because it competes poorly in the petri dish against other fecal organisms. Although *H. pylori* has frequently been amplified by PCR from saliva and dental plaque, it has seldom been cultured. Vomitus has been inadequately studied to date. Environmental sources (including water, animal reservoirs, and even flies) have also been touted by some as the source of infection.[43,44] With the exception of non-human primates (a rare exposure for humans), however, *H. pylori* has not been cultured from any sources in the environment. Moreover, the lack of regulatory genes in *H. pylori* suggests that the organism would have difficulty adapting to environments outside its natural human host.[17] Needless to say, more studies are critical in order to understand this very important aspect of *H. pylori* epidemiology.

EPIDEMIOLOGICAL EVIDENCE FOR A LINK BETWEEN *H. PYLORI* AND NONCARDIA GASTRIC CANCER

It has been known for decades that noncardia gastric cancer typically arises in the setting of chronic gastritis. When *H. pylori* was first discovered to cause gastritis, many scientists immediately became interested in the organism as a potential cause of stomach cancer. By deductive reasoning, because *H. pylori* caused the vast majority of chronic gastritis, it was concluded that the organism was a possible "carcinogen."

The simplest studies evaluating this association were "ecologic" studies that correlated rates of *H. pylori* infection in different populations with rates of gastric cancer in those same populations. The two largest and best of these studies were a Chinese study, reported in 1990,[45] and the Eurogast study, reported in 1993.[46] In the first of these, investigators found a significant correlation between *H. pylori* prevalence and cancer mortality in 46 rural counties in China (correlation coefficient = 0.4; $P = 0.02$). In the Eurogast study, *H. pylori* prevalence and gastric cancer rates (incidence and mortality) were compared in 17 populations in 13 countries (Algeria, Japan, the United States, and 10 countries in Europe). Again, a significant correlation was observed between infection and cancer rates. Interestingly, however, some countries fell out of the pattern observed for the overall group. For example, Algeria and the United States were found to have disproportionately low incidences of cancer considering their prevalences of *H. pylori*. Thus, the correlation between *H. pylori* prevalence and gastric cancer incidence has some important deviations from the norm.

Temporal studies have also indicated a correlation between trends in *H. pylori* prevalence and trends in cancer incidence. As gastric cancer rates have been declining over time, so has *H. pylori* incidence.[36,37]

Other epidemiological studies evaluating the role of *H. pylori* in cancer fall into one of two categories: either retrospective case-control studies or prospective, nested-case-control studies. The retrospective studies evaluate whether *H. pylori* is more common in cancer patients than in persons without cancer. Unfortunately, many of these studies have been hampered by serious problems of bias. Control subjects were often poorly selected and analyses were often not adjusted for known confounders such as socioeconomic status and age. Primary tumor sites within the stomach were often not distinguished. Moreover, there appear to be intrinsic flaws to this type of study design when evaluating the role of *H. pylori* in cancer. *H. pylori* appears to thrive only in normal gastric epithelium. As the stomach becomes more and more abnormal in its progression to cancer, *H. pylori* infection appears to diminish in quantity and may disappear entirely.[47–49] Thus, biopsies obtained from a stomach cancer or from surrounding abnormal tissue may not contain *H. pylori*, despite its prior or coincident presence in nondiseased sections of the same stomach. This problem in sampling the gastric mucosa will not be observed in controls who do not have cancer or cancer precursors. Furthermore, cancer patients may have reduced antibody response to *H. pylori* either due to underlying illness or to the diminishing load of organisms in the stomach. Cancer patients may also have received antibiotics for intercurrent illness that might temporarily inhibit detection of infection. These biases would all tend to mask an association between infection and cancer. Yet, despite the many biases, *H. pylori* has been significantly linked to cancer in a large proportion of studies. Two meta-analyses of all case-control studies permit us to estimate a pooled measure of risk and to evaluate the reasons for study result heterogeneity.[50,51] In a meta-analysis performed by Hunt and colleagues, 6 (43%) of 14 retrospective studies linked *H. pylori* to cancer.[50] Similarly, Eslick and Talley reported that 15 (45%) of 33 studies (including the nested studies described below) identified a significant association between *H. pylori* and cancer.[51] In both meta-analyses, infection increased the risk of cancer approximately twofold, with the pattern being similar for diffuse- and intestinal-type tumors. Both meta-analyses concluded that the quality of the individual case-control studies was the best predictor of its final conclusions; the best-designed studies found the strongest associations between infection and disease.

The strongest epidemiological evidence for an association between *H. pylori* and cancer comes from a series of eight prospective case-control studies (Table 14.1).[52–59] These studies all capitalize on the existence of stored serum from well-characterized populations that were being followed over time. In each study, antibodies for *H. pylori* were sought in

Table 14.1 Prospective (Nested) case-control studies of
Helicobacter pylori and gastric cancer

Population (ref)	Mean years follow-up	Cases infected (%)		Controls infected (%)	Odds ratio	95% CI
UK (men) (53)	6	20/29	(69)	54/116 (47)	2.8	1.0–8.0
California (52)	14	92/109	(84)	66/109 (61)	3.6	1.8–7.3
Hawaii (men) (54)	13	103/109	(94)	83/109 (76)	6.0	2.1–17
Sweden (55)	5	46/56	(82)	110/224 (49)	5.0	2.2–11.5
Finland[a] (57)	5	73/84	(87)	121/146 (83)	2.5	1.1–5.6
Japan[b] (56)	8	41/45	(91)	170/225 (76)	3.4	1.2–9.9
Taiwan (59)	3	20/29	(69)	130/220 (59)	1.6	0.7–2.6
China (58)	2	47/87	(54)	146/261 (56)	1.2	

[a]Evaluated IgA titers rather than IgG titers. The odds ratio for IgG (1.5) was not statistically significant.
[b]When adjusted for pepsinogen levels (a marker for atrophic gastritis), *H. pylori* was no longer significantly associated with cancer. This may indicate that *H. pylori* and atrophic gastritis are in the same causal pathway.

banked sera from people who, months to years after serum donation, developed gastric cancer; banked sera from age- and gender-matched controls who had not developed cancer over the same time period were also tested. There are two advantages to these studies when compared with retrospective case-control studies. First, the serum titers are not biased by the coexistence of cancer in the cases. Second, the prospective design assures that the infection came before the malignancy. Six of the nested studies (two from the United States, three from Europe, and one from Japan) showed a significant association between *H. pylori* and cancer. *H. pylori* was linked to both diffuse- and intestinal histologic types of cancer. Only noncardia cancers, however, were related to infection; in none of these studies was an association between *H. pylori* and cancer of the cardia or gastroesophageal junction noted. Moreover, subsequent meta-analysis of these papers suggests that *H. pylori* protects against gastric cancer in this portion of the stomach (personal communication, D. Forman). This finding, if confirmed, has the potential to countermand current exhortations for global *H. pylori* eradication.[60]

Two of the nested-case-control studies, both from Asia and both with short periods of patient follow-up, showed nonsignificant elevation of risk due to *H. pylori* infection. This may reflect the same phenomenon seen in the retrospective studies. as one progresses toward cancer, antibodies in serum disappear. Thus, the shorter the term of follow-up, the less likely the study will be to find a significant effect. In combined data from three studies, there was no link between cancer and infection in the subgroup of subjects with fewer than 5 years of follow-up; in the same studies, however, if subjects had been followed up for more than 10 years, *H. pylori* increased the risk of cancer eightfold.[61] This latter figure probably represents a better estimate of the true risk of cancer associated with infection.

Because *H. pylori* has a more inflammatory phenotype (that with the pathogenicity island—marked by CagA antibodies—and VacA expression) and less inflammatory phenotypes, two groups later reanalyzed their nested-case-control data to examine the role of strain type in disease outcome.[62,63] Among infected people only, subjects who were CagA-positive had a two- to threefold higher risk of cancer than those without CagA antibodies. When persons with CagA-positive *H. pylori* infection were compared with those without *H. pylori* infection, they were found to have almost a 10-fold higher risk of cancer.[63] Those subjects with CagA-negative *H. pylori* infection did not have a significantly higher risk of cancer than uninfected subjects. Interestingly, in one study, those subjects with CagA infections had higher risks of both intestinal and diffuse-type cancers; those with CagA-negative infections had a markedly increased risk of diffuse-type cancers but no increased risk of intestinal-type cancer.[63] This suggests that *H. pylori* causes the two cancers by different mechanisms and that inflammation may be critical in carcinogenesis of intestinal-type tumors but is not a prerequisite for diffuse-type disease.

In 1994, the aggregate of epidemiological studies described here led the International Agency for Research on Cancer (IARC), a branch of the World Health Organization, to declare *H. pylori* a Group I carcinogen, a definite cause of cancer in humans.[64] This conclusion caused some controversy for both scientific and semantic reasons. In particular, it must be remembered that *H. pylori* and gastric cancer occur with high frequency in populations of lower socioeconomic status. It is plausible that a third factor related to both socioeconomic status and *H. pylori* actually causes the malignancy. Statistical methods can be used to limit this confounding, but epidemiological studies can never completely exclude this possibility. Also, the IARC conclusions fostered debate over the meaning of the terms "carcinogen" or "cause." The vast majority of people infected with *H. pylori* do not develop cancer. Thus, many argued, *H. pylori* is not a true carcinogen and, rather than being a cause of cancer, is merely a cofactor for disease. But despite this argument, the IARC conclusions are now widely accepted for a number reasons. First, the epidemiological studies are remarkably consistent despite the many populations studied and the many different types of study design. Second, the associations between *H. pylori* and cancer are very strong, with relative risks considerably higher than those observed in most studies of infection-related cancer (hepatitis B and liver cancer being one exception). Third, there appears to be a dose-response relationship between *H. pylori* and disease in that the strains that are the most inflammatory appear to maximally increase the risk of malignancy. Fourth, *H. pylori* is a plausible cause of cancer because it is a cause of chronic inflammation; chronic inflammation has been linked to cancer in almost all organs in which it occurs. Fifth, there are laboratory and clinical studies that demonstrate putative mechanisms by which *H. pylori* could lead to mutagenic damage (described more fully below). Finally, the semantic argument about cofactor versus cause is spurious. There are very few "sufficient" causes of cancer. Even smoking—one of the strongest risk factors for malignancy known—leads to cancer in only a small minority of those exposed. Yet, if we were to call smoking a cofactor rather than a cause, it would mute its singular health importance. The same could be said for *H. pylori* infection. Thus, although the IARC declaration has had its detractors, the basis for their conclusions appears well reasoned.

PUTATIVE MECHANISMS FOR *H. PYLORI*±INDUCED CARCINOGENESIS

H. pylori infection causes lifelong inflammation of the gastric mucosa. Inflammation, in turn, results in formation of reactive oxygen and nitrogen oxide species (ROS and RNOS) that have the potential of causing mutation (see Chapter 2). In addition, infection causes aberrations in gastric physiology including loss of gastric acidity (hypochlorhydria), alterations in gastric hormone levels, and abnormal processing of antioxidants. These, too, in the right circumstances, may foster carcinogenesis. Finally, *H. pylori* causes epithelial cell proliferation—a known promotor of malignancy (see Chapter 3)—and a corresponding increase in apoptosis. Independently or together, these factors all may contribute to formation or selection of mutated cells and the development of gastric cancer (Figure 14.3).

Inflammation, Oxidative Damage, and Mutation

H. pylori infection causes both chronic and acute inflammation in the gastric mucosa; this inflammation is related to both host and bacterial factors. IL-8 produced by epithelial cells in response to infection appears to be a primary mediator of neutrophil and macrophage influx into the gastric mucosa.[28] The phagocytic cells, in response to *H. pylori* antigens and secreted proteins, are then activated to release reactive oxygen species (ROS) that are detectable with chemiluminescence.[65] These three factors—IL-8, neutrophil and macrophage density, and chemiluminescence—directly correlate with one another. Moreover, together, they all correlate with the density of organisms present on the mucosal surfaces.[66–68] Epithelial cells, too, are thought to release ROS in direct proportion to *H. pylori* density.[69]

As described in Chapter 2, ROS can either directly cause mutation or can react with other chemical species to form highly mutagenic compounds. One extensively studied marker of oxidative damage by ROS is 8-hydroxy-2'-deoxyguanosine (8HdG), an adduct that if unrepaired leads to G→T transversions.[70] The gastric mucosa of *H. pylori*–infected adults

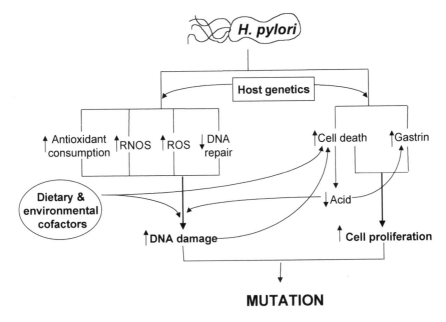

MUTATION

Figure 14.3. In the model shown, *H. pylori*±induced carcinogenesis comprises two primary processes: DNA damage and cell proliferation. These processes are interrelated through apoptotic cell death caused by DNA damage and through hypochlorhydria caused by loss of acid-generating cells (hypochlorhydria enhances formation of mutagenic *N*-nitrosamines). Genetic characteristics of the host and of the bacterium undoubtedly modify the occurrence and progression of these processes.

and children has higher amounts of 8HdG than does the mucosa of those without infection.[71,72] Moreover, 8HdG levels in the gastric mucosa return to baseline after antibiotic therapy, confirming a specific role for infection in the formation of this mutagenic adduct.[71] It is not necessary, however, to impute elevations in 8HdG solely to increased production of ROS. Deficiencies in DNA repair could also cause oxidative adducts to accumulate in the gastric mucosa. In support of this latter mechanism, one study showed that *H. pylori* infection is associated with decreased amounts of excised 8HdG in the urine.[73] One possible explanation for low urinary levels in the face of high mucosal levels is that the DNA repair system for excising 8HdG is deficient. Although further studies must be done to confirm deficiency in DNA repair, this finding conforms with observations in other inflammatory conditions. In vivo, patients with autoimmune arthritides, such as rheumatoid arthritis, have been noted to have deficient DNA repair in circulating lymphocytes.[74] Even more consonant with the *H. pylori* findings are the noted deficiencies in the repair enzyme O^6-alkylguanine-DNA-alkyltransferase with chronic *Schistosoma haematobium* infection of the urinary bladder (see Chapter 12).[75] Deficiency in O^6-

alkylguanine-DNA-alkyltransferase allows the adduct O^6-methyldeoxyguanosine to collect in tissues, increasing the likelihood of mutation and malignant transformation.

In vitro and in vivo studies have also documented increased production of nitric oxide associated with H. pylori.[77,78] Nitric oxide, a relatively reactive species, can induce mutagenic damage directly or by combining with other chemicals to form highly mutagenic species such as peroxynitrite or N-nitrosamines (see Chapter 2). The end result of this process is most likely to be deamination of cytosine and C → T transitions. Macrophages and neutrophils exposed to H. pylori preparations—including preparations with and without LPS—exhibit augmented expression of inducible nitric oxide synthase (iNOS).[78–80] Several investigators have also noted higher expression of iNOS in the stomachs of rats treated with intragastric ammonia; this finding suggests that H. pylori urease, by splitting urea into carbon dioxide and ammonia, plays a role in iNOS production.[81] In human experiments, Mannick and colleagues found iNOS expression to be high in subjects with H. pylori infection and atrophic gastritis.[82] Of interest, these investigators also documented increases in nitrotyrosine—a marker for RNOS-induced damage—in the mucosa of infected patients. As was seen with ROS, both iNOS expression and nitrotyrosine content in the gastric mucosa abated significantly after elimination of infection with antibiotics. Diminutions in iNOS and nitrotyrosine were also observed, but to a lesser degree, when the diets of infected subjects was supplemented with an antioxidant, β-carotene, and an antinitrosating agent, ascorbic acid. Finally, nitric oxide has been found to inhibit one DNA repair enzyme, formamidopyrimidine–DNA glycosylase; this enzyme repairs 8HdG adducts in bacteria.[76]

Alterations in Gastric Physiology

Parietal cells deep in the oxyntic mucosa of the body (corpus) of the stomach produce gastric acid. Stimuli for acid release include histamine, calcium, acetylcholine (the neural stimulus of acid secretion), and the gastric hormone, gastrin.[83] Gastrin, which is produced in the antrum of the stomach, is released in response to intraluminal protein, neural stimuli (including gastrin-releasing peptide) and hormonal stimuli. Additionally, its secretion depends on intraluminal gastric acidity; when luminal pH is less than 2.5 to 3.0, release of the hormone is suppressed. Regulation of acid output is not the sole function of gastrin, however. For unknown reasons, gastrin also stimulates epithelial cells to proliferate, particularly within the gastric antrum.[84] Trophic effects of gastrin can also be observed in colon and in lung.

H. pylori infection has diverse effects on these physiologic processes. Normally, H. pylori prefers to live in parts of the stomach with neutral pH. As such, under normal physiologic conditions, it shuns the gastric body where acid is produced and confines itself to the gastric antrum (the non–acid-secreting portion of the stomach). There, it lives beneath the mucus gel, shielded from intraluminal acid. Paradoxically, however, antral *H. pylori* stimulates gastrin release and augments acid secretion, at least postprandially.[85,86] This type of response, while restricting the hospitable zone for the organism, may precipitate duodenal ulcer disease, particularly in people with other predisposing factors for ulcers (for example, family history, cigarette smoking, or use of nonsteroidal anti-inflammatory agents).

In a substantial subset of people, however, particularly in developing countries, *H. pylori* infection involves not only the antrum but also the body of the stomach (pangastritis); in still others, infection involves the body almost exclusively (corpus-predominant gastritis). These forms of infection are also characterized by focal destruction of the gastric glands in the antrum (where gastrin is produced) and the corpus (where acid is produced)—a condition termed multifocal atrophic gastritis.[87] It is not known what determines the ability of *H. pylori* to colonize the body in some hosts. Some investigators speculate that body involvement is a function of duration of infection, with people infected in childhood most likely to have corpus gastritis as adults.[83,88] Other scientists maintain that the ability of *H. pylori* to colonize the body is determined by host genetic factors.[89] Still others postulate that cofactors such as diet and nutrition are the critical determinants of the site of *H. pylori* infection.[90] Whatever the truth may be, extension of *H. pylori* into the body coincides with glandular destruction, loss of acid-secreting ability (hypochlorhydria), and an increased likelihood of developing cancer.[91]

Hypochlorhydria has the potential for contributing to carcinogenesis in five ways. First, hypoacidity fosters chemical reactions involved in the formation of mutagenic N-nitrosamines from intraluminal nitrites.[92–94] N-nitrosamines are epidemiologically linked to gastric cancer. Second, hypoacidity decreases intraluminal concentrations of vitamin C.[94] Ascorbic acid (one form of vitamin C) is an antioxidant and a strong inhibitor of N-nitrosation. In the normal stomach, ascorbic acid is actively secreted into the gastric lumen, resulting in concentrations in the gastric juice far higher than those in the tissues or blood.[95] In the setting of *H. pylori* infection and corpus gastritis, however, ascorbic acid levels in the gastric juice plummet. If hypochlorhydria is also present, ascorbic acid levels drop further, a finding that is reversible with acid stimulation.[96] Thus, corpus gastritis and its associated hypochlorhydria increase formation of mutagens and reduce the ability to combat them. Third, hypochlorhydria causes feedback secretion of gastrin.[97] Gastrin, in turn, causes proliferation of epithelial cells.[98] Two studies indicate that hypergastrinemia is a strong risk factor for subsequent development of gastric adenocarcinoma, independent of the presence of *H. pylori* infection.[99,100] This association was somewhat more pronounced for tumors of the body than the antrum (Parsonnet, unpublished data), an expected finding because the trophic effects of gastrin are limited to the oxyntic mucosa.[101,102] Fourth, hypochlorhydria appears to allow *H. pylori* to grow more extensively into the gastric body. This topographical expansion has been particularly well documented in patients who are receiving proton pump inhibitors (PPIs) — medications that block the hydrogen–potassium ATP pump and shut down acid secretion.[103–105] Consequently, the acid-secreting glands of the body become more and more atrophic, potentially perpetuating acid suppression even after PPI use ceases.[106] Fifth, some investigators speculate that hypoacidity allows overgrowth of nitrate-fixing bacteria that can convert nitrates into nitrites and foster formation of N-nitrosamines.[4,107] This hypothesis derived from observations in patients who developed cancer following partial gastric resection for ulcer disease. With the exception of this small subgroup of patients, however, there is little support for the bacterial overgrowth hypothesis.

Thus, the physiologic effects of *H. pylori* on the stomach would appear to predispose infected people to cancer. These physiologic effects alone are probably not sufficient, however, to induce malignancy. Acid inhibitory therapies that mimic the degree of acid suppression observed in *H. pylori* infection have been used for decades. Interestingly, however, there is no evidence in humans or in animals that drug-induced acid suppression leads to malignant transformation of the gastric epithelium.[108–110]

Cell Proliferation and Cell Death

Cell proliferation increases the risk of cancer by increasing the number of cells that are dividing and are therefore susceptible to DNA damage. Mutation resulting from DNA damage is prevented by DNA repair enzymes or by shutdown of the cell cycle and programmed cell death (apoptosis). Although this system is highly efficient, it is not perfect. Thus, having an increased number of cell divisions will invariably result in a higher rate of mutation (see Chapter 3).

Hyperproliferation of gastric mucosal cells in *H. pylori*–infected people has been amply documented. In virtually all in vivo studies of *H. pylori* gastritis—regardless of the method used to document cell proliferation (immunohistochemical quantification of the proliferation-associated antigen, Ki-67; labeling of proliferating cell nuclear antigen; bromodeoxyuridine labeling; flow cytometry)—the proliferative compartment is expanded.[111–113] This proliferative effect is particularly prominent in patients infected with the CagA-positive phenotype of *H. pylori*[114] and in those with advanced preneoplastic lesions (atrophic gastritis, incomplete intestinal metaplasia, and dysplasia).[115–117] When *H. pylori* is infection is cured with antibiotics, cell proliferation declines dramatically.[111,112,118]

Because mucosal hyperproliferation with *H. pylori* infection is not accompanied by a massive buildup of cells (e.g., formation of adenomas), it must be appropriately balancing cell loss. This cell loss may occur either by necrosis or by apoptosis. *H. pylori* infection does damage cells and probably directly causes cell death. Known cellular toxins include VacA, urease, ammonia, and products of the inflammatory process such as monochloroamine.[119-121] With the resultant cytotoxicity, a hyperproliferative response would be required to maintain an intact mucosa. Apoptosis is also increased with infection, however, indicating not only augmented necrosis but also genetic damage in surviving cells.[122,123] Not surprisingly, this increase in apoptosis coincides with accumulation of p53 within cells of the epithelial surface.[123] Thus, hyperproliferation may be a necessary response to compensate for both necrotic and apopotic death. Interestingly, patients with the CagA-positive phenotype of *H. pylori* have increased cell proliferation but apoptosis does not increase correspondingly.[114] This can be interpreted in two ways. $CagA^+$–$VacA^+$ *H. pylori* may induce higher rates of necrotic cell death than other forms of infection. Necrotic death of damaged cells may then obviate the need for apoptosis. Peek and colleagues, however, postulate that the discordance between proliferation and apoptosis indicates an inability of the gastric mucosa to compensate for DNA damage.[114] If this discordance in surface epithelial cells reflects events in the stem cell population, one could envision a higher risk of mutation and cancer. Much more work is required, however, to confirm this hypothesis.

How *H. pylori* may induce apoptosis remains a subject of active inquiry. Several in vitro studies indicate that the organism directly precipitates apoptosis. In one study, incubation of *H. pylori* with a gastric cancer cell line resulted in decreased epithelial cell growth and DNA synthesis, and increased apoptosis.[124] The addition to the cultures of inflammatory cytokines commonly found in the mucosa of *H. pylori*–infected people (i.e., tumor necrosis factor–α and interferon gamma) markedly potentiated these effects. Also using tissue culture, Chen and colleagues showed that the effect of *H. pylori* on apoptosis could be abrogated if the organisms were not permitted to contact the cells directly, suggesting that direct binding is a requirement for initiation of apoptosis.[125] They additionally reported that *H. pylori* binding induced Bak, a member of the Bcl-2 family that enhances apoptosis. Yet, it remains unknown whether these in vitro events similarly occur in vivo and whether gastric epithelial stem cells would respond in a similar manner as gastric cancer cell lines. In rats, application of *H. pylori* lipopolysacchoride to the mucosal surface precipitates apoptosis, not only in the surface epithelium but in the gastric necks where stem cells reside.[126,127] In infected humans, too, the zone of apoptosis appears to extend deeper in the mucosa than in uninfected humans.[122] It is too early to say, however, whether any of these findings has clinical significance in the induction of cancer.

Mutations in Gastric Cancer

Various mutations have been identified in gastric cancers. These mutations differ in the intestinal and the diffuse types of disease, suggesting that the etiologies of these two tumors also differ. Because *H. pylori* has been linked equally strongly to both tumor types, it falls to reason that infection may be implicated in mutagenesis by several distinct mechanisms.

Mutations in *p53* are seen in 40% to 65% of gastric cancers, making this the most common of the known cancer-associated mutations in the stomach.[128–131] These mutations are significantly more common in intestinal-than in diffuse-type cancers, however, and can also be found in precancerous conditions to intestinal-type cancers, such as intestinal metaplasia (incomplete type) and dysplasia.[132,133] In contrast, when *p53* mutations do occur in diffuse tumors, they tend to be late events. Within gastric cancers, the site of *p53* mutation can be quite variable. In over 50% of intestinal-type-tumor cases (over 90% in some studies), the *p53* mutations appear as G:C→A:T transitions at CpG sites[128,129,134]; these CpG mutations have been related statistically to the coincident presence of *H. pylori* infection in the mucosa.[128] This makes intuitive sense, for CpG mutations are thought to be mediated by oxidative damage, such as that induced by inflammation. Mutations at other sites in *p53* in intestinal tumors have been linked statistically to dietary factors, such as high nitrite intake.[128] Risk factors for *p53* mutations in diffuse tumors have not been similarly studied.

Microsatellite instability from mismatch repair deficiency, the next most common genetic abnormality observed in gastric cancers, is also more common in intestinal than in diffuse tumors.[135,136] One result of microsatellite instability—frameshift mutation in transforming growth factor–β II receptor—prevents the inhibition of cell growth normally mediated by transforming growth factor–β, thus giving mutated cells a proliferative advantage.[137] Other mutations seen with some frequency in intestinal-type tumors occur in the *MCC* and *APC* genes and in the epidermal growth factor receptor genes, *erb*B-2 and *erb*B-3.[138] In diffuse tumors, mutations in the K-*sam* oncogene and in the epithelial-cadherin gene occur more frequently.[12] Mutations in *ras* are rarely seen in intestinal tumors but have been reported in 10% of diffuse tumors.[129,139,140] It remains to be seen how any of these mutations is correlated with *H. pylori* infection or with inflammation.

ANIMAL MODELS FOR *H. PYLORI* INFECTION AND CANCER

Laboratory research in *H. pylori*–induced carcinogenesis has been hampered by the lack of good animal models. Although numerous *Helicobacter* species infect animals, *H. pylori* naturally infects only humans and nonhuman primates. Unfortunately, animal infections with other *Helicobacter* species do not mimic all aspects of human *H. pylori* infections. For example, the gastric *Helicobacter* found in mice and cats, *H. felis*, does not attach to the gastric epithelium; adhesion to gastric epithelial cells is thought to be a critical factor in *H. pylori* pathogenesis. Other *Helicobacters* exclusively infect the colon or biliary system. Although it has been possible to "force" *H. pylori* infection into mice and rats, these animals do not manifest significant gastritis. Moreover, mice are a particularly bad species for cancer research because they rarely develop gastric adenocarcinoma (much of the stomach has a squamous epithelium), even when treated with potent chemical carcinogens. Rhesus monkeys are naturally infected with *H. pylori* but both the expense and the longevity of these animals makes cancer experimentation impractical. Despite these problems, however, models in mice, ferrets, monkeys, and gerbils may provide some useful information on *Helicobacter* carcinogenesis.

In 1992, an unusual outbreak of hepatitis and hepatocellular carcinoma occurred in a national animal laboratory.[141] Although, at first, the epidemic was suspected to be caused by an environmental toxin, extensive investigation revealed the causative agent to be a previously unrecognized *Helicobacter* species, *H. hepaticus.* This organism causes low-grade infection of intrahepatic bile canaliculi of most mouse strains but hepatic carcinoma in males of the A/JCr strain particularly.[142,143] A/JCr males infected with *H. hepaticus* develop chronic hepatitis with necrosis and proliferation of hepatocytes and bile ducts; over time hepatic adenomas and carcinomas occur.[144] When treated with a single dose of a tumor initiator, N-nitrosodimethylamine (NMDA), infected male mice express cyclin D at higher levels than do mice without infection.[145] A consequent higher rate of cell turnover could explain the accelerated development and the multiplicity of liver tumors observed in these animals. Like gastric epithelial cells in *H. pylori*–infected humans, liver cells in male mice with *H. hepaticus* contain higher amounts of 8HdG than do cells in control mice, suggesting an important role for ROS in mutation and cancer.[146] But, whereas the ROS that cause DNA adduct formation in *H. pylori* infection are thought to derive from inflammatory cells, the ROS in *H. hepaticus*–infected livers appear to be produced by phase I enzymes in the liver parenchymal cells. Mutations observed in the mice also differ from those in humans; the most common oncogenic mutation in human gastric cancers, *p53* mutations, have never been identified in this mouse model.[147] Thus, although the *H. hepaticus* model will certainly continue to provide fascinating insights into carcinogenesis, fundamental differences between hosts, sites of infection, and organisms may limit its applicability to human disease.

Preliminary experiments with *H. mustelae* infection indicate that this species may be a gastric mutagen in its natural host, the ferret. Most ferrets harbor *H. mustelae*—a pathogen that bears many similarities to *H. pylori*—in their stomachs.[148] *H. mustelae* attaches to the gastric mucosa in a manner similar to that of *H. pylori*, and, like the latter, also causes chronic inflammation, hypochlorhydria, and elevations in serum gastrin. Ferrets with *H. mustelae* develop gastric atrophy frequently and gastric adenocarcinoma on rare occasion.[149] Gastric cancer occurs consistently, however, when infected animals are exposed to the mutagen *N*-methyl-*N*-nitro-*N'*-

nitrosoguanidine (MNNG).[150] Whether MNNG-induced tumors would occur with lower frequency in uninfected animals has yet to be demonstrated.

Rhesus monkeys naturally harbor *H. pylori* and *H. heilmanii*; these organisms are so common, it is difficult to identify animals that are infection free. In the few *H. pylori*–free animals that have been studied, however, inoculations of the organism can cause persistent infection similar to that seen in humans.[151] Although a significant proportion of inoculations result in either no infection or transient infection, animals that become persistently infected develop gastritis and may progress to atrophic gastritis.[152] The type of gastric response that occurs in monkeys appears to be determined by characteristics of both the host animal and the infecting organism.

Mongolian gerbils may eventually prove to be the best animal for studying *H. pylori* carcinogenesis. These animals, which are readily infectable with *H. pylori*, develop both gastritis and gastric ulceration when infected.[153] Mongolian gerbils also readily develop gastric adenocarcinoma in response to exogenous mutagens. Preliminary data suggest that when compared with exogenous mutagens alone, the combination of exogenous mutagens and *H. pylori* infection markedly increases the likelihood of tumor development.[154] Although much is yet to be learned about this model (for example, it is unknown whether *H. pylori* attaches to the gerbil gastric mucosa, whether inflammation correlates with cytotoxin production, or whether tumors have mutational similarities to human tumors), thus far it appears to show promise.

WHY SOME AND NOT OTHERS

One of the most perplexing questions with respect to *H. pylori* and gastric adenocarcinoma is why, when half the world's population is infected, only a few get cancer. Just 1% of infected people suffer this misfortune. That a minority develops malignancy, however, should not be too surprising. Most people who smoke don't get lung cancer. Most people who contract *Mycobacterium tuberculosis* don't get tuberculosis. In fact, it is quite rare that an exposure uniformly gives rise to disease. But to prevent gastric cancer, it is important to understand why the majority escapes malignancy and a scattered few do not. Furthermore, the patterns of gastric cancer must be understood in the context of all *H. pylori*–related diseases. In particular, it has been observed that people who have duodenal ulcer disease, a common outcome of *H. pylori* infection, have a lower risk of gastric cancer than the average population.[155] Why should two diseases caused by the same organism rarely occur in the same individual?

It is simplest to address this last question first. Duodenal ulcer disease occurs exclusively in people who are capable of producing normal or high amounts of gastric acid. Thus, the gastric acid secretion pathway must be intact. Gastric cancer occurs predominantly in people who have deficient production of gastric acid. Indeed, in many people who have gastric cancer, the acid-secreting cells of the stomach have been destroyed by atrophic gastritis. This distinction—high acid for ulcers, low acid for cancer—provides a clean dichotomy for why the two diseases occur in relatively distinct populations.

It remains to be explained, however, why some people with *H. pylori* infection retain acid-secretion capacity whereas others do not. Currently, there are four hypotheses for this variability from person to person: (1) the infecting organisms are genetically different; (2) the hosts are genetically different; (3) the circumstances when infection initially occurred are different; and (4) exposures to environmental cofactors are different. There is support for each of these hypotheses.

H. pylori Strain Type

H. pylori is genetically diverse. In unrelated individuals, identical *H. pylori* strains are rarely, if ever, seen.[156] Even within families, strains frequently differ.[157] Unfortunately, little is yet known about the clinical significance of these strain differences. However, as mentioned previously, epidemiological studies indicate that strains containing the *H. pylori* pathogenicity island engender increased risk for intestinal-type gastric cancer when compared with strains that do not contain this gene cassette. Similarly, in prospective studies, *H. pylori*–infected people with CagA antibodies are two times more likely to progress from nonatrophic gastritis to atrophic gastritis than are *H. pylori*–infected people without these antibodies.[158]

Strains with the pathogenicity island are not evenly distributed across populations. For example, one study found high prevalences of CagA-positive strains in populations of Peru and Thailand but not of China, New Zealand, the Netherlands, or Canada.[159] In a study conducted in the United States, CagA antibodies were more common in *H. pylori*–infected blacks (79.4%) than in *H. pylori*–infected Hispanics or whites (63.8% and 50 percent, %).[160] It is not certain, however, whether these differences in prevalence of the various *H. pylori* strains translate into differences in disease incidence. Moreover, the data on *H. pylori* strain type cannot explain the observed dichotomy between peptic ulcer disease and gastric cancer because CagA-positive strains appear to increase risk of both of these processes.

Human Genotype

Several human genetic factors have been linked to *H. pylori* carcinogenesis. Glutathione-S-transferase-μ (GSTM1) is one of several glutathione-S-transferases that conjugates and detoxifies carcinogenic compounds. In some, but not all, studies, people who have the GSTM1 null genotype have been found to be at higher risk for gastric cancer than those with a functional GSTM1 gene.[161,162] When GST genotype was evaluated in conjunction with *H. pylori* infection, the null genotype of GSTM1 was significantly more common in infected cancer patients than in infected people without cancer (65.7% vs. 37.1%; $P < .05$).[163] Moreover, *H. pylori*–infected cancer patients were more likely to have the null genotype than were cancer patients without infection (65.7% vs. 31.3%; $P < .05$). This suggests that the combination of *H. pylori* and GSTM1 genotype may magnify cancer risk.

McColl and colleagues have postulated that the acid response to *H. pylori* is also genetically determined. They observed that first-degree relatives of patients with gastric cancer had a muted acid response to gastrin stimulation and higher rates of atrophic gastritis.[89] However, similar acid responses among relatives may indicate that family members have similar *H. pylori* strains or similar circumstances of *H. pylori* exposure, rather than a hereditary predisposition to hypochlorhydria. Azuma and colleagues reported that the human leukocyte antigen HLA type DQA1*0102 was less common among subjects with atrophic gastritis and gastric cancer than among infected subjects without these conditions. Other investigators have reported different HLA genotypes in duodenal ulcer and in cancer patients but have not related these types to *H. pylori* infection.[164] Additional human genetic factors that are being explored in relation to infection include ABO blood group type, Lewis blood group type, and mucin genotype.[165–169] Any of these genetic factors could predispose infected hosts to one disease outcome and prevent another. Much more work needs to be conducted on these factors, however, before their role in *H. pylori*–related diseases is established.

Circumstances of Acquiring Infection

For most cancers that succeed inflammation, duration of the inflammatory process correlates directly with cancer risk. This has been particularly well shown for hepatocellular cancer and hepatitis B, epidermoid cancer and chronic osteomyelitis, and colon cancer and ulcerative colitis.[170–172] The same is probably true of *H. pylori* infection; the longer the period of infection, the higher the likelihood of cancer. That duration of infection is important conforms with the multistep model of carcinogenesis, in which time is required for the numerous genetic "hits" to occur that ultimately precipitate cancer. Thus, people who are infected with *H. pylori* in childhood would have a greater chance of acquiring all the genetic mutations required for cancer during their lifetime than those who are infected in adulthood. Although it is commonly believed that almost all infection worldwide is acquired in childhood, making this age dichotomy irrelevant,[90] this is not necessarily the case. Infection models from Europe and from the United States suggest that the average age of acquiring infection is increasing over time.[36,37] This may, in part, explain both the decline in cancer rates in these parts of the world and the increasing age at which cancer occurs.

It is also plausible that, in addition to providing for a longer duration of infection, the child's stomach offers a different physiologic milieu in which infection can occur. These physiologic differences, too, could contribute to infection outcome. The few endoscopic studies comparing children and adults that have been performed indicate that histologic patterns of infection differ by age. Children tend to have less acute inflammation and more prominent lymphoid follicles than do adults.[173] One study also indicated that in developing countries, children are more likely than adults to have *H. pylori* extend to the corpus of the stomach,[174] suggesting a greater likelihood of hypochlorhydria in children. This may explain why even with antral gastritis, duodenal ulceration is a rare response to childhood *H. pylori* infection.[173] Although it is difficult to prove that age at infection influences disease outcome, some circumstantial data support this hypothesis. In a study from Hawaii, infected people with gastric cancer tended to have been younger children in large families compared to infected people without cancer; in contrast, infection in duodenal ulcer disease was not associated with birth order.[175] Youngest children tend to acquire enteric infections early in childhood, whereas oldest or only children acquire infections later; this supports a role for early childhood acquisition of *H. pylori* in disease outcome. Note, however, that these data are circumstantial at best and require further corroboration.

Environmental Cofactors for Infection

Graham argues that age at which cancer patients and noncancer patients acquire infection is too difficult to study and is ultimately irrelevant.[90] Instead, he maintains that childhood malnutrition and infectious diseases are the critical factors in establishing the path that infection follows. By causing hypochlorhydria, these processes would allow *H. pylori* to extend its domain into the gastric corpus, thereby initiating the chain of events that leads to malignancy many years down the line. In the absence of malnutrition or infection, *H. pylori* would remain confined to the antrum, and intraluminal acid levels would remain normal or high. Unfortunately, there are as yet no data to support this intriguing hypothesis. Although many studies report hypochlorhydria in malnourished children, these studies were conducted before the discovery of *H. pylori*; in the absence of careful investigation, one cannot distinguish whether *H. pylori*–related corpus gastritis is the cause or the effect of malnutrition-related hypochlorhydria. There is even less concrete evidence that concurrent infection allows *H. pylori* to progress. Unfortunately, because of the difficulty in conducting intensive investigations in children, most of whom have no symptoms referable to the stomach, it may be quite difficult to collect the data necessary to confirm or refute this hypothesis.

There are other known risk factors for gastric cancer, however, that could potentially interact with *H. pylori* to magnify disease risk. The most extensively studied environmental exposure leading to cancer is diet. It is widely accepted that diets high in salt and nitrates increase cancer risk; diets rich in fresh fruits and vegetables, on the other hand, protect against gastric cancer.[4] Because *H. pylori* both induces nitric oxide formation (potentially fostering the formation of N-nitroso compounds from intraluminal nitrites) and destroys intraluminal ascorbate, it is plausible that the combination of infection and diet is synergistically more potent than either factor alone in causing cancer. Cigarette smoking may also alter the outcome of *H. pylori* infection.[176,177] A small proportion of gastric adenocarcinomas appear to have clonal integration of Epstein-Barr virus (see Chapter 7).[178,179] No studies evaluating the joint effects of *H. pylori* and EBV have yet been conducted.

Summary of Cancer Outcome Variability

For cancer to occur, several genetic mutations typically must be extant. These mutations may not be uniform from person to person. Different combinations of mutations could lead to different types of tumors in different individuals. In any specific case of cancer, the precise mechanism by which each of the sundry mutations occurred may never be known. All the above factors—*H. pylori* strain type, host genetics, circumstance of infection, and infection cofactors—could contribute in varying proportion to each individual case. Given the multiplicity of cancer pathways, it becomes important to focus not on any specific causal chain of events, but rather on the disease risk factors that are amenable to intervention within particular populations.

PREVENTION OF *H. PYLORI*±RELATED GASTRIC CANCER

There are three possible ways that *H. pylori*–related gastric cancer could be prevented. First, infection itself could be prevented by either interrupting transmission pathways or by vaccinating uninfected people. Second, infected people could be treated with antibiotics or a therapeutic vaccine and their infections cured. Third, because *H. pylori* is rarely, if ever, sufficient in itself to cause cancer, the cofactors for cancer could be ameliorated and cancer prevented by this less direct route. Each of these approaches has its pros and cons.

Primary Prevention of Infection

The prevalence of *H. pylori* infection in the United States, Europe, and Japan has decreased dramatically over the past century, with estimates of this decline ranging from 26% to 52% per decade.[36,37,180,181] The disappearance of *H. pylori* has occurred without any specific public health interventions directed against the organism. Moreover, the decreased prevalence of infection cannot be attributed to widespread use of antibiotics; mathematical models suggest that the decline antedated the 1950s when these drugs became widely available. Ultimately, the reason the organism is disappearing is not known. It is possible that the current dip represents a low point in the organism's natural cycle and that the lapse is only temporary. It is more plausible, however, that improvements in nutrition, household sanitation, and household crowding caused this dramatic change.

This fortuitous disappearance of *H. pylori* implies that primary prevention of infection is not only possible, but is easily achievable as countries improve their socioeconomic conditions. Improving the general standard of living may be sufficient to prevent both *H. pylori* infection and other enterically transmitted organisms that exact such a heavy health toll worldwide. Of course, it is also possible that current trends will not continue unabated. Mass migrations of people due to economic hardships can easily change the epidemiology of infectious agents. Even smaller events, such as the broader use of daycare centers for children, could reverse current trends. But, all told, the epidemiological information to date gives little need for pessimism.

Should the current rate of decline continue unabated, *H. pylori* could disappear from some populations entirely within the next few generations (M. Tsugawa, personal communications). For many people, however, this will not happen soon enough; a large number will die of *H. pylori*–related infection, particularly in developing countries, before the organism loses the war of attrition. One way to accelerate the organism's demise is to prophylactically immunize uninfected people. Currently, several oral and intranasal vaccines provide protective mucosal immunity against *H. pylori* in mice These vaccines include *Salmonella typhimurium* recombinants that express *H. pylori* urease[182,183] and recombinant *H. pylori* proteins (urease, cytotoxin, or catalase), each given with immunogenic adjuvants.[184,185] No vaccine has yet proved efficacious in humans, however, and there is reason for caution. Some of the damage caused by *H. pylori* may result from an autoimmune response, so vaccination actually could induce the chronic inflammatory response that it is intended to avert.[185]

Unfortunately, the elimination of *H. pylori* may not be purely beneficial. In the past year, several studies have indicated that *H. pylori* infection may protect against development of adenocarcinomas of the gastric cardia and gastroesophageal junction.[186] Although, on a global scale, these forms of cancer currently represent only a small portion of gastric malignancies, their apparent increase in frequency is of concern. To date, the protective association between *H. pylori* and cardia cancers is poorly understood. It is plausible that the association is spurious and that infection is only a marker for some other adverse exposure. It is hard to remain sanguine about the elimination of *H. pylori*, however, while this issue remains unresolved.

Secondary Prevention–Treatment of *H. pylori* Infection

H. pylori infection is curable with antibiotic therapy. There is, as yet, minimal evidence, however, that eradication of infection can halt the chain of events leading to gastric cancer. Nonetheless, even if antibiotics prevent a small percentage of cancers (e.g., 20% to 30%), screening and treatment of *H. pylori* could be a cost-effective strategy to prevent malignancy in American adults.[187,188] In high-risk groups, such as Japanese-Americans, screening and treatment of *H. pylori* could be cost-effective at even lower levels of treatment efficacy. Because of the risks of widespread antibiotic use, however, screening and treatment programs are unlikely to come into practice unless well-conducted clinical trials support their use. Such trials are currently under way and are of two types. The first type entails randomizing tens of thousands of infected people to *H. pylori* therapy or placebo and following the subjects for gastric cancer incidence over 10 to 20 years. Such studies are now being conducted in Europe and China.[189] If treatment proves effective in reducing cancer rates, these studies would provide the most definitive proof that *H. pylori* causes malignancy and that screening and treatment are warranted. Unfortunately, these studies are extremely expensive to undertake and require many years. Furthermore, after considerable time and expense, there is no guarantee that the number of subjects studied, the rate of cancer occurrence, or the rate of *H. pylori* infection will be large enough to achieve sufficient statistical power.

A second and simpler type of study involves randomizing subjects with gastric preoplastic conditions to *H. pylori* therapy or placebo and monitoring the progression or regression of these conditions. Such studies of "intermediate biomarkers" for cancer require less time and fewer subjects than the cancer prevention studies described above, but also produce less definitive results. Even if preoplastic conditions melt away with antibiotic therapy, cancer could still occur unabated. Several large, randomized trials of preoplastic lesions are currently under way throughout the world.[189] Small case series that looked at regression of preoplastic conditions have yielded mixed results.[190–193] The most intriguing study thus far has been a nonrandomized trial of *H. pylori* eradication in Japanese patients who had early gastric cancer extirpated by local resection of the mucosa.[194] In this study, patients who were additionally treated with anti–*H. pylori* antibiotics had no tumor recurrence whereas those who did not receive antibiotics had the expected recurrence rate of 10%. This suggests that *H. pylori* eradication not only can prevent cancer but can do so at a very late stage in tumor development.

In the absence of conclusive data, clinicians are in a quandary about what to do to help their *H. pylori*–infected patients. Many are treating patients whom they consider to be at "high risk" for cancer. Such high-risk patients might include those with a family history of stomach cancer, with a diagnosis of intestinal metaplasia, or those from an ethnic group with high rates of stomach cancer. Another indication for therapy, according to some clinicians, is the long-term use of PPIs. Kuipers and colleagues showed that *H. pylori*–related gastritis progresses to atrophic gastritis in the setting of prolonged PPI use.[106] They postulated that by causing atrophic gastritis and prolonged hypochlorhydria, PPIs might predispose users to malignancy. Although this hypothesis has not been proved (indeed, some claim the opposite to be the case), some practitioners now treat all *H. pylori*–infected patients before initiating PPI therapy, with the hope of preventing cancer.

Secondary Prevention–Cofactors for Cancer

Although treating *H. pylori* infection would seem a logical approach to preventing gastric malignancy, there are other risk factors for the disease that could be addressed instead. In particular, eating a diet rich in fruits and vegetables or supplemented with multivitamins could decrease gastric cancer incidence. The advantage of this strategy is that it might also prevent other diseases besides stomach cancer. Cigarette smoking has also been linked to gastric tumors,[176] and, once again, elimination of this cofactor could benefit many organ systems besides the stomach.

SUMMARY

In the very few years since its discovery, remarkable strides have been made in understanding *H. pylori* infection as it relates to one of the world's most common and fatal malignancies—gastric cancer. Yet many critical questions remain. Much more needs to be done to understand the pathogenesis of tumor development. Piecing together this process would provide insights not only into gastric malignancy but into other inflammation-related cancers as well. The mode of transmission of *H. pylori* needs to be elucidated to prevent its continued spread, particularly in developing countries. But, most importantly, we need to decide whom to treat. We are not yet to the point where we can confidently resolve to eliminate all *H. pylori* infection from the globe as we did with smallpox. There are too many unanswered questions to risk such a strategy. Yet neither can we cavalierly ignore the many people whose lives might be saved by a short course of antibiotics. In the United States, the decision about whom to screen and treat has become a personal one, between physician and patient. Fortunately, the next decade should witness an explosion of new data that will help to resolve these thorny issues.

REFERENCES

1. Murray CJ, Lopez AD. Mortality by cause for eight regions of the world: Global Burden of Disease Study. Lancet 1997;349:1269–1276.

2. National Cancer Institute. SEER Cancer Statistics Review, 1973–1994 (Online). http:/www-seer.ims.nci.nih.govPublications/CSR7395. Bethesda: National Cancer Institute;1997.

3. Coleman MP, Esteve J, Damiecki P, Arslan A, Renard H. Trends in Cancer Incidence and Mortality. Lyon: International Agency for Research on Cancer; 1993:193–224.

4. Howson C, Hiyama T, Wynder E. The decline in gastric cancer: epidemiology of an unplanned triumph. Epidemiol Rev 1986;8:1–27.

5. Murray CJ, Lopez AD. Alternative projections of mortality and disability by cause 1990–2020: Global Burden of Disease Study. Lancet. 1997;349:1498–504.

6. Parkin DM, Muir CS, Whelan SL, Gao YT, Ferlay J, Powell J. Cancer Incidence in Five Continents. Lyon: International Agency for Research on Cancer; 1992:301–353.

7. Rios-Castellanos E, Sitas F, Shepard NA, Jewell DP. Changing pattern of gastric cancer in Oxfordshire. Gut 1992;33:1312–1317.

8. Wang HH, Antonioli DA, Goldman H. Comparative features of esophageal and gastric adenocarcinomas: recent changes in type and frequency. Hum Pathol 1986;17:482–487.

9. Salvon-Harman JC, Cady B, Nikulasson S, Khettry U, Stone MD, Lavin P. Shifting proportions of gastric adenocarcinomas. Arch Surg 1994;129:381–388; discussion 388–389.

10. Lauren P. The two histological main types of gastric cancer: diffuse and so-called intestinal type carcinoma. Acta Pathol Microbiol Scand 1965;64:31–49.

11. Correa P, Cuello C, Duque E, et al. Gastric cancer in Colombia. III. Natural history of precursor lesions. J Natl Cancer Inst 1976;57:1027–1035.

12. Becker KF, Atkinson MJ, Reich U, et al. E-cadherin gene mutations provide clues to diffuse type gastric carcinomas. Cancer Res. 1994;54:3845–3852.

13. Munoz N, Connelly R. Time trends of intestinal and diffuse types of gastric cancer in the United States. Int J Cancer 1971;8:158–64.

14. Fukao A, Tsubono Y, Tsuji I, Hisamichi S, Sugahara N, Takano A. The evaluation of screening for gastric cancer in Miyagi Prefecture, Japan: a population-based case-control study. Int J Cancer 1995;60:45–48.

15. Blot WJ, Li JY, Taylor PR, et al. Nutrition intervention trials in Linxian, China: supplementation with specific vitamin/mineral combinations, cancer incidence, and disease-specific mortality in the general population. J Natl Cancer Inst 1993;85:1483–1492.

16. Marshall BJ. History of the discovery of C. pylori. In: Blaser MJ, ed. Campylobacter pylori in gastritis and peptic ulcer disease. New York: Igaku-Shoin; 1989:7–23.

17. Tomb JF, White O, Kerlavage AR, et al. The complete genome sequence of the gastric pathogen Helicobacter pylori. Nature 1997;388:539–547.

18. Parsonnet J. Helicobacter. In: Gorbach SL, Bartlett JG, Blacklow NR, eds. Infectious Diseases. Philadelphia: WB Saunders; 1998:1952–1961.

19. Lee A, Fox J, Hazell S. Pathogenicity of Helicobacter pylori: a perspective. Infect Immun 1993;61:1601–1610.

20. Boren T, Normark S, Falk P. Helicobacter pylori: molecular basis for host recognition and bacterial adherence. Trends Microbiol 1994;2:221–228.

21. Clyne M, Drumm B. Absence of effect of Lewis A and Lewis B expression on adherence of Helicobacter pylori to human gastric cells. Gastroenterology 1997;113:72–80.

22. Clyne M, Drumm B. Adherence of *Helicobacter pylori* to the gastric mucosa. Pediat Gastroenterol 1997;11:243–248.[Abstract]

23. Segal ED, Falkow S, Tompkins LS. *Helicobacter pylori* attachment to gastric cells induces cytoskeletal rearrangements and tyrosine phosphorylation of host cell proteins. Proc Natl Acad Sci USA 1996;93:1259–1264.

24. Mobley HL. *Helicobacter pylori* factors associated with disease development. Gastroenterology 1997;113:S21–S28.

25. Eaton KA, Brooks CL, Morgan DR, Krakowka S. Essential role of urease in pathogenesis of gastritis induced by *Helicobacter pylori* in gnotobiotic piglets. Infect Immun 1991;59:2470–2475.

26. Hazell SL, Mendz GL. The metabolism and enzymes of *Helicobacter pylori*: function and potential virulence effects. In: Goodwin CS, Worsley BW, eds. *Helicobacter pylori*: Biology and Clinical Practice. Boca Raton, Fla: CRC Press; 1993:115–42.

27. Ernst PB, Crowe SE, Reyes VE. How does *Helicobacter pylori* cause mucosal damage? The inflammatory response. Gastroenterology 1997;113:S35–S42; discussion, S50.

28. Crabtree JE. Gastric mucosal inflammatory responses to *Helicobacter pylori*. Aliment Pharmacol Ther 1996;10 (suppl 1):29–37.

29. Appelmelk BJ, Negrini R, Moran AP, Kuipers EJ. Molecular mimicry between *Helicobacter pylori* and the host. Trends Microbiol 1997;5:70–73.

30. Xiang Z, Censini S, Bayeli PF, et al. Analysis of expression of CagA and VacA virulence factors in 43 strains of *Helicobacter pylori* reveals that clinical isolates can be divided into two major types and that CagA is not necessary for expression of the vacuolating cytotoxin. Infect Immun 1995;63:94–98.

31. Censini S, Lange C, Xiang Z, et al. cag, a pathogenicity island of *Helicobacter pylori*, encodes type I-specific and disease-associated virulence factors. Proc Natl Acad Sci USA 1996;93:14648–14653.

32. Xiang Z, Censini S, Bayeli PF, et al. Analysis of expression of CagA and VacA virulence factors in 43 strains of *Helicobacter pylori* reveals that clinical isolates can be divided into two major types and that CagA is not necessary for expression of the vacuolating cytotoxin. Infect Immun 1995;63:94–98.

33. Cover TL, Glupczynski Y, Lage AP, et al. Serologic detection of infection with cagA+ *Helicobacter pylori* strains. J Clin Microbiol 1995;33:1496–500.

34. Smith KL, Parsonnet J. *Helicobacter pylori*. In: Evans A, Brachman P, eds. Bacterial Infections of Humans. New York: Plenum Publishing Corp; 1998:337–353.

35. Parsonnet J. The incidence of *Helicobacter pylori* infection. Aliment Pharmacol Ther 1995;9(suppl 2):45–52.

36. Parsonnet J, Blaser MJ, Perez-Perez GI, Hargrett-Bean N, Tauxe RV. Symptoms and risk factors of *Helicobacter pylori* infection in a cohort of epidemiologists. Gastroenterology 1992;102:41–46.

37. Banatvala N, Mayo K, Megraud F, Jennings R, Deeks JJ, Feldman RA. The cohort effect and *Helicobacter pylori*. J Infect Dis 1993;168:219–221.

38. Malaty HM, Graham DY. Importance of childhood socioeconomic status on the current prevalence of *Helicobacter pylori* infection. Gut 1994;35:742–745.

39. Replogle ML, Glaser SL, Hiatt RA, Parsonnet J. Biological sex as a risk factor for *Helicobacter pylori* infection in healthy young adults. Am J Epidemiol 1995; 142:856–863.

40. Eurogast Study Group. Epidemiology of, and risk factors for, *Helicobacter pylori*

infection among 3194 asymptomatic subjects in 17 populations. Gut 1993; 34:1672–1676.

41. Malaty HM, Engstrand L, Pedersen NL, Graham DY. *Helicobacter pylori* infection: genetic and environmental influences. Ann Intern Med 1994;120:982–986.

42. Megraud F. Transmission of *Helicobacter pylori*: faecal-oral versus oral-oral. Aliment Pharmacol Ther 1997;9(suppl 2):85–92.

43. Hopkins RJ, Vial PA, Ferreccio C, et al. Seroprevalence of *Helicobacter pylori* in Chile: vegetables may serve as one route of transmission. J Infect Dis 1993; 168:222–226.

44. Klein PD, Graham DY, Gaillour A, Opekun AR, O'Brian Smith E, Gastrointestinal Physiology Working Group. Water source as risk factor for *Helicobacter pylori* infection in Peruvian children. Lancet 1991;337:1503–1506.

45. Forman D, Sitas F, Newell DG, et al. Geographic association of *Helicobacter pylori* antibody prevalence and gastric cancer mortality in rural China. Int J Cancer 1990;46:608–611.

46. Eurogast Study Group. An international association between *Helicobacter pylori* infection and gastric cancer. Lancet 1993;341:1359–1362.

47. Masci E, Viale E, Freschi M, Porcellati M, Tittobello A. Precancerous gastric lesions and *Helicobacter pylori*. Hepatogastroenterology 1996;43:854–858.

48. Osawa H, Inoue F, Yoshida Y. Inverse relation of serum *Helicobacter pylori* antibody titres and extent of intestinal metaplasia. J Clin Pathol 1996;49:112–115.

49. Genta RM, Graham DY. Intestinal metaplasia, not atrophy or achlorhydria, creates a hostile environment for *Helicobacter pylori*. Scand J Gastroenterol 1993;28:924–928.

50. Huang J, Sridhar S, Chen Y, Hunt RH. Meta-analysis of the relationship between *Helicobacter pylori* seropositivity and gastric cancer. Gastroenterology 1998;114:1169–1179.

51. Eslick GD, Talley NJ. *Helicobacter pylori* infection and gastric carcinoma: a meta-analysis. Gastroenterology. 1998;114:A592[Abstract]

52. Parsonnet J, Friedman GD, Vandersteen DP, et al. *Helicobacter pylori* infection and the risk of gastric carcinoma. N Engl J Med 1991;325:1127–1131.

53. Forman D, Newell DG, Fullerton F, et al. Association between infection with *Helicobacter pylori* and risk of gastric cancer: evidence from a prospective investigation. Br Med J 1991;302:1302–1305.

54. Nomura AMY, Stemmerman GN, Chyou P, Kato I, Perez-Perez GI, Blaser MJ. *Helicobacter pylori* infection and gastric carcinoma in a population of Japanese-Americans in Hawaii. N Engl J Med 1991;325:1132–1136.

55. Siman JH, Forsgren A, Berglund G, Floren CH. Association between *Helicobacter pylori* and gastric carcinoma in the city of Malmo, Sweden. A prospective study. Scand J Gastroenterol 1997;32:1215–1221.

56. Watanabe Y, Kurata JH, Mizuno S, et al. *Helicobacter pylori* infection and gastric cancer: a nested case-control study in a rural area of Japan. Dig Dis Sci. 1997;42:1383–1387.

57. Aromaa A, Kosunen TU, Knekt P, et al. Circulating anti-*Helicobacter pylori* immunoglobulin A antibodies and low serum pepsinogen I level are associated with increased risk of gastric cancer. Am J Epidemiol 1996;144:142–149.

58. Webb PM, Yu MC, Forman D, et al. An apparent lack of association between

Helicobacter pylori infection and risk of gastric cancer in China. Int J Cancer. 1996;67:603–607.

59. Lin JT, Wang LY, Wang JT, Wang TH, Yang CS, Chen CJ. A nested case-control study on the association between *Helicobacter pylori* infection and gastric cancer risk in a cohort of 9775 men in Taiwan. Anticancer Res 1995; 15:603–606.

60. Graham DY. Can therapy even be denied for *Helicobacter pylori* infection? Gastroenterology 1997;113:S113–S117.

61. Forman D, Webb P, Parsonnet J. *H. pylori* and gastric cancer. Lancet 1994; 343:243–244.

62. Blaser MJ, Perez-Perez GI, Kleanthous H, et al. Infection with *Helicobacter pylori* strains possessing cagA is associated with an increased risk of developing adenocarcinoma of the stomach. Cancer Res 1995;55:2111–2115.

63. Parsonnet J, Friedman G, Orentreich N, Vogelman J. Risk for gastric cancer in persons with CagA positive and CagA negative *Helicobacter pylori* infection. Gut. 1997;40:297–301.

64. IARC Working Group on the Evaluation of Carcinogenic Risks to Humans. *Helicobacter pylori*. In: Schistosomes, Liver Flukes and *Helicobacter pylori*: Views and Expert Opinions of an IARC Working Group on the Evaluation of Carcinogenic Risks to Humans. Lyon: International Agency for Research on Cancer; 1994:177–240.

65. Davies GR, Simmonds NJ, Stevens TR, et al. *Helicobacter pylori* stimulates antral mucosal reactive oxygen metabolite production in vivo. Gut 1994;35: 179–185.

66. Davies GR, Banatvala N, Collins CE, et al. Relationship between infective load of *Helicobacter pylori* and reactive oxygen metabolite production in antral mucosa. Scand J Gastroenterol 1994;29:419–424.

67. Zhang Q, Dawodu JB, Etolhi G, Husain A, Gemmell CG, Russell RI. Relationship between the mucosal production of reactive oxygen radicals and density of *Helicobacter pylori* in patients with duodenal ulcer. Eur J Gastroenterol Hepatol 1997;9:261–265.

68. Zhang QB, Dawodu JB, Husain A, Etolhi G, Gemmell CG, Russell RI. Association of antral mucosal levels of interleukin 8 and reactive oxygen radicals in patients infected with *Helicobacter pylori*. Clin Sci (Colch) 1997;92:69–73.

69. Bagchi D, Bhattacharya G, Stohs SJ. Production of reactive oxygen species by gastric cells in association with *Helicobacter pylori*. Free Radical Res 1996;24: 439–450.

70. Cheng KC, Cahill DS, Kasai H, Nishimura S, Loeb LA. 8-Hydroxyguanine, an abundant form of oxidative DNA damage, causes G→T and A→C substitutions. J Biol Chem 1992;267:166–172.

71. Hahm KB, Lee KJ, Choi SY, et al. Possibility of chemoprevention by the eradication of *Helicobacter pylori*: oxidative DNA damage and apoptosis in *H. pylori* infection. Gastroenterology 1997;92:1853–1857.

72. Baik SC, Youn HS, Chung MH, et al. Increased oxidative DNA damage in *Helicobacter pylori*-infected human gastric mucosa. Cancer Res 1996;56:1279–1282.

73. Witherell HL, Hiatt RA, Replogle M, Parsonnet J. *Helicobacter pylori* infection and urinary excretion of 8-hydroxy-2-deoxyguanosine, an oxidative DNA adduct. Cancer Epidemiol Biomarkers Prev 1998;7:91–96.

74. Harris G, Asbery L, Lawley PD, Denman AM, Hylton W. Defective repair of O(6)-methylguanine in autoimmune diseases. Lancet 1982;2:952–956.

75. Badawi AF, Cooper DP, Mostafa MH, et al. O6–alkylguanine-DNA alkyltrans-ferase activity in schistosomiasis-associated human bladder cancer. Eur J Cancer 1994;30A:1314–1319.

76. Wink DA, Laval J. The Fpg protein, a DNA repair enzyme, is inhibited by the biomediator nitric oxide in vitro and in vivo. Carcinogenesis 1994;15:2125–2129.

77. Rachmilewitz D, Karmeli F, Eliakim R, et al. Enhanced gastric nitric oxide synthase activity in duodenal ulcer patients. Gut 1994;35:1394–1397.

78. Wilson KT, Ramanujam KS, Mobley HL, Musselman RF, James SP, Meltzer SJ. *Helicobacter pylori* stimulates inducible nitric oxide synthase expression and activity in a murine macrophage cell line. Gastroenterology 1996;111:1524–1533.

79. Shapiro KB, Hotchkiss JH. Induction of nitric oxide synthesis in murine macrophages by *Helicobacter pylori*. Cancer Lett 1996;102:49–56.

80. Tsuji S, Kawano S, Tsujii M, et al. *Helicobacter pylori* extract stimulates inflammatory nitric oxide production. Cancer Lett 1996;108:195–200.

81. Konturek SJ, Konturek PC, Brzozowski T, Stachura J, Zembala M. Gastric mucosal damage and adaptive protection by ammonia and ammonium ion in rats. Digestion 1996;57:433–445.

82. Mannick EE, Bravo LE, Zarama G, et al. Inducible nitric oxide synthase, nitrotyrosine, and apoptosis in *Helicobacter pylori* gastritis: effect of antibiotics and antioxidants. Cancer Res 1996;56:3238–3243.

83. Parsonnet J. *Helicobacter pylori* in the stomach—a paradox unmasked. N Engl J Med 1996;335:278–280.

84. Walsh JH. Role of gastrin as a trophic hormone. Digestion 1990;47(suppl 1):11–16; discussion, 49–52.

85. Mulholland G, Ardill JE, Fillmore D, Chittajallu RS, Fullarton GM, McColl KE. *Helicobacter pylori* related hypergastrinaemia is the result of a selective increase in gastrin 17. Gut 1993;34:757–761.

86. Moss SF, Calam J. Acid secretion and sensitivity to gastrin in patients with duodenal ulcer: effect of eradication of *Helicobacter pylori*. Gut 1993;34:888–892.

87. Ruiz B, Correa P, Fontham ET, Ramakrishnan T. Antral atrophy, *Helicobacter pylori* colonization, and gastric pH. Am J Clin Pathol 1996;105:96–101.

88. Sonnenberg A. Temporal trends and geographical variations of peptic ulcer disease. Aliment Pharmacol Ther 1995;9 (suppl 2):3–12.

89. el-Omar E, Oien K, El-Nujumi A, et al. Prevalence of atrophy and hypo-chlorhydria is high in gastric cancer relatives and related to *H. pylori* status. Gastroenterology 1998;114:A2419.[Abstract]

90. Graham DY. *Helicobacter pylori* infection in the pathogenesis of duodenal ulcer and gastric cancer: a model. Gastroenterology 1997;113:1983–1991.

91. el-Omar EM, Oien K, El-Nujumi A, et al. *Helicobacter pylori* infection and chronic gastric acid hyposecretion. Gastroenterology 1997;113:15–24.

92. You WC, Zhang L, Yang CS, et al. Nitrite, N-nitroso compounds, and other analytes in physiological fluids in relation to precancerous gastric lesions. Cancer Epidemiol Biomarkers Prev 1996;5:47–52.

93. Pignatelli B, Malaveille C, Rogatko A, et al. Mutagens, N-nitroso compounds and their precursors in gastric juice from patients with and without precancerous lesions of the stomach. Eur J Cancer 1993;29A:2031–2039.

94. Mowat C, Carswell A. Omeprazole lowers gastric juice ascorbic acid and ele-

vates gastric juice nitrite concentrations. Gastroenterology 1998;114:A236. [Abstract]

95. Sobala GM, Schorah CJ, Sanderson M, et al. Ascorbic acid in the human stomach. Gastroenterology 1989;97:357–363.

96. O'Connor HJ, Schorah CJ, Habibzedah N, Axon AT, Cockel R. Vitamin C in the human stomach: relation to gastric pH, gastroduodenal disease, and possible sources. Gut 1989;30:436–442.

97. Feldman M. Gastric secretion in health and disease. In: Sleisenger MH, Fordtran JS, eds. Gastrointestinal Disease. 4th ed. Philadelphia: WB Saunders; 1989:713–734.

98. Walsh JH. Role of gastrin as a trophic hormone. Digestion. 1990;47 (suppl 1):11–16; discussion 49–52.

99. Parsonnet J, Kim P, Yang S, Orentreich N, Vogelman JH, Friedman GD. Gastrin and gastric adenoacarcinoma: a prospective evaluation. Gastroenterology 1996;110:A574.[Abstract]

100. Hansen S, Vollset SE, Ardill JES, et al. Hypergastrinemia is a strong predictor of distal gastric adenocarcionoma among *Helicobacter pylori* infected persons. Gastroenterology. 1997;112:A575.[Abstract]

101. Hansen OH, Pedersen T, Larsen JK, Rehfeld JF. Effect of gastrin on gastric mucosal cell proliferation in man. Gut 1976;17:536–541.

102. Hakanson R, Sundler F. Trophic effects of gastrin. Scand J Gastroenterol Suppl 1991;180:130–136.

103. Sakaki N, Arakawa T, Katou H, et al. Relationship between progression of gastric mucosal atrophy and *Helicobacter pylori* infection: retrospective long-term endoscopic follow-up study. J Gastroenterol 1997;32:19–23.

104. Logan RPH, Walker MM, Misiewicz JJ, Gummett PA, Karim QN, Baron JH. Changes in the intragastric distribution of *Helicobacter pylori* during treatment with omeprazole. Gut 1995;36:12–16.

105. Xia H, Kalantar J, Eslick GD, et al. Anti-secretory drugs increase corpus gastritis but only in the presence of *Helicobacter pylori* infection. Gastroenterology 1998;114:A335.[Abstract]

106. Kuipers EJ, Lundell L, Klinkenberg-Knol EC, et al. Atrophic gastritis and *Helicobacter pylori* infection in patients with reflux esophagitis treated with omeprazole or fundoplication. N Engl J Med 1996;334:1018–1022.

107. Correa P, Haenszel W, Cuello C, Tannenbaum S, Archer M. A model for gastric cancer epidemiology. Lancet 1975;2:58–60.

108. Moller H, Nissen A, Mosbech J. Use of cimetidine and other peptic ulcer drugs in Denmark 1977–1990 with analysis of the risk of gastric cancer among cimetidine users. Gut 1992;33:1166–1169.

109. Colin-Jones DG, Langman MJ, Lawson DH, Logan RF, Paterson KR, Vessey MP. Postmarketing surveillance of the safety of cimetidine: 10 year mortality report. Gut 1992;33:1280–1284.

110. La Vecchia C, Negri E, D'Avanzo B, Franceschi S. Histamine-2-receptor antagonists and gastric cancer risk. Lancet. 1990;336:355–357.

111. Lynch DAF, Mapstone NP, Clarke AMT, et al. Cell proliferation in *Helicobacter pylori* associated gastritis and the effect of eradication therapy. Gut 1995;36: 345–350.

112. Murakami K, Fujioka T, Kodama R, Kubota T, Tokieda M, Nasu M. *Helicobacter pylori* infection accelerates human gastric mucosal cell proliferation. J Gastroenterol 1997;32:184–188.

113. Fan XG, Kelleher D, Fan XJ, Xia HX, Keeling PW. *Helicobacter pylori* increases proliferation of gastric epithelial cells. Gut 1996;38:19–22.
114. Peek RM, Moss SF, Tham KT, et al. *Helicobacter pylori* cagA+ strains and dissociation of gastric epithelial cell proliferation from apoptosis . J Natl Cancer Inst 1997;89:863–868.
115. Yabuki N, Sasano H, Tobita M, et al. Analysis of cell damage and proliferation in *Helicobacter pylori*-infected human gastric mucosa from patients with gastric adenocarcinoma. Am J Pathol 1997;151:821–829.
116. Abdel-Wahab M, Attallah AM, Elshal MF, et al. Cellular proliferation and ploidy of the gastric mucosa: the role of *Helicobacter pylori*. Hepatogastroenterology 1997;44:880–885.
117. Fraser AG, Sim R, Sankey EA, Dhillon AP, Pounder RE. Effect of eradication of *Helicobacter pylori* on gastric epithelial cell proliferation. Aliment Pharmacol Ther 1994;8:167–173.
118. Cahill RJ, Sant S, Hamilton H, Beattie S, O'Morain C. *Helicobacter pylori* and increased cell proliferation: a risk factor for cancer. Gastroenterology 1993; 104:A1032.[Abstract]
119. Fiocca R, Luinetti O, Villani L, Chiaravalli AM, Capella C, Solcia E. Epithelial cytotoxicity, immune responses, and inflammatory components of *Helicobacter pylori* gastritis. Scand J Gastroenterol Suppl 1994;205:11–21.
120. Dekigai H, Murakami M, Kita T. Mechanism of *Helicobacter pylori*-associated gastric mucosal injury. Dig Dis Sci 1995;40:1332–1339.
121. Smoot DT. How does *Helicobacter pylori* cause mucosal damage? Direct mechanisms. Gastroenterology 1997;113:S31–34.
122. Moss SF, Calam J, Agarwal B, Wang S, Holt PR. Induction of gastric epithelial apoptosis by *Helicobacter pylori*. Gut 1996;38:498–501.
123. Jones NL, Shannon PT, Cutz E, Yeger H, Sherman PM. Increase in proliferation and apoptosis of gastric epithelial cells early in the natural history of *Helicobacter pylori* infection. Am J Pathol 1997;151:1695–1703.
124. Wagner S, Beil W, Westermann J, et al. Regulation of gastric epithelial cell growth by *Helicobacter pylori*: evidence for a major role of apoptosis. Gastroenterology. 1997;113:1836–1847.
125. Chen G, Sordillo EM, Ramey WG, et al. Apoptosis in gastric epithelial cells is induced by *Helicobacter pylori* and accompanied by increased expression of BAK. Biochem Biophys Res Commun 1997;239:626–632.
126. Piotrowski J, Piotrowski E, Skrodzka D, Slomiany A, Slomiany BL. Induction of acute gastritis and epithelial apoptosis by *Helicobacter pylori* lipopolysaccharide. Scand J Gastroenterol 1997;32:203–211.
127. Piotrowski J, Skrodzka D, Slomiany A, Slomiany BL. *Helicobacter pylori* lipopolysaccharide induces gastric epithelial cells apoptosis. Biochem Mol Biol Int 1996;40:597–602.
128. Palli D, Caporaso NE, Shiao YH, et al. Diet, *Helicobacter pylori*, and p53 mutations in gastric cancer: a molecular epidemiology study in Italy. Cancer Epidemiol Biomarkers Prev 1997;6:1065–1069.
129. Hongyo T, Buzard GS, Palli D, et al. Mutations of the K-ras and p53 genes in gastric adenocarcinomas from a high-incidence region around Florence, Italy. Cancer Res. 1995;55:2665–2672.
130. Poremba C, Yandell DW, Huang Q, et al. Frequency and spectrum of p53 mutations in gastric cancer—a molecular genetic and immunohistochemical study. Virchows Arch 1995;426:447–455.

131. Starzynska T, Marsh PJ, Stern PL. p53 overexpression as a marker of malignancy in gastric biopsies. Surg Oncol 1993;2:321–324.

132. Gomyo Y, Osaki M, Kaibara N, Ito H. Numerical aberration and point mutation of p53 gene in human gastric intestinal metaplasia and well-differentiated adenocarcinoma: analysis by fluorescence in situ hybridization (FISH) and PCR-SSCP. Int J Cancer 1996;66:594–599.

133. Ochiai A, Yamauchi Y, Hirohashi S. p53 mutations in the non-neoplastic mucosa of the human stomach showing intestinal metaplasia. Int J Cancer 1996;69:28–33.

134. Renault B, van den Broek M, Fodde R, et al. Base transitions are the most frequent genetic changes at P53 in gastric cancer. Cancer Res 1993;53:2614–2617.

135. Shinmura K, Sugimura H, Naito Y, Shields PG, Kino I. Frequent co-occurrence of mutator phenotype in synchronous, independent multiple cancers of the stomach. Carcinogenesis 1995;16:2989–2993.

136. Strickler JG, Zheng J, Shu Q, Burgart LJ, Alberts SR, Shibata D. p53 mutations and microsatellite instability in sporadic gastric cancer: when guardians fail. Cancer Res 1994;54:4750–4755.

137. Myeroff LL, Parsons R, Kim SJ, et al. A transforming growth factor beta receptor type II gene mutation common in colon and gastric but rare in endometrial cancers with microsatellite instability. Cancer Res 1995;55:5545–5547.

138. Wu MS, Shun CT, Wang HP, et al. Genetic alterations in gastric cancer: relation to histological subtypes, tumor stage, and *Helicobacter pylori* infection. Gastroenterology 1997;112:1457–1465.

139. Lee KH, Lee JS, Suh C, et al. Clinicopathologic significance of the K-ras gene codon 12 point mutation in stomach cancer: an analysis of 140 cases. Cancer 1995;75:2794–2801.

140. Ranzani GN, Renault B, Pellegata NS, et al. Loss of heterozygosity and K-ras gene mutations in gastric cancer. Hum Genet 1993;92:244–249.

141. Ward JM, Fox JG, Anver MR, et al. Chronic active hepatitis and associated liver tumors in mice caused by a persistent bacterial infection with a novel Helicobacter species. J Natl Cancer Inst 1994;86:1222–1227.

142. Fox JG, Li X, Yan L, et al. Chronic proliferative hepatitis in A/JCr mice associated with persistent Helicobacter hepaticus infection: a model of helicobacter-induced carcinogenesis. Infect Immun 1996;64:1548–1558.

143. Nyska A, Maronpot RR, Eldridge SR, Haseman JK, Hailey JR. Alteration in cell kinetics in control B6C3F1 mice infected with Helicobacter hepaticus. Toxicol Pathol 1997;25:591–596.

144. Canella KA, Diwan BA, Gorelick PL, et al. Liver tumorigenesis by Helicobacter hepaticus: considerations of mechanism. In Vivo 1996;10:285–292.

145. Diwan BA, Ward JM, Ramljak D, Anderson LM. Promotion by Helicobacter hepaticus-induced hepatitis of hepatic tumors initiated by N-nitrosodimethylamine in male A/JCr mice. Toxicol Pathol 1997;25:597–605.

146. Sipowicz MA, Chomarat P, Diwan BA, et al. Increased oxidative DNA damage and hepatocyte overexpression of specific cytochrome P450 isoforms in hepatitis of mice infected with Helicobacter hepaticus. Am J Pathol 1997;151:933–941.

147. Sipowicz MA, Weghorst CM, Shiao YH, et al. Lack of p53 and ras mutations in Helicobacter hepaticus-induced liver tumors in A/JCr mice. Carcinogenesis 1997;18:233–236.

148. Fox JG, Otto G, Murphy JC, Taylor NS, Lee A. Gastric colonization of the ferret with *Helicobacter* species: natural and experimental infections. Rev Infect Dis 1991;13 (suppl 8):S671–S680.

149. Fox JG, Dangler CA, Sager W, Borkowski R, Gliatto JM. Helicobacter mustelae-associated gastric adenocarcinoma in ferrets (Mustela putorius furo). Vet Pathol 1997;34:225–229.

150. Fox JG, Wishnok JS, Murphy JC, Tannenbaum SR, Correa P. MNNG-induced gastric carcinoma in ferrets infected with Helicobacter mustelae. Carcinogenesis 1993;14:1957–1961.

151. Dubois A, Fiala N, Heman-Ackah LM, et al. Natural gastric infection with *Helicobacter pylori* in monkeys: a model for spiral bacteria infection in humans. Gastroenterology 1994;106:1405–1417.

152. Dubois A, Berg DE, Incecik ET, et al. Transient and persistent experimental infection of nonhuman primates with *Helicobacter pylori*: implications for human disease. Infect Immun 1996;64:2885–2891.

153. Tatematsu M, Yamamoto M, Shimizu N, et al. Induction of glandular stomach cancer in *Helicobacter pylori*-sensitive Mongolian gerbils treated with *N*-methyl-*N*-nitrosourea and *N*-methyl-*N*'-nitro-*N*-nitrosoguanidine in drinking water. Jpn J Cancer Res 1998;89:97–104.

154. Tokieda M, Honda S, Fujioka T, Moriuchi A, Nasu M. *N*-methyl-*N*'-nitro-*N*-nitrosoguanidine induced gastric carcinoma in Mongolian gerbils infected with *Helicobacter pylori*. Gastroenterology 1998;114:A690.[Abstract]

155. Hannson L, Nyren O, Hsing AW, et al. Risk of stomach cancer in patients with gastric or duodenal ulcer disease. N Engl J Med. 1996;335:242–249.

156. Akopyanz N, Bukanov NO, Westblom TU, Berg DE. PCR-based RFLP analysis of DNA sequence diversity in the gastric pathogen *Helicobacter pylori*. Nucleic Acids Res 1992;20:6221–6225.

157. Wang JT, Sheu JC, Lin JT, Wang TH, Wu MS. Direct DNA amplification and restriction pattern analysis of *Helicobacter pylori* in patients with duodenal ulcer and their families. J Infect Dis 1993;168:1544–1548.

158. Kuipers EJ, Perez-Perez GI, Meuwissen SG, Blaser MJ. *Helicobacter pylori* and atrophic gastritis: importance of the cagA status. J Natl Cancer Inst 1995;87: 1777–1780.

159. Perez-Perez GI, Bhat N, Gaensbauer J, et al. Country-specific constancy by age in cagA+ proportion of *Helicobacter pylori* infections. Int J Cancer 1997; 72:453–456.

160. Parsonnet J, Replogle M, Yang S, Hiatt R. Seroprevalence of CagA-positive strains among *Helicobacter pylori*-infected, healthy young adults. J Infect Dis 1997;175:1240–1242.

161. Katoh T, Nagata N, Kuroda Y, et al. Glutathione S-transferase M1 (GSTM1) and T1 (GSTT1) genetic polymorphism and susceptibility to gastric and colorectal adenocarcinoma. Carcinogenesis 1996;17:1855–1859.

162. Deakin M, Elder J, Hendrickse C, et al. Glutathione S-transferase GSTT1 genotypes and susceptibility to cancer: studies of interactions with GSTM1 in lung, oral, gastric and colorectal cancers. Carcinogenesis 1996;17:881–884.

163. Ng EK, Sung JJ, Ling TK, et al. *Helicobacter pylori* and the null genotype of glutathione-S-transferase-mu in patients with gastric adenocarcinoma. Cancer 1998;82:268–273.

164. Go MF. What are the host factors that place an individual at risk for *Helicobacter pylori*-associated disease? Gastroenterology 1997;113:S15–S20.

165. Hallstone AE, Perez EA. Blood type and the risk of gastric disease. Science. 1994;264:1386–1388.
166. Boren T, Falk P, Roth KA, Larson G, Normark S. Attachment of *Helicobacter pylori* to human gastric epithelium mediated by blood group antigens. Science 1993;262:1892–1895.
167. Sipponen P, Aarynen M, Kaariainen I, Kettunen P, Helske T, Seppala K. Chronic antral gastritis, Lewis(a+) phenotype, and male sex as factors in predicting coexisting duodenal ulcer. Scand J Gastroenterol 1989;24:581–588.
168. Mentis A, Blackwell CC, Weir DM, Spiliadis C, Dailianas A, Skandalis N. ABO blood group, secretor status and detection of *Helicobacter pylori* among patients with gastric or duodenal ulcers. Epidemiol Infect 1991;106:221–229.
169. Yamashita Y, Chung YS, Sawada T, et al. F1 alpha: a novel mucin antigen associated with gastric carcinogenesis. Oncology 1998;55:70–76.
170. Payne RJ, Nowak MA, Blumberg BS. Analysis of a cellular model to account for the natural history of infection by the hepatitis B virus and its role in the development of primary hepatocellular carcinoma. J Theor Biol 1992;159:215–240.
171. Stewenius J, Adnerhill I, Anderson H, et al. Incidence of colorectal cancer and all cause mortality in non-selected patients with ulcerative colitis and indeterminate colitis in Malmo, Sweden. Int J Colorectal Dis 1995;10:117–122.
172. Wening JV, Stein M, Langendorff U, Delling G. Chronic osteomyelitis and cancer of the fistula. Langenbecks Arch Chir 1989;374:55–59.
173. Mitchell HM, Bohane TD, Tobias V, et al. *Helicobacter pylori* infection in children: potential clues to pathogenesis . J Pediatr Gastroenterol Nutr 1993;16:120–125.
174. Queiroz DM, Rocha GA, Mendes EN, et al. Differences in distribution and severity of *Helicobacter pylori* gastritis in children and adults with duodenal ulcer disease. J Pediatr Gastroenterol Nutr 1991;12:178–181.
175. Blaser MJ, Chyou PH, Nomura A. Age at establishment of *Helicobacter pylori* infection and gastric carcinoma, gastric ulcer, and duodenal ulcer risk. Cancer Res 1995;55:562–565.
176. Tredaniel J, Boffetta P, Buiatti E, Saracci R, Hirsch A. Tobacco smoking and gastric cancer: review and meta-analysis. Int J Cancer 1997;72:565–573.
177. Kurata JH, Nogawa AN. Meta-analysis of risk factors for peptic ulcer. J Clin Gastroenterol 1997;24:2–17.
178. Moritani S, Kushima R, Sugihara H, Hattori T. Phenotypic characteristics of Epstein-Barr-virus-associated gastric carcinomas. J Cancer Res Clin Oncol 1996;122:750–756.
179. Osato T, Imai S. Epstein-Barr virus and gastric carcinoma. Semin Cancer Biol 1996;7:175–182.
180. Roosendall R, Kuipers EJ, Buitenwerf J, et al. *Helicobacter pylori* and the birth cohort effect: evidence of a continuous decrease of infection rates in childhood. Am J Gastroenterol 1997;92:1480–1482.
181. Replogle ML, Kasumi W, Ishikawa KB, et al. Increased risk of *Helicobacter pylori* associated with birth in wartime Japan. Int J Epidemiol 1996;25:210–214.
182. Gomez-Duarte OG, Lucas B, Yan ZX, Panthel K, Haas R, Meyer TF. Protection of mice against gastric colonization by *Helicobacter pylori* by single oral

dose immunization with attenuated *Salmonella typhimurium* producing urease subunits A and B. Vaccine 1998;16:460–471.

183. Corthesy-Theulaz IE, Hopkins S, Bachmann D, et al. Mice are protected from *Helicobacter pylori* infection by nasal immunization with attenuated *Salmonella typhimurium* phoPc expressing urease A and B subunits. Infect Immun 1998;66:581–586.

184. Radcliff FJ, Hazell SL, Kolesnikow T, Doidge C, Lee A. Catalase, a novel antigen for *Helicobacter pylori* vaccination. Infect Immun 1997;65:4668–4674.

185. Czinn SJ. What is the role for vaccination in *Helicobacter pylori?* Gastroenterology 1997;113:S149–S153.

186. Chow W, Blaser MJ, Blot WJ, et al. An inverse relation between *cagA+* strains of *Helicobacter pylori* infection and risk of esophageal and gastric cardia adenocarcinoma. Cancer Res 1998;58:588–590.

187. Parsonnet J, Harris R, Hack HM, Owens DK. Modelling cost effectiveness of *Helicobacter pylori* screening to prevent gastric cancer: a mandate for clinical trials. Lancet. 1996;348:150–154.

188. Fendrick AM, Chernew M, Hirth RA, Scheiman JM. Clinical and economic effects of *H. pylori* screening to prevent gastric cancer. Annu Meet Int Soc Technol Assess Health Care 1997;13:67. [Abstract]

189. Forman D. Lessons from ongoing intervention studies In: Hunt RH, Tytgat GNJ eds. Helicobacter pylori: Basic Mechanisms to Clinical Care, 1998. Dordrecht; 1998:354–361.

190. Ciok J, Dzieniszewski J, Lucer C. *Helicobacter pylori* eradication and antral intestinal metaplasia—two years follow-up study. J Physiol Pharmacol 1997;48 (suppl 4):115–22.

191. Maconi G, Lazzaroni M, Sangaletti O, Bargiggia S, Vago L, Porro GB. Effect of *Helicobacter pylori* eradication on gastric histology, serum gastrin and pepsinogen I levels, and gastric emptying in patients with gastric ulcer. Am J Gastroenterol 1997;92:1844–1848.

192. Forbes GM, Warren JR, Glaser ME, Cullen DJ, Marshall BJ, Collins BJ. Long-term follow-up of gastric histology after *Helicobacter pylori* eradication. J Gastroenterol Hepatol 1996;11:670–673.

193. van der Hulst RW, van der Ende A, Dekker FW, et al. Effect of *Helicobacter pylori* eradication on gastritis in relation to cagA: a prospective 1-year follow-up study. Gastroenterology 1997;113:25–30.

194. Uemura N, Mukai T, Okamoto S, et al. Effect of *Helicobacter pylori* eradication on subsequent development of cancer after endoscopic resection of early gastric cancer. Cancer Epidemiol Biomarkers Prev 1997;6:639–642.

15

Helicobacter pylori: A Model for Extranodal Lymphoma

PETER G. ISAACSON

Non-Hodgkin's lymphoma (NHL) comprises a clinicopathogically heterogeneous group of tumors whose classification has long been and, to a certain extent, continues to be a source of controversy. The emergence of more effective means of therapy for NHL in the 1960s and 1970s led to a certain urgency to define more precisely the pathology of the disease entities that differed in their optimum response to the various treatment modalities. Responding to this need, Rappaport, in 1966, proposed the first clinically relevant classification of NHL.[1] Following the dramatic advances of the 1960s in knowledge of lymphocyte biology, the groups of Lukes and Collins in the United States[2] and of Lennert in Germany[3] showed that the pathology of different NHL closely recapitulated the histological and immunophenotypic features of different components of lymph nodes; they formulated the first biologically rational classifications of NHL that, happily, served to increase the clinical relevance of classifying these tumors.

As the classification of NHL developed, increasing emphasis was placed on the histologic, cytologic, immunophenotypic, and functional relationships between the various neoplasms and the normal lymph node. Such was the enthusiasm of hematopathologists for this new science that they almost completely overlooked the fact that a substantial proportion (25% to 40%) of NHL arise from extranodal sites.[4,5] These sites include other primary lymphoid organs, such as Waldeyer's ring and the spleen; nonlymphoid organs that contain a substantial lymphoid component, such as the intestines; and organs devoid of lymphoid tissue, such as the brain.

In 1983 Isaacson and Wright,[6] in describing two cases of low-grade gastrointestinal lymphoma, speculated that the histologic and behavioral properties of these lymphomas were more akin to those of mucosa-associated lymphoid tissue (MALT) than to those of lymph nodes. Subsequent studies showed that other low-grade extranodal lymphomas exhibited similar properties,[7,8] and the term MALT lymphoma was suggested for this group of tumors. The close relationship between these lymphomas and MALT was further reinforced by immunohistological analyses of Peyer's patches, which are the predominant component of MALT.[9] In particular, low-grade MALT lymphoma cells share many properties with the population of marginal-zone B cells that is present in Peyer's patches.[10]

GASTRIC LYMPHOMA

Gastric lymphoma is by far the most common member of the MALT lymphoma group. As such, it is one of the most common extranodal lymphomas[4]; in its own right, however, it is a comparatively rare tumor accounting for between 1% and 7% of all gastric malignancies.[11,12] Several recent studies, however, have suggested that the incidence is increasing.[13–15] Changing criteria for diagnosis, particularly following the proposal of the MALT lymphoma concept, could explain a portion of this increase, but several careful population-based studies have provided evidence for a true increase in incidence.[16] There is, too, considerable geographic variation in the incidence of gastric lymphoma, which seems, for example, to occur with particular frequency in northeastern Italy.[17]

Gastric lymphoma is most common in people over 50 years of age, and the male to female ratio is approximately 1.5 to 1. The clinical presentation and endoscopic findings in low-grade gastric MALT lymphoma are more suggestive of chronic gastritis or of peptic ulcer disease than of a neoplasm. In most cases, the lymphoma is confined to the gastric wall (stage 1_E), with involvement of gastric lymph nodes (stage 11_E) in a minority of cases. In this respect, gastric lymphomas differ markedly from comparable low-grade B-cell lymphomas arising in lymph nodes: The latter tend to be widely disseminated early in their course.[18]

The histological features of low-grade gastric lymphoma closely recapitulate those of the Peyer's patch (Figure 15.1).[8,9] The neoplastic cells infiltrate the marginal zone around and between reactive B-cell follicles and invade the epithelium of isolated glands to form the characteristic lymphoepithelial lesions. These latter structures are thought to be the neoplastic equivalent of the so-called lymphoepithelium, an epithelium infiltrated by B cells, typified by the epithelial dome over Peyer's patches, which is a defining feature of MALT. Certain histologic features suggest that the lymphoma cells are immunoresponsive; these features include the presence of scattered transformed cells, plasma cell differentiation, and the phenomenon known as follicular colonization.[19] Plasma cell differentiation is usually maximal beneath the surface epithelium and suggests that the lymphoma cells may be responding to an antigen in the

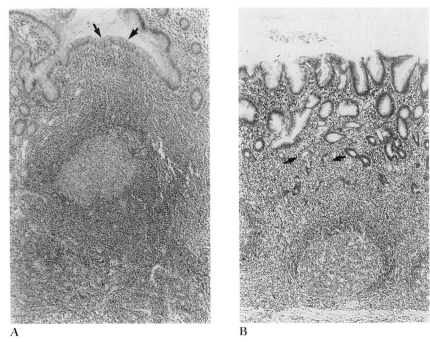

A   B

Figure 15.1. (A) Peyer's patch comprising lymphoid follicle with a broad marginal zone. A lymphoepithelium formed by B cells infiltrating the dome epithelium is indicated by the arrows. (B) Low-grade B-cell gastric MALT lymphoma comprising a reactive B-cell follicle surrounded by an infiltrate in the marginal zone that invades individual glands to form lymphoepithelial lesions (arrows).

gastric lumen or in the epithelium itself. Follicular colonization, whereby the neoplastic B cells specifically colonize reactive follicle centers, is thought possibly to be analogous to the movement of marginal-zone B cells into the follicle center; such movement has been shown to occur in rodent spleens after antigenic stimulation.[20]

The clinical course of low-grade gastric MALT lymphoma is remarkably indolent.[21] The tumor remains localized to the stomach and gastric lymph nodes for prolonged periods that may comprise several years. Peripheral dissemination to the bone marrow and to other sites occurs infrequently and then only late in the course of the disease.

The favorable clinical course of low-grade gastric MALT lymphoma has led to speculation that the tumor is not a truly malignant neoplasm, and terms such as pseudolymphoma have been suggested as more appropriate for this lesion. However, low-grade gastric MALT lymphoma fulfils the requirements for the definition of a malignant neoplasm. It is a monoclonal B-cell proliferation[22] that exhibits a variety of clonal cytogenetic abnormalities,[23] of which trisomy 3 is the most common.[24] Moreover, low-grade

B-cell gastric lymphoma is invasive and is capable of disseminating, which it does, frequently to regional lymph nodes and less frequently to distant sites.[25,26]

Gastric lymphoma often presents as a high-grade tumor when its manner of presentation and clinical course are much more typical of malignant disease and are similar to gastric carcinoma. The histologic features of high-grade B-cell gastric lymphoma are not distinctive; in many, but not all, cases, residual foci of low-grade MALT lymphoma can be found, implying that a low-grade lymphoma has transformed.[27] In addition, high-grade gastric B-cell lymphoma shares certain genetic properties with low-grade MALT lymphoma, including the absence of t(18;14), which is present in up to one third of nodal high-grade B-cell lymphomas, and an increased frequency of trisomy 3. Many, if not most, cases of high-grade gastric B-cell lymphoma therefore can be considered to be high-grade MALT lymphomas, and will share any etiologic factors implicated in the pathogenesis of the low-grade disease.

HELICOBACTER PYLORI AND GASTRIC LYMPHOMA–INDIRECT LINKS

The history of *Helicobacter pylori*, its identification, its bacteriological properties, and its role in the pathogenesis of chronic gastritis and gastric adenocarcinoma have been summarized in Chapter 14. The suggestion that there might be a link between *H. pylori* infection and gastric lymphoma was engendered by the realization that although the stomach is the most common site of MALT lymphoma, the gastric mucosa is normally devoid of any organized lymphoid tissue. Several groups have, however, shown that the hallmark of the immune response to *H. pylori* is the accumulation of organized lymphoid tissue comprising B-cell follicles and a surrounding lymphoplasmacytic infiltrate in the gastric mucosa[28–30] indeed, the presence of B-cell follicles in gastric mucosa is virtually pathognomonic of *H. pylori* infection. A recent study of the lymphoid infiltrate induced by *H. pylori* has shown that these B-cell follicles are associated with an adjacent lymphoepithelium (Figure 15.2).[31] Infection by *H. pylori*, therefore, results in the accumulation of MALT in the gastric mucosa.

If the explanation for the occurrence of MALT lymphoma in the stomach lies in the accumulation of MALT as a result of *H. pylori* infection, then *H. pylori* should be present in the gastric mucosa of patients who have this tumor. Wotherspoon and associates[31] examined histologic sections of gastric-mucosa biopsies and gastric resections from 110 patients who had gastric lymphoma; they identified *H. pylori* in 102 (92%) of these patients.

Epidemiological studies have further reinforced the association between *H. pylori* and gastric lymphoma. Circumstantial evidence was pro-

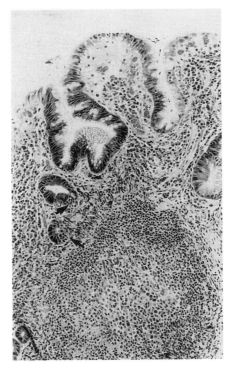

Figure 15.2. Chronic follicular gastritis due to *Helicobacter pylori*. Adjacent to the lymphoid follicle is a lymphoepithelium formed by B cells infiltrating the epithelium of individual glands (arrows).

vided by Doglioni and colleagues[17] who showed that the incidence of gastric lymphoma in a small community (Feltre) in northeastern Italy was 12 or 13 times that in comparable communities in Britain. The prevalence of *H. pylori* infection in endoscopy patients in Feltre was estimated to be approximately 85% compared to 40% to 50% in the three British communities studied. More definitive evidence has been provided by the study of Parsonnet and colleagues.[32] In a nested case control analysis, these authors showed that patients who had gastric lymphoma were sixfold more likely to have been infected previously with *H. pylori* than were matched controls who had non-gastric lymphoma.

Given the evidence that *H. pylori* infection is associated with the development of both gastric carcinoma and lymphoma, we might expect that these two tumors would occur simultaneously with a frequency greater than that due to chance alone. Although this hypothesis has not been formally tested, there are numerous case reports of both tumors occurring coincidentally in the same patient.[33] Of greater significance is the recent report from a single center in Japan of nine cases of coincident gastric carcinoma in a series of 233 cases of gastric lymphoma.[34]

ANTIGENIC STIMULATION AND GROWTH OF LOW GRADE B-CELL LYMPHOMA

The observations summarized here point to a prominent role for *H. pylori* in the pathogenesis of gastric lymphoma, and lead naturally to speculation that the presence of the organism may have an effect on the growth of the lymphoma itself. In this regard, there are several lines of evidence that suggest that the growth of low-grade B-cell gastric lymphoma may be influenced by a local antigen. As outlined on page 410, some of the histological features of low-grade gastric MALT lymphoma—including the presence of transformed blasts, plasma cell differentiation and follicular colonization—are consistent with the tumor being subject to antigenic drive. Moreover, all the accessory cells necessary for an immune response are also present within the tumor.

The curious tendency for low-grade gastric lymphoma to remain localized to the stomach for prolonged periods could be explained by such a phenomenon: Even if the lymphoma cells gain access to the peripheral circulation and hence to distant sites, which they surely must do, they will fail to grow there in the absence of the antigen. This possibility would explain the findings in a case of gastric lymphoma in which investigators identified neoplastic cells in the splenic marginal zone using anti-idiotypic antibodies, yet found no clinical, histologic, or molecular evidence of lymphoma growth in the spleen.[35]

More direct evidence that antigens—and, more specifically, bacteria—may play a role in the growth of MALT lymphoma, although not gastric lymphoma, has been obtained from clinical studies of patients with immunoproliferative small intestine disease (IPSID), which is a distinctive variety of MALT lymphoma. It has been known for many years that in patients with early stages of this disease, sterilization of the small intestine with antibiotics may lead to regression of the lymphoma.[36,37] If, as seems likely in the light of the evidence summarized above, antigenic drive is important for the growth of low-grade gastric lymphoma, then—taking IPSID as an example—the antigen is likely to be an infectious organism. The only pathogenic organism known to occur with any regularity in the stomach is *H. pylori*.

H. PYLORI AND THE GROWTH OF LOW-GRADE MALT LYMPHOMA

When unsorted cells from cases of low-grade primary B-cell gastric lymphoma are cultured under standard conditions, they characteristically die within 5 days. However, in three cases studied, when heat-killed whole-cell preparations of certain strains of *H. pylori* were added to these cultures, clustering and proliferation of tumor cells were observed.[38] The three different cases of gastric lymphoma were each stimulated optimally by three different clinical strains of *H. pylori*. This finding reflects the extreme strain variability of *H. pylori*[39] and hence of differences in the profile of *H. pylori*–derived molecules to which the patients had been exposed before gastrectomy. Proliferation of the tumor cells was associated with expression of interleukin-2 (IL-2) receptors and release of tumor cell–derived immunoglobulin (Ig) and IL-2 into the supernatant. In contrast with the gastric lymphomas, low-grade MALT lymphomas of the salivary gland and thyroid, and a nodal lymphocytic lymphoma, all of which responded to control mitogens, did not respond to any of the strains of *H. pylori*. The removal of T cells from the crude cell suspensions of gastric lymphomas before culturing the cells abrogated all indices of activation induced by the inclusion of *H. pylori* in the cultures.

These experiments suggest either that the MALT lymphoma B cells were directly responsive to *H. pylori* but required T-cell help to make a proliferative response, or that *H. pylori* stimulated intratumoral T cells, which in turn provide help for tumor cell proliferation.

H. pylori induces a significant local humoral response. It was considered possible, therefore, that the Ig expressed and secreted by the lymphoma might recognize *H. pylori* antigens. Researchers investigated the specificity of tumor cell Ig by preparing mouse–human heterohybridomas and human–human hybridomas as a source of tumor-derived Ig.[40,41] In the four cases reported to date, the tumor Ig was found to recognize distinct autoantigens, including follicular dendritic cells, basement membrane, IgG, and epitopes associated with IgA and IgM. There is evidence that antibodies to *H. pylori* antigens may cross-react with human autoantigens.[42] Studies using murine monoclonal antibodies have shown clearly cross-reactivity between epithelial antigens and *H. pylori*; cross-reactivity between the heat shock proteins of *H. pylori* and of humans have also been observed and may serve as a basis for autoimmunity.[43] However, there was no evidence of cross-reactivity of lymphoma-derived Ig with *H. pylori* antigens under any of the conditions tested[40,41]

Given that gastric MALT lymphoma cells are not stimulated by *H. pylori* directly through the antigen receptor, the possibility that the lymphoma is stimulated by *H. pylori* via an alternative undefined route was investigated. Since the B cells clearly needed T-cell help to respond to *H. pylori* in the experiments using the whole cell suspension derived from the tumors,[38] investigators replaced the T cells by cross-linking CD40, using CD40-coated Lmtk-CDw32 cells.[44] This cross-linking allowed the properties of the B cells to be studied in the absence of T cells. Addition of *H. pylori* strains that clearly stimulated the whole-tumor–derived cell suspension in the earlier experiments failed to increase the proliferation of tumor cells maintained in culture by cross-linking CD40. Therefore, *H. pylori* do not stimulate gastric MALT lymphoma B cells directly.

The tumor cells do not appear to be directly stimulated by *H. pylori*, so researchers have examined the tumor-infiltrating T cells.[45] The strain specificity of the whole-tumor-cell populations proved invaluable in these studies, because it allowed a strain of *H. pylori* that stimulated the tumor in earlier studies of the unsorted tumor cell suspension to be compared with a strain that did not. Using an EBV-transformed B-cell line produced with the patients own splenic B cells to present the *H. pylori* strains to tumor-infiltrating T cells, Hussell and colleagues noted that the specificity for strains of *H. pylori* resided in the tumor-infiltrating T-cell population. Interestingly, splenic T cells from the same patient did not respond to the stimulating strain of *H. pylori*, demonstrating that the *H. pylori*–responsive T-cell population was local. This finding provides a highly plausible explanation for the observation that low-grade gastric MALT lymphomas remain localized to the stomach for long periods: The lymphomas are dependent on activated T cells, which, although present in abundance at sites of *H. pylori* infection, are unlikely to be present outside the stomach and, possibly, outside of the gastric lymph nodes.

Because T cells can provide help for B cells both by provision of a high cytokine environment and through contact, antibodies to the ligand for CD40 (CD40L) were titrated into unsorted cell suspensions from a gastric lymphoma, to block contact between CD40 and its ligand, which is essential for T-cell help for B-cell proliferation and Ig secretion.[46] The addition of anti-CD40L inhibited B-cell clustering and reduced B-cell proliferation, showing that B cells require contact-dependent help from the tumor-infiltrating T cells. Supporting this observation, Hussell found that transferring cytokine-containing supernatants from proliferating cultures to isolated tumor B cells did not support proliferation of the tumor cells.

Although the specificity for strains of *H. pylori* appears to reside in the tumor-infiltrating T-cell population in the cases studied, the progenitor B cell of the malignant clone must have some property that results in its uncontrolled proliferation in the presence of T-cell help. This property could be either a genetic alteration (trisomy 3?)[24] resulting in growth advantage, or an abnormal biological property of the cell, such as the ability to recognize autoantigen.

ERADICATION OF *H. PYLORI* AND REGRESSION OF LOW-GRADE GASTRIC MALT LYMPHOMA

In the light of the circumstantial histologic evidence that the growth of low-grade gastric MALT lymphoma is influenced by antigen, and of the more substantive experimental evidence summarized above, Wotherspoon and associates evaluated the effect of eradicating *H. pylori* in clinical cases of gastric lymphoma.[47] Six patients (three females and three males) in whom primary low-grade gastric MALT lymphoma (stage 1_E) and *H. pylori* infection had been diagnosed with endoscopic biopsy were selected for the study. In five of the six, molecular analysis using the polymerase chain reaction (PCR) had confirmed a monoclonal B-cell population in the lesion. In all patients, the lymphoma had not given rise to an identifiable

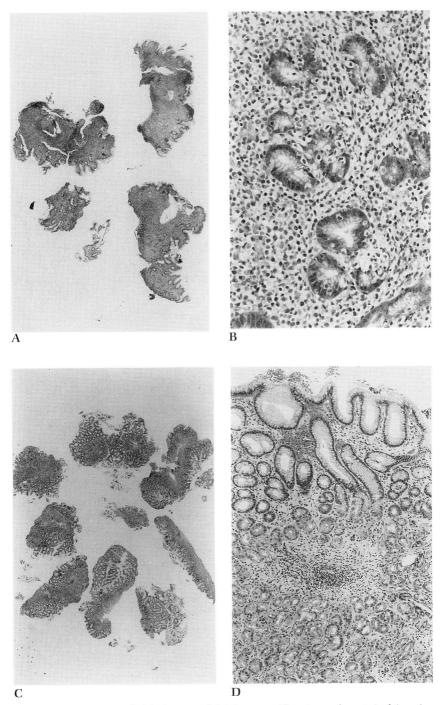

Figure 15.3. (A) and (B): low and high magnification of gastric biopsies from a patient with a low-grade MALT lymphoma and *H. pylori* infection. (C) and (D): repeat gastric biopsies from same case after eradication of *H. pylori*. There are single small lymphoid infiltrates but no evidence of lymphoma.

tumor mass and was thus thought to represent early disease. After the diagnostic biopsy, the patients received amoxicillin and metronidazole, either with tripotassium dicitrobismuthate (five patients) or with omeprazole (one patient). Repeat posttreatment biopsies were performed at regular intervals, and each was evaluated for the histologic changes of lymphoma, for the presence of *H. pylori*, and for any molecular evidence of a monoclonal B-cell population. In all six patients, *H. pylori* was successfully eradicated and complete remission of the lymphoma was achieved as judged on endoscopic, histologic, and molecular grounds (Figure 15.3).[47,48] Studies of further cases[48,49] have shown similar results except that in some cases, molecular evidence of the presence of monoclonal tumor cells has persisted in the absence of any histologic evidence of disease.

Several independent groups[49–52] have now confirmed that eradication of *H. pylori* may induce remission in cases of low-grade B-cell lymphoma of the stomach. As work has progressed, a number of questions have arisen relating to the interval between *H. pylori* eradication and remission of the lymphoma, the likely duration of the induced remission, the relevance of persistent "molecular disease," the effect of *H. pylori* eradication in more deeply invasive lymphomas, and the effect of relapse or reinfection by *H. pylori*. It is also important to clarify whether the growth of low-grade gastric MALT lymphomas can become independent of *H. pylori* and whether high-grade gastric lymphomas could respond to this novel form of therapy.

In most cases, some degree of histologic response to treatment of the *H. pylori* infection has been evident 2 to 3 months after eradication of the organism. This has not necessarily meant complete histologic regression, which has taken as long as 22 months in one case (Isaacson, unpublished data). In practical terms, if the appearances of the biopsy are consistent with ongoing regression of lymphoma, then provided that *H. pylori* remain undetectable, it is probably worthwhile to wait for up to 12 months before proceeding to another form of therapy. The initial group of six patients with gastric lymphoma treated by antibiotic eradication of *H. pylori* have now been followed up for 36 months. All have remained free of disease, but in one patient a faint monoclonal band detectable with PCR has reappeared in the absence of histologic evidence of disease.[48] A single case has also been reported in which lymphoma was treated by eradication of *H. pylori* serendipitously; this patient has remained in remission for 7 years.[53]

In some cases of low-grade gastric MALT lymphoma, eradication of *H. pylori* leads to complete endoscopic and histologic regression of disease, but PCR shows persistence of the neoplastic clone.[49] This finding probably is a reflection of the half-life of neoplastic lymphocytes and plasma cells, which is at present unknown. However, prolonged follow-up in two such cases has shown disappearance of these molecular changes 12 and 28 months after complete histologic regression.[49]

Almost all reported cases of gastric lymphoma treated successfully by eradication of *H. pylori* have consisted of flat mucosal lesions, and the inference has been that these lesions are probably superficial and restricted to the mucosa. More deeply invasive tumors are likely to produce elevated tumor masses. The use of techniques such as endoscopic endosonography is necessary to assess accurately the depth of invasion of these larger tumors; the results of treatment of cases staged in this way are still awaited. A single case has been reported in which a large ulcerated gastric lymphoma that penetrated the submucosa was treated successfully by eradication of *H. pylori*.[52] A related question is whether gastric lymph node involvement, which may be present even when the lymphoma is restricted to the mucosa, will respond to eradication of *H. pylori*, and the same question applies to distant foci of disease.

Reinfection of the stomach following successful eradication of *H. pylori* is thought to occur uncommonly. When *H. pylori* organisms do reappear in the stomach, they do so almost always as the result of unsuccessful eradication therapy and recrudescence of the original infecting organism. There are two reports of this phenomenon leading to rapid relapse of lymphoma. In a single case (Isaacson, unpublished data), relapse occurred after treatment with both combination chemotherapy and *H. pylori* eradication; this relapse was associated with reappearance of *H. pylori*, and complete regression was achieved by eradication of the organism for the second time. Clearly, patients successfully treated for gastric lymphoma by *H. pylori* eradication must be kept under close surveillance for any evidence of relapse of their *H. pylori* infection.

It is difficult to conceive that in those cases of low-grade MALT lymphoma that have disseminated beyond the immediate gastric environment, the growth of the tumor remains dependent on antigenic drive provided by *H. pylori*. That loss of this dependency may occur has been shown in one case studied in vitro (Spencer and Isaacson, unpublished). Tumor cells from this case proliferated spontaneously in culture, to the extent that any enhanced proliferation after the addition of *H. pylori* would have been masked. In this particular case, t(1;14) had been demonstrated in the lymphoma cells.[23] Interestingly, cells from a low-grade MALT lymphoma of the lung with this translocation[54] exhibited similar behavior. These preliminary findings suggest that loss of response to *H. pylori* may represent a genetic change associated with progression of gastric MALT lymphoma. In this context, however, it is worth noting that in one of the cases studied in vitro by Hussell and associates,[38] tumor cells derived from a secondary focus of lymphoma in the small intestine responded to stimulation by strain-specific *H. pylori*.

The histologic evidence for antigenic drive that characterizes low-grade gastric MALT lymphoma is lost in high-grade B-cell gastric lymphoma. This, together with the findings in one case studied in vitro by Hussell and associates,[38] suggests that high-grade gastric lymphomas will not respond to eradication of *H. pylori*. Nevertheless, the presence of associated low-grade MALT lymphoma in many cases suggests that it is prudent to eradicate *H. pylori* as part of the treatment of high-grade gastric lymphoma.

SUMMARY AND CONCLUSIONS

The evidence summarized in this chapter suggests the following scheme for the pathogenesis of gastric lymphoma. The first step is accumulation of lymphoid tissue (MALT) in response to infection of the stomach by *H. pylori*. In rare instances, this lymphoid infiltrate contains cells with a growth advantage, possibly due to a genetic change (perhaps trisomy 3). The result is a monoclonal lymphoproliferative lesion that is responsive to *H. pylori*–driven T-cell help. Further genetic changes [such as t(1;14)] may lead to escape from T-cell dependency and ultimately to transformation to high-grade lymphoma.

Low-grade B-cell gastric lymphoma is the paradigm for the entire group of MALT lymphomas, members of which occur in a wide variety of extranodal sites. It is likely that the growth of this group of lymphomas is governed by a series of different antigens, many of which might, like *H. pylori*, be microbiological. These agents await identification.

REFERENCES

1. Rappaport H. Tumors of the hematopoietic system. In: Atlas of Tumor Pathology, Section 3: Fascicle 8, Washington DC: US Armed Forces Institute of Pathology.
2. Lukes RJ, Collins RD. New approaches to the classification of the lymphomata. Br J Cancer 1975;31(suppl 2):1–28.
3. Lennert K, Mohri N, Stein H, Kaiserling E. The histopathology of malignant lymphoma. Br J Haematol 1975;31(suppl 1):193–198.
4. Freeman C, Berg JW, Cutler SJ. Occurrence and prognosis of extranodal lymphomas. Cancer 1972;29:252–260.
5. Otter R, Bieger R, Kluin PM, et al. Primary gastrointestinal non-Hodgkin's lymphoma in a population-based registry. Br J Cancer 1989;60:745–750.
6. Isaacson P, Wright DH. Malignant lymphoma of mucosa-associated lymphoid tissue: a distinctive type of B-cell lymphoma. Cancer 1983;52:1410–1416.
7. Isaacson P, Wright DH. Extranodal malignant lymphoma arising from mucosa-associated lymphoid tissue. Cancer 1984;53:2515–2524.
8. Isaacson PG, Spencer J. Malignant lymphoma of mucosa associated lymphoid tissue. Histopathology 1989;11:445–462.
9. Spencer J, Finn T, Isaacson PG. Human Peyer's patches: an immunohistochemical study. Gut 1986;27:405–410.
10. Spencer J, Finn T, Pulford KAF, Mason DY, Isaacson PG. The human gut contains a novel population of B lymphocytes which resemble marginal zone cells. Clin Exp Immunol 1985;62:607–612.
11. Dragosics B, Bauer P, Radaszkiewic T. Primary gastrointestinal non-Hodgkin's lymphomas: a retrospective clinicopathologic study of 150 cases. Cancer 1985; 55:1060–1073.

12. Weingrad DN, Decosse JJ, Sherlock P, Straus D, Lieberman PH, Filippa DA. Primary gastrointestinal lymphoma: a 30–year review. Cancer 1982;49:1258–1265.
13. Sandler RS. Has primary gastric lymphoma become more common? J Clin Gastroenterol 1984;6:101–107.
14. Severson RK, Davis S. Increasing incidence of primary gastric lymphoma. Cancer 1990;66:1283–1287.
15. Hayes J, Dunn E. Has the incidence of primary gastric lymphoma increased? Cancer 1989;63:2073–2076.
16. Pinotti G, Novario R, Berrino F, et al. Primary gastric non-Hodgkin's lymphoma in a population-based registry. Hematologica 1992;77:405–412.
17. Doglioni C, Wotherspoon AC, Moschini A, de Boni M, Isaacson PG. High incidence of primary gastric lymphoma in Northeastern Italy. Lancet 1992; 339:834–835.
18. Isaacson PG, Norton AJ. Extranodal Lymphomas. Edinburgh, London, Madrid, Melbourne, New York, Tokyo: Churchill Livingstone; 1994.
19. Isaacson PG, Wotherspoon AC, Diss T, Pan L. Follicular colonization in B-cell lymphoma of mucosa-associated lymphoid tissue. Am J Surg Pathol 1991; 15:819–828.
20. MacLennan ICM, Liu YJ, Oldfield S, et al. The evolution of B-cell clones. Curr Top Microbiol Immunol 1990;159:37–63.
21. Cogliatti SB, Schmid U, Schumacher U, et al. Primary B-cell gastric lymphoma: a clinicopathological study of 145 patients. Gastroenterology 1991; 101:1159–1170.
22. Spencer J, Diss TC, Isaacson PG. Primary B cell gastric lymphoma: a genotypic analysis. Am J Pathol 1989;135:557–564.
23. Wotherspoon AC, Pan LX, Diss TC, Isaacson PG. Cytogenetic study of B-cell lymphoma of mucosa-associated lymphoid tissue. Cancer Genet Cytogenet 1992;58:35–38.
24. Wotherspoon AC, Finn TM, Isaacson PG. Trisomy 3 in low-grade B cell lymphomas of mucosa associated lymphoid tissue (MALT). Blood 1995;85:2000–2004.
25. Diss TC, Peng H, Wotherspoon AC, Pan LX, Speight PM, Isaacson PG. Brief report: a single neoplastic clone in sequential biopsy specimens from a patient with primary gastric mucosa-associated lymphoid tissue lymphoma and Sjogren's syndrome. N Engl J Med 1993;329:172–175.
26. Montalban C, Castrillo JM, Serano M, et al. Gastric B-cell mucosa-associated lymphoid tissue (MALT) lymphoma: clinicopathological study and evaluation of the prognostic factors in 143 patients. Ann Oncol 1995;6:355–362.
27. Chan JKC, Ng CS, Isaacson PG. Relationship between high-grade lymphoma and low-grade B-cell mucosa-associated lymphoid tissue lymphoma (MALToma) of the stomach. Am J Pathol 1990;136:1153–1164.
28. Wyatt JI, Rathbone BJ. Immune response of the gastric mucosa to *Campylobacter pylori*. Scand J Gastroenterol 1988;23:44–49.
29. Stolte M, Eidt S. Lymphoid follicles in the antral mucosa: immune response to *Campylobacter pylori*. J Clin Pathol 1989;42:1269–1271.
30. Genta RM, Hamner HW, Graham DY. Gastric lymphoid follicles in *Helicobacter pylori* infection: frequency, distribution, and response to triple therapy. Hum Pathol 1993;24:577–583.
31. Wotherspoon AC, Ortiz-Hidalgo C, Falzon MR, Isaacson PG. *Helicobacter pylori-*

associated gastritis and primary B-cell gastric lymphoma. Lancet 1991;338: 1175–1176.

32. Parsonnet J, Hansen S, Rodriguez L, Gelb AB, Warnke RA, Jellum E, Orentreich N, Vogelman JH, Friedman GD. *Helicobacter pylori* infection and gastric lymphoma. N Engl J Med 1994;330:1267–1271.

33. Wotherspoon AC, Isaacson PG. Synchronous adenocarcinoma and low-grade B-cell lymphoma of mucosa associated lymphoid tissue (MALT) of the stomach. Histopathology 1995;27:325–331.

34. Nakamura S, Akazawa K, Yao T, Tsuneyoshi M. Primary gastric lymphoma. Cancer 1995;76:1313–1324.

35. Spencer J, Diss TC, Isaacson PG. A study of the properties of a low-grade mucosal B-cell lymphoma using a monoclonal antibody specific for the tumor immunoglobulin. J Pathol 1990;160:231–238.

36. Gilinsky NH, Novis BH, Wright JP, Dent DM, King H, Marks IN. Immunoproliferative small-intestinal disease: clinical features and outcome in 30 cases. Medicine 1987;66:438–446.

37. Ben-Ayed F, Halphen M, Najjar T et al. Treatment of alpha chain disease: results of a prospective study in 21 Tunisian patients by the Tunisian-French Intestinal Lymphoma Study Group. Cancer 1989;63:1251–1256.

38. Hussell T, Isaacson PG, Crabtree JE, Spencer J. The response of cells from low-grade B-cell gastric lymphomas of mucosa associated lymphoid tissue to *Helicobacter pylori*. Lancet 1993;342:571–574.

39. Akopyanz N, Bukanov NO, Westblom TU, Berg DE. PCR based analysis of DNA sequence diversity in the gastric pathogen *Helicobacter pylori*. Nucleic Acids Res 1992;20:6221–6225.

40. Hussell T, Isaacson PG, Crabtree JE, Dogan A, Spencer J. Immunoglobulin specificity of low-grade B cell gastric lymphoma of mucosa associated lymphoid tissue. Am J Pathol 1993;142:285–292.

41. Greiner A, Marx A, Heesman J, Leebman J, Schmausser B, Muller-Hermelink HK. Idiotype identity in a MALT-type lymphoma and B cells in *Helicobacter pylori* associated chronic gastritis. Lab Invest 1994;70:572–578.

42. Negrini R, Lisato L, Zanella I, Cavazzini L, Gullini S, Villanacci V, Poiesi C, Albertini A, Ghielmi S. *Helicobacter pylori* infection induces antibodies cross reacting with the gastric mucosa. Gastroenterology 1991;101:437–445.

43. Macchia G, Massone A, Burroni D, Covacci A, Censini S, Rappuoli R. The hsp60 protein of *Helicobacter pylori*: structure and immune response in patients with gastroduodenal disease. Mol Microbiol 1993;9:645–652.

44. Banchereau J, De Paoli P, Valle A, Garcia E, Rousset F. Long term human B cell lines dependent on IL-4 and antibody to CD40. Science 1991;251:70–72.

45. Hussell T, Isaacson PG, Crabtree JE, Spencer J. *Helicobacter pylori* specific tumor infiltrating T cells provide contact dependent help for the growth of malignant B cells in low-grade gastric lymphoma of mucosa associated lymphoid tissue. J Pathol 1996;178:122–127.

46. Grabstein KH, Maliszewski CR, Shanebeck K, Sato TA, Sprigg MK, Fanslow WC, Armitage RJ. The regulation of T cell-dependent antibody formation in vitro by CD40 ligand and IL-2. J Immunol 1993;150:3141–3147.

47. Wotherspoon AC, Doglioni C, Diss TC, Pan L, Moschini A, De Boni M, Isaacson PG. Regression of primary low-grade B-cell gastric lymphoma of mucosa associated lymphoid tissue after eradication of *Helicobacter pylori*. Lancet 1993;342:575–577.

48. Wotherspoon AC, Doglioni C, de Boni M, Spencer J, Isaacson PG. Antibiotic treatment for low-grade gastric MALT lymphoma. Lancet 1994;343:1503.

49. Savio A, Franzin G, Wotherspoon AC, Zamboni G, Negrini R, Buffoli F, Diss TC, Pan L, Isaacson P. Diagnosis and post-treatment follow up of *Helicobacter pylori* positive gastric lymphoma of mucosa associated lymphoid tissue: histology, PCR or both? Blood 1996:87:1255-1260.

50. Roggero E, Zucca E, Pinotti G, et al. Eradication of *Helicobacter pylori* infection in primary low-grade gastric lymphoma of mucosa-associated lymphoid tissue. Ann Intern Med 1995;122:767–769.

51. Bayerdorffer E, Neubauer A, Rudolph B, et al. Regression of primary gastric lymphoma of mucosa-associated lymphoid tissue type after cure of *Helicobacter pylori*. Lancet 1995;345:1591–1594.

52. Weber DM, Dimopoulos MA, Anandu DP, Pugh WC, Steinbach G. Regression of gastric lymphoma of mucosa-associated lymphoid tissue with antibiotic therapy for *Helicobacter pylori*. Gastroenterology 1994;107:1835-1838.

53. Blecker U, McKeithan TW, Hart J, Kirschner BS. Resolution of *Helicobacter pylori* associated gastric lympho-proliferative disease in a child. Gastroenterology 1995;109:973–977.

54. Wotherspoon AC, Soosay GN, Diss TC, Isaacson PG. Low-grade primary B-cell lymphoma of the lung. an immunohisto-chemical, molecular and cytogenetic study of a single case. Am J Clin Pathol 1990;94:655–660.

16

Bacterial Infection
and Colon Cancer

DAVID B. SCHAUER

Much of the knowledge about the molecular and genetic basis of cancer has been gained through the study of colon cancer. These advances have been facilitated by the high frequency of the disease and the resulting abundance of clinical specimens in the Western world, as well as by the fact that certain inherited syndromes predispose to colonic neoplasia. A working model for colon carcinogenesis has been developed,[1] and studies on spontaneous and induced colon tumors in animals, coupled with studies on familial and sporadic colon cancer in people, have confirmed and extended the role of each of the component genes in this multistep process. Characterization of the genetic changes that occur in colon carcinogenesis do not necessarily indicate their etiology. Clearly, some individuals are at high risk for colon cancer because of inherited germ line mutations, such as *APC* gene mutations in familial adenomatous polyposis[2] and mismatch-repair-gene mutations in hereditary nonpolyposis colon cancer.[3,4] However, the genes involved in both of these syndromes act in a recessive manner at the cellular level, and a second, somatic event is necessary for the development of tumors. Furthermore, these hereditary cancer syndromes account for less than 1% and less than 6% of all colon cancer cases, respectively, and it has been estimated that no more than 20% of all colon cancer cases are hereditary.[5] What then is the etiology of acquired genetic change in colon cancer?

A simple view of colon carcinogenesis, shaped partly by studies of chemically induced rodent skin tumors, is that genotoxic carcinogens are ubiquitous in the environment, and that mutant cells, initiated by these chemicals, can be promoted by various environmental factors to become neoplastic. The diet is a rich source of carcinogens, tumor promoters, and mutagens, but none of these substances have been correlated with risk of colon cancer. Paradoxically, it has been suggested that populations that eat diets with the highest levels of preformed genotoxic agents tend to be those with the lowest colon cancer rates.[6] To rationalize this apparent contradiction, Aries and colleagues postulated that colon cancer is caused by a metabolite produced *in situ* by bacterial metabolism of some benign substrate.[7]

The human large intestine contains one of the most complex microbial ecosystems in nature. About 10^{14} bacterial cells are present in the colon of any given individual, consisting of hundreds of species, greater than 99% of which are anaerobes. The predominant organisms are *Bacteroides, Bifidobacterium,* and *Eubacterium* species; anaerobic gram-positive cocci, *Clostridia,* enterococci, and various species of Enterobacteriaceae are also common.[8,9] Dietary components that are not digested and absorbed from the small intestine pass into the colon. This organic material includes nonstarch polysaccharides (i.e., fiber), and resistant starch, which represent usable energy sources for the microbes. In addition to these dietary carbohydrates, endogenous polysaccharides from mucus and bile acids that escape enterohepatic circulation are also metabolized by colonic bacteria. It appears that secondary bile acids, as well as short-chain fatty acids (the end products of bacterial carbohydrate metabolism), can influence cell proliferation and may play a role in tumor promotion. There is also evidence that resident colonic bacteria can enzymatically activate procarcinogens. Finally, infection with pathogenic bacteria can increase epithelial cell proliferation, and can lead to infiltration of the colonic mucosa with inflammatory cells. Reactive products from these cells, including oxygen free radicals and nitric oxide, can contribute to epithelial cell proliferation and may themselves be genotoxic. Thus, a more complex picture begins to emerge of environmental factors, acting in concert with host genetic factors, leading to colon cancer (see Figure 16.1). There is yet no definitive proof that bacteria cause colon cancer. However, several lines of evidence from epidemiological data, intervention studies, clinical studies, and animal model studies suggest that bacterial infection does play a role in colon carcinogenesis.

EPIDEMIOLOGY AND GLOBAL DISEASE BURDEN

Colorectal cancer is one of the most common malignancies in Western society. Approximately two thirds of the estimated total of 570,00 new cases each year will occur in the developed world, which represents only one quarter of the world population.[10] It is the third most frequent type of malignancy in the world; only cancers of the lung and the stomach are more common in men, and only cancers of the breast and the cervix occur more frequently in women.[11] "Large bowel cancer" comprises at least three kinds of disease, each with different incidence and mortality parameters in different geographic locations, and with distinct male-to-

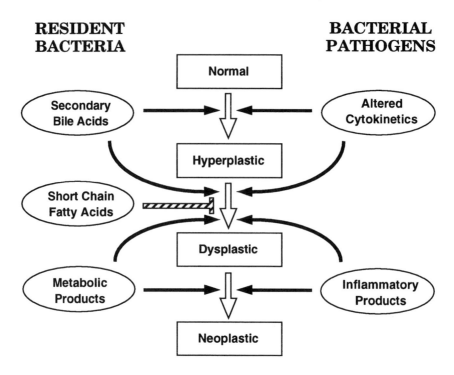

RESIDENT BACTERIA

BACTERIAL PATHOGENS

Normal

Secondary Bile Acids

Altered Cytokinetics

Hyperplastic

Short Chain Fatty Acids

Dysplastic

Metabolic Products

Inflammatory Products

Neoplastic

Figure 16.1. Model for bacterial effects on progression from normal colon epithelium to colon cancer. Resident bacteria (left side) produce secondary bile acids, which contribute to epithelial cell hyperplasia and dysplasia, and metabolize procarcinogens to carcinogens, which contribute to dysplastic and neoplastic changes. Resident bacteria also produce short-chain fatty acids that protect against dysplastic change. Bacterial pathogens (right side) can alter epithelial cytokinetics, resulting in hyperplasia and, perhaps, dysplasia. Bacterial pathogens can also induce an inflammatory response, the products of which may be mutagenic and may contribute to dysplastic and neoplastic changes.

female ratios. In areas of the world where large-bowel cancers are infrequent, the disease usually manifests in the ascending (right-side segment) of the colon. In regions where the disease has a higher incidence, the cancer is often found in the descending (left-side segment) of the colon and in the rectosigmoid junction.[12] Rectal cancer—that is, cancer that is situated within 8 centimeters from the anus—appears to be different from either of the colon cancer presentations as far as risk factors are concerned.[12] The male-to-female incidence ratio of colon cancer is near unity, whereas it is approximately 1.5 for rectal cancer.[10] Rectal cancer is also more common in some populations at low risk for colon cancer, and alcohol intake appears to be a risk factor for rectal cancer, but not for colon cancer.[10] Because of these differences, and because there is significantly less contact with luminal and surface-associated bacteria in the rectum compared to the colon, the remainder of this chapter will consider only cancer of the colon.

Age-adjusted colon-cancer rates are generally higher in developed countries than in the developing world.[11] Incidence is high, with a rate of approximately 20 to 30 per 100,000, in the United States, Canada, Australia, and in western and northern Europe. There is a low incidence, ranging from 1 to 5 per 100,000, in Africa and the Indian subcontinent, as well as in many parts of China. In general, the global incidence of colon cancer is rising, although there are a few notable exceptions. Europe has seen a widespread increase in the incidence of colon cancer, more marked in eastern than in western countries. However, the incidence in some eastern European populations, such as in Romania and in rural areas of Poland, has remained low. Across Asia there is an order-of-magnitude difference in the incidence of colon cancer. The greatest increases have been in Japan, where low rates in the 1960s have given way to rates comparable to those in other developed countries. In Central and South America, the incidence of colon cancer is rising steadily in most populations. In the United States, there have been increases in most male populations, but increases have generally been less marked among females. Mortality is not rising as rapidly as incidence, and in some populations, such as the United States, Canada, Sweden, and the European Community, it is falling steadily.[10] Early detection seems to contribute, at least in part, to increasing incidence coupled with a general decline in mortality in the developed world.[13] However, variable trends, particularly among different ethnic groups in the same area, suggest that rising incidence rates are not exclusively an artifact of changes in diagnostic practices.[10]

Significant differences in the risk of developing colon cancer have also been noted in subpopulations exposed to the same gross environmental conditions. Seventh Day Adventists[14] and members of the Church of Latter Day Saints in the state of Utah[12,15] have a lower incidence of colon cancer when compared to the general population in North America. Furthermore, in low-risk population groups, colon cancer occurs more frequently in individuals who are in a higher socioeconomic class, and who eat a more Western (i.e., high fat, low fiber) diet.[16] Many studies have demonstrated that first-generation immigrants from parts of the world with low colon cancer incidence to regions with higher incidence rapidly acquire the increased risk associated with the place to which they migrate.[12,17–20]

Historically, the distinct differences in incidence and mortality as a function of geographic residence and of migration from a region of low risk to a region of higher risk led to the hypothesis that lifestyle was associated with disease incidence. In particular, it became apparent there was a marked difference in presumed dietary-fat intake between populations in Western countries and in Japan.[8,12,21] In Western countries with a high incidence of colon cancer, populations obtain 40% to 45% of their daily caloric intake from fat (both saturated and unsaturated), or about 130 to 150 grams of fat per day. In contrast, the traditional dietary fat intake in Japan accounts for 10% to 15% of calories, more of it being unsaturated because it is derived from fish oils.[12] The recent increase in colon cancer incidence in Japan is likely to be attributable to a change from the more traditional diet to a western diet.

An interesting exception to the higher rates in the West was observed in rural Finland, where the incidence of colon cancer was approximately the same as in populations consuming a traditional Japanese diet. In the Finnish population, total fat intake was similar to that found in other Western countries, and most of it was saturated fat, coming primarily from dairy products.[12] Reddy and colleagues have suggested that this exceptional situation could be accounted for by the fact that people in rural Finland consume a diet rich in fat, but also high in cereal fiber.[22] In addition, heavy consumption of dairy products may also result in higher intake of calcium, which has been shown to reduce the activity of bile salts.[12] In another noted exception, Mormons in Utah were found to have a typical American dietary pattern, but they also consumed cereal products and bread made from stone-ground grain with a high fiber content; the control U.S. population consumed baked goods made with more refined flours.[12] Seventh Day Adventists in the United States have a lower incidence of colon cancer than the general population, probably because, as vegetarians, they consume a diet low in fat and high in fiber. Thus, diet appears to have a major effect on colon cancer incidence. It appears to be the bacteria in the large intestine, however, that transform dietary fat and fiber into factors that influence colon cancer risk.

BILE ACIDS

The liver synthesizes two bile acids—cholic acid and chenodeoxycholic acid—which are secreted in the bile as glycine or taurine conjugates. Their function is to emulsify fat in the duodenum and to permit the digestion and absorption of fat from the small intestine. The conjugated bile acids are well ionized in the duodenum and are usually referred to as bile salts. Because of their hydrophilicity, they are not passively absorbed from the bowel but rather are actively transported from the terminal ileum. More than 95% of the bile acids are reabsorbed and return to the liver via the hepatic portal vein, resulting in efficient conservation by means of the enterohepatic circulation. The bile salts are then resecreted for a further enterohepatic cycle. The bile-salt pool undergoes six to 12 cycles per day; the number of cycles increases in parallel with dietary fat intake. The 2% to 5% of the bile acids that are not absorbed, which amounts to an average of 20% of the bile-acid pool per day, are lost from the small intestine and reach the colon, where they become substrates for bacterial metabolism. The colonic bacteria carry out two major reactions on the bile salts. First, free bile acids are released by deconjugation of the amino-acid molecule on the carboxyl group. The second major reaction is 7–dehydroxylation to yield deoxycholic and lithocholic acids from cholic and chenodeoxycholic acids, respectively. The free bile acids are poorly ionized and lipophilic. Deoxycholic acid is absorbed from the colon by passive diffusion to some degree, but lithocholic acid is almost insoluble and little is reabsorbed.

Bile acids were initially studied as potential carcinogens because of their structural similarity to polycyclic aromatic hydrocarbons.[8,21,23] Studies in the 1970s demonstrated that the secondary bile acids deoxycholic and lithocolic acid, but not the primary bile acids cholic and chenodeoxycholic acid, are potent tumor promoters in rodents.[24] That is, they increase the number and reduce the latency period of both preneoplastic and neoplastic lesions following a sub-threshold dose of an initiating carcinogen. Feeding high-fat diets also results in an increased fecal bile acid concentration and a higher tumor incidence. Animals on a diet in which 40% of calories derive from fat excrete approximately 12 milligrams of bile acids per gram of stool, compared to animals on a low-fat diet (with 10% of calories from fat), which excrete approximately 4 milligrams per gram of feces.[12] High concentrations of fecal bile acids cause colonic bacteria to produce larger amounts of 7-α-dehydroxylase, the enzyme involved in conversion of primary to secondary bile acids.[21] Thus, a high-fat diet enhances both the formation and the bacterial degradation of bile acids, which exert a promoting influence on colon tumors.

Human epidemiological evidence also suggests that diet is an important factor in colon carcinogenesis. Although numerous dietary components have been identified as potential carcinogens, secondary bile acids are perhaps most strongly implicated in the process.[25] Populations that have a high incidence of colon cancer and consume a high-fat diet excrete more secondary bile acids, and have higher fecal concentration of these compounds, than do control populations.[6,21,26] Although population studies show a consistent relationship between colon cancer and both dietary fat and fecal bile acid concentration, case-control studies are less convincing. Most case-control studies, however, suffer from a number of serious flaws. These flaws include the failure to exclude cases with hepatic metastasis, which may reduce bile-acid output; and the failure to match controls for symptoms and for hospitalization, both of which affect appetite and diet, and thus bile-acid output.[6]

The mechanism by which secondary bile acids promote tumor formation remains poorly defined. These agents can disrupt the integrity of the cell membrane of colonic mucosal cells and cause direct mucosal damage, as evidenced by changes in colonic histology. The resulting cell loss stimulates compensatory cell renewal, increasing the fraction of cells in S phase, and possibly increasing the number of target cells for spontaneous and induced mutations.[26] Alternatively, secondary bile acids may act by activating protein kinase C, a serine and threonine kinase that has been proposed to regulate cell proliferation and tumor promotion[27]. Protein kinase C is a calcium- and phospholipid-dependent enzyme. The endogenous ligand of protein kinase C is diacylglycerol. An important source of diacylglycerol is the hydrolysis of phosphatidylinositol-4,5-biphosphate by phopholipase C. Luminal bile acids in the colon may interact in the presence of bacterial phospholipase C to produce dicylglycerol.[28] Diacylglycerol is a potent tumor promoter in mouse skin[29] and may have similar activity in the colon. Diacylglycerol has been detected in normal human fecal samples, and is derived at least in part from the action of intestinal bacteria. It has also been suggested that deoxycholic acid may stimulate proliferation by triggering the local release of prostaglandin E_2 from colonic enterocytes.[26]

If secondary bile acids are involved in colon carcinogenesis, then several prevention strategies should be available. They include decreased dietary fat, increased cereal fiber, supplements of calcium, and supplements to acidify the colon.[6] The rationale for decreasing dietary fat is to decrease bile-acid secretion and subsequent loss from the ileum, thus decreasing the concentration of secondary bile acids in the colon.[6] Cereal fiber has proven stool-bulking properties, and may also decrease the concentration of colonic secondary bile acids.[6] Calcium supplements offset the tumor-promoting effects of bile acids, most likely by reducing the latter's solubility.[6] Acidification decreases bacterial dehydroxylation of bile acids, and also enhances the precipitation of the secondary bile acids that are formed. Usually, acidification can be achieved with a readily metabolizable carbohydrate, such as lactulose; however, this goal is typically incompatible with stool bulking.[6]

SHORT-CHAIN FATTY ACIDS

The bacteria in the colon, and the anaerobes in particular, are saccharolytic. They obtain their energy by fermenting carbohydrates that escape enzymatic digestion in the small intestine.[30] Most of this carbohydrate is dietary fiber in the form of nonstarch polysaccharides, but it also includes resistant starch, and endogenous polysaccharides from mucus and from shed epithelial cells.[31] The most important end products of bacterial carbohydrate breakdown are the short-chain fatty acids acetate, propionate, and butyrate.[31] Together, they are produced at a rate of at least 300 millimoles per day.[32] The ratio of fatty acid by-products is determined by the sugar composition of carbohydrate. Fermentation of xylose tends to yield butyrate, glucose yields propionate, and uronic acids produce acetic acids.[32] Butyrate is preferentially taken up by colonic epithelial cells, where it is actively metabolized to produce energy. It is an important energy source for the colonocytes, and it is metabolized in preference to glucose or glutamine.[32] Propionate and acetate are also rapidly taken up by these cells, but are translocated across the basolateral membrane into the portal hepatic circulation, where they may have effects distant from the site of their production.[31]

All three major short-chain fatty acids stimulate proliferation of normal colonic epithelium.[31] The proliferation is physiologic, in the sense that it is limited to the basal-crypt compartment and does not cause expansion of the proliferative zone—a change that is considered to be a preneoplastic biomarker.[31] Conversely, in colon-tumor cell lines, butyrate, and, to a lesser degree, propionate inhibit cell proliferation and induce a more differentiated phenotype.[32] Hyperproliferation in human colonic biopsies, induced in vitro by incubating specimens from the proximal colon or from the rectosigmoid colon with deoxycholic acid, is blocked by the addition of butyrate.[31] In vivo studies demonstrate that dietary-fiber supplementation leads to increased butyrate levels, which are associated with reduced colonic proliferation and lowered tumor mass in rats after treatment with the carcinogen dimethylhydrazine.[32] Thus, the balance of protective factors such as short-chain fatty acids and of detrimental factors such as secondary bile acids may determine carcinogenic outcome in the human large bowel.[31]

In a self-renewing tissue such as the colonic epithelium, the regulation of cell number must be strictly controlled to ensure that the rate of new cell production balances the rate at which cells undergo growth arrest, apoptosis, or exfoliation (see Chapter 3). Butyrate induces apoptosis in colon-tumor cell lines, although some cell lines are relatively more resistant.[32] The mechanism by which butyrate induces apoptosis is unclear, but it has been proposed that hyperacetylation of histones, and the resulting changes in chromatin structure, may lead to altered gene expression and to modification of the accessibility of the chromatin to DNases.[32] Butyrate also targets the cytoskeleton, modifying microfilament and microtubule assembly.[32] Propionate can also induce apoptosis, although it is less effective than butyrate.[32] Acetate is the least effective fatty acid, but it does induce apoptosis at concentrations of 40 millimoles per liter. In the colon, typical molar ratios of acetate:propionate:butyrate are 57:22:21, and the concentration of acetate in the colonic contents may reach 60 millimoles per liter; therefore, the concentrations of acetate required for apoptosis may be physiologic.[32]

ACTIVATION OF PROCARCINOGENS

Hepatic metabolism is generally oxidative, often involving the activation of compounds by the addition of molecular oxygen. Metabolism by the colonic microflora is generally reductive, often using the same compounds as terminal electron acceptors. In addition, while the liver is actively conjugating compounds to molecules such as glucuronic acid and sulfate, the bacteria in the colon efficiently deconjugate these compounds as soon as the compounds reach the colon via the bile. Thus, from a chemical perspective, the colonic microflora tend to reverse the metabolism of the liver, often resulting in reabsorption of compounds that were originally directed toward excretion. Consequently, we must always consider the colonic microflora when we study "host" metabolism of endogenous or exogenous compounds—particularly those compounds that may cause human cancers.[33]

Although there is no direct evidence that colonic bacteria cause colon cancer in humans, data do show that the intestinal microflora can perform reactions that generate carcinogens.[9] A good example of the carcinogenic potential of colonic bacterial enzymes relates to the naturally occurring compound cycasin, which is found in the seed and the root of cycad plants, such as the tropical fern.[8,9,21] When cycasin is fed to normal rats, the animals develop colon tumors; however, the compound is completely inactive when given orally to germ-free rats.[8,9,21,34] Cycasin is a glycoside, and bacteria perform hydrolysis of its β-glycosidin linkage to obtain the sugar for energy. The aglycone methylazoxymethanol, which is the active carcinogen, is coincidentally released.[9] This type of hydrolysis is one of the best-known examples of bacterial activation of procarcinogens.[9,21]

Other hydrolysis reactions involve a variety of glycosidases, the most important of which appear to be β-glucuronidase and β-glucosidase.[9,21,33] Glycosides enter the gut primarily from the diet, largely as plant flavanoids, and from the liver, as compounds that have been detoxified by glucuronide formation and subsequently secreted into the bowel via the bile.[9,21] On a per-cell basis, *Escherichia coli* and *Clostridium* species have the highest β-glucuronidase activity, whereas *Lactobacillus* and *Bifidobacterium* species have the lowest.[9,21] For β-glucosidase, *E. coli* has the lowest activity and *Bacteroides* species and *Streptococcus faecalis* have the highest.[9] Bacterial β-glucuronidase seems to play an important role in the activation of procarcinogens. This enzyme has a wide substrate specificity and can consequently hydrolyze many different glucuronides.[21] Although variations in diet appear to exert little effect on the bacterial composition in the colon, the metabolic activities of the microflora have been shown to be labile and to be influenced greatly by dietary factors.[9] β-glucuronidase activity has been studied in volunteers on high-animal-fat and on nonmeat diets. Higher fecal enzyme activity was noted in subjects on the high-animal-fat diet,[35] and a shift from a high-animal-fat diet to a nonmeat diet was associated with a decrease in fecal β-glucuronidase activity.[9]

Bacterial nitroreductase and azoreductase are responsible for reducing aromatic nitro and azo compounds to aromatic amines. These latter compounds are mutagens, especially following hepatic microsomal activation.[30] Reduction of aromatic nitro groups is a complex reaction that involves the addition of six electrons. The intermediates include a nitro free radical, a nitroso group, and an N-hydroxy group, all of which have been implicated as genotoxic compounds.[9] Bacteria can also add a nitroso group to secondary amines, producing carcinogenic nitrosamines, which have been detected in human bowel contents.[36] Bacteria can use nitrite, produced through the reduction of dietary nitrate by many common microbial species, as the nitrosating agent in this reaction.[9] Most of the artificial coloring additives used in the food, printing, and textile industries are dyes that contain a single azo bond.[9,21] These water-soluble dyes are not absorbed well from the intestine and are subject to bacterial action in the colon.[21] Bacterial microflora can reductively hydrolyze the azo bond to form substituted aromatic amines, a group of compounds that also are well-established carcinogens.[9,21]

Several chemicals have been isolated from fried or broiled proteinaceous foods that belong to a novel class of heterocyclic amines. These chemicals include 2-amino-3-methylimidazo-(4,5-*f*)quinoline (IQ), 2-amino-3,4-dimethylimidazo(4,5-*f*)quinoline (MeIQ), 2-amino-3,8-dimethylimidazo(4,5-*f*)quinoxaline (MeIQx), and 2-amino-1-methyl-6-phenylimidazo (4,5-*b*)pyridine (PhIP). Normally, these compounds require activation in the liver before becoming potent mutagens or carcinogens. However, the IQ subclass (e.g., IQ and MeIQ) can be activated in the colon by *Eubacterium* and *Clostridium* species via anaerobic hydration–dehydgrogenation at position 7 of IQ, yielding 7-hydroxy-IQ, which is directly mutagenic in bacterial mutagen assays.[33]

Another class of potent, direct-acting genotoxins that is detected in the feces of most persons consuming normal Western diets is the fecapentaenes. These compounds are highly sensitive to oxidation. In fact, they are inactivated by liver microsomal preparations normally added to bacterial mutagen assays to activate compounds by oxidation.[9,21] The structures of the fecal mutagens were first described in 1982,[37] and were confirmed independently the following year.[38] The compounds—(S)-3–(1,3,5,7,9-dodecapentaenyloxy)-1,2-propanediol and the corresponding tetradeca homologue—are called fecapentaene-12 and fecapentaene-14, respectively.[9] Feces contain up to several milligrams of fecapentaenes per kilogram, and the compounds are stable under strict anaerobic conditions.[21] They are produced in the colon by *Bacteroides* species from polyunsaturated ether phospholipids known as plasmalopentaenes. The biological role of the precursor molecules is not known, but it has been suggested that they could function as antioxidants.[33] Although there is no direct evidence that the fecapentaenes or the 7-hydroxy "IQ" compounds influence colon cancer risk, the potency and the prevalence of these bacterial metabolites is a cause for concern.[33]

If some bacterial enzymes do contribute to the risk of human colon cancer, then suppressing these activities may decrease the production of tumor promoters and decrease the activation of procarcinogens.[39] Dietary intake of fermented milk containing *Lactobacillus acidophillus* has been shown to reduce the counts of putrefactive bacteria such as coliforms and to increase the counts of Lactobacilli in the intestine.[39] Several lines of evidence support the tumor-inhibitory properties of lactic acid bacteria. *Lactobacillus* species produce antitumor substances that have been shown to be components of the bacterial cell wall.[40] There is also epidemiological evidence that rural Finns, who are among the highest consumers of dairy products and who have a decreased colon cancer incidence, have increased counts of fecal *Lactobacillus* species.[41] Recent studies have shown that feeding a particular strain of *Lactobacillus casei* before and during carcinogen treatment leads to a significant reduction in colon tumor incidence and a 65% reduction in colon tumor burden in dimethylhydrazine-treated rats on a 20% corn oil diet.[42] Even when fed to rats on a low corn oil diet, which yields half as many tumors, the *L. casei* strain caused a 48% reduction in tumor burden compared to control animals. This finding suggests that lactic acid bacteria may act independent of secondary bile acids, although the exact mechanism remains unclear.

PATHOGENIC BACTERIA AND EPITHELIAL CELL PROLIFERATION

Alterations in the cytokinetics of the colonic epithelium occur in familial adenomatous polyposis,[43,44] in individuals who have had sporadic adenomas[44,45] or colon cancers,[44–46] and in patients with idiopathic inflammatory bowel disease.[47,48] All these diseases are associated with an increased frequency of colon cancer. The grossly normal-appearing mucosa of these patients has increased epithelial cell proliferation. The hyperproliferation is associated with the presence of dividing cells in the upper third of the crypts, which are not observed in the mucosa of normal subjects.[49] Similar exaggerated epithelial proliferation with expansion of the proliferative compartment occurs in the colon of laboratory mice infected with the pathogenic bacterium *Citrobacter rodentium*.[50]

Infection of laboratory mice with *C. rodentium*—previously designated *C. freundii* biotype 4280[51] but now recognized to be a separate *Citrobacter* species[52]—causes transmissible murine colonic hyperplasia. The disease is characterized by a self-limiting hyperproliferative state in the descending colon, secondary inflammation, rectal prolapse, and variable mortality.[53] The hyperplastic state promotes chemically induced colon tumors.[54] A 70% incidence of early neoplastic lesions after dimethylhydrazine administration is observed in uninfected mice after 3 months of treatment; infected animals have comparable incidence and severity of lesions after only 1 month of treatment.[54] There is no evidence that infected mice develop tumors in the absence of carcinogen treatment.

Following oral inoculation of laboratory mice with *C. rodentium*, bacteria are first observed attaching to colonic enterocytes between 2 and 4 days after inoculation.[55] The number of *C. rodentium* organisms increases to reach maximal density between 7 and 10 days after inoculation.[56] Maximal mucosal hyperplasia, on the other hand, occurs approximately 2 weeks after inoculation.[55] By this time, the number of *C. rodentium* organisms in the colon is decreasing. Between 4 and 6 weeks after inoculation, the organism is no longer present in the colon.[56] Interestingly, studies with oral neomycin sulfate have shown that treatment on the second day after inoculation results in eradication of the organism but does not prevent the induction of colonic hyperplasia.[56] The duration of infection between 2 and 10 days after inoculation does correlate with the degree of hyperproliferation, however. In the absence of treatment, the hyperplasia gradually regresses and eventually resolves approximately 45 days after inoculation.[56]

The mechanism by which *C. rodentium* induces mucosal hyperplasia is not fully understood. Bacterial attachment is associated with intimate contact between the bacteria and the apical surface of the colonic enterocytes, cytoskeletal rearrangements within the epithelial cells, and dissolution of the microvillus brush border.[55,57] These changes have been called attaching and effacing lesions,[58] and are characteristic of human enteropathogenic *E. coli* and enterohemorrhagic *E. coli* infections. The bacterial genes necessary for formation of attaching and effacing lesions are present on a pathogenicity island of chromosomal DNA, approximately 35 kilobases in length.[59] The genes on the pathogenicity island code for an outer membrane adherence protein called intimin,[60] a specialized type III secretion system,[61] and several secreted proteins.[62] It appears that export of these bacterial products leads to tyrosine phosphorylation of host-cell proteins[63] and to the mobilization of intracellular free calcium.[64] The exact relationship between these signal-transduction events and induction of a hyperproliferative state remains to be determined.

Savidge and associates have characterized the cytokinetics in the small-intestine mucosa of five children with enteropathogenic *E. coli* infection.[65] Compared to those of controls, crypts from infected children were 1.6 times longer and had 2.2 times greater labeling index. These changes are comparable to those in the colonic mucosa of *C. rodentium*–infected mice, which exhibit 2.0 times longer crypts with 1.6 times greater labeling index in moderate cases and up to 2.7 times longer crypts with 2.2 times greater labeling index in severe cases.[50] Despite the fact that different methods were used to label proliferating cells in the *E. coli* study and the *Citrobacter* study, the alterations are remarkably similar. Perhaps even more telling is that other disease states in the small intestine of children that were found to be associated with crypt elongation and increased labeling index, including celiac disease and giardiasis, do not significantly expand the proliferative compartment.[65] That is to say, labeled cells are not found outside of the lower third of the crypt, which is the normal proliferative zone. Expansion of the proliferative compartment, as seen in enteropathogenic *E. coli* infection and in *C. rodentium* infection in mice, may be a better marker for colon cancer risk than hyperproliferation that remains confined to the normal proliferative zone. Questions remain about the extent to which enteropathogenic *E. coli* colonize the large intestine, and whether enterohemorrhagic *E. coli*, which does colonize the ascending colon, can cause similar alterations of epithelial cytokinetics. It may be that infection with certain bacteria results in expansion of the prolifera-

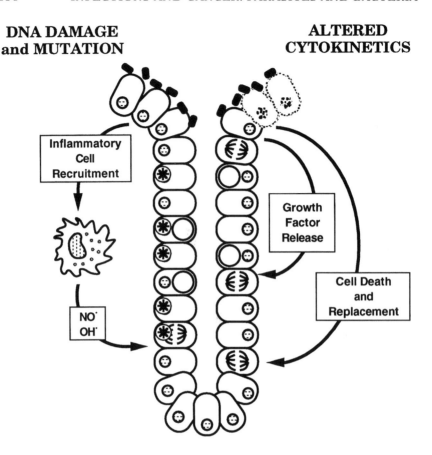

Figure 16.2. Possible mechanisms by which pathogenic bacteria contribute to the development of colon cancer. Bacterial interaction with epithelial cells may lead to the recruitment and activation of inflammatory cells, which in turn release mutagenic products, including nitric oxide (NO·) and hydroxyl radical (OH·). These products may damage epithelial cell DNA and lead to mutation (✻). Bacterial interaction with epithelial cells may also result in cell death and compensatory renewal or cellular release of growth factors, resulting in hyperproliferation and expansion of the proliferative zone. These changes may provide a promoting effect on colon cancer development. Infection with a given bacterial pathogen may be associated with genotoxicity, or altered cytokinetics, or both.

tive compartment, thus increasing the risk of colon cancer (see Figure 16.2). Other pathogens may be associated with increased mitotic activity in response to the loss of surface colonocytes, but without expansion of the proliferative compartment; this may have little or no effect on colon cancer risk.

Expansion of the proliferative compartment and increased colon cancer risk have been documented in a few other hyperplastic conditions associated with bacterial infection. In a report by Williams and colleagues, the aromatic-amine carcinogen 3,2'-dimethyl-4-aminobiphenyl (DMAB) was administered to Syrian hamsters.[66] Previous studies had demonstrated that this carcinogen causes urinary bladder tumors but not colon tumors in hamsters (although it does cause colon tumors, as well as urinary bladder tumors, in rats). The presence of atypical proliferative enterocolitis in the hamsters enhanced the carcinogenic effect of the chemical and led to the development of tumors in the small intestine and in the colon.[66] The causative agent of the hyperproliferation was not determined. Perhaps the most common cause of proliferative enteritis in hamsters is infection with *Lawsonia intracellularis.*[67] This obligate intracellular bacterial pathogen has been previously referred to as an intracellular *Campybylobacter*-like organism (ICLO), but taxonomic studies indicate that the organism is related to members of the *Desulfovibrio* genus.[68] *L. intracellularis*-infected hamsters exhibit mucosal hyperplasia, often associated with goblet cell loss. The DMAB-treated hamsters had increased numbers of goblet cells in association with mucosal hyperplasia. These changes are probably more consistent with chronic *Clostridium difficile* infection.[69] However, the presence of *L. intracellularis* and/or *C. difficile* was not documented. The mechanisms by which *L. intracellularis* or *C. difficile* induce mucosal hyperplasia are not fully understood. The pathogenesis of these conditions are likely to be distinct, given that the former is an intracellular parasite of enterocytes and the latter is an extracellular toxin-producing organism. In any case, it is apparent that diverse bacterial species can cause colonic epithelial hyperplasia that may, in turn, increase the incidence of neoplastic disease.

PATHOGENIC BACTERIA AND MUCOSAL INFLAMMATION

An important feature of active inflammatory bowel disease—a condition known to increase the risk of colon cancer—is the presence of activated inflammatory cells in the bowel. Oxygen free radicals produced by macrophages and neutrophils may cause mutations in epithelial cells by multiple mechanisms (see Figure 16.2 and Chapter 2).[70] Investigators are also considering the possibility that nitric-oxide synthesis by these same professional phagocytes may produce somatic mutations by the reaction of nitrogen oxides with amines to produce carcinogenic nitrosamines.[71] Nitrite formation and activated inflammatory cells were originally associated because of the observation that when *E. coli* lipopolysaccharide is injected into rats, urinary excretion of nitrite and nitrate increases 10-fold.[72] The source of nitrite was shown to be activated macrophages,[73] which produce nitric oxide by inducible nitric oxide synthase.[74] There is good evidence that nitrite is produced during active—but not during quiescent—inflammatory bowel disease by inflammatory cells in the lamina propria, perhaps leading to the formation of N-nitroso compounds and nitrosamines.[71,71a]

There is also abundant evidence that pathogenic bacteria can elicit an inflammatory response in the colon. Some of the better known causes of infectious colitis include *Shigella* species and enteroinvasive *E. coli*, *Campylobacter* species, and *C. difficile* (pseudomembranous colitis). It seems plausible that chronic infection could contribute to the risk of colon cancer. Indeed, the chronic inflammatory state induced by administration of dextran sulfate sodium to hamsters for 180 days results in the development of tumors.[75] However, a complicating factor is that chronic inflammation in the colon often is associated with epithelial hyperplasia. For example, administration of degraded carrageenan in the drinking water of rats induces colitis, but also increases the labeling index of epithelial cells in the proximal and distal colon almost two-fold.[76] Thus, the independent contributions of inflammation and hyperplasia to malignant transformation are hard to delimit. It is interesting, however, that nonsteroidal anti-inflammatory drugs are negatively associated with colon cancer risk in people,[77,78] and are able to reduce the frequency of premalignant and malignant lesions in chemically induced rodent colon cancer models.[79] Further studies are under way to dissect the independent role of inflammation in the pathogenesis of colon cancer.

SUMMARY

Colon cancer is a multifactorial disease, involving both genetic and environmental factors. Epidemiological studies, intervention studies, clinical studies, and studies with animal models suggest that bacteria may play a role in colon cancer, but so far definitive proof is lacking. The consequences of interactions between the host and bacteria (both normal microflora and pathogens) are also complex, and involve both genetic and environmental factors. Bacteria rarely affect a single aspect of host biology; instead, they can alter histology, cell kinetics, cell metabolism, immune response, and so on. The most obvious changes may not be the most relevant for cancer risk. An example of this complexity is the set of changes that occurs in human inflammatory bowel disease. Chronic inflammatory bowel disease in the colon is known to increase the risk of colon cancer.[80] The etiology of inflammatory bowel disease is unknown, and remains controversial. Some investigators have postulated that the condition is caused by a specific microbial pathogen: others believe that it is an inappropriate reaction to ubiquitous luminal antigens. Although colon cancer in patients with inflammatory bowel disease accounts for a small percentage of the total number of cases of this malignancy, the pathophysiology of this disease provides insight into the mechanisms by which bacterial infection might lead to colon cancer.

Patients who have inflammatory bowel disease with total colonic involvement for more than 10 years were examined for fecal bile-acid concentrations.[6] Increased fecal bile-acid concentration correlates with increased severity of epithelial dysplasia. It also correlates with the presence of larger adenomas, suggesting that secondary bile acids may be involved in adenoma growth, but perhaps not in adenoma formation.[6] Epithelial-cell proliferation in inflammatory bowel disease is abnormal, the pattern being similar to that found in other premalignant states: expansion of the proliferative compartment and proliferation of surface epithelial cells. These abnormalities persist even when the disease is under good clinical control and the mucosa is minimally inflamed.[81] Active inflammatory bowel disease is associated with increased rectal nitrite levels, suggesting enhanced production of nitric oxide and formation of N-nitroso compounds.[71] Any and all of these effects, which have also been observed with bacterial infection, may contribute to colon cancer risk in chronic inflammatory bowel disease.

The complex environment of the human colon contains a multitude of factors that have the potential to affect cancer development. Perhaps no factors are more influential than the resident bacterial microflora in health, and infectious bacterial pathogens in disease (see Figure 16.1). By various stratagems, bacteria alter exogenous and endogenous compounds. They directly and indirectly modulate epithelial-cell growth, cell death, and genotoxicity. These activities would appear to be intimately related to colon cancer risk, but conclusive evidence will come from additional laboratory and epidemiological studies.

Acknowledgements

Research in my laboratory is funded by grants CA63112 and DK52413 from the National Institutes of Health.

REFERENCES

1. Fearon ER, Vogelstein B. A genetic model for colorectal tumorigenesis. Cell 1990;61:759–767.
2. Miyoshi Y, Ando H, Nagase H, et al. Germ-line mutations of the *APC* gene in 53 familial adenomatous polyposis patients. Proc Natl Acad Sci USA 1992;89: 4452–4456.
3. Fishel R, Lescoe MK, Rao MRS, et al. The human mutator gene homolog MSH2 and its association with hereditary nonpolyposis colon cancer. Cell 1993;75:1027–1038.
4. Leach FS, Nicolaides NC, Papadopoulos N, et al. Mutations of a *mutS* homolog in hereditary nonpolyposis colorectal cancer. Cell 1993;75:1215–1225.
5. Rossi SC, Srivastava S. National Cancer Institute workshop on genetic screening for colorectal cancer. J Natl Cancer Inst 1996;88:331–339.
6. Hill MJ. Bile flow and colon cancer. Mutat Res 1990;238:313–320.
7. Aries C, Crowther JS, Drasar BS, Hill MJ. Degradation of bile salts by human intestinal bacteria. Gut 1969;10:575–577.
8. Simon GL, Gorbach SL. The human intestinal microflora. Dig Dis Sci 1986; 31:147S–62S.

9. Goldin BR. In situ bacterial metabolism and colon mutagens. Ann Rev Microbiol 1986;40:367–393.

10. International Agency for Research on Cancer. Cancer Incidence in Five Continents. Volume VI. Lyon: International Agency for Research on Cancer; 1992.

11. International Agency for Research on Cancer. Trends in Cancer Incidence and Mortality. Lyon: International Agency for Research on Cancer; 1993.

12. Weisburger JH, Horn CL. Human and laboratory studies on the causes and prevention of gastrointestinal cancer. Scand J Gastroenterol 1984;19(suppl 104):15–26.

13. Bonneux J, Barendregt JJ, Looman CWN, van der Maas PJ. Diverging trends in colorectal cancer morbidity and mortality: earlier diagnosis comes at a price. Eur J Cancer 1995;31A:1665–1671.

14. Phillips RL, Garfinkel L, Kuzma JW, Beeson WL, Lutz T, Burton B. Mortality among California Seventh-Day Adventists for selected cancer. J Natl Cancer Inst 1980;65:1097–1107.

15. Enstrom JE. Cancer risk among Mormons in California during 1968–75. J Natl Cancer Inst 1980;65:1073–1082.

16. Wynder EL. The epidemiology of large bowel cancer. Cancer Res 1975;35:3388–3394.

17. Staszewski J, Haenszel J. Cancer mortality among the Polish-born in the United States. J Natl Cancer Inst 1965;35:291–297.

18. Haenszel W, Kurihara M. Studies of Japanese migrants. I. Mortality from cancer and other diseases among Japanese in the United States. J Natl Cancer Inst 1968;40:43–68.

19. McMichael AJ, Giles GG. Cancer in migrants to Australia: extending the descriptive epidemiological data. Cancer Res 1988;48:751–756.

20. Grulich AE, McCredie M, Coates M. Cancer incidence in Asian migrants to New South Wales, Australia. Br J Cancer 1995;71:400–408.

21. Gorbach SL, Goldin BR. The intestinal microflora and the colon cancer connection. Rev Infect Dis 1990;12(suppl 2):S252–S261.

22. Reddy BS, Cohen LA, McCoy D, Hill P, Weisburger JH, Wynder EL. Nutrition and its relationship to cancer. Adv Cancer Res 1980;32:237–345.

23. Kay RM. Effects of diet on the fecal excretion and bacterial modification of acidic and neutral steroids, and implications for colon carcinogenesis. Cancer Res 1981;42:774–777.

24. Narisawa T, Magadia N, Weisburger J, Wynder EL. Promoting effect of bile acids on colon carcinogenesis after intrarectal instillation of N-methyl-N'-nitro-N-nitrosoguanidine in rats. J Natl Cancer Inst 1974;53:1093–1097.

25. Garewal H, Bernstein H, Bernstein C, Sampliner R, Payne C. Reduced bile acid-induced apoptosis in "normal" colorectal mucosa: a potential biological marker for cancer risk. Cancer Res 1996;56:1480–1483.

26. Nagengast FM, Grubben MJAL, van Munster IP. Role of bile acids in colorectal carcinogenesis. Eur J Cancer 1995;31A:1067–1070.

27. Steinbach G, Morotomi M, Nomoto K, Lupton J, Weinstein IB, Holt PR. Calcium reduces the increased fecal 1,2–sn-diacylglycerol content in intestinal bypass patients: a possible mechanism for altering colonic hyperproliferation. Cancer Res 1994;54:1216–1219.

28. Morotomi M, Guillem JG, LoGerfo P, Weinstein IB. Production of diacylglycerol, an activator of protein kinase C, by human intestinal microflora. Cancer Res 1990;50:3595–3599.

29. Yuspa SH, Poirier MC. Chemical carcinogenesis: from animal models to molecular models in one decade. Adv Cancer Res 1988;50:25–70.

30. Roberton AM. Roles of endogenous substances and bacteria in colorectal cancer. Mutat Res 1993;290:71–78.

31. Scheppach W, Bartram HP, Richter F. Role of short-chain fatty acids in the prevention of colorectal cancer. Eur J Cancer 1995;31A:1077–1080.

32. Hague A, Elder DJE, Hicks DJ, Paraskeva C. Apoptosis in colorectal tumor cells: induction by the short chain fatty acids butyrate, propionate and acetate and by the bile salt deoxycholate. Int J Cancer 1995;60:400–406.

33. Van Tassell RL, Kingston DGI, Wilkins TD. Metabolism of dietary genotoxins by the human colonic microflora; the fecapentaenes and heterocyclic amines. Mutat Res 1990;238:209–221.

34. Laqueur GL, McDaniel EG, Matsumoto H. Tumor induction in germfree rats with methylazoxymethanol (MAM) and synthetic MAM acetate. J Natl Cancer Inst 1967;39:355–371.

35. Reddy BS, Weisburger JH, Wynder EL. Fecal bacterial β-glucuronidase control by diet. Science 1974;183:416–417.

36. Thompson M. Aetiological factors in gastrointestinal carcinogenesis. Scand J Gastroenterol 1984;19(suppl 104):77–89.

37. Hirai N, Kingston DGI, Tassell RLV, Wilkins TD. Structure elucidation of a potent mutagen from human feces. J Amer Chem Soc 1982;104:6149–6150.

38. Gupta I, Baptista J, Bruce WR, et al. Structures of fecapentaenes, the mutagens of bacterial origin isolated from human feces. Biochemistry 1983;22:214–245.

39. Rafter JJ. The role of lactic acid bacteria in colon cancer prevention. Scand J Gastroenterol 1995;30:497–502.

40. Sekine K, Toida T, Saito M, Kuboyama M, Kawashima T, Hashimoto Y. A new morphologically characterized cell wall preparation (whole peptidoglycan) from Bifidobacterium infantis with a higher efficiency on the regression of an established tumor in mice. Cancer Res 1985;45:1300–1307.

41. International Agency for Research on Cancer, Intestinal Microecology Group. Dietary fibre, transit time, faecal bacteria, steroid, and colon cancer in two Scandinavian populations. Lancet 1977;2:207–211.

42. Goldin BR, Gualtieri LJ, Moore RP. The effect of Lactobacillus GG on the initiation and promotion of DMH-induced intestinal tumors in the rat. Nutr Cancer 1996;25:197–204.

43. Lipkin M. Phase 1 and phase 2 proliferative lesions of colonic epithelial cells in diseases leading to colon cancer. Cancer 1974;34:878–888.

44. Lipkin M, Blattner WA, Gardner EJ, et al. Classification and risk assessment of individuals with familial polyposis, Gardner syndrome and familial nonpolyposis colon cancer from [³H]dThd-labeling patterns in colonic epithelial cells. Cancer Res 1984;44:4201–4207.

45. Maskens AP, Deschner EE. Tritiated thymidine incorporation into epithelial cells of normal-appearing colorectal mucosa of cancer patients. J Natl Cancer Inst 1977;58:1221–1224.

46. Romagnoli P, Filipponi F, Bandettini L, Brugnola D. Increase of mitotic activity in the colonic mucosa of patients with colorectal cancer. Dis Colon Rectum 1984;27:305–308.

47. Biasco G, Lipkin M, Minarini A, Higgins P, Miglioli M, Luigi B. Proliferative and antigenic properties of the rectal cells in patients with chronic ulcerative colitis. Cancer Res 1984;44:5450–5454.

48. Deschner EE, Winawer SJ, Katz S, Kahn E. Proliferative defects in ulcerative colitis patients. Cancer Invest 1983;1:41–47.

49. Deschner EE. Cell proliferation and colonic neoplasia. Scand J Gastroenterol 1988;23(suppl 151):94–97.

50. Barthold SW. Autoradiographic cytokinetics of colonic mucosal hyperplasia in mice. Cancer Res 1979;39:24–29.

51. Barthold SW, Coleman GL, Bhatt PN, Osbaldiston GW, Jonas AM. The etiology of transmissible murine colonic hyperplasia. Lab Anim Sci 1976;26:889–894.

52. Schauer DB, Zabel BA, Pedraza IF, O'Hara CM, Steigerwalt AG, Brenner DJ. Genetic and biochemical characterization of *Citrobacter rodentium* sp. nov. J Clin Microbiol 1995;33:2064–2068.

53. Barthold SW, Coleman GL, Jacoby RO, Livstone EM, Jonas AM. Transmissible murine colonic hyperplasia. Vet Pathol 1978;15:223–236.

54. Barthold SW, Jonas AM. Morphogenesis of early 1,2–dimethylhydrazine-induced lesions and latent period reduction of colon carcinogenesis in mice by a variant of *Citrobacter freundii*. Cancer Res 1977;37:4352–4360.

55. Johnson E, Barthold SW. The ultrastructure of transmissible murine colonic hyperplasia. Am J Pathol 1979;97:291–314.

56. Barthold SW. The microbiology of transmissible murine colonic hyperplasia. Lab Anim Sci 1980;30:167–173.

57. Schauer DB, Falkow S. Attaching and effacing locus of a *Citrobacter freundii* biotype that causes transmissible murine colonic hyperplasia. Infect Immun 1993;61:2486–2492.

58. Moon HW, Whipp SC, Argenzio RA, Levine MM, Giannella RA. Attaching and effacing activities of rabbit and human enteropathogenic *Escherichia coli* in pig and rabbit intestines. Infect Immun 1983;41:1340–1351.

59. McDaniel TK, Jarvis KG, Donnenberg MS, Kaper JB. A genetic locus of enterocyte effacement conserved among diverse enterobacterial pathogens. Proc Natl Acad Sci USA 1995;92:1664–1668.

60. Jerse AE, Yu J, Tall BD, Kaper JB. A genetic locus of enteropathogenic *Escherichia coli* necessary for the production of attaching and effacing lesions on tissue culture cells. Proc Natl Acad Sci USA 1990;87:7839–7843.

61. Jarvis KG, Girón JA, Jerse AE, McDaniel TK, Donnenberg MS, Kaper JB. Enteropathogenic *Escherichia coli* contains a specialized secretion system necessary for the export of proteins involved in attaching and effacing lesion formation. Proc Natl Acad Sci USA 1995;92:7996–8000.

62. Kenny B, Finley BB. Protein secretion by enteropathogenic *Escherichia coli* is essential for transducing signals to epithelial cells. Proc Natl Acad Sci USA 1995;92:7991–7995.

63. Rosenshine I, Donnenberg MS, Kaper JB, Finlay BB. Signal transduction between enteropathogenic *Escherichia coli* (EPEC) and epithelial cells: EPEC induces tyrosine phosphorylation of host cell proteins to initiate cytoskeletal rearrangement and bacterial uptake. EMBO J 1992;11:3551–3560.

64. Baldwin TJ, Ward W, Aitken A, Knutton S, Williams PH. Elevation of intracellular free calcium levels in HEp-2 cells infected with enteropathogenic *Escherichia coli*. Infect Immun 1991;59:1599–604.

65. Savidge TC, Shmakov AN, Walker-Smith JA, Phillips AD. Epithelial cell proliferation in childhood enteropathies. Gut 1996;39:185–93.

66. Williams GM, Chandrasekaran V, Katayama S, Weisburger JH. Carcinogen-

icity of 3-methyl-2-naphthylamine and 3,2′-dimethyl-4-aminobiphenyl to the bladder and gastrointestinal tract of the Syrian golden hamster with atypical proliferative enteritis. J Natl Cancer Inst 1981;67:481–488.

67. McOrist S, Gebhart CJ, Boid R, Barns SM. Characterization of *Lawsonia intracellularis* gen. nov., sp. nov., the obligately intracellular bacterium of porcine proliferative enteropathy. Int J Syst Bacteriol 1995;45:820–825.

68. Fox JG, Dewhirst FE, Fraser GJ, Paster BJ, Shames B, Murphy JC. Intracellular *Campylobacter*-like organism from ferrets and hamsters with proliferative bowel disease is a *Desulfovibrio* sp. J Clin Microbiol 1994;32:1229–1237.

69. Ryden EB, Lipman NS, Taylor NS, Rose R, Fox JG. *Clostridium difficile* typhlitis associated with cecal mucosal hyperplasia in Syrian hamsters. Lab Anim Sci 1991;41:553–558.

70. Cheng KC, Cahill DS, Kasai H, Nishimura S, Loeb L. 8-hydroxy-guanine, an abundant form of oxidative DNA damage, causes G→T and A→C substitutions. J Biol Chem 1992;267:166–172.

71. Roediger WEW, Lawson MJ, Radcliffe BC. Nitrite from inflammatory cells—a cancer risk factor in ulcerative colitis? Dis Colon Rectum 1990;33:1034–1036.

71a. Singer II, Kawka DW, Scott S, Weidner JR, Mumford RA, Riehl TE, Stenson WF. Expression of inducible nitric oxide synthase and nitrotyrosine in colonic epithelium in inflammatory bowel disease. Gastroenterology 1996;111;871-885.

72. Wagner DA, Young VR, Tannenbaum SR. Mammalian nitrate biosynthesis: incorporation of $^{15}NH_3$ into nitrate is enhanced by endotoxin treatment. Proc Natl Acad Sci USA 1983;80:4518–4521.

73. Hibbs JB, Taintor RR, Vavrin Z. Macrophage cytotoxicity: role for L-arginine deiminase and imino nitrogen oxidation to nitrite. Science 1987;235:473–476.

74. Marletta MA, Yoon PS, Iyengar R, Leaf CD, Wishnok JS. Macrophage oxidation of L-arginine to nitrite and nitrate: nitric oxide is an intermediate. Biochemistry 1988;27:8706–8711.

75. Yamada M, Ohkusa T, Okayasu I. Occurrence of dysplasia and adenocarcinoma after experimental chronic ulcrative colitis in hamsters induced by dextran sulphate sodium. Gut 1992;33:1521–1527.

76. Deschner EE. Cell turnover and colon tumor development. Prev Med 1987;16:580–585.

77. Greenberg ER, Baron JA, Jr. DHF, Mandel JS, Haile R. Reduced risk of large-bowel cancer among aspirin users. J Natl Cancer Inst 1993;85:912–916.

78. Giovannucci E, Rimm EB, Stampfer MJ, Colditz GA, Ascherio A, Willett WC. Aspirin use and the risk for colorectal cancer and adenoma in male health professionals. Ann Intern Med 1994;121:241–264.

79. Eberhart CE, Dubois RN. Eicosanoids and the gastrointestinal tract. Gastroenterology 1995;109:285–301.

80. Levin B. Inflammatory bowel disease and colon cancer. Cancer 1992;70:1313–1316.

81. Serafine EP, Kirk AP, Chambers TJ. Rate and pattern of epithelial cell proliferation in ulcerative colitis. Gut 1981;22:648–652.

INDEX

acetaldehyde as biomarker in alcoholic hepatitis, 63

acetate production by colonic bacteria, 430–431

acetylkynurenine as bladder carcinogen, 332

N-acetyl-L-cysteine (NAC), glutathione-level control by, 67, 69

acidic fibroblast growth factor (aFGF), expression in Kaposi's sarcoma, 221

aconitase, inactivation of, 46

acyclovir, 223

adenomatous polyps
  cell proliferation in, 95
  DNA replication in, 92

adenovirus(es)
  cyclin interaction with oncoprotein of, 120
  E1B of, 168–169
  role in respiratory illness, 110–111

adherence factors, 25

adult T-cell leukemia (ATL), from HTLV-1, 289–309

aflatoxin
  as carcinogen, 90, 102, 233–234, 241, 248, 250
  as risk for hepatocellular carcinoma, 359
  schistosomiasis activation of, 334

Africa
  Burkitt's lymphoma in, 107, 184–185
  Epstein-Barr virus in, 192
  hepatitis viruses in, 269
  hepatocellular carcinoma in, 240–241, 250
  HTLV-1 in, 292
  Kaposi's sarcoma in, 209, 211
  nasopharyngeal carcinoma in, 186
  schistosomiasis and bladder cancer in, 318

African Americans
  gastric cancer in, 372
  H. pylori infections in, 377–378, 391

aging
  as cause of cancer, 3–4
  mutation increase during, 36

AIDS. *See also* HIV
  Burkitt's lymphoma with, 186

  genetic alterations in, 139, 145
  immunosuppression in, 109, 131, 133
  Kaposi's sarcoma in, 99, 112, 207, 212–214, 221
  lymphomas in. *See* AIDS lymphomas
  p53 mutations in, 197

AIDS lymphomas, 132, 138–146
  Epstein-Barr virus role in, 183–184, 190, 209
  interleukin role in, 142–145
  primary effusion type, 209
  of T cells, 191

AirS/BarA, as *E. coli* sensor protein, 25

alcoholic hepatitis
  biomarkers in, 62–63
  as cancer risk factor, 62, 94, 233, 241, 252, 269
  inflammation role in, 62, 94

aldehydes
  genotoxicity of, 53, 57
  from lipid oxidation, 59, 70

alkylation, inappropriate, DNA damage from, 92

O^6-alkylguanine-DNA-alkyltransferase in bladder-cancer tissue, 325–326, 383

alpha 1 antitrypsin deficiency, as cancer risk factor, 94, 233, 234

alpha-proteobacteria, as pathogens, 22–23, 24

American Association of Cancer Research, 10

amines
  carcinogenic, 433
  genotoxicity of, 56–57
  hypochlorous acid reaction with, 44

3-amino-1-methyl-5*H*-pyridol[4,5-*b*]indole in studies of liver tumors, 334

β-aminopropionitrile (BAPN) use in schistosomiasis therapy, 336

anal cancer in HIV-positive men, 164

androgenic-anabolic steroids, as carcinogens, 233–234

angiofollicular lymphoid hyperplasia. *See* Castleman's disease

angiogenesis
  as host response, 26
  interleukin promotion of, 221–222